Threads

Better Court than Coroners

Memoirs in a Duty of Care

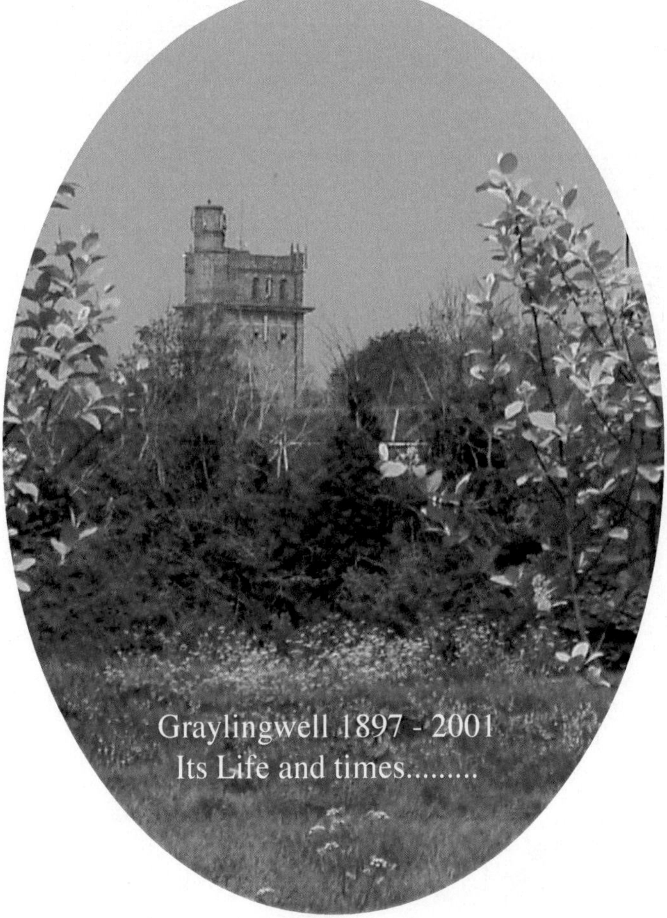

Graylingwell 1897 - 2001
Its Life and times.........

A Personal Account
by
Barone Hopper

First limited edition — 2011

Published by:
PV Publications
26 Sandfield Avenue
Littlehampton
West Sussex.
BN17 7LL

email: info@baronehopper.co.uk
web: http://www.baronehopper.co.uk

Printed by:
Ashford Colour Press
Unit 600 Fareham Reach
Fareham Road
Gosport
Hants
PO13 0FW

ISBN: 978-0-9569910-0-3

Better Court Than Coroners

Memoirs in a Duty of Care

Vol I

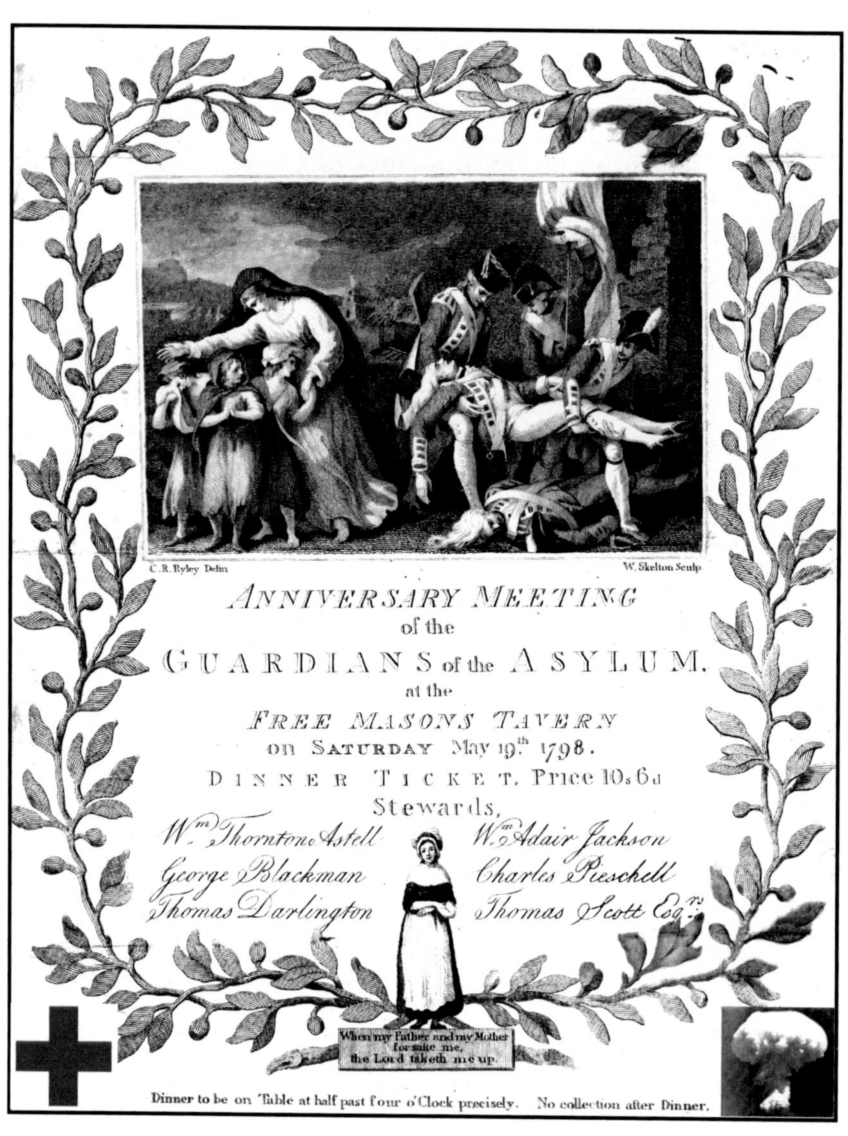

Guardians of the Asylum. 1798

Acknowledgements

A few (among many) good people who (directly or indirectly) contributed to these personal *Memoirs* - between the 1960s and early 2000s, from oral and written correspondence:

Patricia *Sara* Hopper, Philip and Christopher Hopper, Emil Hopper. *Amanda* Russell Hopper. Mathew Thomas. Maud Susie Dolan (nee Hopper nee Manton). Lillian Collier (nee Manton), James, Arthur, and the *Manton* family. Basil Boxall (Graylingwell Admin). Brenda Wild (RMN). Dr. Brian Vawdrey (Psychiatry), George Pople (MWO). W.P. Izzard (Nurse Tutor). Cicely Bartram and Vera Goodall (OT). Christopher Doman (Chichester Solicitor). Chris and Alison Rudkin (for support). Rosemary and Bill Corner (Social Work and Probation). Carol Jones (Nurse). David Cushing (PNO). Rhoda Platt (SNO). Dr. (Prof) Lionel Haward (Forensic Psychology. Univ Surrey). Dr. Hugh Franklin (Bio-chemist) and Winifred Franklin. RMN Charge Nurses and Sisters - Mrs. Wanstell, Mrs. Weeks, Mrs. Vincent, Mrs. Macdonald, Mrs. Connolly (and family of -), Bob Wanstall, Norman Weeks, Leo Lunny and George Stevenson. Psychiatrists, Drs - Michael Matthews, Jack Scrivener, John Towers, John Morrisey, Norman Capstick, Angus McPherson, Doros Pallis, Mary Rice, Julia Wilkinson, Tom Pastor (Psychiatry), and Dr. Chris Haffner (Wessex Unit Child Psychiatry). Drs - Rollin, Martin Roth, Peter Sainsbury and, Jim Jenkins (Graylingwell MRC Psychiatry). Bill Reavley, Roy Curtis, Brenda Mumford, (Psychology). Johnny White (Graylingwell Head gardener).Hugh Weston (Engineer). Steve Bruce (Artist). Robert and Beryl Graves, and Colin Wilson (Lit). Rear-Admiral Ronald Oldham and artist Marjorie Ingledon (Fourth Way. Upper Dicker). Watkins of Cecil Court London. Peter Pettit Lecturer (Reading Univ). Dr. (Prof) Peter Nolan Phd. (Birm'n and Stafford Univ's). Les and Peggy Chalk (Welfare and SSD). Joy King and Sean Wilson (MH Res Care). Peter Cooke (WSCC SSD. Editor). John Munro (WSCC SSD. Editor). Rosemary Harvey (Curator. *Heatherbank* Museum. Glasgow). Mandy Hart (Chi Museum), Dr. Pauline Buzzing (Chi Archives), and thank you to WSCC Chichester Archives staff, helpful during the 1980s - who published a little of my *History* ... Vera Searle (nee Lewington. Nurse in 1919 & 1920s). Les Dicker (Dispensary boy 1919 to be a Deputy Chief Male Nurse). Ronald and Molly Green and Molly Hunt (nee Green). John Donnabie (CPN). Patricia Alldridge (Curator, Bethlem Royal Hospital and Maudsley Hospital Museum). Thank you to *all* curators and Staff of numerous UK psychiatric hospitals who sent material in early 1980s. Judith Glover (Historian). Mr Paddy G Driscoll (Graylingwell Admin). Mrs. Paddy Donnelly (Secretary, Personal Ass't to Chief Executive). Mick Jenner (Admin). Keith Hollister (Admin), AA Jackson (Admin), David Grace (Admin), A.J. Browne (Admin). Special thanks to Dame Alison Munro OBE (Chichester Health Authority and Graylingwell Chairperson 1982-1988 - who was most encouraging in correspondence with me to compile a Social History). Sir Patrick Symons (First Chairman of the to be new *Trust*, in late 1990s, to replace the old Graylingwell management) - who too, was most helpful - it was at the time of Graylingwell's Centenary in 1997 (about my booklet and half-hour documentary on Graylingwell); I briefly corresponded with, and met, Mr Gerald Le Blount Kidd who chatted about his father, the hospital's first Medical Superintendent, and witness to the first world war's exodus of Graylingwell's patients in 1915. Not to be forgotten. Many ex- *patients* who related uncounted anecdotes but, whose names are withheld - to protect patients' confidentiality. Special mention (latter years of The Project) of Admin Basil Boxall who after a twenty-years gap gave up many hours over several years checking up *the facts* names et cetera (with his wife Pat's blessing). And in an age of *Computer* I am especially grateful to Alan Betts Computer Consultant (polymath), who gave incredible help maturing this work. And thank you to Mr Lee Cooke for assisting in technical presentation of *Better Court Than Coroners* ... Barone Hopper. 2009.

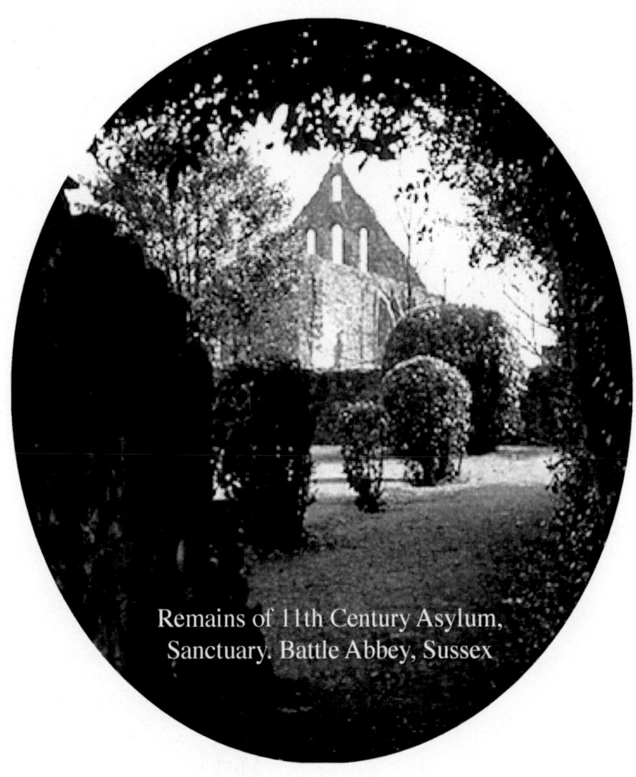

Remains of 11th Century Asylum, Sanctuary. Battle Abbey, Sussex

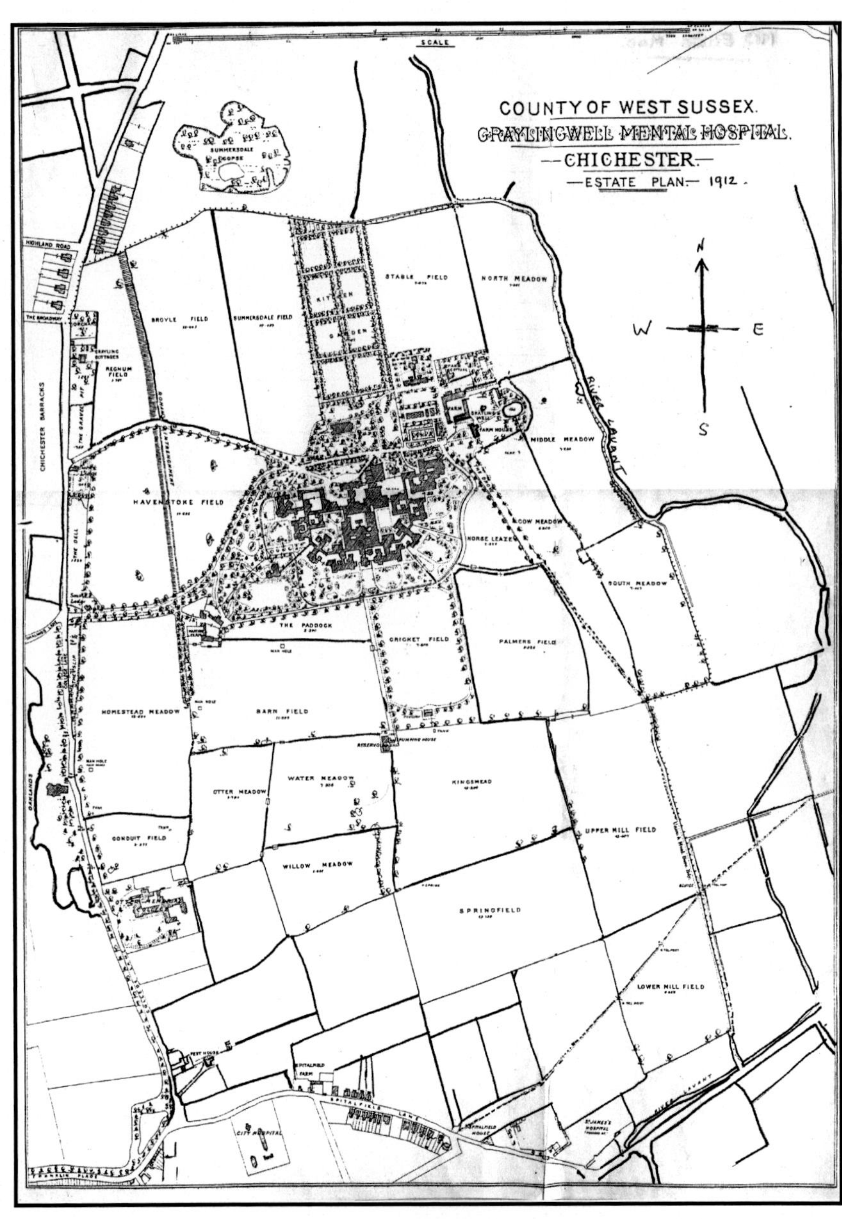

Graylingwell Estate Plan. 1912

Better Court than Coroners, Memoirs in a Duty of Care

Memoirs of a three-year passage whilst working in a Long-stay Psychiatric Hospital during the 1960s and Seventies. Subject being - a Duty Of Care. By: Barone Hopper Registered Mental Nurse (RMN); Diploma in Psychiatric Child Care (Dip Psy. CC); Certificate of Qualification in Social Work (CQSW); Diploma in Social Work (Dip SW); Approved Social Worker (ASW); Mental Welfare Officer (MWO).

Synopsis. For over thirty years I have been collating Social History, daily life, during one century in a late Victorian built long-term English psychiatric hospital (aka asylum). The work includes my own experience, supported by staff colleagues, as a student in the 1960s, and subsequently as Registered Mental Nurse and generic Senior Mental Health Social Worker, working in Graylingwell Hospital and Sussex Community at large. It is an austere, sometimes dramatic, mostly routine *duty-of-care* history of *day-to-day* workings of *any* closed similar old long-term caring institution. Throughout the work, I am observer *and* one inquiring participant.

The record includes memories of long past staff, civilian and ex- military-service psychiatric patients. Thirty-plus years recording personal memories given in debates with practitioners working (or who had worked) in one or more of our long-stay mental hospitals. A Primary Source. Many of my informants date back to their working in the early 20th century — persons employed on site in (mostly European) Military, Health and Welfare care institutions. Narrative threads woven into the uneven script include administrators, cleaners, clerks, cooks, doctors, engineers, mental-welfare-officers, nurses, occupational-therapists, painters, pharmacists, philosophers, physicists, porters, psychologists, psychoanalysts, psychiatrists, relieving officers and social workers, volunteers and ward-orderlies — even a 1940 hospital shepherd and his family (who lived on the hospital estate) and, of course, our patients.

The Book is written in Two Parts. A narrative with personal memories, aided by considerable research and observations - including self-observation. And a detailed *Appendix*, contained in Volume II, as background, which includes - one hundred years of Graylingwell's year-by-year Social History in chronological abstracts; its life and times; topography; tithe maps; and numerous illustrations with b&w and coloured photographs. And many collated and captioned contemporary forms and interviews taken from transcripts of personal field and hospital surveys; the whole together, are testimonies, of my own and older colleagues (living and many, since deceased) - like a Topsy compendium. A way of life no longer existant.

CONTENTS :

Chapter Four — Chilgrove One Ward

Chapter Five — Bramber Two Ward

Chapter Six — Nausea

Chapter Seven — Night Duty

Chapter Eight — Summersdale Villa

Preface

This book is *not* a sensational expose of institutional abuse - it *is* about hospital patients and their carers. I feel I should add that this work makes *no* claims to be a complete picture of psychiatric life, or pretence to own special knowledge of patient care. The bulk of the book, in all its anecdotes, cameos, and incidents, is about sick people and their carers: about adjustment, self-exploration - and *the* conundrum - ruminant of human existence.

It would be lovely to recall only tales of a happy often humorous place and to depict numerous scenes wholly without dour sickness, death or unhappy disorder - even of occasional chaos. Despite this fact it is *not* my intention to compliment historic myths that this long-stay psychiatric hospital institution was a place of Gothic horror - it was not!

TO THE
ASYLUM
I hope you
won't think me
foolish

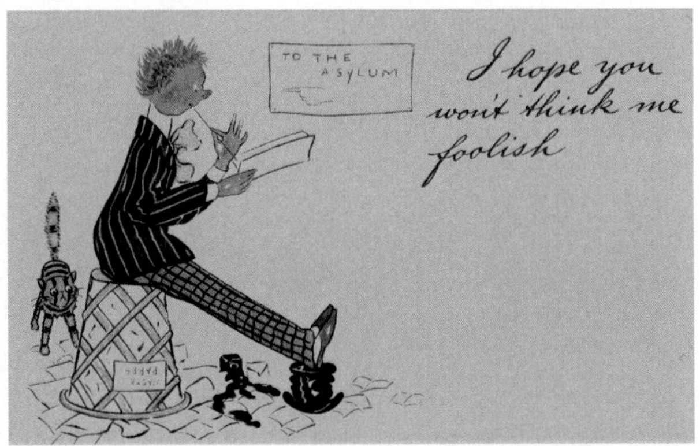

TO THE ASYLUM . H. Cowham. Raphael Tuck 'Series 1271' (nd) c1906.

At all times a refuge, asylum and place of healing, it was for many long-stay residents - their home. The subject matter of this collection is singularly un-attractive, in sickness, poverty and suffering; but ... and it deserves emphasis, ' Getting better, though often a painful affair is along with the passing view of our Sanctuary's inhabitants - is essentially a good thing. ...'

It was the time of the post-war Beat Generation and, especially, the benign period of *The Flower People* and *Peace Movements* - all to shortly fall ; peace petals fallen as Vietnam and events in Northern Ireland and USA bred much more vociferous movements and politically motivated pressure groups of the 1960s and 1970s.

Dramatis Personae

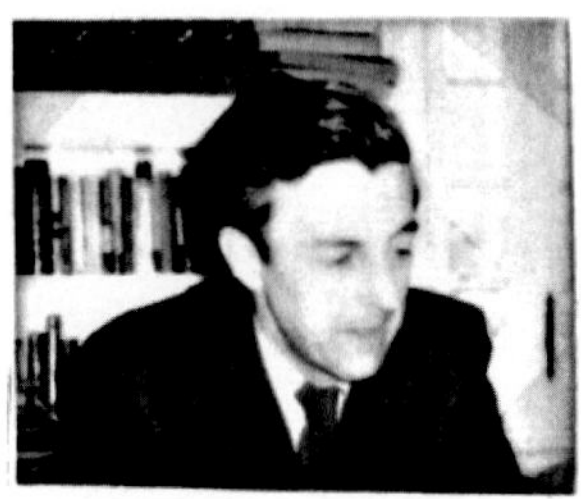

Basil J Boxall (aka Admin Baz). Graylingwell Patients' Affairs and Medical Records Officer, from 1950. (See, magazine, *The Hospital,* Sept. 1971.)

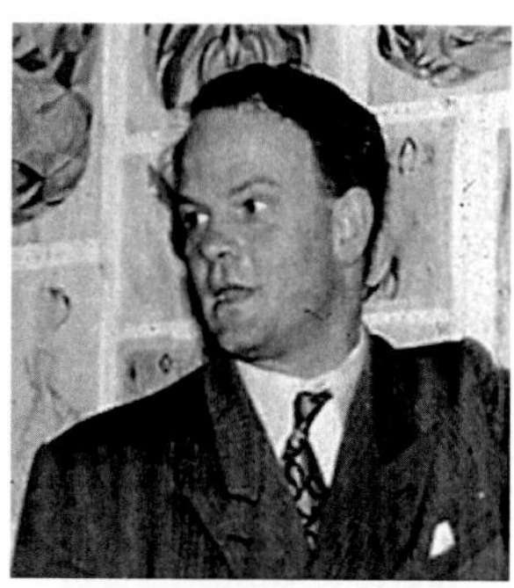

Dr Brian Vawdrey (aka Dr Joyce). Ex-Major RAMC : Graylingwell Consultant Psychiatrist & Psychoanalyst (Dr Ernest Jones a predecessor), at Graylingwell & The Acre in 1960s.

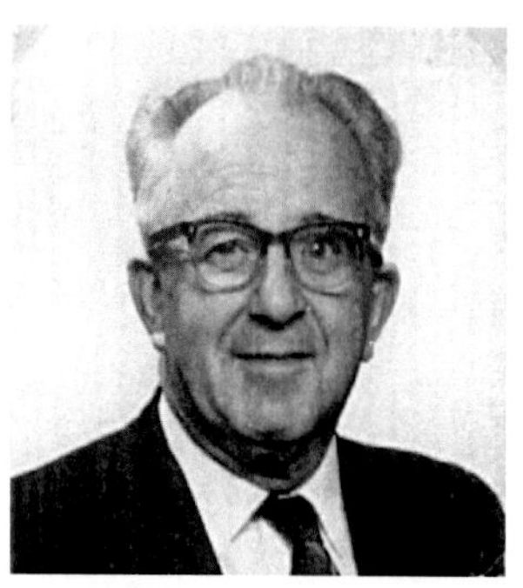

George Pople (aka MWO George) Poor Law Relieving Officer from 1931 and, West Sussex Mental Welfare Officer in 1960s.

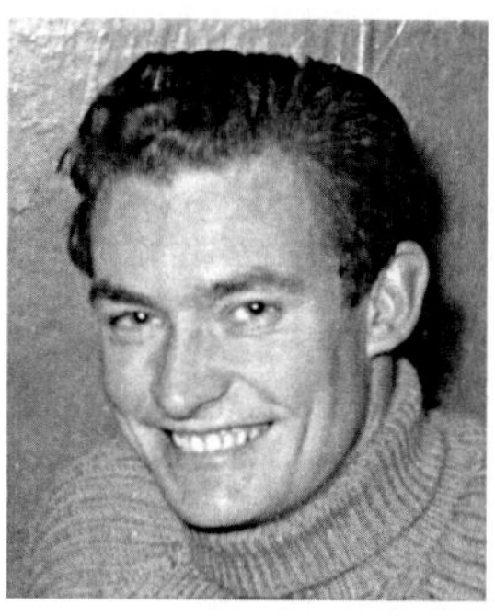

Barone Hopper (aka Barry). Charge Nurse. RMN student 1967-1970. Senior Social Worker.and Mental Welfare Officer. West Sussex.1971-2000.

Substantial memoirs (testimonies) were contributed as oral and written transcripts from taped interviews, conducted in 1981, with Basil Boxall, Dr Brian Vawdrey, George Pople (who contributed a lengthy autobiography, entitled *40 Years on The Parish,* unpublished) and Mental Welfare Officer Barone Hopper.

Chapter One
The Front Entrance

'... life is made up of ever so many partings welded together. '[1]
Charles Dickens. Joe to Pip. Great Expectations. 1861.

30th September, 1967

Entrance—War Years—Evacuation—Orphanage—Christmas Island—Graylingwell

Front Entrance

I was on duty. Student alone. Left in-charge of *the* whole male acute psychiatric locked ward. In confrontation with one angry, fractious patient, attacking another, but docile patient.

'What's up John? What's the problem?'

Moments ago I'd signalled to Geoff, our young brown-coated ward-orderly, to take two frightened patients away from the dormitory back towards the crowded day-room. We were the only two staff presently on duty in the ward. The Charge Nurse was on his day off. His deputy, our staff nurse, was out on an important errand.

Bramber Two John was one of our most disturbed patients and, stone-faced, was brandishing a chair above the head of Manny, a helpless fellow patient, lying down on his own bed. Poor Manny, but two nights ago he had witnessed his sleeping neighbour attacked by this man, a disturbed tall John. There were a lot of people named John in the hospital, patients and staff, colloquially our patient was known as Tall John.

'Tell me about it. Come on John. All right?'

I had a re-assuring smile (I hoped) on my face as I reached down to a petrified Manny. Slowly and gently, I lifted him up off the bed, and directed him off towards the day-room. He was still staring up at a now bemused Tall John. Inside myself I suppressed rank fear.

Only seconds had elapsed since my arrival at the bedside and other patients' departure from the scene to the lounge. Geoff knew to ring for help from The Office. John answered, menacing - a flat petulant tone.

'Manny wouldn't give me a fag... '

A few seconds silence...

'Would you like *me* to get *you* a cigarette, John?'

'Yes please Barry.'

Tension dissolved as he lowered the chair to the floor.

'I'd have been all right if Manny had given me a fag Barry,' Tall John mumbled *sotto-voce* as, shuffling, he followed me down the dormitory. As we approached the ward office, Geoff emerged from the day-room to open the entrance door to two white-gowned staff sent up by The Office - to help out.

What had brought me into *this* line of work? Incident over, as I walked back into the day-room I thought what am I *doing* here ... on a *locked* ward in this asylum, a long-stay psychiatric hospital in the mid 1960s? ... Twenty years past and more had past since my early years in a lonely wartime childhood. Tangled roots ... threads tenuous, sparse and brittle in a cigarette card genealogy.

I'd been moved *at least* a dozen times, since my birth in 1937 at a Mill Hill, Hendon, nursing home. Father departed (whatever sad reasons) in early 1940s. I was evacuated, parentless, because I only lived with my mother until 1942, and was not with her again until mid-1951. On the 4th August 1955 I was then called up for National Service. My younger brother was born in 1938 (he emigrated to Cape Town in 1964). Aged three he was in Millwall Hospital when it was bombed, and later, he was sent *alone* up north to Yorkshire; as I had earlier been evacuated *alone* to Heston Middlesex (later Heathrow), by Hounslow, in 1942. We were displaced, separated, as infants from mid-'42, as well as from our mother, then a wartime London bus-conductor (clippie) and single parent. Bro and I did not 'meet' again for some years; indeed, we did not know of each other's existence until he joined me in The Orphanage in Summer 1945. I was eight, he was just seven. And then the stranger he was to me disappeared into a distant house called Brooklands in Wray Park Road. Decades later when we chatted about that time, he recalled we could not understand each other's laconic introductions at all. He had been living up north with foster parents somewhere in Yorkshire, and I had been moved about the south, variously in north London, Middlesex, south Wales and Reigate in Surrey with no idea what I must have sounded like to him.

So as a family we had been broken-up, evacuated in 1939 as one of the several moves between 1937 and '44. Moved from nearby Elstree Film Studios where father, and my namesake, Australian and American (with comedians Olsen and Johnson) vaudeville artiste, had worked. Down and back again to London off the old Ballspond Road, where the 1940 blitz demolished our lodgings. I wonder what happened to Mrs. Clements, our landlady, at One

Baxter Grove? I was twice evacuated up to Northampton. Blitz over! Back down again to the fractured shrapnel of London in '42 Homerton E8 at a busy London Transport cafe, sited next to the bus station and opposite a string of barrage balloons in Victoria Park. Then but an infant, I can still easily recall seeing those huge grey flying elephantine balloons.

And on recall, I can still smell escaped gas and the frequent awful effluent from bomb craters, shrapnel-fractured gas mains and open sewage pipes from jagged holes in our roads; piles of playground rubble and blown-out windows from a local dense wood of many broken homes. I collected still warm shiny, jagged, sharp metal pieces out of the gutters and off of the pitted pavements (proud and boasting of 'finds' to my infant peers). Exploratory playtime games amongst broken glass amid the ruins, splintered timber and shredded burnt bricks. Early memories: a five year old evacuee held up in someone's arms at 37 Church Road Heston hearing night-time guns; searchlights, a lone parachutist descending in a stark white sudden beam of light. Flames! And the noise! The cacophony of war! Hide and seek; hiding as instructed under a bed when the air-raid siren sounded until collected and moved downstairs, and huddled under a table, held within a metal caged Morrison shelter placed in the centre of the blessed Esaus, frontroom sanctuary until the wailing song of the all clear. Four, five and six years old. Wartime normality. I would know no personal domestic family home for twelve years of my early life. But of course there were *The Homes*[2].

From the age of just seven years, settled early in 1944 for seven long summers, I lived in an austere large Orphanage[3] with other, orphan or single-parent, abandoned children, at that charitable institution known as the Spurgeon's Orphan Homes. There I lived among two hundred or more wartime children. Girls lived on one side, boys on the other.

In Summer '44, Spurgeon Homes' children were interrupted at play due to numerous invading busy metal bodies. I watched those long silver missiles passing by overhead, standing mesmerised on 'The Huts' concrete square playground. They were 1944 unmanned Nazi doodlebugs; the V1 silent, flying bombs; and more destructive, soft droning V2 rockets, with swift tails seen as suddenly they dropped like silent meteorites, the enemy dealing sudden death in our midst. We orphanage kids were soon marched out. I remember it well, crocodile *en masse* in the middle of Holmsdale Road. We were again evacuated in haste; moving from Reigate railway station to Swansea in South Wales. I to

Gogregrieg. We returned to Surrey under bunting saying 'Welcome Back' - in Spring 1945.

On a pleasant occasional Saturday afternoon perambulation in the 1940s, we children were sometimes, unescorted, allowed to adventure out into the nearby town of Redhill and stroll onto Earlswood Common. As we approached the waste of the Redhill Common boundaries we avoided one area purposely, like the plague, skirted that section more out of conscious fear (of the unknown) than for any other logical reason. The tabooed area housed a large asylum, mostly hidden behind high brick walls and a boundary of thick green foliage. As young children it was rumoured that you could only get in by a Green Ticket, whatever that was. Once you were in there you would disappear ... forever. That graphic image, retained in my memory, was later reinforced when the Surrey Earlswood Asylum's towering brick buildings could be seen more clearly from the steam driven Southern Railway trains, moving slo' to-and-fro' - between the Brighton and Victoria terminals.

One Spring day in 1944 (before evacuation), after gazing up at a noisy airforce-duel dog-fight over the nearby South Down hills, three of us small boys, standing on a mound of soft clay (which we prized for a plasticine), looked across a *ha-ha* trench, over our home's perimeter fence, across to Oak Road, and beyond over a similar wooden palisade into another enclosed space, where an abundance of loud happy infants' laughter could be heard. They could *not* see it, for they were in, as a raised board faced Oak Road across from us advertised, an enclosed Sunshine Home For Blind Children. Together, we three six and seven year olds, estranged by war; lived and survived in institutions, and did not yet know the word. Equally unknown to us those anonymous blind children and ourselves — were each other's realities. Since separating from my mother, we rarely saw her in the early years; but in the postwar years my bro and I saw her for one Saturday afternoon per calendar month (missing one from time to time) called (as in all institutions) Visiting Day. Each Sunday after morning church we were instructed to write a letter to someone - a relative if we had one. But we did not personally know our mother's address, only that it was somewhere in North London. The carers had possession of such details.

When some time in 1946-7, two older boys ran away (out of adventure rather than out of fear but an evasion). My bro and I (then 8 and 9 years old) admitted that we had nowhere to run to, and anyway our mother couldn't have us, so what was the point of bunking off? Fortunately there was no cruelty by caring staff. One Hut 12 housemaster, Mr G., a young, arrogant, athletic. Dickens like character, Wackford Squeers the bully, had severely whacked my brother Mick and myself, and many other young children but, found out, was sacked for excess use of the willow cane and general face-slapping and too frequent other sadistic punishments - but G. was an exception to the rule. As kids we had identities but were known by numbers (as HM Forces) rather than by name. I recall being 72 (at eight years old) and later 56 and 14. Before leaving the orphanage and Reigate Grammar School, just 14 years old, in July 1951, I was No.2.

If I never experienced anything, then, I believed what I first read or heard from others on a subject: especially, if it was presented in a dramatic popular image. This was in the 1940s and early 1950s when I was so young and slow to grow up, and immature. In that austere bunkered little world of mine I found it chocka with comic book images, including fun and lampoon images on lunacy. Certainly, such sad aspects of humanity were frequently caricatured to purposely deny, to hide, potential taboo horrors such as the ugly realities of war, loneliness, and madness. Years later 1960s Sunday magazine supplements and other liberal media helped to breakdown, in some measure, those former loveless boyhood times and prejudices, sufficient for me to be able to eventually work and serve in a sanctuary aka the asylum and a long-term hospital, Graylingwell.

I gave in my notice in early 1967 to my employers, the Press and Information Bureau (P& I dept.) at the new London Victoria Scotland Yard. I had been previously based at old New Scotland Yard, (our then ground floor room located next door to a waiting space for hardened media crime reporters and, close by, a grim small police Black Crime Museum). The Press Bureau daily monitored incoming, often awesome and tragic, forensic events experienced about the great London metropolis. (I recall awful pics of the Sixties Torso murder dredged from the Thames like a Dickens' plot and Blake's prison escape, and occasional shootings in cold blood of our London bobbies.) No more would I, as a civvie clerical assistant, be scanning thirty plus newspapers each morning, to mark up and remove for the daily Met's press cuttings (added to from the cutting agencies packages). This folio was intended for heads of all departments starting at the top, Sir Joseph Simpson (a giant of a man I sometimes passed in the lift, impressive in his full uniform - an august presence indeed). I was responsible (via our civvie mandarins the PIO and SEO) for the Met Police cuttings' distribution from the hierarchical top of the list, the commissioner, down to the (seemingly) out-on-limb secret SO12 (Special Branch) annexe. On completion of this round I would attend to the current intake of wanted press passes. Before leaving, I was moved upstairs to work out my notice, in the Met's own General Orders library section until the end of August. I had attended a successful interview at Graylingwell down at Chichester in early May, but I nearly never made it — to Graylingwell, that is, where I was due to start training in September.

During 1965-67 with John (a clerical colleague), when I was employed at New Scotland Yard, I joined the Royal Army Medical Corps as a reservist to become a member of the part-time Territorial Army at a branch based at Harrow in Middlesex. Subsequently, at the time of my formal entry at Graylingwell as an RMN student, I was still enrolled in the RAMC. It was customary in the TAVR to attend occasional weekend exercises and attend a mandatory annual fortnight away on medical training, whether at home or abroad. In the summer of 1967 our RAMC contingent was committed to fly out to Germany for a post-nuclear exercise. I had never been in an aeroplane before, and we departed from Heathrow on a propelled (military I think) aircraft. I was fortunate to sit adjacent to a window overlooking a wing where I could observe the nebulous spin of two propellers. About ten minutes or so out and I saw one propeller splutter and stop altogether. Then alarm, as on the other side another propeller stalled. Over the tannoy our captain reassured us that due to technical faults (the remaining two props were fine) we were returning to the airport. After some delay we embarked on an alternative craft to fly to a small German airfield at Tempelhof (or was it Gatow?). As part of the army exercise we were later well strapped into a helicopter (another first for me). I recall gazing out down through the open door at speeding tanks in spirals, engaged in their own exercise.

Our allocated task was to receive casualties from a nuclear zone. In June 1967 at an RAMC TA camp thermonuclear decontamination tent in Germany we had to learn how to separate out the 'walking wounded' from the more serious injuries, and anticipate who would be first to be flown out from the casualty station. We had to learn something about the injuries themselves from burns and blisters and visceral evidence of known radiation sickness, contagious dangerous toxic radioactive exposure *per se*. All the likely types of casualty after or during a battle, with unspecified nuclear weapons included. Suddenly we were interrupted as all our senior NCOs were called over to a tent where a conflab took place with our officers. After their return, looking rather grim, we sat as a group huddled together with our own two staff sergeants.

It was explained that a war had broken out in the Middle East between Israel and Egypt. And it was possible that if it escalated, we (meaning the British) might become involved, even by default. Tiger, one of our Staffs, cautioned us that he remembered as a young squaddie attending a similar territorial exercise in 1939 — and not returning home for six years. But of course it was the infamous Six Day War. Ironic. Whilst stationed on that coral atoll of Christmas Island (now part of *Kiribati* the Gilbert Islands) ten years ago, I recall the tragic Suez conflict taking place and having a similar crisis briefing from officers and NCOs.

On return home to Blighty, shortly before Sara, our infants and I moved down south into West Sussex. Our RAMC Territorial Army Reserve contingent had a follow up visit after TAVR training in June 1967 in Germany, to D block Netley Asylum, (part of the military hospital, built at Southampton at the time of the Crimea war and opened in 1863).[4] Netley (aka Victoria Hospital, one of two military hospitals in Hampshire), was a massive building, where I experienced a lengthy visit to a filled male psychiatric ward and chatted awhile with a Senior psychiatric nurse, a regular RAMC warrant officer, and spoke briefly with several bedridden patients - anonymous peace-war (aka conflict!) mind damaged war veterans. The foregoing events are presented as a prelude to my being a three-year student state Registered Mental Nurse at Graylingwell Hospital — somewhat as an anti-climax.

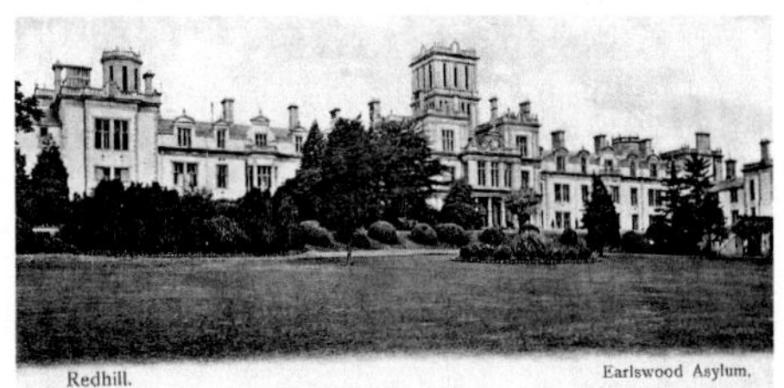

1908. Feeble-minded, Suitable For Treatment, were placed in the Royal **Earlswood Asylum,** Redhill, Surrey (built 1855). Dr. J.Langdon Down (Downs' Syndrome) its first Medical Superintendent. Earlswood accomodated idiots, Mentally Subnormal, and Educated Subnormal (ESN). (Graylingwell, however, made use of its own Sanatorium.) Earlswood closed down on March 31st 1997, its residents re-housed in the community; site converted to 'luxury apartments' and general housing.

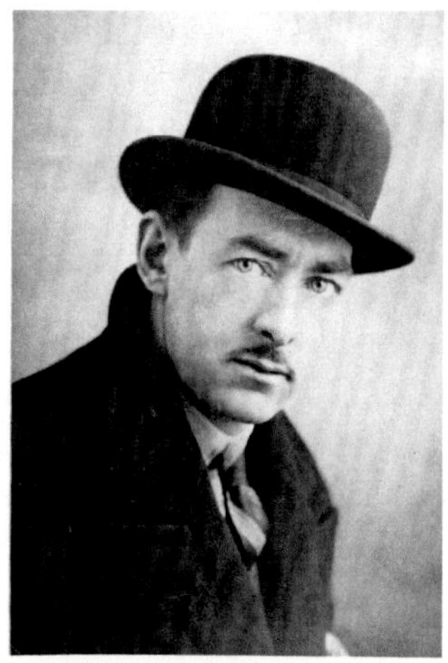

My unknown father, a **mystery,** (*his* father was Johanan William Hopper an Austrian artist, who had emigrated to Australia sometime c.1900 - or before?). My father's name Barone Ernst Hopper, above (b.1902- d.1972): Australian or N.Z. born. Lifetime in circus, USA's vaudeville (as Ole Olsen & Chic Johnson) artiste: & latter years a stage-designer at Elstree in England. Pic circa.**1940.**

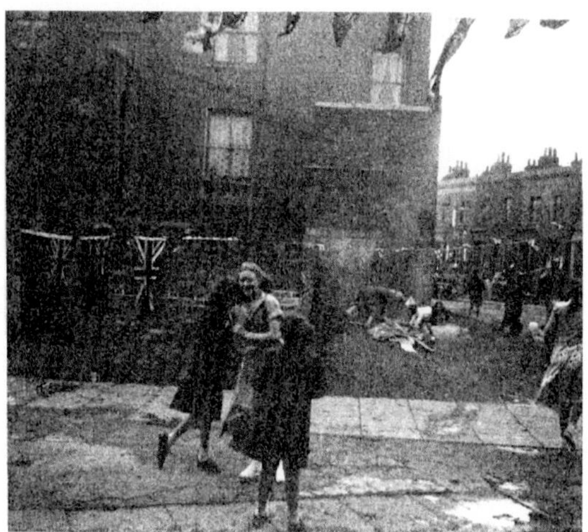

1940.Site of our last home: London Blitz kids; but away, we'd recently evacuated (evacuees for 12 years;1939 -1951), when our home was totally destroyed by fire during the '40 blitz : this was, No 1 Baxter Grove off Wall Street & Ballspond Road, Islington. Pic of it as empty brown-site at Coronation celebrations in 1953. This whole area in London N1 demolished in 1960s - replaced by post-war flats.

BOMBED-OUT

Aerial blitzkrieg adds a new problem to the million worries of war—the problem of these bombed out of home. Where can they get shelter, food, a bed? Some areas know the answer. Others don't.

Picture Post. Vol.9.No2. p9, October 12th.**1940.**

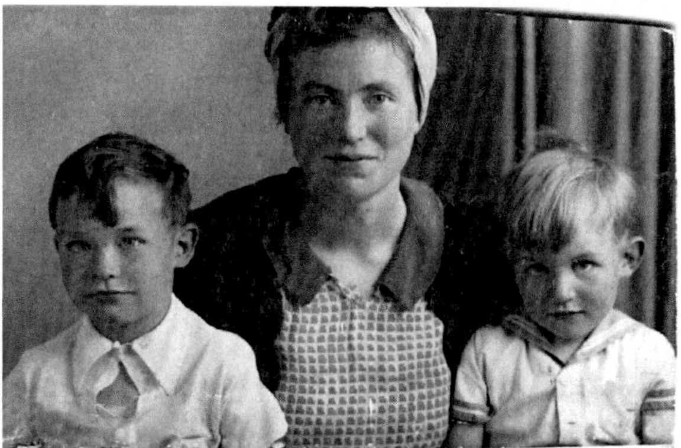

1942. Homeless. **Centre,** mother Maude Susie Hopper (nee Manton, years later, new surname Dolan). **Left,** author, Barone Carl Hopper age 5yrs 3mths. - **Right**, bro Emil Moody Hopper. A rare pic. On back of photo stamped June 4th - bro was 3 yrs old on June 3rd. This was time of yet another family wartime breakup as I was (again), separated, and evacuated fostered out to Heston Middlesex (for a while). 1944 I moved into an orphanage. My infant bro Emil, would also be evacuated - without mother - but alone up-north to Yorkshire ... till Summer 1945, when he too entered the orphanage, and joined me at Reigate.

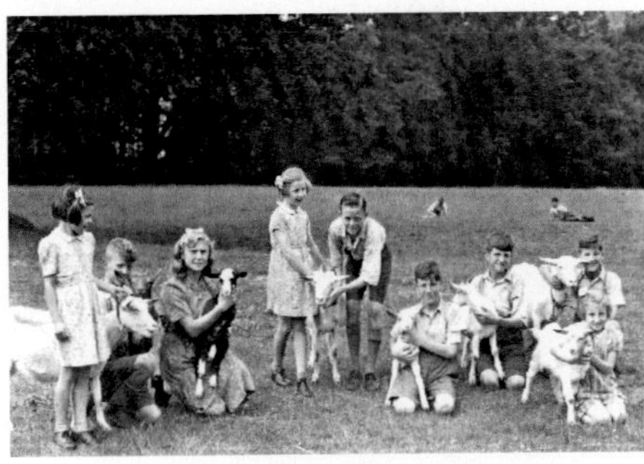

1946. Spurgeon's Orphan Homes in Reigate Surrey. Boys lived on one side of grounds - girls on the other. Photo a posed united pic with other kids, taken on girls side down in front of St. David's house. Bro and I would eventually leave The Homes in July 1951.

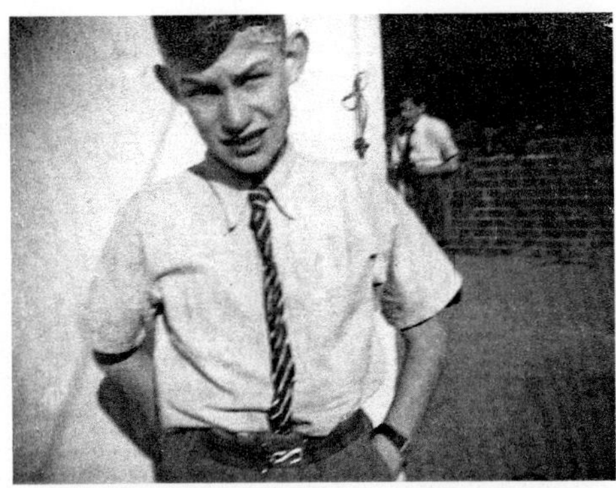

1950. In Spurgeon's Orphan Homes. My bro Emil posing in The Huts Yard (yards away from where in 1944, I had stood alone, and watched overhead doodle bugs & V2s; and again subsequently evacuated with other children to South Wales - and, on return, my bro joining me in The Homes in Summer of 1945).

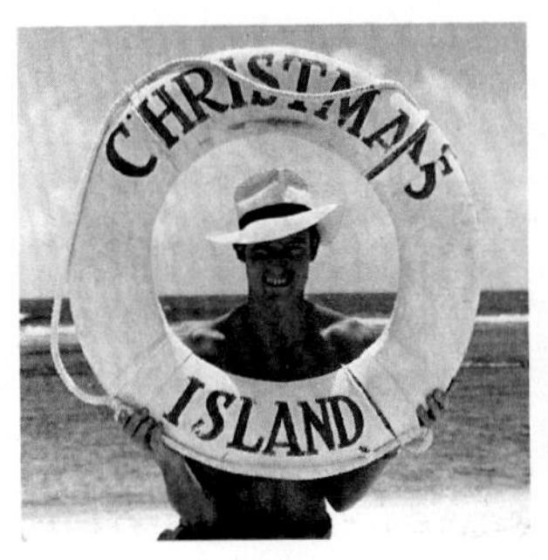

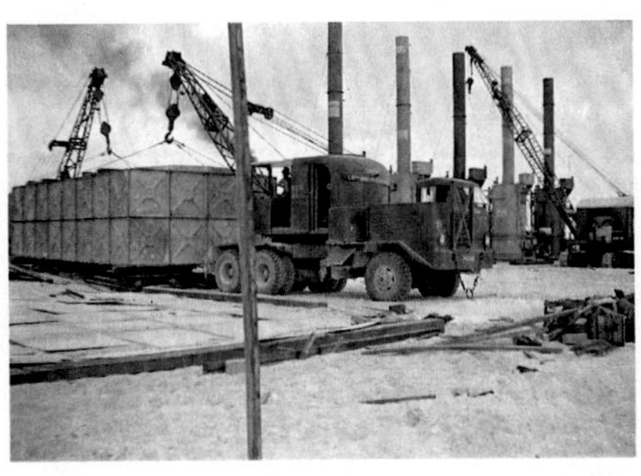

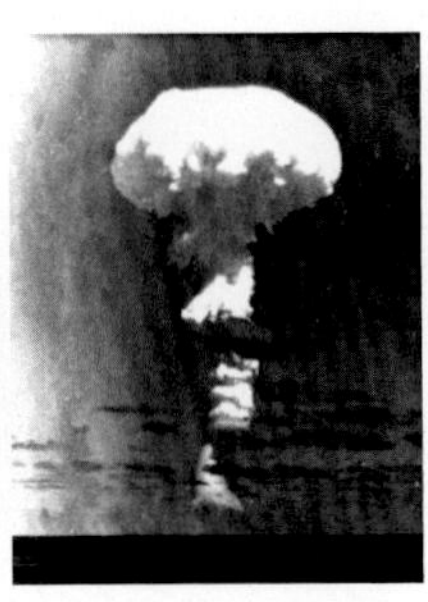

1957. Left. Me. ... **Right.** H Bomb... One of British servicemen stationed on Christmas Island in the Mid-pacific 1956-7. **Middle** photo shows sappers of 28 Field Engineer Regiment constructing a large Distillation Plant to receive surrounding salt waters of the Pacific - no fresh water to be had on the coral island. Fortunately we troops were assured that we're safe from all and any exploded 'clean' (triggered above ground or above sea - ie not 'dirty' bombs - sic), experimental H bomb thermonuclear detonations. And, were told ; "You are perfectly safe from any after-effects from even minimal exposure afterward radiation effects.' (Hmm !) Lucky! ... I missed MUCH bigger H bombs yet to be exploded (with radiation), in the months and years ahead: some - over the island itself. All stationed personnel would know nothing about deadly, later possibilities of ingested Ionised toxic matter. ... I later, married in 1964, two children - and entered Graylingwell Hospital as a student psychiatric nurse in September 1967: Ten years on. ...

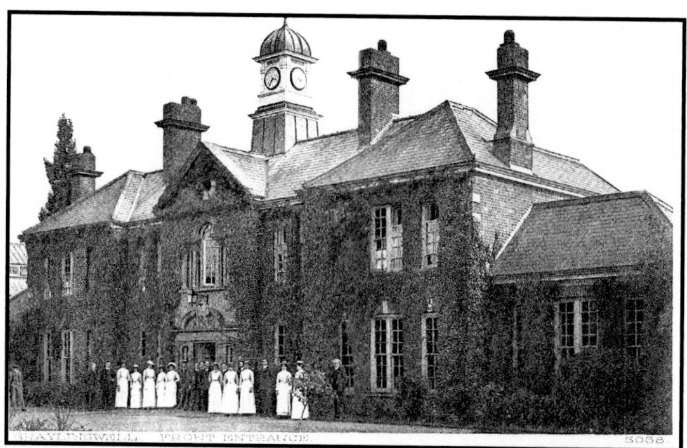

1909. Graylingwell Hospital *Front Entrance* — photo from post card.

1960s. Nurse Training School with our Graylingwell nurse tutor, ex RAMC, to front. Source, Graylingwell brochure, early 1960s.

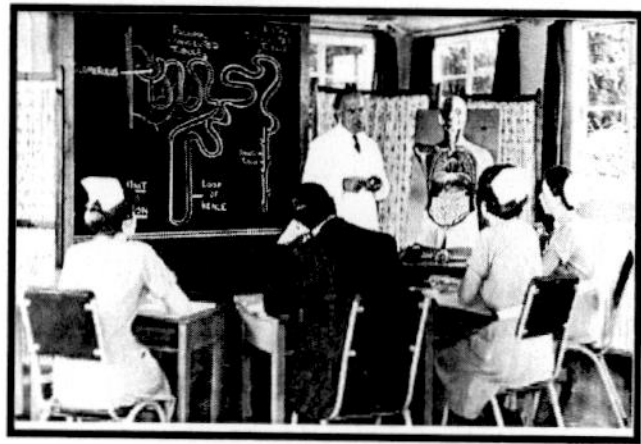

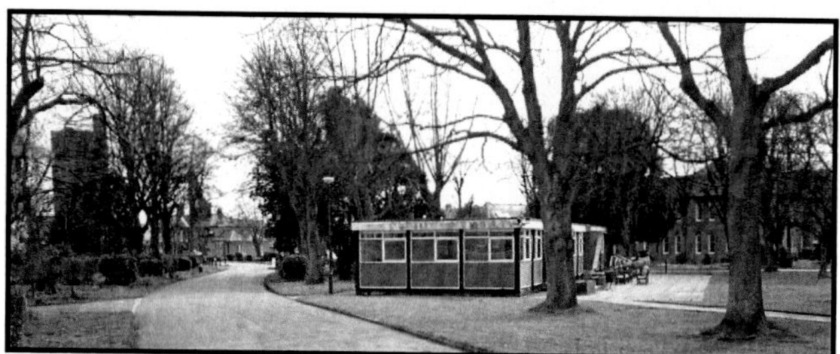

1980. Panorama from Summersdale Road. Naunton Pavilion café on Havenstoke parkland. Photo by author.

Graylingwell Hospital

Sunday, 3 September, 1967

Autumn, early afternoon, a wet, dark, sunless day: a lone figure, anxiety hidden and under control, I descended awkwardly, weighed down with baggage, from the green Southdown double-decker bus at a northeast Chichester crossroads bus-stop, adjacent to the hospital entrance.

Westward, at the junction of the Broyle and Wellington Roads, was a walled-in Royal Military Police barracks (Roussillion) the site of an old gallows. Oakwood Park was across the road from the old peninsular Napoleonic barracks where, Don Quixote would have relished the sight of the two windmills that once stood there. The Festival Theatre now built on this parkland.

South of the bus-stop, down a slope, was Love Lane — since re-named College Lane. The Bishop Otter Teachers' Training College (now Chi University) was halfway down its length, where a small running stream showed a ditch on its east side. A hundred-plus yards further down, and close to the road was the site of an old pest house hospital where, in the 18th century, smallpox patients and other deemed anti-socially diseased people were cloistered. Earlier, pest houses were known as leper or lazar houses — then early hospitals.

Nearby, off Spitalfield Lane, was St. Richard's Hospital, built in 1939, which had been constructed on part of the ancient St. James Leper Hospital site; the lands were owned by the See of Chichester, in the medieval period. The leper hospital (one of four in Chichester), off the Westhampnett Road, was built in the 12th and 13th century with its own adjacent small church sanctuary and out-houses. Seventeenth century surviving archives disclose the early leper house supporting 'local cripples, *the insane*, and other incurables'. But as for the physically well but unemployed...

Across the road, opposite the site of the 19th century pest house off Love Lane, were the rear grounds of a Chichester workhouse. This building dated from the charity of Cawley, a regicide in the mid-seventeenth century, who established a poor house (Cawley's Almshouse), outside the city's northern gate on parish wasteland. Within this later-designated workhouse grounds, labour-yard poor-law staff gave food to the needy, in exchange for an obligatory period of work, under the watchful eye of a parish overseer.

Clearly for centuries, here in Chichester, West Sussex, as indeed benignly throughout the land, with its one-time twelve-thousand and more local such parishes, statutes provided for the poor, sick and unemployed together with its unfortunate deemed lunatics.

North of the bus-stop was Summersdale copse, in the Parish of Lavant. The local Sussex Southdown low chalk-hills area well-known to notables, past and present, including William Blake of Felpham, visiting poet William Cowper, Rudyard Kipling and Anna Sewell, Tickner Edwardes, the Powys brothers, Mervyn Peake and Simon Brett of Burpham (who was living in John Cooper Powys early 20th Century Residence) — to name a few. Above, on the upper slopes of the hills, could be seen the Goodwood Estate's racecourse. And below, on the lower slope of the downs, out-of-sight, but within easy walking distance, was Goodwood, the site of an old racing car circuit and site of a small airfield (once RAF Westhampnett). Eastward was the hospital grounds, which was my destination - Number 9, College Lane, formerly known as the West Sussex County Asylum, opened in 1897 for needy pauper lunatics.

The *West Sussex Gazette,* a champion of the new hospital from the outset, supported the needs of the staff and inmates. In the edition of July 13th 1899,[5] quoting from the first *Annual Report* (1897—1898), contributed by the Asylum's superintendent - the local newspaper said:

> "Dr. Kidd has especial pleasure in recording the resolution of this committee to allow the institution to be called, for unofficial purposes, 'Graylingwell Hospital.' Modern buildings erected for the care and treatment of the mentally afflicted aim at combining the elements of a home with those of a hospital, but as long as they continue to be saddled with the term 'asylum', so long will the unfortunate patients have to endure the dreaded stigma inseparably associated with the same. When it is once recognised that these institutions are special hospitals for the scientific treatment of a particular disorder, a great step will have been made towards accomplishing the disorder, a great step will have been made towards accomplishing the destruction of this stigma, the application of which at present constitutes a pitiless aggravation of a very pitiful affliction ..."

The superintendent's recorded facts (accepting there may be rotten apples in any barrel), exposed the gothic myth that all Victorian hospitals and caring institutions were cruel and vindictive by their very existence. And for me, on entry, the long stay hospital in the 1960s sustained a home (albeit austere) and hospital for people who, whatever an individual's history, were unable to personally survive in day-to-day normal life, or be coped with by family or friends within their local community. I wanted to learn and be of some service.

The Chichester bus moved on up to Summersdale and the low hills. The departing vehicle seemed slow and sluggish, like a huge hump-backed glistening Tenniel green-caterpillar out of *Alice In Wonderland*, spraying mud gutter rain-water and crushed browned Autumn leaves in its wake. As I entered the main hospital open driveway, I passed the South Lodge, a small gate-house but, without any gate — on my left. There was a gate still there in the early Nineteen fifties; a large white one, outside the South Lodge Main Entrance to the drive, registering the grounds as private rather than an open right of way (in the 1950's, it was closed for one day a year). At some stage, during this time, it was taken down for a repair, and not replaced.

In front of The Lodge in 1967 stood a signpost that advertised *Graylingwell Hospital and Day Hospitals. West Sussex Area Health Authority. Chichester District*. The wooden-plank sign-board painted in blue and gold had the Sussex shield motif of six Martlets painted above the text. On the left side of the ascending driveway, and at each side of the tandem pathway, stood tidy spaced trees which wove symmetrical lines; horse-chestnut on my left and lime trees on my right, snaking the half-mile hospital drive.

Each tree was a patient sentinel.

A large area of grass parkland extended on the immediate left, with a noticeable concave sloping earthwork forming a small green trench — as if some creature had one-time burrowed its way northward across the field. Across the drive, vaguely to the right, I could just see an assortment of tall red brick buildings behind trellis trees, iron-railings, gardens and grassland — but, no high boundary brick-walls.

'Gotta cigarette, sir?'

Stepped in front of me, blocking my progress, was a large corpulent man. The rain was pouring off his hat-less head. He was wearing an ill-fitting black plastic mackintosh, which reached down onto an over large pair of Wellington boots. (Ouch! and what did I look like to him?) He waited, eyes hooded by the wet cape of long unkempt hair; like the tree behind him, dark and statuesque, he stared blankly at me, awaiting a reply.

'Eh, er — erm. Sorry...!' I spluttered in staccato cadence. 'I don't smoke...' Muttered in truth and intended good manners. Before any further exchange could ensue the man stepped back against the water black tree trunk, under its insufficient umbrella of leaves and, as I moved on, he about turned, leaned back against the bark — and appeared to no longer see me. I left him looking back down the pathway from which I had just emerged. A few paces on I again looked back, but he had disappeared. Curious; was he a patient? A vagrant? He could hardly have been a member of staff. Whoever he was, he was no apparition.

The hospital report of 1898 gave initial statistics of 202 male and 239 female patients safely in their charge. No out-patients in those days. Dr. Harold Kidd said:

" Of the total number of those discharged, 24 were sent out as recovered."

And this was in the first year! Not bad for a believed closed institution to which the *scientifically* certified were believed to be condemned:

" ... Calculated in proportion to the admissions, excluding transfers, this represents 22.9 per cent which is a satisfactory result year's working..."

On guard, the good doctor reassured the Chichester public-at-large that only the really insane were allowed to remain in their charge in the asylum, and added, in respect of:

"Malingering... Whatever any doubt was entertained as to the stability of the patient's mind, the discharge was made subject to absence for four weeks, or longer ...."

(Under the 1890 Lunacy Act, if a patient remained AWOL for 28 days they could be discharged. But, re-admitted as a new admission if detained, and found certifiable. Subsequent Mental Health Acts in the twentieth century would repeat this 28 days survival clause.) Dr. Kidd added:

" There have been no re-admissions ...."

Vigilant, he further informed the press:

" One patient, however, was brought back under the following circumstances. A.W., alias M., was admitted in August 1897, with a history of having been sent to various asylums four or five times during the preceding three years. Whenever discharged, he contrived to get himself re-admitted, either by committing some such action as undressing himself in the street, or by performing some wanton deed of mischief in such a way that suspicion, but no actual proof, should fall upon him, and when arrested, feigned madness. He was a constant source of anxiety to the police, and expense to the ratepayer. After being kept under observation for some months, he was ordered to be discharged in August 1898. A few days afterwards he was brought back to the asylum with the statement that he had attempted to commit suicide by placing himself upon the railway line. It was obvious that he was *malingering*, and he ultimately admitted that he had acted deliberately, so as to be brought back to the asylum. He stated that as there was no train due, he placed himself upon the line, having seen a signalman nearby and knowing that he would be observed , and any chance of harm happening to him prevented. Under these circumstances he was cautioned by the committee chairman and ordered to be discharged as 'not insane'. Within a few days he deliberately set fire to some stacks, and contrived to be taken up in the neighbourhood on suspicion. This time, however, he was promptly committed for trial at the Lewes Assizes, and on conviction sentenced to eight years' penal servitude." [6]

In retrospect, it appeared obvious that, anonymous A.W's clinical details on his reception would have been recorded somewhere, and kept in one of the early pig-skin bound *Case books. (*And undoubtedly is still there — untraced. — somewhere in Chichester county archives). If, following re-admission, he was again certified, the case note would have had two photographs attached (one on admission another at discharge; the hospital Dispensary took and processed these identity pictures). This procedure continued until or about the first world war when Graylingwell was re-designated one of fifteen or so war hospitals. Thus on admission a patient was designated clinically, *scientifically* insane or not: in need of an alienist ... or not.

Why A.W. in 1897—8 should have been in such a suicidal state (and it was a crime to make such an attempt until 1961), was not recorded as a viable need; a prognosis for help indicating a clear disability: but not punishment for his suffering?Was a relieving officer (social worker) called upon?

What, why, is the The Unconscious, unconscious! Freud and Breuer's *Studies in Hysteria* — first published in Germany in 1893 — and Freud's (free association) seminal *The Interpretation of Dreams* in 1900, [7] suggested the *living* unconscious (inner space) *as a source*, naming the *intangible*, unknowable (unspeakable) - really does exist! But, dreams and hysteria, at the turn of the century, appeared, it seemed, to most laymen and specialists alike; the stuff and nonsense of ancient alchemy and astrology, and The Occult (para-psychology) as lunacy and horror stories. Meanwhile, Graylingwell, for their 441 lunatic patients care and treatment, listed only two qualified Doctors in the 1899 stats, Dr. Kidd and his Assistant Dr. Steen. In the pre-morbid Occupations of the patients admitted to the asylum in that year were two sailors and four soldiers — listed in Table XII of the 1898 Annual Report.

It was tragic. In the local *West Sussex Gazette* [8] in its July 13th 1899 edition, a short footnote read : 'The other day an army pensioner, who went scathless through Rorke's Drift, killed himself by lying down in front of a railway train. He had previously made an unsuccessful attempt to end his life by cutting his throat. He had better have fallen before the Zulus.'

Making further connections the Anglo-Zulu battle had been fought over twenty years before, during January 1879: I had in 1967 seen and enjoyed the heroics of Rorke's Drift in the fictional 1964 film Zulu and would later read eye-witness accounts, collated by the South African journalist Duncan C.F. Moodie's 1879 contemporary work *Moodie's Zulu War.* [9] The latter work included an official report by witness Lt. R.M. Chard. R.E. on the recent action. At the rear of the book, in the Appendices, was a complete list of the combatants at Rorke's Drift.[10] A hundred or so of Chard's comrades — officers, N.C.O.s and men — fought in the uneven battle; it was estimated that there were 3,000 or more Zulu warriors.

Who was that un-named suicide (a neurasthenic - war casualty?) of 1899. Was he on sapper Lt. Chard's '79 list of participants, - or was this source anonymous; as in the W.S.G. jotting - was he indeed an untreated *later* casualty of that *heroic* event?

And was he referred to Graylingwell?

At my own beginning in Graylingwell in 1967, I was readily *sensitive* to its latent history, sensitive to those, known and unknown, mentally afflicted that were referred to by Dr. Kidd in his first annual report. I joined my own impressions, threads and traces; phantoms and ghosts; shadows and glyphs, in and about the grounds: gelled with their residue of recorded memories — in *Case notes* — in paperwork in press records, presently residing in 1960s *Patients Affairs* archives, located in a small loft over the hospital's medical records (previously a provisions store before conversion). Momentarily I lost previous concentration, but the ghost wind and cutting rain, acting as a catalyst, again increased my pace. I passed no other person, though a Morris black-car splashed by and disappeared into the grey-mist veil ahead.

Marked by a high castellated red-brick tower on a low-crest of the road, and viewed through the watery veil emerged a gaunt tower-like Peake castle like Gormenghast, or motte-and-bailey Tolkien Isengard. The tower could be perceived as a place of learning, a sanctuary for those in need of care — and its carers. A mist-hidden mulberry grove asylum for resident monks — mystics of a Sarmoun Brotherhood high-up in a faraway Afghan Hindu Kush. On a clear day this water tower mist-free was easily seen from Tangmere — several miles east of the hospital estate. Adjacent to The Tower was the main building and the front entrance. Suddenly, I was at my destination.

A crescent-shaped tarmac driveway with a one-way entrance and exit, a matching green-island directly opposite the front entrance. The island a well cared for garden of trees and flower beds, several seats *in situ.* Adjacent to the front entrance, cobbled with a layer of small stones, shingle noisily crunched as I approached its wide double-door. This late Victorian building was clothed in substantial thick green ivy, part of which was draped over the doorway — a thick moustache about its face. Over the heavy white painted door with its large polished brass door handle was the West Sussex shield with its six Martlets cast above the lintel, an icon-like protective mark. This had as its provenance, its historic pedigree as an Asylum dating back, in common law, and statute, to the fourteenth century called:

> The law of the PREROGATIVA REGIS, dated, A.D. 1323 - 4. Anno 17 Edw.2. ft. CAP.IX & CAP.X.

This is an early English statute which ensured provision in establishing a duty of care contract for selected disabled subjects, offering sanctuary, a named person was authorised as or by the reigning sovereign — the titular head of state. It was a man-created Law [11] which, taken as a natal right, ascribed royal lineage as divine — or won by battle — which gave the reigning monarch jurisdiction '*over the estates of idiots or natural fools*'. And, bound him or her to find '*necessaries*' for any person '*that beforetime hath had his wit and memory and, should 'happen to fail of his wit.'* I remained unclear as to the probable fate of all other monarch's (titular head) owned citizens, who as subjects possessed *no* estate but, would meet the physiological deficits that might advise such a diagnosis — to find *necessaries.*

The hospital was in the 1960s — as all state institutions, still under the benign *living* legal auspicious of The Royal Prerogative, viz our government was deemed responsible for all hospital residents, as I then believed on my entrance into the caring profession at Graylingwell Hospital. But unknown as yet to me, the Prerogative, was undergoing rank *political* changes as to what body and *who* was to be responsible for the *helpless* in the country; or so recent media appeared to reassure its trusting public. In fact I was wrong. The recent *Mental Health Act,1959,*[12] had already repealed this medieval statute — at least Chapters xi and xii, of that act; but I would learn of this conundrum later.

The medieval statute and related innumerable Acts that followed over the next 600 plus years was enacted to protect interests of those deemed sick, needy and disordered — the patients; certified, voluntary, subsequently informal patients — whether resident or outpatients. Not always including its caring staff, who may or may not be protected in law and, who were accountable to their employers, the local parish authorities in most cases. I was joining this community of hundreds of staff carers at the psychiatric hospital.

Above the lintel of the front entrance was a substantial raised carved half-circle, over which mid-centre a glass covered lamp was extended, covering the main entrance. Perpendicularly and above the lamp, over the doorway, an ornate tall colonnaded window, a third eye, watched me, as it observed all new and established entrants alike. At the top was headed a triangular roof section enclosing a small inset window — the whole-unit raised out and forward of the long grey-tiled extended roof.

Centrally on the roof top was a mounted cupola dome with a three-sided clock, above which stood a wrought-iron weather-vane - with a clearly observed, carved 1896 inscription, marking the date of the hospital's building completion. Graylingwell was formally opened in 1897. This was not of course just coincidence: 1897 was also the date of Queen Victoria's Diamond Jubilee. And in great style both events were elaborately celebrated, as a new millennium drew closer, to the turn of the new century.

On the right side of the doorway a large polished brass doorbell was seated; after pressing it as I entered the building. It felt as though I had pressed the nipple of an electric starter button of a vast but silent, mechanical machine. Out of the wind and rain I discovered an area echoing silence in stark contrast to the elements outside.

The front entrance hall and corridor floor was laid in a soft bright red carpet. The side-walls, or rather the lower half wall was papered in a wood grain and wood beading nailed on top. Above was a bright white ceiling — a warm entrance to any potential resident or visitor. Behind the glass-panel 'Enquiries', was a telephone switchboard kiosk. Inside on the immediate right sat a bespectacled young lady, the duty receptionist. Her long dark hair hung down partially across her welcome smiling face above a taut crisp well-filled embroidered white blouse. The rest of her form was properly hidden behind a wood business counter, as she peered through the glass at me.

'Good Lord ... you're drenched aren't you ?'

It was rather obvious, but equally clear that she was being kind and sympathetic to me, a complete stranger. This casual act made me feel not only warm but welcome. I smiled back at her, and relaxed. 'Please, could you direct me to the main Nursing Office ?'

'Certainly. You go down to the bottom of this passage. Turn left. And then first right, you will find it half way down that corridor on your left. You can't miss it.'

'Thank you.'

Drenched, I paddled my way down the corridor, and noticed side rooms marked by tacked on door labels; doctors' rooms; waiting rooms; and toilets - men, women, staff. A single unoccupied phone booth door was open, with visible debris on its square floor. On my way I passed two middle-aged ladies who appeared to be in some slight disagreement ... 'Sister said I *can* do it.' A hard accent on the cadence, possessive. Their dresses seemed very colourful; their dressed hair bound with psychedelic mauve and purple colours. I assumed they were wearing Sunday best.

As I approached the nursing office, a notice signposted its rooms, I observed a tall, well-built young man in a flowing unbuttoned white coat and grey trousers, disappearing round the bend, to the right, at the bottom of this narrow corridor. On the door marked Reception, a footnote underneath the text said 'All visitors and nurses please report to this office', I knocked, a little gingerly. 'Come in,' a loud but cheerful voice replied.

The middle-aged well dressed lady in a blue blouse and grey skirt was the Duty S.N.O. (senior nursing officer), who introduced herself as Mrs. Vatson. Seeing me a little puzzled, she explained. ' Senior nurse administrators wear civvies on most occasions; and generally, we only wear uniform if on duties about the wards. All nurse grades above that of charge nurse and sister mostly dress in civilian clothing. Medical staff wear white coats or civilian clothing — as they choose.'

As I was expected, I was quickly re-directed to staff quarters. I reckoned the speed I was turned around had something to do with a small pool of rainwater about my feet.

My temporary home was a minute bedroom located above a staff restaurant. Its window looked out upon an enclosed quadrangle-yard with an overgrown grass area enclosing several irregular shaped flower-beds, bordered by incomplete meandering broken paving. I later learnt that the singular locked male acute ward was on the opposite side. My own single room was a minute neophyte's cell.

Stripping off my sodden clothing I examined the space — nondescript, two-foot-six inches bed with bedding supplied, small wardrobe, chest of drawers and a single chair. The window had green curtains including a half-net. And, blessed, there was a single radiator below the window ledge which supplied central heating.

I changed into in a thick sweater and a pair of casual grey trousers, after a brisk towelling down. Closing the door behind me, I realised the room was one of half-a-dozen for *Male Staff Only.* A tacked-on notice at the doorway into this area emphasised this significant fact. These minute rooms — or cells — were located over the staff restaurant.

A bathroom and toilet was placed at the end of the narrow corridor, close to the doorway, off which the six rooms were located. I looked in and observed a large solid but chipped, deep white-enamelled vessel with raised side-handles. This large bath was a reminder of a past local public-baths facility I was acquainted with in Church Street, Stoke Newington in north London N16. They were near my then very first *real* home, at 139 Dynevor Road, a small terraced house, without a bathroom and an 'outside' toilet, to which I'd first moved to out of Spurgeon's Orphan Homes back in July 1951 after fourteen long years mostly being in the care of others. The small mid-terraced house had considerable bomb ruins surrounding it. I recall a weekly visit to local public baths cost sixpence. This included a clean towel and small tablet of soap. I then joined a long queue with other men and boys.

About teatime, not long after four o'clock, I descended the short flight of echoing concrete steps into the corridor. The Graylingwell staff restaurant entrance was but a few yards along to my right. On entry it was empty of other members of staff — and so quiet. I could hear the sound of the still beating rain up against the nearby windows. The staff restaurant displayed about a dozen or so, square laid tables.

A lone young waitress appeared from behind me and asked what I wanted. I selected an egg-on-toast with bread-and-butter and a pot-of-tea from the daily printed menu placed on each table — interesting. At the bottom of the text a line recorded that the menu had been printed at the hospital's own printing department, which was in fact about a hundred or so yards away situated next to the hospital bakery on one side, and an upholstery workroom on the other side. I was impressed. Clearly the hospital was self-sufficient with numerous facilities. Just how large a Community it was I had yet to divine.

The waitress blended with the so clean neat and symmetrical laid-tables, covered with immaculate pressed white table-cloths. Perhaps it was my placid mood that seemed to emphasise the quietude about the room, and in its location, in this very large caring institution. As my first ritual in the hospital, this so small everyday event of eating a meal, as a new resident, gave a distinct ambience, a purposeful dignity, to the occasion.

As she served me the waitress said 'Good afternoon' and enquired as to if I were a new staff member. I confirmed the probably obvious, though not necessarily so, fact. She replied, laconically, as if to reassure me. 'Welcome. This is a really *good* hospital.' Duty done, she about-turned, and moved on — presumably, to attend other duties beyond this room.

I sipped my tea and mused on the newness of it all before looking further about the room. To my surprise, in a corner behind me I observed a dark young man, apparently finishing *his* tea. And, we two were the *only* persons in the dining- room. He was smartly dressed, certainly compared to my own rather casual appearance.

We caught each others' eye and grinned inanely at each other. In that almost church quiet, we were too shy, too polite, to presume any introduction. I returned to the egg-on-toast recalling that surely I had seen him a few hours ago? He had been a few yards in front of me as I left the Chichester railway station; he was getting into a taxi as I had set off to walk to the nearby bus station. So ... was he too a new intake student?

Nowhere to go at this time, I hesitated to explore the hospital interior as I did not yet know my boundaries, and what was formally out-of-bounds. Indeed I would feel quite intrusive in going into relative forbidden places; and besides, the still falling rain further inhibited going outside for any exploratory walks.

I returned to my room to finish unpacking. There were few clothes to put away so I stacked my books on the top of the chest of drawers. Early evening I sought out the telephone kiosk I had noticed on my arrival. I was to telephone Sara, who was staying with her parents in Lancing with our two infants Paul and Kit, whilst we sought our own accommodation.

As I walked back from the telephone I passed in the corridors, a few people who I assumed from their physical postures but lax walking pace — and snatches of overheard conversation — were possibly visiting relatives on their way back home. I passed two other people who seemed at home, exchanging a little noisy communication which, to me, identified them as resident patients.

It was the end of my first day at the psychiatric hospital as a first year student and I expected to sleep well. I felt content — it has been a good beginning.

Putting my book down, extinguishing the light, the last sound I heard before going off to sleep was the distinct sound of breaking glass from across the quadrangle, followed by a loud but muffled voice shouting out some demand or other.

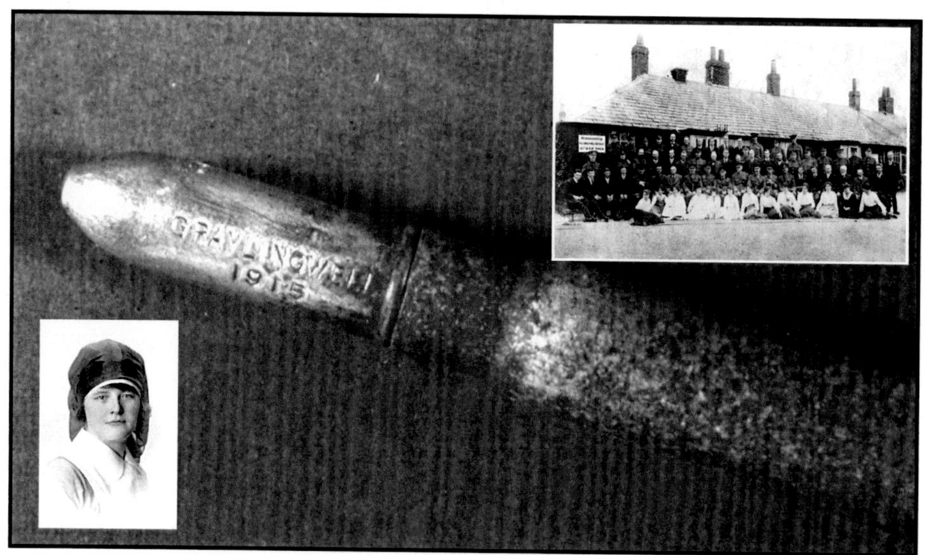

1915. Graylingwell War Hospital souvenir bullet, dated 1915. Donated by postwar nurse Vera Lewington (later Searle) who first worked during the war, as a seventeen year old clerk, in a 35th R.D.R. area (Chichester) recruiting office at nearby army barracks, based at Summersdale, north Chichester. Vera then trained as a nurse for the insane. As a 19 year old probationer nurse, she was later informed by the hospital authority it was forbidden for ladies to visit the nearby soldiers that were stationed at the old Napoleonic (Roussillion) barracks. She married a qualified Graylingwell nurse, leaving as a charge nurse in 1926 as, then, no *married* couple could be employed as nursing staff.

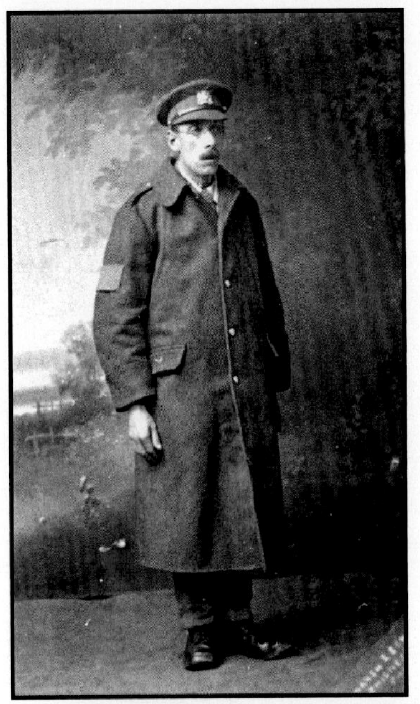

1916. First World War soldier patient posed in Graylingwell War Hospital. Note square patch on his greatcoat. (Photo by Marsh & Sons, Chichester.) **Below:** Graylingwell Military Hospital, Ward Sisters. (Photo, Marsh)

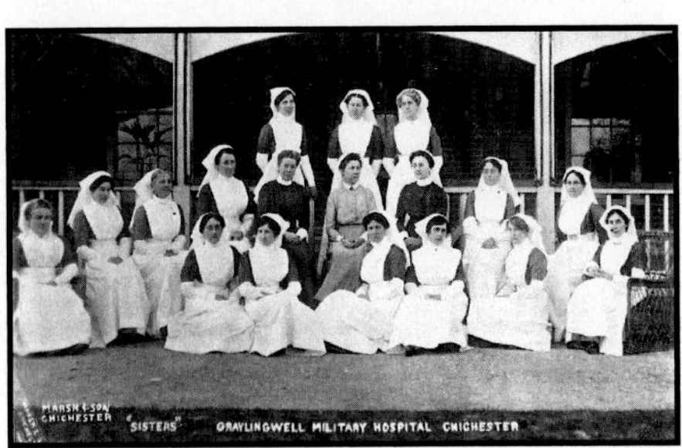

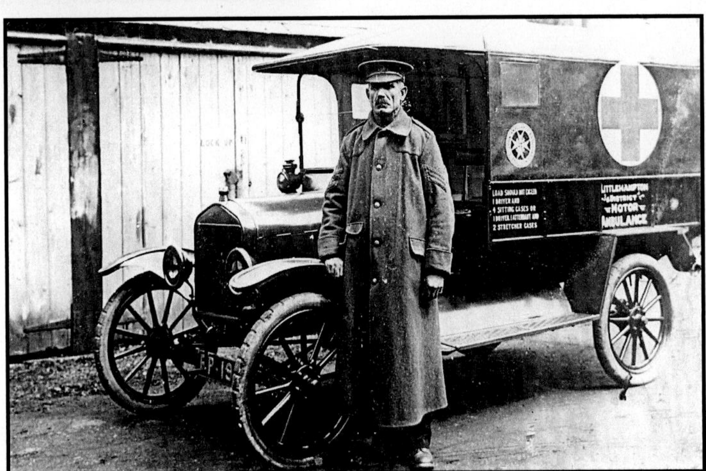

1915.First World War Ambulance and driver for Littlehampton and District. This vehicle would certainly have paid numerous visits to and from Graylingwell War Hospital. In 1915, Martin's Farm had completed structural alterations for motor ambulances - and stallage for seven extra cows. (Photo source, Jack Thompson.)

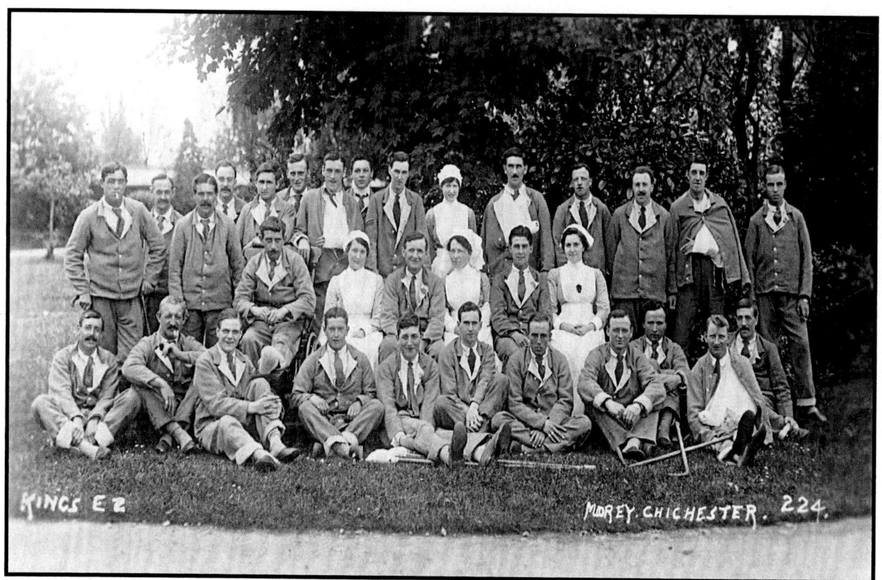

1915. Graylingwell War Hospital (c.1915 - pre-Somme). Patients & staff of King's E2 Ward. Back of photo the following ; Back row - Blois (?). Middle row (L to R) Pearl, Nurse Gray, Pte. Short, Nurse Blacklock, Clarke, Nurse Holmes. Front row. 1234 then Pte Blood, Pte. Edwards.

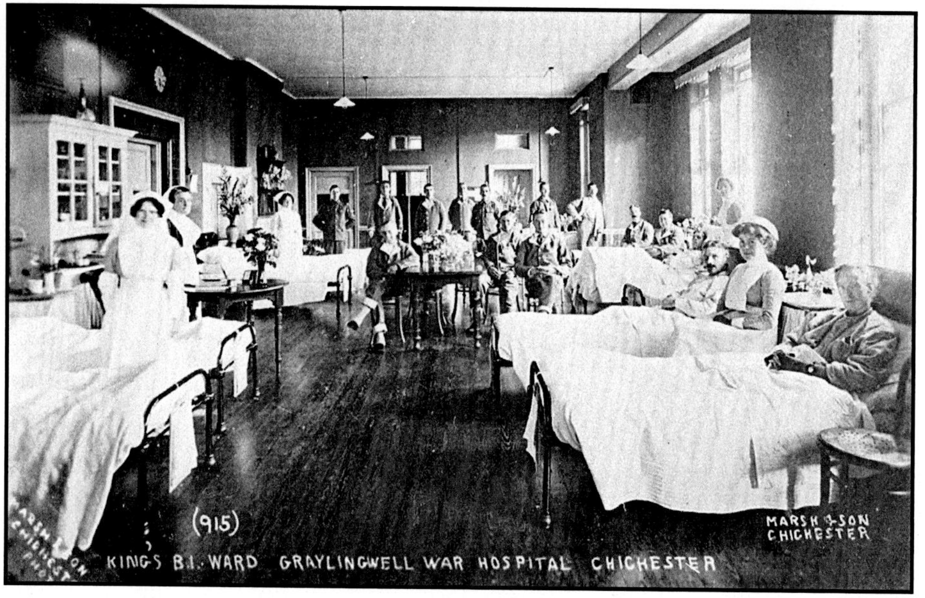

1915. Graylingwell War Hospital King's B1 Ward. Later known as Male Bramber One Ward. I noticed the dormitory ward fabric little changed in the 1960s - fifty years on.

Chapter Two
Intake

' Dear Boy. History must be accompanied with Chronology, as well as Geography or else one has but a confused notion of it, for it is not sufficient to know what things have been done, which History teaches us, and where they have been done, which we learn by Geography, but one must know when they have been done, and that is the particular business of Chronology.'[1]
Lord Chesterfield. Letters To His Son. Sept. 15th 1739.

4th September to 6th October 1967

Intake—School—Syllabus—Admin Baz—Grand Tour—Villas—Superintendent—Graylingwell War Hospital 1915—The Somme—Baggage—Water Tower—Sandown—Dr. A.J. Cronin—Not Bedlam—Memories—Diary Notes—Classification—Watershed 1946—To Wards

Intake
Monday, 4th September 1967

There were five students in our intake meeting for the first time in The Office, three women and two men (the other man was my 'distanced friend' from the restaurant who I glimpsed en route to the hospital). We confronted each other, aware that our small group was to study as registered mental nurses. We were all dressed casually, because our hospital uniforms would not be ready until we had been measured for them by the hospital's own tailor.

We realised how important this initial meeting was, and sheepish grins passed across our bemused faces ... 'Hi ... new student ... ? '

Muted introductions. God ... how banal, the real sounded.

No time for enquiries of each other as we were directed out towards the school, through the front entrance. A signpost alongside the entrance to the North Drive directed us towards Summersdale Villa ward and the school behind it. The rain had stopped and, though overcast, it was dry. As we walked I noticed a number of male patients working leisurely amongst the lush green garden beds alongside the drive. A thick-rubbered two-wheeled trolley lay half off the road, half-filled with weeds and bric-a-brac.

The girls walked in front; Harry and I chatted as we walked behind. His Christian name was long and biblical — his surname sounded more French than African — and during that first exchange *he* asked if I would call him Harry (Barry was my long-used aka). And so, nicknamed already, we introduced ourselves to the others as *'I-Barry-he-Harry*' (to our joint amusement). Harry emanated a strength and dignity permeated by a distinct shyness. A tall handsome African, he was new to this country having only flown in from Ghana the day before. His excellent English reminded me guiltily of my own lack of fluency of other tongues.

School

We followed a crescent drive behind Summersdale Villa and on our right, just visible behind several trees and bushes, saw two low white pre-fabricated buildings. These two pre-fabs reminded me of numerous similar wartime low dwellings that abounded in the war-torn London ruins of my early youth (many *temporary* post-war prefabs had survived well into the 1960s). The Nurse Training School hut was on our left, and a second separate hut, then designated as a patients' Art Department, on the right. A narrow pave-stone pathway led off the concrete drive and into the school - which was used for any non-ward teaching. The building, L-shaped, provided three large rooms and a number of minute office cells and storerooms, as well as two separate toilets and a wash area with kettle heating facilities.

One large room provided clinical instruction, a hospital bed fully made, with a table and chair. Around the sides of the room in glass-cabinets or placed in cream-painted wooden drawers was a host of clinical apparatus, including large and small syringes, with boxes of enclosed needles — each coloured differently for size identification. Several drawers were full of bandages, cotton-wool-balls, and various sterilized kits ready for instant use. Apparatus was self-evident for male or female catheterisation for post-operative patients (or otherwise inhibited men or women). Also, neatly stacked to the sides were other as yet unidentified items and wooden equipment. On the walls were various charts — urine, litmus colour instant identification, a chart on the uses and abuses of insulin and a diagrammatic poster on the use of a triangular bandage. A large scale map of West Sussex was also visible.

Moving out of the clinic area we entered a minute compact library, with a number of tables and chairs to the front. To the west, through the library window, we saw in one large field several horses grazing. And over a low hedgerow, and across Wellington Road, could be seen the Barracks of the Royal Military Police, behind its own high red-brick wall. In all, surely, the school hut housed a microcosm of essential nurse education facilities to be found within most hospitals throughout the world.

Back out of the library we moved into the other part of the L-building to the largest room, which was the lecture room of the school. A large revolving blackboard was set away from a wall on its own frame on castors, and was prominent at the front. Overhead, a small cinema-screen was tightly rolled up into a ceiling fitting. In front of the blackboard, some four feet away, was one of four rows of three unpretentious wooden desks, with a tubular chair with a red plastic covered surface behind each. A mounted skeleton (dubbed Jane) resided in a corner recess, with a white modesty coverlet. At the other end of the lecture room another doorway led southwards and out. Adjacent, behind vegetative green facings, was the towering red-brick structure rear of Summersdale.

Just inside the doorway a small room was boxed off. It was the office cell of the principal nursing tutor and his colleague who was another Male Nursing Tutor. The school's windows were curtained with dark green fabric, and below the window sills were wall-radiators for winter heating. The walls were, not surprisingly, painted in white. The otherwise bare floor was of an immaculate red-tiled brick, for no carpet or scattered mats were to be seen in this room. The building was clean and sterile in its thoroughness. As we soon would learn, this complemented the whole vast hospital complex, and reflected clean, well-cared-for patients and hospital estate. The pre-fab school was where the Nurse Caretakers were trained, and our intake group would spend considerable time within its tiny, but welcome, sanctuary rooms.

Our casual tour of the School completed, a man emerged from the office and introduced himself to us as the hospital's principal nursing tutor. Mr Watkinson was a middle-aged man, slightly balding with a prominent nose, sharp intelligent grey-eyes, short stature and broad-shoulders. He was smartly dressed in a full-length white uniform coat — starched clean and pressed, this garment was worn over customary, but then obligatory, charcoal-grey-suit, white-shirt and narrow Windsor knotted grey tie — with polished plain black shoes. This, we learnt, was the formal hospital uniform for all male nursing staff. Female staff wore one shade of blue nursing uniform, dependent on the type of course they were on — Pupil Nurse, Cadet Nurse or Registered Mental Nurse student (or whether Staff Nurse or Sister-Charge Nurse). Nursing Officers dressed noticeably in civilian clothes though the male nursing staff, of whatever grade, mostly wore their grey suit as uniform.

Mr Watkinson asked if we were settled in all right. And whether we had had time to become acquainted with each other. 'After all', he reminded us, 'You will be together quite a deal over these next three years - if you do stay the course.' We acknowledged that we had only less than half-an-hour before met each other at the Office and needed time for better introductions all round. For the first-time we sat, self-conscious, a little uncomfortably, at the desks in the lecture room. Our Tutor stood before us — as he would presumably many, many times ahead.

'Before I outline the Course to you all, I think it would be better if we spoke a little about ourselves. Become better acquainted. This I hope will make you all feel a bit more relaxed,' the Tutor began. I pondered how many times, throughout one's lifetime, one experienced such introductions — and, eventually, departures.

We acknowledged by nodding our heads and looked to him for introductions. The girls sat in the front with Harry and I to the back, but close behind the others. We spent a while talking about ourselves, our background, districts we came from, marital-state, and general aspirations and expectations. Two girls were from Sussex. One was from Chichester; a tall girl who was dark haired, with thick rimmed glasses, dressed in casual white sweater and black skirt. She was aged 23 years, single, with some auxiliary nursing experience, and her name was Audrey. Next to Audrey was Rose, a smaller, older woman of twenty-eight years, pretty, with short fair hair and round face, dressed in a green dress. She was married with two infant children, and her husband was an engineer. Rose's mother-in-law looked after the children when Mum or Dad were not at home. Rose presently lived in Bognor Regis. On the other side of Rose sat the youngest of our group, twenty-year- old Sally, a pretty, dark-haired, lean-built girl who had travelled down from Nottinghamshire. Her father had agreeably driven down from Nottingham and they arrived early that morning. Sally was dressed colourfully in a patterned blouse and skirt. She was unmarried and had no nursing experience but, from the outset Sally bubbled with enthusiasm where-as we other older colleagues were somewhat guarded in our disclosures — at this time.

Harry next, spoke quietly, slowly, explaining that because he had arrived at Heathrow airport only the day before, this event was quite a strange experience for him. He declared that he was twenty-five years old, single and one of three children. His father, who at one time was a senior Civil Servant in Ghana but more recently had been an accountant, had died quite recently. We all commiserated with him. Till several weeks before, Harry had been on a course of further education back home. He was smooth featured, with dark skin, close curled dark hair, six feet tall, medium build, and smartly dressed in a dark suit and tie.

And last, I introduced myself. Of similar build and height to Harry - but the oldest at thirty-years old, married with two infant children. I then lived within the hospital grounds, whilst looking locally for more suitable accommodation for my family — who were staying with my in-laws. Audrey and Rose lived outside the hospital. Harry, like myself, lived on the hospital estate. Mr Watkinson concluded this introductory session by explaining his principal role, his expectations as our instructor; and his expectations of us as mature committed RMN candidates. His qualifications, he informed us, were state, Registered Mental Nurse (RMN); general, State Registered Nurse (SRN); Diploma of Nursing Studies; and various other teaching qualifications.

Our tutor warmed to our group as a body, and reiterated that we would be attending the School full-time for the first six weeks, culminating in an elementary internal Preliminary Examination — to appraise our progress and attitudes to date. Much of our time during these weekdays would be in guided tours of the various departments and wards within the hospital grounds.

As student RMNs we would be prepared for two principal GNC — General Nursing Council — external examinations. The first formal examination was due at the end of the first year — known as the Intermediate Examination, this would include a considerable amount of physiological questions, in line, to a point, with our alternative student colleagues in the general nursing field. At one time both RMNs and SRNs attended the same preliminary examinations. Only later, after this generic background, did specialised finals differ in presentation. Our second and principal examination would be the state *Registered Mental Nurse* qualification.

The final exam would be taken at the conclusion of three years service. But, preceding the external examinations, there would be internal hospital examinations — failures may make three attempts at their final RMN but, if unfortunate will be re-appraised as a State Enrolled Nurse (SEN). Periodic ongoing tests, ward-based examinations and clinical assessments would also be taking place. In the third year an internal exam would conclude (the last hurdle) the Community Care Block — and to the Final ...

Syllabus

Our initiation into what constituted ward-based, normal day-to-day work activities happened when Mr Watkinson disappeared for a moment, and reappeared with five small red books - one for each of us. Together we read the front-cover carefully, and examined the contents. 'These are your work records — one for each of you.' Mr Watkinson said. It read :

SYLLABUS of Subjects for Examination and RECORD of Practical Instruction and Experience for the Certificate of MENTAL NURSING. 1964.

The illustrated document, its red cover embossed with gold lettering, was issued by The General Nursing Council for England and Wales. Opening it up, the white page repeated the cover script, with several additions. The first related to the exact contents of the publication and stated that it — 'May not be reprinted or reproduced either in whole or in part without the sanction of the Council'. Entries were to be made for Name of Student Nurse, Date of entry to Training and, allocated, GNC. Index Number. The text of this vital document to individual training was introduced by a Preface; and a description of examinations described *The Syllabus...*

Section I - A comprehensive introduction to the Study of Mind and Body.
Section II - On Principles and Practice of Psychiatric Nursing including First Aid. The text covered history, administration, ethics, Ward Management, and especially a number of sub-headings and numerous details and facets of Patient Care and Nursing Procedure.
Section III - In depth - Psychopathology, Psychiatry and Psychiatric Treatment; and Legal and Administrative aspects related to all aspects of Patient Care.

The rest of the syllabus covered the above sections with each item, as learned by the student, to be individually checked off by a sister or charge nurse (and signed by them as verification), counter-signed by the student — and finally acknowledged by the classroom tutors signature. It was all very thorough and reminded us why we were there to learn. At the rear of this syllabus and record, the following indicated our, to be, involvement in community care and introduction to other professionals in the field of caring for sick and needy. Educational Visits gave nine headings (with room for additions) covering visits to out-patient clinic, observation wards, resettlement training centre, juvenile or adult court, hospital for the mentally subnormal, child guidance clinic, psychiatric unit for children, remand home and visits to patients' homes...

Times and Treatment, along with training and variation of attitudes and philosophy of care, were reflected in the final section of the Syllabus. A new printed sheet covered up an earlier text which headings were still visible beneath, reminding that this section was to record the amount of *mandatory* weeks to be spent in each area of patient care. The partially hidden text read: *Admission Ward - Geriatric patients - Long stay patients with disturbed behaviour - Neurotic patients - Convalescent patients - Occupational and Industrial Unit - Other experience please specify.*- The superimposed and presumably contemporary 1960s text sub-headings now read:

Newly admitted and short stay patients
Medium and long stay patients
Physically ill patients
Geriatric patients
Occupational and Industrial Unit
Night duty (specify experience)
Other experience (please specify).

At the end of the three-year RMN training in September 1970, when all experience was completed, the work-book would be countersigned by the head of nurse training school. The red document reflected how detailed the areas of our training would be. What it could not, and would not, record was each of our own unique spheres of experience — extra-mural studies, and how they might personally change or affect us generally, as finally trained Psychiatric Nurses. A separate notebook, diary or journal would be the nearest to such a personal record — to include extra-curriculum interests.

Mr Watkinson allowed us a quarter of an hour or so to peruse the record books, then again gained our attention. And, matter of factly, outlined the days programme. 'I appreciate this hospital and its large rambling enclosed grounds will be difficult for you to find your way around for a while. So I suggest we start our visits this afternoon after lunch. I will start by introducing you to several of the out-buildings, away from the main building. First we'll visit Kingsmead which is presently in use as an experimental day hospital. This unit provides a community health service which allows a number of patients to attend for out-patient day-treatment, and return home each evening. It is open five days a week. Afterwards I shall introduce you to Sandown house, an experimental alcoholic unit, which specialises in *Therapeutic Community Care*. You will learn more about this later on.'

'Initially selected patients attend for a course of treatment for twelve weeks, and as individuals contribute in running all domestic activities in that milieu. But, first we must go over to the Main Building to collect your individual ward keys. Oh!' he paused, admitted an afterthought. 'Have each of you got one of the *Nurse Training School* green booklets? You should have had one sent on to you before arrival. You will find it quite useful - and self-explanatory.' We nodded our heads. My copy was on the desk. It needed a better map of the grounds — an aerial photograph of the site was included. I mused... where am I *now*?

At a gesture we rose from our seats and departed for the main building, I chatted with Rose on the way over. She admitted that she had wanted to be a student nurse for years and had already worked in other hospital departments. It was approaching dinnertime and the driveway was inundated with staff and patients making their way back to their own wards — most patients returning from occupational or industrial therapy areas.

Admin Baz

Mr Watkinson led us into one of the administrative offices situated opposite the main general nursing office (with which we were already becoming familiar). It was explained to us by the clerk across the wooden counter barrier that these keys were expensive to replace — about ten pounds each, a large sum. Our tutor added that not so many years ago if any nurse lost their key they would experience instant dismissal from their post. The most helpful clerk explained that there were three types of ward key, large iron-wrought jigsaws — a male key for the male nursing staff to open only the male wards on the male side of the hospital complex, a female key, for female staff, operating on the female wards and finally a master-key to open all wards, only to be used by a chosen few of the senior nursing and medical administration. We got the message — and signed.

The admin clerk informed us that, in future, our salary payslips would be collected from here at the end of each month, and any pay queries would be personally dealt with through this office. Our P64s and other formal papers had earlier been handed in to the office — as practised with all new staff posts. The most efficient clerk, a member of the patients affairs department, was a lean dapper, all-smiling (for real) agile gentleman, first name Basil, popularly known as Baz. I would come to be acquainted with him in this office, and about the wards, and on numerous future occasions in hospital and later in the community at large, he was a mine of information.

From here onwards I knew the clerk as *Admin Baz.* His work was crucial in the general administration of hospital wards and patients legal issues, and meant he could often be encountered on the phone or frequently on his visits to the wards staff and patients; talking to other office staff about hospital affairs such as Supplies or the hospital's financial affairs, and staff pensions and communications — outside the hospital community these personnel seldom had contact, experience of the hospital patients and ward culture.

Grand Tour

Mr Watkinson excused himself as we left the administration office, and arranged to meet us all after dinner time back at the school. Together as a group we departed for lunch at the restaurant, feeling already united as a benign unit.

On the way back after lunch we studied a large diagrammatic black and white map of the hospital, hung on a wall at the bottom of the main entrance hallway. It was one of those *'You Are Here'* location maps. At first glimpse the main building looked like a cut-out, resembling an x-ray of a huge butterfly. The front entrance was the head; the Eastergate block was north west, with other male wards further west. Slightly ahead, at its north east, *opposite* side top corner was the Fawcett and Edgeworth female block, and directly to the east the other female wards — right side of the body. Bottom left, south west, an extended leg identified a covered way to Graylingwell House, the male nurses home: Bottom right, another leg was cut by a roadway and, outside, Richmond Villa at its south east foot. Below the main building and to the south of Richmond Villa was another detached building – identified as Kingsmead Villa.

Sandown House, the alcoholic unit, was next to and in front of Sherwood House and day nursery, with the Roman Catholic chapel in one corner of its block. These detached buildings were in the north east corner of the hospital grounds, across lawns and trees to the front of the main entrance. Summersdale Hospital was situated to the north west, with the nurse training school behind it. Already briefed to visit Kingsmead and Sandown, we located these buildings and the training school. Arriving back at the school, Mr Watkinson soon turned us around — as we made for the Kingsmead villa.

Despite studying the fixed map, we all felt lost, without a real clue as to the best route to take. Our Tutor suggested we should walk right through the Main Building corridors and emerge out at the Richmond Villa covered way — which preceded it. It seemed a long dark journey through the winding maze of corridors and fire-doors, despite the pleasant light-tan paint adorning its tube like walls and clean bright green lino-tiles upon the floor. Mr Watkinson continued his mechanical tour.

'Below this corridor, the Engineers inform me, lies a duplicate subterranean chain of corridors carrying all the plumbing and other essential piping facilities.' We marvelled at the largeness of this late Victorian Pavilion edifice. It was without opulence, but certainly no ugly complex. The Hospital was built as The West Sussex Asylum — to use current colloquialism, purpose built. The architects. Blomfield and sons, had taken a great deal of trouble to give it the huge airy space, sanctuary, and security which was needed for the numerous patients and caretaking staff.

Electricity supplies were introduced into the asylum in 1897, in combination with gas mantles. Initially, the wards had no electric points available, for they were not viable and would certainly have been unsafe. In fact, all wards relied on small iron *coal* stoves till a very late date; gas-jet urns for heating water were introduced into ward kitchens in the 1950s. Prior to that time tea urns, as all heated food, had to be taken manually to all wards and offices.

In the heart of Islington, London N1 my maternal grandparents had resided in an early 19th century minute terraced one-time bricklayer labourers cottage. This was at 2 Baxter Grove, off Wall Street and the Ballspond Road, and it survived the 1940 blitz — whilst down the Grove at No.1, lodgings of my mother and our family were flattened by said blitz. I recall rare visits out of the orphanage as a child and seeing the gas mantles and oven being lit by tapers and swan vesta matches kept on the mantelpiece, so comfort modernisation and *then* state of the art utilities of Graylingwell back in the late 1890s was *well* appreciated.

Few people passed by in the corridors. It was now two-thirty in the afternoon and the majority of staff and patients were occupied on site where they were supposed to be. Patients' afternoon work fixed between two o'clock, after dinner-time and three-thirty. Our tea-break was set for four o'clock in the staff restaurant. All patients' meals were served on their own wards. Mr Watkinson, once more garbed in his crisp white coat, walked ahead of us at a brisk pace. I chatted with Sally and Rose on the way to our destination. Sally was bubbling, her distinct Nottinghamshire dialect adding more colour to her conversation. Rose and I mostly listened, adding occasional comment. Harry and Audrey accompanied our principal tutor just ahead.

Turning a bend in the main corridor we abruptly led off to our right, through semi transparent thick polythene fire-proof doors and fastened back main metal doors, into the South East leg — the narrow covered way, with Richmond Villa and Kingsmead Villa clearly signposted by the doorway. I turned my collar up as we turned right into the driveway as a light rain began to fall. It was only a short walk to isolated Kingsmead. Beyond it, not more than two hundred yards way, the hospital sports and social club house was pointed out to us. Across the driveway was an unmistakable cricket field with a large iron-roller to one side, with its inevitable cricket pavilion seen across the far side of the Hospital's sports grounds. South was St. Richard's Hospital visible in the background.

The southern driveway completely encircled the sports field. The main building and its ward gardens and trees dominated the northern view behind. In the immediate South nestled the small city of Chichester, its foundations and port dating back long before any invading Romans built their walls. The spire of Chichester Cathedral was clearly visible, its sharpened pencil towering above the city's southern serrated skyline. Lines of trees and patchwork fields, with occasional other outbuildings, were marked apart by distinct hedgerows to the east and west. The river Lavant [2], reduced to a sunken brook, circled east of the hospital grounds and over and under around Chichester, en-route for the harbour via sunken ditches. Kingsmead Villa had a short gravel driveway of its own, its small car park (once enclosed gardens) adjacent to a corner of the surrounding macadam road around the cricket field.

Entering Kingsmead Villa we were immediately aware of considerable noise, music was being played somewhere in a room upstairs. A charge nurse in his white coat emerged from an office and gently signalled an apparently satisfied male patient off to one of the ground floor rooms. For the next twenty minutes or so we were introduced to, it seemed, dozens of busy occupied rooms; each apparently with a staff member. Unless garbed in white coat, or an already familiar blue dress if a nurse or auxiliary, it was often difficult to tell who was staff and who was the patient. It was patiently explained to us by the charge nurse that the Villa block was being used as a day hospital. This enabled patients to return to their homes for each evening and weekend.

The unit had been open for its present use about ten months. One of the present treatment programmes was designed for desensitizing individuals suffering from various phobias — pathological fears which reduced their self-reliance to an almost negligible amount (and were often symptomatic of other more deep-seated fears and anxieties). One art therapy room, with a Dansette machine playing Elvis in one corner, was in use during our introductory visit. Whilst impressed with the numerous activities, energy and enthusiasm of the Charge Nurse and his staff, we felt our distance, more as visitors than soon-to-be-involved student participants. Patients, at this very early introduction to our work, we felt, were even more remote.

It was early days.

Villas

On leaving the building we found it was still raining. Despite the inclement weather we agreed to walk outside, around the main outer driveway — around the Southern periphery of the Main Hospital building. Mr Watkinson reminded us that all Villas were built in direct response to the liberal 1930 *Mental Treatment Act* which allowed individuals in the community to undergo a period of treatment and rest *without* any need for certification, i.e. informal admissions. The patients we had witnessed at the Kingsmead Villa were perhaps typical of this group. Any one of its patients could significantly be a close relative, next door neighbour or friend — given an aggregate of stress, or bereavement, any individual amongst us is so vulnerable. He had clearly followed this rota for intake students and visitors many times, as he gave further topographical and historical information, and continued in his monotone commentary, to describe buildings and features within the grounds. We stopped midway, faced northward, and gazed back at the wide vista of the main building.

'With separate fronting, up that short driveway, you can see the accommodation for a doctors' residence — It's on the first floor. On the ground floor is a small dispensary, and a room used by the visiting hospital dentist. You can see the top of the main hall to the rear. The medical officer's residence links up with its driveway and this south road, between the west side of the cricket field, the two fields of the paddock, and Barn Field - which takes its place name from the former Martin's Farm, or rather what remains of it, which is over there.'

Mr Wilkinson pointed to the end of this S shaped winding concrete driveway. On the corner bend, ahead of us, on our walk was a small complex of farm buildings. They sat next to a clump of trees — two abreast, on the estate border and adjacent to College Lane. The Martin's Farm tall trees were planted in line with an noticeable earthwork which I had noticed on entering the Hospital grounds. Of historical significance — part of an ancient entrenchment perhaps.

Our Tutor continued, 'The carriageway to the Doctors' Quarters was originally planned as the main entrance. It's used nowadays as a rear entrance, and ambulances draw up at this back entrance where horse carriages used to disembark. It might explain the ornate gardens and trees in the landscape immediately to its front. You can see two small fountains, no longer functioning, one in front of Anderson and another in front of Amberley.' An ornate monkey-puzzle tree, next to each fountain was included among the variety of trees and flower beds of the two airing courts. All the wards were spread out left and right of the M.O.s quarters: Males to the left and Female wards to the right.

Moving on and we passed Martin's Farm on our left, and on our right, Amberley, Bramber and Chilgrove blocks. Asylum planners had labelled wards alphabetically from the foci of the Doctors' Residence — again, the suggestion of the one-time possible, intended Front Entrance, the 1897 wards as male and female A.B.C.D. residential blocks. But even before the main building was completed, the Chichester based visiting committee had faced the fact that the capacity of the asylum was already woefully under the required number of beds. Statistics for the new asylum had been kept, since 1893, following the County of West Sussex compliance with recent 1890 Lunacy laws. They accepted responsibility for *all* its registered pauper lunatics and began a singular Admissions and Discharges Book under the heading of West Sussex County Asylum in 1893.

But, potential inmates for the new asylum were widely scattered about the country, with outstanding 'contracts' made with other county asylums, (who too were having to juggle their statistics and contracts) and private licensed houses. There was also the added responsibility, under the Poor Laws, for housing chronic — deemed incurable — diagnosed pauper lunatics in the large West Sussex parish workhouses. In 1895, the visiting committee reported on progress of the new Chichester Asylum - in the local West Sussex Gazette:

> 'West Sussex Asylum. A Long Expected Report. Amount Of Contract. Comparison With Estimates. In these circumstances your committee have endeavoured to arrange for other Asylums receiving the patients, but have been unable to find accommodation. They, therefore, reported the matter to the Commissioners In Lunacy, who, however, are not able to name any Asylum where there would be room to receive the cases, and who are of the opinion that the only practicable course will be to make arrangements for the admission

> of some of the chronic patients into a Workhouse under Section 26 of The Lunacy Act, 1890, with the consent of The Local Government Board and The Commissioners. Consequently your Committee are about to make preliminary enquiries of The Board Of Guardians on the subject commencing with those in West Sussex.'

By law, only *certificated* insane could be admitted into the new 1890s public asylums. This remained so, until the instrumentation of the far-reaching *1930 Mental Health Acts*; fuelled by horrors of *The Great War* attrition — what a misnomer (inadequate facilities for treating shell-shocked, suffering from conditions such as retrograde amnesia, conversion-hysteria (many via Netley Military Hospital at Southampton) casualties, and many thousands of neurasthenic (nervous) breakdowns, which were instigated by the traumas of those war years, exacerbated by gross fiscal poverty, class politic ignorance, and prejudice). *Non-certified* indigent idiots — the feeble-minded — and those branded with a lack of *moral fibre* imbeciles (to quote early shell shock diagnostic terms) who remained resident and destitute on the workhouse wards — their keep paid for out of parish rates. This classification would soon overflow, by default, numerous clinical NYD shell-shocked war casualties into local parish Workhouse casual wards. [3]

New extension building work in the asylum, which was commenced in October 1899, planned to house 300 new patients, 200 female and 100 male. The same month, in 1899, an *Annual Report* would record the 'Calling out of Army Reserve men to join the colours caused the hospital to lose services of nearly half of male staff.' — which was the South African Boer War. The new female E block opened in July 1901; and the male E block opened on January 1902, but the construction of the Main Building extensions was not without its problems (as work had been delayed due to a labour strike).

The retrospective 1900 *Annual Report* recorded a manpower staff shortage in the hospital, and in its expansion workforce (which had a depleted building labourers' team of workers). I was reminded of Trade Union strikes about in early 20th century as described by Robert Noonan (aka Robert Tressell) in his classic *The Ragged -Trousered Philanthropists* [4]. Noonan was an artist and house painter who after various wanderings resided in Hastings about 1902, where he worked part-time for local builders and wrote in his spare time. He completed his work but died of tuberculosis in 1911.

The abridged version of Noonan's book appeared in 1914 but, a full version wasn't published till 1955. The substance of his work - Trade Union discord and wage' appraisals — coincided around the time of local labour discord (I am not inferring one as cause of the other, rather, a reflection upon the socio-economic climate of the time, in that first year of the new century), which encouraged a local labour strike at Graylingwell on the First of January in 1900. Contemporary photographs were taken of the striking building labourers in the Graylingwell grounds — after the strike was resolved, the pictures were posed outside the recently completed new extension blocks - spades an' all. A reminder of those not so far off, earlier Asylum days - and the Nineteenth century ...

Superintendent

We returned to the main south drive, also referred to as the Farmhouse Road. A significant building, opposite Havenstoke Parkland, was signposted down a short driveway. At its end a cul-de-sac emerged, from a covered tubelike brick passage linked to the main building by a symbiotic umbilical cord; its origin located between the male B and C blocks. The corridor then terminated in a detached male nurses' home. This building was originally the Nineteeth century asylum residence of the first superintendent, Dr Kidd, his family, and servants, long before the coming of the National Health Service. I saw tall soldier trees around this late-nineteenth-century elite carriage driveway surrounded the one-time taboo island. Medical superintendent of the *new* asylum, Dr. Harold Kidd, was appointed on the First of October in 1896. This fact gleaned from our Principal Tutor made me think hard about welfare provisions available throughout the whole of the Nineteenth century.

Graylingwell War Hospital, 1915

When writing in *War Gossip* magazine for a children's publication (and anxious civilian public waiting at home to receive wartime casualties), and accepting a non-combatant's rank ignorance, an un-named 1855 journalist wrote:

> 'To most of us the sensation of living in a time of war is altogether new and unfamiliar; for there was nothing in the campaigns against the Afghans, the Caffres or the Burmese, to bring the fact so palpably home to us as what we have seen and heard within the past twelve months. For my part, I can remember seeing the public dinner in the streets to celebrate the peace after the battle of Waterloo, a sight, perhaps, the better impressed on my memory by some one giving me a lump of pudding, as my father carried me in his arms along the sidewalk. And when I grew older, and could read about the long years of hostilities which cost England so vast an amount of men and

money, and Napoleon his empire, it was to me a never-ceasing source of wonder that my parents had lived through such a terrible war. On winter evenings, when the day's work was over (asked) "Now tell us all about the war, And what they killed each other for." '[5]

I found the foregoing 1855 retrospect on the end of the Napoleonic wars not written in the aftermath of the Great War 1914-1918, but post-Waterloo, a personal anecdotal recollection of being a child in 1815, and adult as a non-combatant at the time of the bloody Victorian Crimea War in the Near East. As to 1855 poor law facilities for surviving Victorian Crimea war wounded, there was, in the main, *only* the formal poor-law out-relief and the post 1834 New Poor Law relieving officer an assistant overseer (social worker); a few county and military asylums, workhouse casual wards. And there was a little charity, like the C.O.S. (Charity Organisational Society) with its wonderful band of lady parish, church based, district visitors (like Louisa Twining and Octavia Hill). But, for most paupers, there was *only* the existing poor laws (often with their so punishing penalties and steered by elected Overseers) for consideration if qualified — including covering the needs of vagrant war veterans, battle-worn traumatised home undead and their associated families.

It was often the local parish church officials, *The Churchwardens*, who proved angels of mercy to both needy parishioners, and the unknown poor sick and wounded, civilians soldiers and seamen rendered homeless (legally criminalised as vagrants); people passing through as starving mostly unclad travellers, found about in their own local community. For many in a postwar climate who could *not* find work or who were by age or infirmity unable to work, and so unemployable, would often be treated as pejoratived malingerers and imprisoned in a House of Correction, Prison or in a new asylum Workhouse.

At the end of the so costly American, and French Napoleonic wars, in 1817, one of our Sussex coast churches at Broadwater (near Worthing), recorded compassion in its *Churchwardens Accounts* (1662-1836) p191, wherein I found the following entries:

'Expenditure. Edw Penfold's separate Account as Churchwarden. ... 1817. March 29th. Relv' 3 wounded seamen ... 6d. April 9th. ditto a Woman & 3 children. ... 6d. Relv' a poor man distressed ... 6d. May 17th. ditto 2 seamen ... 6d. June 7th. Rel'd a Poor Man on the road. ... 1s. July 5th. Rel'd a Poor Man on the road. ... 6d.'

This charity was possible before the introduction of the New Poor Law of 1834 when the new Town Hall would replace many of the church based vestry meetings of Churchwardens and Overseers of the poor; and of officials owed fiscal duties of care towards the poor of the parish - and vagrants (unable to provide for their own needs) passing through the local parish boundaries. And, one hundred years on from 1815...

Still the *same* old poor laws in operation during The Great War. ... And the same shameful treatment of many casualties (not at all, all); many sick veterans wrongfully branded as wilful malingerers — if they were distressed for over two weeks duration. I learnt that as the lead weight of the Crimean war's cost in human casualties became apparent, a new military hospital, *The Victoria* (after Queen Victoria who had a special interest in its erection), was built to receive battle casualties; built nearby old Netley Abbey, close to the waterside with its long pier for docking close to Southampton Docks; very much in demand during the Boer War ... and during the Great War. Also at nearby Gosport, Portsmouth, was the Naval Haslar hospital (built 1753 rebuilt 1818, this replaced an earlier, but smaller, *Fortune* naval hospital built 1713). At the time of the Crimea *Haslar* offered 2,000 beds. *Netley* (the Royal Military Hospital of Victoria), at the time of its opening as the Victoria Hospital in 1863, had a total of 138 wards housing 1065 beds.The Hampshire military hospitals, with at least 3,000 beds, would prove inadequate during the forthcoming Great War and so throughout the country, numerous improvised facilities were opened up (Sussex *Graylingwell* in 1915 a collective over 1,000 beds). Invaluable military hospitals continued to serve the distant Afghan wars; Zulu War; Boer War; and, two horrendous World War's casualties — product of the awesome savage (so-called scientific) Nineteenth and Twentieth century war campaigns. Notably, Graylingwell served them well - with distinction.

The country in 1914 was ill-prepared for so many military casualties statistics, and too few hospital facilities, for these new war-damned. The industrial *Great War* formally began 4th August 1914. The so-called 'phoney' war existing into 1915. H.G. Wells (1866-1946) author of *War of the Worlds* (1896) and *War in the Air* (1904), contributed a series of articles endorsing a just conflict, which he believed would 'disarm' Germany in three months — his optimistic articles published in a booklet titled *The War That Will End War.* [6] In' *The Sword of Peace* [7] an *optimistic* Wells said:

> 'Europe is at war! The monstrous vanity that was begotten by the easy victories of '70 and '71 has challenged the world, and Germany prepares to reap the harvest Bismarck sowed.'

France had previously been defeated (and Paris occupied), by Prussians, in the 1870-1871 campaign and again occupied in *The Great War* trenches of 1914-1918 — then, again, in the Second World War. Freedom censored amid the black tissue of Goebbels' lies and successful black propaganda. Vichy unfree, enslaved (as most of Europe) by the new military world order, enforced by Nazi occupation (Great Britain and America were *not* occupied). *Three* generations, grandparents, parents and children, experienced three bloody wars and dire invasions — uninvited foreign occupation of their country — in one lifetime.

In reading, and interviews with colleagues, in the 1960s, I was convinced European Nazi occupation, especially as found by inmates of concentration camps, and experiences of Vichy citizens, had contributed to Jean Paul Sartre's (1905-80), existential works of philosophy, essays, plays and novels —reflected in his *Roads to Freedom* trilogy of anti-hero novels. [8] Sartre (perhaps unwillingly?) subsequently, contributed, clinical and media growth, of postwar anti-psychiatry literature: (R.D. Laing, Sartre, and forensic *anti-psychiatry.*) And how this anti-war lexicon thread influenced selection, diagnosis and treatment classification in media, and duty of care at psychiatric hospitals and clinics, (including 1970s Graylingwell hospital), during the latter Twentieth century, and the ultimate, inevitable, breakup of long stay hospitals. But, back in the early years of the Nineteenth century, like the label *malingering*, being designated *poor* (as paupers, working class, labouring classes, et cetera), had sadly, long been a pejorative to elite Establishment (not so to the Church); and, the often not intentioned, use of multiple lists of *Statistics* was unhelpful in its dehumanising the subjective content of these sources of information.

The Great War was *not* over by Christmas 1914 as H.G. Wells and the media expected. The indecisive stalemate of the contenders, German central powers, versus the British French and allies, precluded an horrendous escalation of *millions* of military and civilian casualties found on both sides - *grossly* unprepared for the consequences and *shell-shocked* (I use it as metaphor) disabled survivors with many, many amnesiac untold tales yet (if ever) to be told. In occupied France Jean Cocteau (1889-1963) artist playwright poet philosopher had been refused *formal* enlistment in 1914, due to ill health, but enlisted as a volunteer in the Red Cross ambulance service at the front. Cocteau, in an autobiography, commentated on the *logistics* with dire irony, on dearth of French medical and transportation resources — and formal attitudes to wanton need (a nation found unprepared, by its country's leaders):

> 'I had just come from Rheims. Everybody was lamenting over the cathedral, while thousands of soldiers, dying of wounds, tetanus, gangrene, and starvation, were being left at the Hospice, without any measures being taken for their evacuation, without treatment and without food.' [9]

A formal circular was sent in 1915 to over fifteen County Asylums in England, Scotland and Wales, including Graylingwell, mandatory instructions from the *General Board of Control - Re: Accommodation for Patients received from active war zones* (a form dated 31st March) to open as a War Hospital (all wards re-named King's Wards on the male side and Queen's Wards on the female side) from 1st April 1915. In the 1960s and Seventies the past Administrative Records of the War Hospital's occupation were *not* to be found by me in the hospital's own Archives. They were expected to be stacked alongside 'unclaimed' baggage deposited over the years, in the Patients Affairs department. I believed the wartime records (of both world wars) were in *The Imperial War Museum* in old Bethlem, Lambeth Road in South London.

Many years later, in 1997, at Graylingwell Hospital's Centenary, I met up with Dr. Harold Kidd's son, Gerald Le Blount Kidd, in the grounds of the hospital. Born at Graylingwell in 1910, a tall elderly kind gentleman, naturalist and published poet [10], he'd travelled from Westerham in Kent. As we sat down on a garden seat set directly across from the building's original asylum front entrance, Mr Blount Kidd described to me his memories of himself, as a young child, standing alongside his father and seeing *outgoing* fleets of charabanc buses emptying the hospital of its resident patients back in 1915 — all except a few patients who went to relatives, and a number who stayed at the farmhouse with the hospital bailiff, Mr Peacock.

Seven hundred and forty seven patients were relocated, among ten other county asylums; Fareham, Wallingford, Portsmouth, Whitecroft, Chartham, Canterbury, Haywards Heath, Hellingly, Barming Heath, and Netherne. And for the next four years Graylingwell was re-designated as a war hospital, until departure of the military authorities, and return of surviving pre-war residents and staff in 1920.

And, of Graylingwell war hospital's first grim intake, an *incoming* 1915 convoy, reported by *The West Sussex Gazette* on 11th May:

> 'Upon leaving the station the crowd outside raised a cheer as each little party of wounded drove away to the hospital. Of the 150 or so first casualties - one third were stretcher cases, brought from Southampton: The convoy contained many from the Highland Regiments.'

Among the festive crowd offering support, outside Chichester railway station, were waiting notables, which included The Mayor of Chichester Councillor S.A. Garland, Esquire and Justice of the Peace. And, from active in khaki to blue-coated war wounded (first of thousands to follow in four terrible years), casualties came from battles at the front. These casualties were from the other ranks (Officers went elsewhere) and how many 'shell shocked' patients? In 1916 casualties came from The Somme to the Chichester' Graylingwell war hospital - via Netley military hospital at Southampton.

The Somme

From our very first meeting, our ex-RAMC tutor, Mr Ilford (I never did know his rank), in 1967 suggested that if any one of us RMN students would really like to explore diagnostic ambiguities, and attitudes to past hysteria, anxiety-neuroses (war neuroses), malingerers (were they really), attempted suicides, et cetera, then it would pay to search and find art and literature produced by persons who had themselves actually fought and lived in those times. 'But I doubt you will find many first hand war memoirs by the rank and file, as most were written by ex-officers or established writers and poets.' And of course he was right. 'Much of it will be anti-war rather than heroic literature.' But of course it was *not* necessary — we were only mandated to read up and memorise named recommended textbooks, like Ackner, for the state exams. He looked at me and smiled, nodding, in sympathy. I thought, he'd already summed me up, and knew I would do just that — though it would take immeasurable time for me to examine this aspect of clinical *and* social history, and in autobiography for authenticity.

I did not need much encouragement to follow this line of research — my own family had been heavily involved in the First and Second World Wars, as well as my own recent military experiences in the 1950s and 1960s, which now led me into research on shell-shock, and the danger of the de-humanising in the use of statisitics in describing the fate of millions of people in wartime.

For example, about the same time that my Grandfather was fighting in the trenches at The Somme one old soldier (writer Ian Hay, 1876-1952), a young officer, a sub, in 1916,[11] carried a WW2 general's baton in his knapsack, and as a Major-General years later, recalled shell-shock casualties in his memoirs:

> 'In The First World War we used to speak of 'shell-shock cases' - men who, though unwounded, had been mentally prostrated for the time being by their battle experiences, and must be soothed, comforted, and rested until nature had resumed control and restored them to their normal faculties. Various specifics were tried not unsuccessfully. I (the writer) retain a vivid recollection of a vast dock-shed in Southampton in July 1916, crowded from end to end with stretchers containing the first contingent of wounded from the First Battle of the Somme. In one corner, somewhat apart from the rest, lay the shell-shock cases. They were attended by a professional mesmerist who had been called in to lull their wandering, unhappy minds, if he could, to some sort of restful oblivion. '[12] (Note use of the term mesmerist in 1916.)

Optimism of an early Victory end of the war (both the Allies *and* Central powers believed that God was with them, and that *their* side would be the victors) disintegrated with reported, horrific, statistics during the first *Battle of The Somme* in 1916. Just on the *first day of the infantry offensive* July 1st the British estimated military casualties [13] were a devastating 57,000 (21,392 killed and missing) — and little ground gained by the slaughter on both sides.[14] Ian Hay was one witness at that large Southampton Docks 'shed' with the arrival of the first batch of Somme casualties — which included *shell-shocked* troops, those suffering amnesia (a not-yet-diagnosed (NYD) injury), and attrition from the recent battle who were awaiting dispersal from Netley to other war hospitals (including Graylingwell and East Preston in West Sussex.)

The Somme highlighted a crossover from blanket optimism to gross horror and much pessimism at its cost in human lives. Back home, propaganda was of a just conclusion in a heroic victory as the media remained in total disbelief and denial. Thousands survived — but in attrition left many mortally undead. I enjoyed a brief literary exchange with Robert Graves (who was in ill health) and his wife Beryl Graves in late 1960s and early seventies. In 1928, friend of Graves, also a Somme' veteran of The Great War, Henry Williamson, author of *Tarka the Otter,* with T.E. Lawrence, author of *Seven Pillars of Wisdom & Revolt of The Desert*, began a lifetime friendship: In Williamson's autobiography, he recorded[15] in diary correspondence with Lawrence, Sassoon-like and ruefully - one decade after the war, he wrotc to him bitterly of those bland statistics:

> 'July the First, anniversary of the opening battle of the Somme ('A Real British Victory at Last,' had cried the London papers. 60,000 British casualties and nearly all back in the old front line before midday, says history) and on July 2 a letter.'

Anonymous Great War attrition, statistics, continued adding up thousands of untreated shell-shocked (aka 'unwounded') combatants. An embarrassment to the government, and military authorities. At first refusing to admit to the attrition caused by then continuous mounds of slaughter. And in propaganda (for the sake of discipline) insisted that if any war casualty, civilian or military, was not diagnosed as clinically insane and admitted into an Asylum for incurables, or designated moral imbeciles and entombed in the parish workhouse. And, if any subsequent shell-shocked wounded patient was unable, or refused to return and again participate in the carnage of the trenches, individuals were to be criminalised and, or branded as coward, imprisoned or be called lunatic (whatever their history). At least, such neglected casualties back at the front on 'light duties' might have been inhumanely dubbed by non-combatant civilians as white-feathered malingerers; strong, broken heroes became weak, exhausted — and disabled — by attrition.[16]

Army authorities instructed its field medical officers that they were *forbidden* [17] to diagnose lower ranks as suffering with shell-shock (*not* like officers war-poets Wilfred Owen and Siegfried Sassoon who were treated for Shell shock in 1917 at Craiglockhart convalescent hospital, SW Edinburgh, now Napier University) from June 1917. Troops in the trenches were *forbidden* to use the word, deny its existence, but use the acronym *NYD* (Not Yet Diagnosed) in casualty reports and statistics. Writer historian and poet veteran Robert Graves feared toxic chemical Gas attacks even more than shells and recorded a military trench *Special Order* that the word Gas should *not* be used in frontline correspondence but, in-denial, the bland word 'Accessory' be substituted for Gas-cylinder and 'severe penalties on anyone who used any word but 'accessory' in speaking of the gas.' [18]

Twenty years on, after the First World War: during the Second World War, whilst the Allies followed the guidelines of the Geneva Convention (bless'im Colonel Blimp), in rank contrast, treatment of the Axis' Nazi concentration camps were, where - *Corporate Murder, dehumanisation* through *genocide* - was mandatory. For example, two only survivors from one 'batch' of a transport *intake (*from one statistic total of 400,000 un-named human beings - who had been recently exterminated), one man said that these corpses were being unburied; and were 'dug up bodies of the Ponari mass graves'; and amongst them, 'one of these two survivors uncovered his mother, three sisters, and their children.' An SS Gestapo soldier, directing this operation, demanded that, in future, 'You are to burn *all* gassed bodies', and informed the two prisoners, that *it is forbidden* to use the words *corpse,* or *victim.* 'These are sub-humans.'

The Gestapo man said, these dead are blocks of wood, shit, with absolutely *no* importance. Anyone who says *corpse* or *victim* will be beaten. The German made them refer to the excavated bodies as *figuren.* That is as puppets, as dolls or as *schmatter*, which meant rags. The polish jew prisoner asked how many figuren there were in the graves (to be dug up). The Head of the Vilna Gestapo told them, quoting bare statistics: 'There are 90,000 people lying there ... and absolutely no trace of them must be left.' [19]

Initially Nazis intended to concentrate in The *Final Solution (*aka holocaust), eliminating all members of the Jewish faith, as sub-humans, in the occupied countries (*including* natural born Germans), but the culled extermination was extended to include any and *all* sub-human undesirables, everyone in the occupied countries, not of diagnosed *pure* Aryan race. This damned policy of death included emptying all mental asylums and gassing all *mentally ill*, physically disabled, homosexuals, communists, trade unionists, journalists, Freemasons, Gypsies, all Jews, Jehovah's Witnesses and *anyone* found opposed, in anyway, to the Nazi Regime. Any owed duty of care was a zero consideration.

I feel it's too facile (however obvious), to identify *all* Germans and Axis partners rank & file, as though all were willing SS Gestapo troops; though obvious, facing The Enemy most often meant kill or be killed. *But* captured prisoners (regardless of race), wounded civilian and military casualties, allowed treating helpless enemy subjects as human beings. Frenchman Andre Gide (1869-1951) known to Cocteau and Sartre, fleeing from Nazi ruled Vichy France to North Africa, noted in his Journal memoirs dated on - 5 December 1942:

> ' The Germans are behaving here, one is forced to admit, with remarkable dignity', (and, in a footnote) 'Ragu told me that when he had to perform an emergency blood transfusion to try to save a seriously wounded English (or American) prisoner, six German soldiers immediately offered themselves.' 20

I was familiar with pacifist [21] Lew Ayres, starring in the 1930 film, script based on German, Erich Maria Remarque's 1929 anti-war novel *'All Quiet On The Western Front.* Remarque described vividly - battle severed limbs:

> 'We see men living with their skulls blown open; we see soldiers run with their two feet cut off, they stagger on their splintered stumps into the next shellhole; a lance-corporal crawls a mile and half on his hands dragging his smashed knee after him; another goes to the dressing-station and over his clasped hands bulge his intestines; we see men without mouths, without jaws, without faces; we find one man who has held the artery of his arm in his teeth for two hours in order not to bleed to death. The sun goes down, night comes, the shells whine, life is at an end.' [22]

Reality. I read of Frenchman, Henri Barbusse, writing in 1915 of his *poilu* trench friend Poterloo, together, out walking in a quiet pastoral scene - when a shell suddenly explodes about them, and in horror sees his friend - disappear:

> ' ... in the second when vaguely, instinctively, I searched for my comrade-in-arms I saw his body rising, upright, black, his two arms fully outstretched and a flame in place of his head!' [23]

Many survivors could be dehumanised, feel inadequate, and encourage mental illness; perhaps unknown, unrealised, untreated and mute in shell-shock! What happened to them? After the war, depicted in still, *silent* graphic black-and-white movies, *Dr. Mabusse* in German Fritz Lang's 1922 epic said, in writing, up on the screen; 'at least 80% of patients in Lunatic Asylums could be cured by Psychoanalysis .' [24]

Surely, wishful thinking; about a fantasy, in theory - statistics - one-to-one *available* psycho-therapy ... in all war hospitals?

But, It was an obscure pre war two 1935 Hungarian *autobiography* that (for me), duly summed up a fuller introduction, on *intake*; whatever side and nationality an identified 1916 combatant was born into. *Unheroic. Real bloody war.* The following awesome anecdote was written from experience by a Doctor in the field, and compliments Robert Graves and his comrades; albeit all Officers *and* other ranks. My grandfather, his bros, cousins, and overseas blood relatives who survived - or died, during The Great War. All *up-front* combatants, who experienced fear of gas (accessory), and effects of shell shock (aka NYD). Albeit all anonymous war-time casualties, caused by chemical warfare, toxins, machine-gun, and hot shrapnel rains. Survivors frozen in shell shock, as continuously arrived, at Southampton Docks and Netley Military Hospital, or other Nerve Hospitals - *en-route* for Graylingwell War Hospital - or other eventual a destination. ... Hungarian Dr. Volgyesi recalled being in action in the field - no decontamination facility available - in his memoirs he recalled :

> ' ... other scenes, too, rise before my mind, forecasting the ghastly picture of future wars. In Okna, for example, on June 4th, 1916, I first experienced the horror of a gas offensive. The Russians attacked with phosgene gas, but with their first attempt was un-successful; the wind blew the greenish gases back to their dug-outs where they hovered, a yard or so from the ground. They were not equipped with gas-masks, since they had been waiting for the wind to turn for weeks, and the offensive only began when the critical moment at last arrived. The wind however turned again and smothered them in clouds of destructive gas. I heard a chorus of death-cries that resounds in my ears to this day. Within a minute or two, not a man remained alive in that part of the Russian dug-outs. But even so, the misdirected offensive claimed its victims among our own soldiers, too. About five hundred Hungarian soldiers were brought to the first-aid station. They had hardly inhaled any gas at all. Merrily they smoked and jested, without a care in the world. But an hour or so later, without any transition, as though at a word of command, they jumped up as one man and after writhing in terrible agony for a few minutes, lay still and lifeless on the ground, one after another, without exception. And I was compelled to look on, unable to do any thing, with my hands folded, while death made havoc among my comrades. Can such a scene be forgotten?' [25]

In 1915 Graylingwell's Medical Superintendent, Doctor - gazetted Lt. Colonel Kidd of the Royal Army Medical Corps (aka RAMC); Voluntary Aid Detachment nurses (aka VAD.); the Red Cross; albeit all asylum staff were waiting to attend the first of to be anonymous (statistics) thousands of casualties to come - from 1915 onward. Notably two 1917 panoramic photographs of Graylingwell War Hospital's compliment of military staff and its body of volunteers - including boy scouts - were taken for posterity (see Appendix). And Numerous sepia postcard photographs of *recovering* wounded were taken during the war years at Graylingwell - similar pictures taken throughout the war in hospitals and convalescent homes about the country.

Admin Baz our sensitive clerk in 1967 retained a nostalgic description, a memory, shared with him of an incident in Graylingwell during those early days of the Graylingwell war hospital:

> 'During the 1950s I was advised of a World War One event that was either witnessed by my informant or his father at the time. It was a fine day and the recent army recruits in their innocence of youth were marched into the grounds of the hospital singing the usual cheerful songs of the day. Earlier in the day a convoy of war wounded had arrived and were placed on stretchers on the grass probably awaiting admission to the allocated wards. As the column neared the wounded, the front ranks had first sight of the realities of war, and gradually the volume of the singing reduced until complete silence apart from the sound of marching feet.'

For many years following both wars, ex-patients and relatives, occasionally, visited Graylingwell hospital - well into the 1960s. And copy sometimes, appeared in the press; recording some of their memories. In collating material for this history I found a huge gap, absence of detailed military data of its workings as a war hospital - about its service patients: I was unsuccessful in finding Graylingwell War Hospital's records in the hospital's archives (I have tried County Archives and Imperial War Museum and Kew Archives with no success to date). In the attic archives amongst Graylingwell Annual Reports (housed over Patients Affairs) I located Budgelike fragments of a May 1920 retrospective Military Report (p.33) dating from March 13th, 1915: To the Secretary of The Board of Control in London.

Since May 1915, specific General Hospitals throughout the country were established as *Neurological Hospitals*, and from April 1916 (pre-Somme) onwards used 'for cases requiring special but not requiring prolonged treatment' - at that time. And this substantial list certainly provided resources for shell-shocked (even if deemed NYD's on admission) for Officers and other ranks. On this list I located: *Near Worthing. East Preston Military Hospital. For other ranks* - operational by June 18th 1916. This was an independent command from that of Graylingwell. And prior to its acquisition was the large 1875 built East Preston Union Workhouse (for Worthing and District): after the war it returned to its original purpose as a workhouse — until being demolished in 1969. And In the 1920 Annual report (p.37), located in our hospital archives was a helpful reference: 'Dr. G.C. Going, of Littlehampton, took charge of an important Surgical Block coming over every day, until his appointment as Officer-in-charge at East Preston which was a great loss to the Hospital.' [26]

At the Handover of the West Sussex County Asylum, to the War Office Department, in 1915, the Main Building of Graylingwell had: 'had provision for 800 patients and was adapted to afford accommodation for 1,000 sick and wounded, but the number was subsequently increased to 1,068. Affiliated to it and working with the Red Cross, were The Royal West Sussex Hospital, Chichester (50 beds), and the Convalescent Hospitals at Littlehampton (60 beds), Bignor (60 beds) and Arundel.(12 beds) And Worthing for a short while (30 beds) With these, and by extension in time of emergency by marquees, extra beds and billets, the hospital accommodation embraced over 1,400 beds.' I wondered if Bignor (where there were Roman remains) was in fact Bognor?

In one modest report [27] Major Maxwell overseered, accommodation for Medical and Surgical cases on the King's side in Graylingwell. Other wartime photos of that period depict servicemen billeted on the Queen's side hospital wards. Maxwell said: 'The bulk of these were sent over from France during the winter months, when fighting was as a rule slack, and climactic conditions rendered men prone to respiratory and rheumatic diseases.'

America entered the war in 1917, subsequent casualties occupied (amongst other locations) *Milton Asylum* as a War Hospital in Portsmouth and Southsea in Hampshire: where, existent, I would work in from 1971-3. In Graylingwell 1918:-' facilities for training were afforded to Officers of the Medical Service of The United States Army. One of the Officers-in-charge Lt. R.H. George, M.C. afterwards in commemoration of the admission of a number of American wounded in 1918, kindly presented the hospital with an American flag, which had been flown in from France, which had been placed in the chapel.'

Despite austere conditions, Care and Treatment must indeed have been superb in the *Graylingwell War Hospital*, as Doctor Maxwell reported: ' less than 0.5% mortality rate in some 29,000 cases.' He felt that the survival rate was ' largely due to the Commanding Officer, Lt. Col H.A. Kidd, RAMC, alike for his very efficient provision for the varying needs of the patients, his wise advice in all questions of difficulty, and to the persistency of his endeavours to obtain anything that was needed from time to time for special methods of treatment. ... In a *Surgical Report.'* [28]

Baggage

The relative, a great nephew of a long deceased elderly patient, had unexpectedly turned up at the Front Entrance hoping to collect some personal belongings and been directed to Patients Affairs, where after an enquiry and considerable search an old still labelled, stencilled army number and name on a padlocked army kitbag had been unburied from a corner pile, and positively identified. Upstairs over the Patients Affairs office in the attic; on the same floor as redundant records and ephemera of the hospital archives. There in isolation was a small store of past belongings in an unclaimed *Boffin* dust-heap, stuff in inevitable decay. I gathered from Baz that the deceased gentleman had served in the armed forces in The Great War, and unknown in the detritus of those long ago days maybe to be found - remnants threads of a past life amongst this so sad baggage. I thought of the proverbial *Lost Property* department of the London Transport whereto much bric-a-brac and past valuables lay - for how long - unclaimed rack upon rack and out of sight and memory?

What did Great War' Kiplingesque trench squaddies earn as reward - in or out of hospital. Each everyman Tommy Atkins who survived hot silver shrapnel *incoming,* as Bruce Bainsfather. [29] ... *Well, if you knows of a better 'ole, go to it . ...* With luck, escaping a low, downwind foggy death, hovering clouds, stinking bogs, and a drowning in mud-filled trenches; lungs filled with chlorine gas, mustard gas, killer phosgene gas. And with luck survive being torn apart, left, a jagged, fragmented body-and-mind shredded by rapid machine-gun fire on barbed wire. Or being evaporated by heavy gun shell and mortar fire. Fell wounded, stretchered into a ragged tent in the field, and transported across the water to enter a U.K. (or German) War Hospital (like Graylingwell) - alive or undead as legacy on return to Blighty.

Many were not prepared, to expire in excessive heatstroke of Mesopotamian fever, flu, cholera or typhoid, shipped back home into a hospital - or sudden death in the battle-field. Lt. Ernst Junger in his memoirs, *Storm of Steel* said, his CO Colonel von Oppen survived four years in the trenches, and was then transferred to Palestine in January 24th 1918 - only to die shortly afterwards of Asiatic cholera at his new posting. Junger also reported the effects on his comrades, invaded by Spanish Influenza in 1918 ; this epidemic claimed many deaths - on both sides. [30] Did surviving veterans (on either side) receive a pension afterwards; or deceased, for dependants. (Apart from the Glory in being a hero to die for freedom, for your President; Kaiser; King or Country. By proxy in a foreign land.)

As everyman Tommy (aka AB 64 Thomas Atkins) ...Thomas Manton of the Middlesex, my grandfather's younger brother, injured after saving the life of his Commanding Officer. Tommy later to die of his wounds in a Norfolk War Hospital in late 1918. (His sister Lillian was informed of this anecdote by a reputed comrade and a witness.) What did *he* and his battleground bros receive as due monetary payment for the hell which was active service in Gallipoli, Mesopotamian heat, and the Western trenches; to save up for back home family - or possibly a sick body ... in need of home care on his return? Grandfather John Walter Manton (buried in the trenches a number of times) and, his bro Thomas: and, sister Lil's husband Arthur Collier (one of the London old pals, eventually to succumb to shell-shock in 1934). And many blood cousins from Australia, Canada, New Zealand and elsewhere (cap badges and a few war medals - left as baggage to my Great Aunt Lil) - all relatives.

My grandfather's *father* (who with *his* father too died in 1856) born 1849 (a widower since 1901), was a veteran of Afghanistan's 1880 battle of *Ahmed Khel,* and the Indian *Second Afghan Campaign.* He died in 1914 *just* before *The Great War* began, leaving five grown-up children, three grownup sons and two daughters. He'd lost a brother in India 'of a fever' in 1883. As my grandfather born in 1885 (d.1966), would lose a brother Thomas in the Great War in 1918; his other bro Sailor George Manton (1891-1945), survived Gallipoli and Mesopotamia. My Grandfather was attested (signed on) in August 1916 - serving with The 47th (London) Infantry Division from 1916-1919 [31] as a rifleman, short training, posted straight to *The Somme, High Wood,* under the Derby scheme of October 1915. He was then aged 31 years, married with five young children ; three daughters (Lillian, Elsie, and Maude, my mother), and two stepsons Alf and Len (Alf the eldest was fifteen). After the war he added three more offspring, 'twins James and Olive - at last a boy, Arthur, in 1921.

I examined my grandfather's *old-pals* wartime paybook (as it was for thousands of other squaddies) : 'Rifleman 373296 James Walter Manton of 1/ 8th (City of London) Battn., The London Regiment (Post Office Rifles). Attested 3.8.16. ' On (*his In-the-field AB 64*). *Active Service* record :- 'Dated 18 Nov. 1916 (under) Rates of - (pay) . Pay ... 1s (one shilling). Deduct Allotment or compulsory Stoppage ... 6d (sixpence). Net Daily Rate - For Issue (of kit) Words ...(net balance) Sixpence.' (Per day for being compulsorily attested into the armed service.) ... He earnt, in the other ranks, Sixpence a day - *after deductions* in 1916. ... But the ongoing war brought a pay rise ...there was added a pasted in sheet into the paybook - it said ... 'issuable to a soldier from the 29th September 1917 '... Well no it wasn't really a raise in *basic* pay. Paybook subheadings included ... 'Regimental Pay (including the extra 3d per day authorised for Warrant and NCOs of certain arms) ... 1s / Proficiency Pay ... 3d / Difference (if any) to make up the minimum under the Army Order ... 3d / *War Pay ... 1d* / Deduct ... Net daily Rate for Issue: 1s 7d / Word ... One Shilling and Sixpence.'

My grandfather John Walter Manton's basic daily earnings (as most squaddies), after deductions, was from 1916-18: One Shilling (aka *The King's Shilling*), and Sixpence *per day*. No guaranteed pension in the offing, due to any wartime misadventure. On balance, Long John Manton (a leg amputated after the war), and surviving comrades, gained - *One Penny a day* - as *War Pay*. One penny for each day's war-service in the battleground trenches - or other active theatre of war. And as one of Sassoon's war poems reminded, the dead : '*Don't count 'em; they're too many. Who'll buy my nice fresh corpses, two a penny.* '[32]

'So what happens to unclaimed stored baggage ...?' I asked Admin Baz.

'It's kept indefinitely. You never know what someone might enquire after - like domestic valuables. Besides ... As you know logistically few people actually die without there being a claimant for any belongings.' He added with knowledge of recent overseas visitors related to the 1915-20 wartime hospital occupation. And visitors from the recent WW2 conflict. Of those thousands of military personnel, out of Regiments from Australia, Canada, New Zealand, and many from Scotland. 'Not long ago though there was a bit of a sort out.' Baz recalled Roy, one of his senior colleagues in the Finance Department had attended a Specialist down from Sothebys the London auctioneers. 'We had these trestle tables laid up with possible valuables from a collection of old bags and cases which had began to decay and needed to be weeded out.'

'What happened to the proceeds Baz?'

'All of it went into the charity fund for rate-aided patients. ... Extra clothes or holiday trips out of the hospital. ... No *state* funds for social needs for indigent you know.' Leaving the office our intake walkabout continued. Harry grinned, pointed out his room in the Staff Residents Home, the converted former Medical Superintendent' Dr. Harold Kidd's house; presently, a residence for single male staff. No room at that inn, for me. - I was placed over the staff restaurant. We passed a few people on the driveway as we walked the full length of the Main Drive - in Asylum days aka The Carriage Drive. ... Again, we passed the water Tower and modern car park - adjacent to the Engineer Workshops.

I was intrigued when Hugh West (who said '*Hope you'll do a history, one day*.') a hospital engineer, showed me a reference book from the hospital archives, which was located nearby over the Patients' Affairs office, entitled: '*The Divining Rod: its History, Truthfulness & Practical Utility*.'[33] It was used by the hospital 1890s well-sinkers and West Sussex planners for the new asylum. At the front of the book's advertisements was included a substantial list of worthies who had made use of its facilities. Among listed subscribers to the book was the name '*Sir Robert Raper, Chichester*'. Admin Baz remarked to me *Raper* was an eminent ex-Mayor of Chichester - about the time of the planning of the new Asylum.

I noted from official records that the West Sussex authority signed The Contract on February 15th 1893 for the purchase of the Grayling Wells Estate from the Ecclesiastical Commissioners for £19. 500. In November 1893 a trial borehole for water on the estate was successfully completed: And in February 1894 a Contract signed with Duke & Ockendon of Littlehampton for sinking a well. ... I envisaged men, about the 19th century Estate, around in 1893, with hazel-twigs to the fore seeking and finding five or so new sink-holes - one marked this 100 foot water tower .

Water Tower

Stating the obvious our flesh is much composed of tidal water and mystic gravity mixed with floating, bonded homeopathic measures of metal components - as all living things : and the 'organic purity' quality of drinking water essential for 'dietetic purposes' to sustain life. Chichester was fortunate with its adjacent chalk made South Down Hills ; Durrington (near Worthing) and Barnham (east of Chichester) were two alternative possible visited sites considered for the new West Sussex Asylum ; and all of the locations - Worthing, Barnham, and Chichester (thickness of chalk 790 feet), are south of the chalky downs - with substantial filtrated underground springs and accessible wells sunk into this white carbonate of lime for its drawn running water - and supplied the Grayling wells.

Graylingwell Tower was erected between 1893 and 1895 ; its height from the ground to the parapet just over 98 feet (with a minute mast one hundred feet) and twenty-nine feet in width. During 1893-95 the well sinkers made three new sites. Three *old* wells already existed - located on an 1879-80 OS (New parish boundaries) Map - they serviced the old farm-yard and its orchards. One well was north of the house in the orchard; Second well was by The Pond - *The Grayling Well* ; And a third well (on the map) south of the house, in the north of the Cow Meadow adjoining The Drove - marked as a tank (it appears) on an 1900 map of the asylum.

In one Geological Survey, [34] two well sites were described, numbered 96 and 97. They appeared to be an 1897 and 1905 evaluation of the same location - yet appear to be given, different map references. Notably there were *no* references to the 1879-80 Ordinance Survey wells marked on the farm estate, and previous Manor of Grayling Wells extant wells, which of course pre-dated the 1897 Tower site. Stone wells and seeping spring waters had existed back to at least Roman and Saxon days - such as the *Groegelinga Wielle*, the Spring of Groegael's People, a tribe of early occupying Saxons. Perhaps pure conjecture but its Saxon link is quite a possibility. [35] Such water sources came down from the high chalk hills, and Lavant rills, which till well into the 20th century, occasionally rose up and flooded the low grounds of the hospital estate. Bald numbers may appear to a reader bland and boring - yet *such* facts, indeed their real substance was destined for the life blood of all patients and staff and farm livestock. Or if polluted was a forensic cause of wanton death - if the analysis of the water and its quality was ill considered.

The following was one such enquiry : 'West Sussex Mental Hospital. Well No. 96. ' (Analysis of water in 1928). 'Parts per 100,000 ... Total solid matters - 31.0. ... / Organic carbon - .02 ... / Organic nitrogen - .005 .../ Nitrogen as nitrates and nitrates (no ammonia) - .467 .../ Chlorine ... 2.1 / Hardness - temporary 19 degrees, permanent 2.2 degrees. / Very slightly turbid.' Edmunds (Ibid), added a footnote (p248), an observation by Sir E.Frankland, dated August, 1895 :

> "This water is of an extremely high degree of organic *purity*, and is, in every respect, of most excellent quality for dietetic purposes. ... The cause of the very slight turbidity ... should be ascertained. It was probably due to recent operations in the well."

Well *turbid* certainly indicated being muddied, no longer quite so clear; and which was certainly being disturbed by the civil engineers' explorations for the Chichester Asylum's water supply. The 1893 trial bore hole was successfully sunk by the Littlehampton firm Messrs. Duke and Ockendon at eighty feet plus ; the castellated Tower marked this site ; a second *new* trial bore was made in the garden-yard by the Restaurant dining-room. And a third bore hole, Hugh a civil engineer informed me, was hidden, somewhere (unknown) in the Engineers' (ex-stable yard) presently, enclosed works yard. The main well sunk below The Tower site was originally stopped at one hundred feet and three inches (in a three inch trial bore) ; the constructed well was ten feet wide externally - with an internal diameter of seven feet.

During its excavation the well sinkers at eleven feet down discovered ten feet in depth of running sand (with surface water) before stiff clay was reached. Due to this obstacle, for eighteen feet down the well shaft was constituted by iron cylinders (like a collar) in order to exclude the seeping of the surface water and prevent earth shift. Well sinkers dug through earth, running-sand, clay, flint, marl - and at the bottom chalk and flint. With the import of this romantic (well I thought so) historical anecdote; I thought of unknown buried - thousands, of now hidden ancient man-made flint-mines ; the exploration of minerals - of diamond emerald gold silver and tin mines and, especially of the deep coal mines, albeit all underground tunnels, water courses and man-hewed sewers - *all* past pre-mechanical built diggings; often most dangerous underground candle-lit tunnels ; even, to the more recent perilous World War Two Prisoner of war camps' escape tunnels, as the deadly three shifting sand tunnels of Tom Dick And Harry used in 1944 for *The Great Escape*. The tragic event was later made into a feature film in 1963.

At the bottom of Graylingwell's 1895 excavation, a horizontal tunnel was built for eighty-one feet three inches in an easterly direction ; and eighty-two feet six inches in a westerly direction ; the tunnel six feet three inches in height and five feet wide with nine inch thick walls and a six inch concrete base. C. Isler & Co. installed an airlift pump which was sunk below the water line to a recorded depth of 428 feet, which greatly helped the situation - but not enough - as was soon realised. Water was located at a depth of sixty-eight feet, and the new well with the addition of the tunnels, initially gave the hospital a storage *capacity* of 31,000 gallons; on flow yielding approximately 1,000 gallons per hour - which with an estimate of forty gallons per head was, at the hospital's 1897 inception, enough for all staff, residents, laundry, cooking, cleaning et cetera. But, all too soon, it was *not* enough, and with the hospital's new extension blocks, by 1904 the Lavant spring flow into the well was well below the Asylum's needs. And so unable to be wholly self-sufficient, the Chichester

City supply supplemented the hospital's needs, with an additional 1,578,000 gallons - for that year. ... And reviewed thereafter.

Close to the water Tower, on the east side of the detached flint stone Church, was a trio of long interlinked pre-fabricated huts with corrugated asbestos roof-sheeting. On a closer look it appeared to be one long-building with an extension - giving it a T shape. These Occupational Therapy huts, we were informed, were opened in 1952. In fact *all* NHS hospital Farms in 1952 were soon to be closed down - altogether. Graylingwell's own farm *formally* closed in 1957 when its livestock was auctioned off at The Market in Chichester. Though fragments of that very successful business and source of Therapies for selected patients still existed - as I would soon discover. Many staff and long-term patients had strong merit memories of those recent days. After all Chichester till lately, had (still did) remained a thriving rural farming community. And had been so for at least two thousand years ...

Sandown

Finally, we walked around a thick hedgerow, behind a number of large Greenhouses and confronted by a charming single-tiered building called Sandown House, with a grass lawn and marked out Croquet hooped course to its front. A small gravelled driveway close to this edifice and exited on the other side. A raised verandah fronted the whole of this closed, isolated building. With a firm historical purpose, as we soon learnt. Sandown was Graylingwell's own internal Isolation Hospital. (this was a statutory requirement in 1897). It had in its life-time, specifically cared for, staff nursed and sheltered young children; housed female incurables - tuberculosis patients, and later GPIs - General Paralysis of the Insane syphilitics - providing sanctuary accommodation for terminal syphilitic patients - until the coming of the life-saving Sulphonides at the end of the Second World War, and no-more GPIs added to statistics in post-war Annual reports.

The Isolation unit had also been used, along with most of the hospital complex, during the First World War, as part of a troops' hospital. And now this building was in the mid-1960s, a new experimental Alcoholic Unit - designated a *Therapeutic Community*. Up a short flight of steps into the bungalow we were led into the Charge Nurse's office on our immediate left. The building appeared to be a large inverted T-shape. The kitchens and dining room to the rear; dormitory bedrooms to one side of the building, and lounge and day room on the other side. Sandown had only been opened for twelve months and was already rated a success story: Its Charge nurse insisted that motivation to recover was perhaps the most vital factor in gauging a patient's prognosis.

'Once An Alcoholic. Always. An Alcoholic.'

Charge introduced the mantra ... 'You see, by definition diagnosed alcoholics face - or rather are *not* able to face - day to day life issues. Just one drink is likely to be one too many. It leads to another. ... And another. ... And another. There is no way an Alcoholic can just drink socially. Our patients are first dried-out - probably on the Main Admission Wards or at Summersdale. This means they stop *all* drinking. And have their bodies built up with nourishment. Vitamin B12 injections are given regularly for a while. And to counter the craving, Heminevrin capsules each day. Potential Sandown patients reside on the Admission Wards. One of the residents will accompany a staff member in interviewing a new resident. They'll then stay ten to twelve weeks, if accepted, by the Closed Group - of Sandown residents. Prospects are questioned as to whether they're *really* interested in giving drink dependency up. Or reveal that other pressures have brought them into hospital - police action, relatives, friends - or threat of job loss - but *not* sufficiently of their own volition. So - most of these unmotivated patients leave the hospital as soon as they dry-out. But sadly - many are almost guaranteed to turn, eventually, once more to drinking. Once an Alcoholic, always an Alcoholic - but, and it's a huge *but* - we *can* teach how to *stay* off the drink ...'

Whilst in the office we were interrupted, albeit politely, several times by residents.

Group work therapy was an essential part of the alcoholics' treatment programme. Relationships with friends and relatives were discussed, In-camera, within the meetings. And after discharge from the hospital, continuous support was offered to the patients once more living in the community: We left Sandown after half-an-hour. Mr Watkinson felt the afternoon was not quite over. And yet again the introductory tour took off - this time for a brief look at Summersdale Hospital itself. ... But this visit was postponed. We'd already seen a good deal of the expanse of Graylingwell Hospital Estate grounds. Aware that a good deal had yet to be explored. And a satiation point temporarily set in - till morning of the following day. ... And finished our first working day.

Tuesday 5th September 1967

The following morning we made directly for the School - commencement at nine o'clock.

Our first elementary lecture launched us into the contents of the red *Syllabus* book. It was a brighter day than our first introduction and limp sunlight filtered into the class-room. We sat down and Mr Watkinson launched into this first formal lecture of the *Syllabus*. ... Standards of Ethical Conduct. This sentence was headed - '*Ethics and expected Attitudes of new staff employed at the hospital.*' : Ethics equated moral principles. The Nurse has a duty to their patients; the Medical Officers; Ward; and to himself or herself as the employed nurse.' Mr Watkinson emphasised that every doctor and nurse had a first duty to the patients' needs. To attend to their present needs and anticipate future needs. He outlined seven points, each noted and written down from the blackboard :

1 Be alert to his or her wishes. To understand the person.
2. Be gentle but firm.
3. Remain cheerful and pleasant in work. Gain patients' confidence. And listen sympathetically.
4. Do not make promises you cannot keep.
5. Patients do not want their affairs generally talked about.
6. Be concerned but avoid over-familiarity with patients.
7. Don't become too involved - cannot judge as well.

We discussed likely attitudes and expectations of new patients. On arrival they are often frightened. The hospital may be experienced as a strange place with threatening strange faces - the experienced nurse expected to appreciate this fact. The patient's relatives are understandably quite anxious and likely to ask lots of questions. Relatives may, along with their patient charges, be resentful against authority and become quite aggressive. More important - listen. To listen ... One must listen, listen, listen. Be sympathetic and appreciate how patients feel - what they *really* see and feel. Not necessarily what *we* expect them to feel. The person *is* more likely to give helpful information about themselves *if* they feel secure.

The student or qualified staff must be cautious of expressing only their own personal opinions - and, should report factual information to the Sister, Charge Nurse or Doctor. And refer the relatives to a person in charge at that time. A nurse works alongside Medical Officers as colleagues. And is expected to be loyal and respectful towards them: On the ward situation - a nurse is expected to be punctual, orderly and economical on duty - and be on time. Method is required in their work. And good fellowship between the nurses should always be attempted, invoked by team work in working together. Concluding that first basic lecture, our Principal Tutor spoke on aspects of The Nurse as an individual with physical and mental health needs of their own. It was always important to retain extra-mural interests - other maintained activities than nursing studies, indeed separate from any formal studies.

Mid-morning tea-break finished and we spoke of many things, topical and nursing. I asked if anyone knew of any accommodation for a married family in the Chichester area? Mr Watkinson, Audrey and Rose, lived in the community, said 'No'. And, of course, Harry and Sally lived in quarters within the grounds like myself and were not likely to hear of anything available. I purchased the local paper later in the week and visited newsagent advertisement boards. How many times I had engineered this exercise before; searching for alternative accommodation. It certainly reflected on activity outside studies - one's own domiciliary needs. The second half of the morning was under way. Settled at our desks. The blackboard became a screeching harpy as the chalk babbled on and on. And as we knew it would become the norm - episodically - for a long time ahead - in our three years to come.

Dr. A.J. Cronin

Before entering study of Mental Nursing, Psychiatry, and psychic cousin Psychology; we covered a brief History of Nursing - as a profession. It was Nightingale's Crimea War origins in her 1860 *Notes on Nursing* that covered the board ... Most about what constituted good basic health and hygiene. We'd all had pre-conceived notions of what defined a trained Nurse. Schooled by the mass-media, press, books, television, films, plays. And personal knowledge of friends, relatives and others who had been nurses - mostly State Registered Nurses - Victorian Angels of Mercy aka Sisters of Charity - who dutifully acted as dedicated hand-maidens to God-head idyllic Doctors in General Hospitals - and Life-or-Death in post-operative surgical wards ... Nothing yet about the do-not-speak of - Psychiatric care.

At this time in the 1960s the nurses and doctors series of the romantic *Doctor Kildare* was at the front of many viewers telescoped TV fantasy images - including Graylingwell staff and residents: But, there was also Dr. Archibald Joseph Cronin (1896-1981) and his amiable Scot's BBC. earthy series *Dr. Finlay's Casebook* (1962-1971), drawn from austere real-life 1920s and 1930s postwar characters introduced in his autobiographical, *Adventures in Two Worlds.*[36] Cronin had, had his medical studies interrupted by his naval service in the first world war ; and to help fund renewed clinical studies secured a temporary medical post at a Glasgow private asylum, the *Lochlea* Insane Asylum, located four miles west of the city of Glasgow. (Chapter Two in his biography). Doctor Cronin had seen much suffering during his naval service. And of Lochlea insane asylum wrote : 'Much has been written of the inmates of mental institutions that is not only bad taste, but also arrant nonsense. ...' And reflected this humanity in subsequent writings.

As students, our experience in and out of hospital wards - as recipient patients - was recognised as dependence on the quality of facilities, and its doctors and nurses. All these factors Mr Watkinson reflected on as a preamble to the blackboard's main utterings. - But, a rider was mightily added, for in truth, Registered Mental Nurses and Psychiatrists are little known by the media ... In most written Histories On Nursing, trained Registered *Mental (*aka Lunatic*)* Nurses (RMNs) were recorded as taboo *Footnotes* - Annondations - and owed origins from Keepers to Attendants to Nurses - with other additional correlations ...

Mental Health Nurses in long-stay Psychiatric Hospitals historically, had had a stronger male statistical complement than their sisterly General Hospitals. It was the changes in clinical treatments and attitudes that seemed to have eroded media views during antiquity. But sadly, staff employees in Asylums and Mental Hospitals were (are?) too often sensationalised as but bullish brutalizers, in an Hogarthian madhouse a Bedlam (aka bedlem the noise), 18th century ' Gothic horror imagery. ... As too its hospital psychiatric patients were, unjustly, often demonised by media and general public.

We were recommended the following, elementary readings, *before* beginning our induction studies. Remembering that all too soon most of our working time as students would be spent actively on the wards:

Aids to Anatomy and Physiology for Nurses by G. Sears. 10s 6d.
Aids to Practical Nursing by M. Houghton.
Bailliere's Nurse's Dictionary by B. Cape 8s 6d
Aids to Psychology for Nurses by A. Altschul 10s. 6d.
Handbook for Psychiatric Nurses by B. Ackner. 27s. 6d.
First Aid The combined manual of St. John's.
Small English Dictionary.
St. Andrews, and The Red Cross 4s. 6d.

Not Bedlam

The afternoon was taken up by a tour of the Female Wards - on one side of the hospital building. Our first impressions were more often at our own embarrassment. In touring as a group, unseen body-less diamond laser-eyes were everywhere, felt boring into us. I personally felt at times uncertain how to return any fixed gaze in unpatronised sympathy. I felt - as we all did - what I was, a very green student - new to this whole scene. This mode of suffering.

So far, practically all the wards we have seen house forty-eight to fifty-two patients. Most wards are full of the elderly, with few staff to nurture their needs. Most of these patients are seen sitting quiet and unmoving, perhaps not dejected but certainly withdrawn. On introduction, a far cry from *Bedlam* images of *Rakes Progress*, or *Marat-Sade* ravings - imaged by outside laymen. Our tutor suggested that generally we can anticipate our chronic patients as 90% sane, and 10% quite unbalanced - and mostly we address the sane portion whilst allowing for any unbalanced reply.

One Female Ward was for *severely disturbed* patients. Moments before our arrival the Ward Sister had experienced a blast from a nineteen-year-old drug addict. Acute psychotics, subnormal patients with psychiatric symptoms (one young patient is only sixteen years old), schizophrenics, a number of whom are unpredictable in their behaviour, manic-depressives, and other diagnosed psychiatric conditions - they are all to be found as residents in this hospital. Social rejects were also found here. What more orthodox (known) medicine in general nursing cannot cater for are subsequently pigeon-holed to a psychiatric term. Numerous old folk have apparently recovered, but no-one will tolerate them outside in the community, so they stay and were cared for as well as facilities allowed.

I spoke with one old lady of ninety-one years of age who came down to Sussex from London just after the Second World War. She came from Streatham, a place I lived in myself for a while. This enabled us to chat about London - and then about her daughter - her grandsons - one in the RAF, and proudly, she related tales of them all to me. I felt flattered - and not a little humbled. Grandmother was but one of all too many around her age abed in this hospital. In the evening I attended a free film show in the Hall for patients and staff. After some study, I finally retired to bed; a temporary bed-sitter, over the hospital restaurant -and - my mind ticked over and over ...

Wednesday, 6th September 1967

This morning we drifted further through Nursing History and Hospital Etiquette. The afternoon consisted of more tours. First stop was an interesting talk given by the Catering Officer in charge of this entire establishment's dietary needs. There are presently a minimum of 1,009 resident patients - and add, every day, at least, one-hundred-and-fifty staff to cater for - each meal time. An estimate of meals to be required each day was based on a census written up as at midnight the previous day.

I was impressed by recent plans to improve upon the hospital budget - and raise the quality of hospital meals - for staff and patients. It should certainly be acknowledged that here in Graylingwell the food was very good indeed; in the restaurant and on the wards. The Catering Officer was hoping to introduce a scheme that would allow all patients a multiple choice of dishes, for all meals. And by cutting wastage to a minimum, only need to order smaller quantities - and a better quality menu. Imagination! Good housekeeping.

We commenced visiting the male wards. There was strict segregation of the sexes for all patients and staff. Males to one half of the hospital (Kings' wards), and the females (Queens wards), the other half of the main building. Even the very large metal keys are of separate designs; one cut for the male side, a different gauge for doors on the female side. But there is a universal key that opens all doors, and copies held by selected staff.

My first male reception ward aka Admission Ward, was called A1 or Amberley One (for there was an Amberley Two Ward overhead). The patients herein are unfortunately too mixed a group in their Charge nurse's opinion. Six of the ward patients are drug-addicts, remanded to the hospital whilst awaiting a court appearance and for treatment under the requirements of Section 26 of the 1959 *Mental Health Act*. Earlier that day several of the addicts had threatened that if more drug-addicts were sent to the ward, they proposed to gang up and raid the cupboards. Charge nurse said they were tightening security on the ward's prescribed drug supplies. Also on the ward were elderly folk, suffering bereavement and depression. Several residents were in acute phases of schizophrenia. And several manic patients - in the manic stage of manic-depressive illness. And a number of new admissions, yet-to-be-diagnosed patients. Old and young, active and inactive, sixteen to sixty-five years old - on this reception ward.

Memories

Up on Amberley Two ward we met Les a retired Charge nurse (he'd retired in February 1960 on Superannuation as Assistant Chief Male Nurse), who was working part-time as a Staff nurse, and described his long-term patients to us. ... As with a number of residents seen on the Female Wards, most persons *seemed* rather quiet and inactive. Staff said he had been a member of staff in Graylingwell Hospital for forty years (away during war years) ; and remarked that most of the men on this ward were *dried-up schizophrenics*. ...

Les said, staff were generally, formally pensioned off from 55 years old - as with Local Authority professions, Civil servants, Armed Forces, Firemen, Teachers and Policemen ; he had seen *many* changes during his duties of care, over these years. 'The biggest' he said 'in just the past twenty years - since the late war. - When I started (1919) There were no treatments - as there are today. ... See those men?' He pointed to a group of shabbily dressed patients. 'Most of them have been here over thirty years. Came here as young boys. And, with no available treatment, their complaints worsened, and eventually, well - they live now in their world as you do independently in yours...'

He gestured to one short stout middle-aged man pacing up and down, up and down, along the same well measured path close to one wall of the ward. 'See, he's having visual hallucinations now' said the Staff. Sure enough you could see his vacant eyes *seeing* something we could *not* see - and with his hands and fingers he was looking up and down tracing pathways in the air above him. 'Yes', Les said in conclusion. 'We were but their Attendants all those years ago. Most Patients would be locked in - day and night.- There were no day-patients then. And food was, in those early days, compared to today, bad; soup one day, stew the next: They were made to pace around the gardens anti-clockwise. And if there was violence on their parts ...'

I would learn a great deal from this retired old soldier and longtime professional: He first entered the asylum as a Dispensary boy aged Fourteen years in 1917, when it was a War Hospital, under the charge of a Mr Yeatman - and of course he knew Lt. Colonel Kidd - before Les' first army call-up in August 1919: and his return in 1930 to train as a fully qualified Mental Nurse. ... More of our oldest serving member of staff - old soldier - later.

Diary Notes
Thursday, 7th September 1967

Morning, and in training school . We again covered a lengthy, Introduction to an History of Psychiatry. ... And afternoon continued the tour ... First we visited two Churches in the Graylingwell grounds : A Church of England and a Catholic Church. And was introduced to two Industrial and Occupational Therapy huts. Industrial Units prepared patients for (or return to) outside industry where, once again ; if they had worked before illness overtook them (aka pre-morbid). After re-training, it was envisaged, they would be able to earn their own livings. Here, presently, they earnt between ten shillings and forty shillings, depending on their progress at therapy. Occupational therapy *per se* was more a physical and mental distraction for long and short term patients, and was not remunerative.

We visited an isolated Gardening Unit where working patients stated their personal likes and dislikes of the larger, Industrial Therapy Unit. In one aspect, this gardening area appeared to be a lone survivor of the till recently Graylingwell Farm grounds which had enabled the hospital to be wholly self-sufficient, providing fresh food for all its residents. The Farm must have also provided an instant livelihood for many patients and dignity - not in anyway a cheap form of labour as unknowingly politicians might appraise, losing sight of recovering patients' personal needs within the asylum.

Gardening and Industrial Unit areas were on the periphery of previous, Nineteenth century farm premises, adjacent to the residential complex on the North-east side of the vast grounds. I was at this time unclear as to the precise fate of the hospital farm which we could see no longer had any livestock about The Estate. An insular community which was up to the mid 1950s self-sufficient but, no longer so in the 1960s. The Graylingwell Well was located in this North eastern corner of the grounds.

What of the previous farm workers ? - Some now worked in the kitchens, others moved into different trades. And presumably any intention to industrially rehabilitate patients who, along with staff, would have worked on the large hospital farm. New rehabilitation therapeutic units of varying description were now to be found. The old farm buildings were converted to Therapeutic training units. ... We visited an interesting Art Studio where patients of all diagnoses were able to express themselves. - This Studio was till recently a large barn on one side of an square cobbled farmyard.

Late afternoon we visited Richmond House (aka Villa), separately housed from the main Graylingwell Block. In long-stay residence were some sixty plus so-called *burnt-out* female patients separated into two wards; these included previously florid epileptics, schizophrenics or gross IQ mentally sub-normal patients. In Richmond Villa, these old ladies, chronic and unacceptable in the community, remained in residence. ... *This was their home.* One tragic case was a lady who came many years ago and who prior to hospital admission, attempted to commit suicide by inhaling coal-gas - accompanied in the act by her sister. One sister succeeded in killing herself . This lady did not, but did permanently damage her brain cells, leaving her unhappily, and unknowingly, severely sub-normal.

Evening after supper, our group attended an extra-curricular lecture. Giving the talk under the direction of doctor and charge nurse was one of the alcoholics from the Sandown Unit. After voluntarily reading an autobiographical account of his life, a brief talk followed and questions were answered. An early valuable insight into one person's whys as to his chronic alcoholism.

Friday, 8th September 1967

Morning. We continued with politic aspects of medicine which related to the psychiatric hospital. This centred around the linear National Health Service and the Ministry of Health, and its scaled breakdown delegating responsibilities. Afternoon, and for just over half an hour we attended the flint built Church of England, where a memorial service was being held for a recently deceased long-serving member of staff.

We then visited another segregated building which housed relatively better patients; that is, ladies who are considered sufficiently able to work out at full-time jobs outside the hospital grounds. An effective hostel within the hospital grounds. Again we found included in this group of old ladies, a number of previously society rejects. Last this day we visited the modern Psychotherapeutic unit of Nightingale Ward. Tastefully furnished, with a thick carpet, smart contemporary wallpaper and comfortable new furniture. Here Group debates with acute neurotics talking out their anxiety causes , ensued. Here we also had tea ...

Saturday, 9th and Sunday, 10th September 1967

For the Intake of six weeks whilst we attend the school we have all weekends off duty. I had not been out of the hospital grounds for the whole week, but did so this weekend.

Monday, 11th September 1967

Morning, and we met our second tutor - Mr Ilford a Second World War RAMC veteran. And enjoyed chit-chat covering everything and nothing in particular. Hints about methods of learning and retention. Only 8% memorized after four days being one example. Afternoon, some tuition on physiology and reactions on the single-cell unit.

Tuesday, 12th September 1967

Still little concrete learning, but then the induction programme has stipulated these first few weeks as but introductory knowledge. Elaborated further on human and single-cell variations. We later enjoyed a lecture by one of the resident Consultant Psychiatrists on the medical hospital administration.

Wednesday, 13th September 1967

Our second tutor Mr Ilford is slowly escalating studies on biology, physiology and psychiatry. Today we expounded upon the human cell structures and visited other locations. Evening, another extra-curricular attendance held in the hospital committee rooms. We found doctors and mental health workers in a debate on schizophrenic patients - and a prediction of recovery among the hospital geriatric patient population.

Thursday, 14th September 1967

The day passed with a minimal knowledge added to our notes. Mr Ilford has rapidly gained our respect and rapport. He has a knack of generating interest in whatever subject. At present we remain in biology and physiology. In the early evening our class decided to get together for a special study session. We enjoyed the meeting and agreed to do it again.

Friday, 15th September 1967

Janet, our skeleton, was out for display, and we related our anatomical knowledge to date ... And aided by the wisdom of Mr Ilford we fleshed out the undressed body of this naughty lady and imagined all her parts: And in creation and decay we addressed the mystery of life itself - how or rather from *where* - in space - does matter in growth emerge into our space, and in *half-life* decay, in new life reform?

Monday, 18th, September 1967

Lectures and films, all allied to basic health, psychiatry, food and hygiene.

Tuesday, 19th September 1967

Highlight today was a fascinating recorded tape lecture by American Psychologist Dr. Murray Banks. This was a very optimistic talk and can be summed up in the three extracted maxims:

> 'Don't chase happiness with a butterfly net.'
> 'Don't keep looking at the hole - look at the doughnut .'
> 'Our cows are not contented - they're always trying to be better.'

Wednesday, 20th September 1967

A film on 'digestive systems' and continuing notes on biology and physiology. Evening - straight from school attended an extra-curriculum lecture debate on Mental Health Workers, and the Hospital and General Mental Welfare Society serving, in the community. Studied ...

Thursday, 21st September 1967

Talk by our Principal Nursing Officer on the Nursing hierarchy - and how the services are distributed throughout the hospital. The PNO is presently our most senior Senior Nursing Officer, having taken over the previously dominant posts of Matron and Chief Male Nurse - within the hospital. Immediately after the PNO's talk we were shown a film on aggressive behaviour at a Psychiatric Hospital. Again, attempting to ascertain why I am determined to work in this quite obviously stress-laden milieu? Whereas the challenge appeals, and there is some later improved wage-earning prospect - at least on completing training - it is to be acknowledged much more basic than economic ... It is of something very worthwhile - and more - more beyond it ...

Friday, 22nd September 1967

Morning a continuation on the body-systems and how they interact. Body ecology. In the afternoon a Youth Social Worker gave us a brief talk with a following discussion. During the evening we again met as a group for a full hour's study ...

Classification

Monday, 25th September 1967

Morning - we expanded upon the origins of current *psychiatric* terms. And the distribution of wards about the hospital. Mr Ilford explained that any *glossary,* only introduces a list of words, and terms, to describe an approximate or differential (bias) diagnosis. Whatever origin, primary diagnosis, at the time of writing, it infers - about a patient : But *please* to remember that here, such glossary is about a human being; and more so, the patient should *not* be dismissed and worse - be but an inevitable *statistic* shifting from one ward to another - or not.

In a reply to : 'Any Questions?' I asked 'Could *you* define the word *Lunatic*: And when was it - to your knowledge - *first* used in the English language?' Mr Ilford answered, clearly aware that I already anticipated the etymology - the lexicon: 'It originated from the old Latin *Luna* meaning the Moon; I believe the word *lunatic* stems from the 13th century Norman-french word *lunatique* ; which originated from old Latin *luniticus* meaning , a sickness - caused by changing phases of the moon - literally meaning 'Moonstruck.'

Mr Ilford paused, smiled. 'Erm. But that's *not* what or why you asked is it? Do you mean its first appearance in a literary or clinical term: Or use in a *legal* definition? Well - I don't *know* a precise answer to that question. I suggest you - in fact all of you, get used to using the school's library, *and* public libraries, for any in depth researches. And Barry I'd be *most* interested in your answer as to when - and - *why* the word *lunatic* was first used in the English language; I know it had a *k* at the end of it as *lunatick.* Shakespeare made good use of it in the late Sixteenth century. You could start with Doctor Johnson's *Dictionary.* ask the Public Library to help you find it out.' (I recalled past visits to the British Museum Library.) 'It is of course a generic term — synonyms 'Insane and Mad'. Anyways, good question. '

Doctor Johnson's *First Edition* of the 1755 Dictionary, was published in two substantial folios, and consisted of 2,300 pages of etymology. [37] I located, the Glossary in a One Volume abridged 1807 edition ; [38] And found the following pure gold entries. I was unable to copy the Greek words :' *Idiot* s. (from Greek). A fool; a natural; a changeling (Sandys). *Idiotism* s. (from Gk.) *Insanable* a. (insanabilis, Latin.) Incurable; irremediable (Making mad. (Shak.). *Insane*. a. (insanus, Latin.) 1. Mad. *Lunacy.* s. (from Luna, Latin the moon.) A kind of madness influenced by the moon ; madness in general (Suckling). *Lunatick.* a. (lunaticus, Lat.). Mad; having the imagination influenced by the moon (Shak.) *Lunatick.* s. A madman (Graunt).'

Amongst Samuel Johnson's 18th century dictionary definitions on being Mad I also found : ' *Mad.* a. (gemaad, Saxon.) 1. Disordered in the mind; broken in the understanding; distracted (Taylor). 2. Expressing disorder. 3. Overrun with any violent or unreasonable desire (Rymer). 4. Enraged; furious (Decay of piety). ... *Madhouse*. s. (mad and house) . A house where madmen are cured or confined. (L'Estange).' On one ambitious trawl of his Dictionary I was astonished to discover: '*Ontologist*. s. (from ontology.) One who considers the affections of being in general, a metaphysician. ... *Ontology*. s. (from Gk.) The science of the affections of being in general; metaphysician.'

Two-and-a-half thousand years ago, Greek philosophers Socrates, and Plato (c.427- c.347 BC) were replete in *their* writings on Madness. In Plato's dialogue with Socrates called *Phaedrus* :(Socrates to Phaedrus) 'I thought you were going to say - and with truth - madly, but that reminds me of what I am about to ask. We said, love is a sort of madness? *Phaedrus:* Yes. *Socrates* : And that there are two kinds of madness, one resulting from human ailments, the other from a divine disturbance of our conventions of conduct.'[39]. This Platonic analogy remained - today, in the Twentieth Century - I thought. ... *divine* equating modern 1890 William James' Psychological - unknown, 'referring *beyond ...*' [40]

There appeared to be no 'bracketed' Eighteenth century Dr. Johnson sources taken out of a *legal* text; an *idiot* was a natural fool; a *lunatick* could be incurable - or cured or confined! And as for *Ontology* (for I am no trained philosopher in Ancient Greek), Johnson's selections (like Plato) pre-dated : Freud Heideggar Husserl Jaspers Jung and Sartrean existentialism; Psychiatry and Psycho -analysis (science of affections) - by two hundred years: There was no deliberate whiff of black witchcraft or sorcery among his literary sources. There was certainly no crass witchery about the distribution of our hospital wards and its classification in providing indoor (or out-relief) sanctuary for suffering in need - whatever clinical or moral diagnosis. On one occasion Admin Baz recalled admitting Ambulance men and Social Workers observing that admission rates were up at times of the full moon. But on checking out this assumption over a twelve month period of full moon dates he found no correlation.

The *West Sussex Asylum* in 1897 poor law administration, dated back to Elizabethan Poor Law of 1601. [41] First administered under the aegis of 'Churchwardens and Overseers' who were 'to be allowed' (permissive not, at first, compulsory), to collect monies from every parish church and facilitate getting able-bodied unemployed paupers back to work ... 'and towards the necessary Relief of the Lame, Impotent, Old, Blind, and such others among them, being Poor, and not able to work, .. :.' which included Idiots lunatics and other ... others.

And in three centuries to follow, growth of population, abundance crop of wars, natural plagues, disasters, and rank industrialisation : *Classification* of who was an *able pauper* and or *indigent sick* - grew. And how to dispose of rather than comprehend and treat the causes (how easy in retro to read such data) : Always itself frail thin and fractious, a body of mostly charitable and punitive, supporting 'outdoor' and under-funded 'indoor' relief resources for sick and needy poor grew ... a sulphurous chimera of toadstools in an erection of bleak Poor Houses, Houses of Correction, Prisons, Workhouses ... and County Asylums: In some form or other each 'resource' with its own internal lazarette, cell, 'infirmary' or other allocated ward for its sickest inmates.

In the wake of the Napoleonic wars, earnest attempts to 'treat' rather than 'dispose' of a battered nation's war casualties led to a revision of the poor laws which culminated in the 1834 Poor Law Amendment Act. [42] Poor Houses were *not* Workhouses or Houses of Correction - per se - but now equate to Care Homes, in Twentieth Century a classification. Initially plans were for local mixed needy in Poor Houses to be re-classified: To separate - able unemployed but destitute; able-bodied (over sixty) aged - from the Sick and demented; another house for Children (cottage homes) Another for indigent *Sick,* et cetera. The 1836 Union of parishes to share their scarce resources. A good and caring proposition.

Intention was to retain for the West Sussex, Westhampnett Union its 'five old poor houses' : a house at Yapton (near Barnham) solely for the aged; the house at Aldingbourne (between Chichester and Arundel) for Children; at Pagham (Selsey Peninsular) for the aged and infirm ; and at Sidlesham (also Selsey Peninsular) the poor house to be unoccupied till: 'The Board should see *what claims* were made for admission to the workhouse. ...' The new Westhampnett Workhouse (as all Unions) was overseered by a local Board of Guardians - this included Relieving Officers who recommended admissions and where possible, home visiting after care. *The House* was 'presided ' over by The Duke of Richmond living at Goodwood up on the South Downs north of Chichester and Westhampnett. [43]

But, Napoleonic post-war economy dictated that all the old small parish cottage-size poor houses be sold off and all residents be moved-out, into to-be infamous - aided by government parsimony, an old converted *large* House, as a Mixed Union Workhouse (workhouse ethic designated in 1728 or so), and former site of an Elizabethan Mansion at Westhampnett (east of Chichester) to share, such scarce resources for its local needy: Converting the poor houses tried ... but failed, as being too expensive. And so the large Union Mixed Workhouses grew and grew , after numerous government poor-law amendments. I was to 'find ' a number of ex-Sussex parish poor houses - sold off during the 19th century as indigent inmates were 'rehoused' in the new mixed Workhouses : the sick in workhouse infirmaries ; and, able-to-work destitute kept off the streets as otherwise *malingering* beggars - worse, criminalised vagrants.

At the close of the Nineteenth Century the newly opened West Sussex Asylum had had considerable exchange with staff and inmates (aka patients), with local Westhampnett Union Workhouse - which was a but a short walking distance from Graylingwell. On record, for example, Medical Superintendent Dr. Kidd had sent assistance to the Workhouse when it experienced a bad fire on the premises. I recall personally, visiting the site of the old Workhouse and previous Elizabethan Manor House in the early 1980s on responding to information from an elderly informant, who recalled an underground tunnel, that linked a number of the old buildings. The Westhampnett site had recently become a waste disposal building unit and no-one in situ had knowledge of where-it-was, though one person was aware of its possible existence - said it was filled in at sometime. I found a length of the original old red-brick garden wall surviving, with a number of old 'leather' nails in its cracks. Remnant of the 1834 Poor Law Act.

In a rare Poor Law Officers' Journal, 1914 pamphlet, titled *Classification in poor-law institutions*, is quoted: 'Since the late Nineteenth Century,' an un-named official wrote; *'Considerable Progress has been made.'* [44] A copy of this Poor Law amendment, was probably, on a shelf in Dr. Howard Kidd's hospital office at this time - at the outbreak of *The Great War* with it shortly to be designated a War Hospital. This well intended official document declared:

> 'It is probably no exaggeration to say that the number of poor persons who require to seek the shelter of the institutions is not likely in the future, save in very exceptional circumstances, to reach the maximum numbers touched in the past, and Guardians' (The Poor Law Union, Local Board of Guardians), 'may therefore with some confidence sketch their plans for the redistribution of their indoor poor throughout existing buildings, with a complete assurance that the accommodation in most houses is more than likely to be more than adequate for their requirements.'

The above formal poor-law statement, was unbelievably, published and distributed, likely including Graylingwell, in 1914. The innocent writer of the foregoing *gaffe* prophecy, had *no way* of anticipating the tragedy already only *months* ahead with the advent of *The Great War* of 1914-18. And the thousands of 'places' that would be needed for many of its shell shocked war casualties. The writer in early Nineteen-fourteen continued, and unaware, quoted that:

> ' The difference between the old and new regulations is more apparent than real.That is compared, for example, to quote experience of The Commissioners of 1834, but eighty years ago, (in 1834 said): In parishes containing a population of from 300 to 800 (of which there are 5,353), the building called the workhouse is described as being usually occupied by 60 or 80 paupers, made up of a dozen or more neglected children, 20 or 30 able-bodied adult paupers of both sexes, and probably an equal number of aged and impotent persons who are proper objects of relief. Amidst these, the mothers of bastard children and prostitutes live without shame, and associate freely with the youth, who have also the example and conversation of the frequent inmates of the county gaol, the poacher, the vagrant, and decayed beggar, and other characters of the worst description. To these may often be added a solitary blind person, one or two idiots, and not infrequently are heard from the rest, the incessant ravings ofsome neglected lunatic. In such receptacles the sick poor are often immured.' [45]

The War Office 1914 *Manual Of Military Law* (King's Regulations), at the outbreak of war, was mandatory and said:

> 'The Army Council, or any officer deputed by them for the purpose, may, if they or he think proper, on account of a soldier's lunacy, cause any soldier of the regular forces on his discharge, and his wife and child , or any of them , to be sent to the parish or union to which under the statutes for the time being in force he appears , from the statements made in his attestation paper and other available information, to be chargeable ; and such soldier, wife, or child, if delivered after reasonable notice, in England or Ireland at the workhouse in which persons settled in such parish or union are received, and in Scotland to the inspector of poor of such parish, shall be received by the master or, other proper officer of such workhouse or such inspector of poor , as the case may be : ...'

As to how designated lunatic servicemen (not deemed white-feathered cowards), who were unable to be returned to The Front - but remained war casualties (aka wounded). At home and still sick - with dependent families. And in certain need of on-going care and attention - to be treated. *Military Law* prescribed:

> 'In England the lunatic shall be sent to the asylum, hospital, house, or place to which a person in the workhouse aforesaid , on becoming a dangerous lunatic, can by law be removed ; and an order of the Army Council or officer under this section shall be of the same effect as a summary reception order within the meaning of the Lunacy Act, 1890, and the like proceedings shall be taken thereon as on an order under this Act.' [46]

As early as 1917 Dr. Grafton. E. Smith, receiving war casualties, referred to the inadequate extant Poor Law & Military System, with deep disgust. [47] He bewailed the fact, that no new patient suffering from shell-shock or any NYD presentation could be *treated* - unless he or she - had private funds. The Poor Law only provided for 1890 *certificated* lunatics into a County Asylum. Initially a new indigent shell-shocked serviceman could be transferred into a workhouse infirmary for two weeks - but then, if not well enough to return to The Front trenches - or taken into care by caring relatives, otherwise, transferred to a County Asylum.

Dr. Grafton Smith quoting a report, of the current Medico-Psychological Association, said:

> "The present system, which compels all persons, except those able to pay adequately for their maintenance, to apply to the Poor Law authorities in order to secure treatment, is unsatisfactory and unjust. In doubtful and undeveloped cases temporary care can be given only in workhouses or Poor Law infirmaries, which, with very few exceptions, lack proper facilities for treatment. A system which artificially creates paupers in order to obtain medical treatment necessarily acts as a deterrent, so that too frequently there is serious and even disastrous delay." Smith commented that : 'This is not locking the stable door after the horse has gone; it is double-locking him thoroughly, expensively and often unnecessarily, in someone else's stable.'[48]

A matter of being in denial.

The Poor Law authorities attempted to improve *Classification* of its indigent inmates, and out-dated early Dickensian Poor Law (aka On The Parish) facilities. But were unable to anticipate the *immediate* needs of an intake of many thousands of 1914-1918 war undead NYD war wounded - and especially those to be with more *chronic* needs. ... Visiting a current Danish system of poor-law institutions, as a member of a Royal Commission, the Rev. F.R. Broomfield of Cardiff observed, on the current Poor Law (1914):

> 'The poor and destitute are divided into three classes :- (a) The friendly afflicted of any age, and those over sixty years of age who are workless. (b) Those whose poverty is a calamity neither associated with crime or laziness, together with the children who are innocent sufferers. (c) Those whose poverty is a crime, being the result of drunkenness, sloth, improvidence, immorality or some related sin.'

Our country's past poor-law catalogues, recipes of human woe, were thus, often remixed, shuffled like a Tarot pack of playing cards, as each social designated '*class*' becomes a topical *problem* - given a label sans humanity : idiots, inebriates; lunatics deemed *incurable* ; murderous insane shuffled off to Broadmoor in Berkshire: 'other' the non-forensic insane into a Licensed Madhouse, or as they opened into new County Asylums from the 18th century. Still in use in Twentieth century local authority 'contracts'.

Courtney Dainton[49] writing on the introduction of the National Heath Service in 1948 (and removal of the Poor Law legal system) - observed that:

> 'Until the middle of the century (nineteenth) there still remained one class of sufferers for whom there was no hospital provision. These were the incurables. Neither the general nor the special hospitals would admit them, and they had to stay in their own homes, a great burden on their families, ...' To which we might add - classified incurable - to linger for being untreatable in poor-law hospital workhouse infirmaries or other classified asylum facilities.'

Anonymous 'harmless' rate-aided *chronic* moral imbeciles, were placed, alongside, many *untreated*, dumped, wartime casualties, (aka pauper idiots and lunatics). And designated pre-classified (non-clinical) wards, in a mixed Workhouse, or similar rate-aided outhouse. A practice continued, well into the Mid-twentieth century. I quote from the legislation:

> 'Asylums — the expression "asylum" includes any workhouse or other building ... It maybe either an "Institution" or a "hospital" ... the asylum has in fact become a specialised workhouse, in which the principle of classification is carried out to its fullest extent. In such circumstances, it would have been better to abolish the distinction. But since that was not done by the Local Government Act, 1929, these sections have to be retained.' [50]

Asylums and Workhouses between the wars were again re-named, re-classified, as *Public Assistance Institutions* (PAI) after 1930 - the *same* poor-law institutions written in another name. General Workhouse wards in the late 19th century, and early Twentieth century were formally classified as (a) Receiving, and vagrant (casual) wards, (b) Aged and infirm males, (c) Able-bodied males, (d) Able-bodied females with nursery at end, (e) Aged and infirm females, (f) Aged married couples (cottages), (g) Lunatics and epileptics, (h) Maternity, (i) Male infirmary (with separate lock and itch wards), (j) Female infirmary, (k) Isolation block. This nomenclature was in official use in the planning of the wards layout back in 1894 — and *is still in use* in the mid-twentieth century classification of hospital wards.

In the earlier quoted 1914 Poor-law pamphlet, specific guide lines were issued as to *how* to treat asylum and hospital and workhouse *rate-aided* persons in any Union funded ward. The recommendations were exampled on a selection of deemed good Union houses about the country; the models in the pamphlet based on permissive legislation (*the Poor Law Acts did not mandate outright cruelty*) to be punitive - a penal workhouse, like a House of Correction - or not so) where the local authority so ordained the classification of accommodation in its buildings. The basic principle was one of being undeserving or deserving poor (note, the derogatory reference to being poor, as malingerers — even felons):

> 'inmates are housed according to their moral grade (see p.15). Only absolute bare necessities for those with only themselves to blame for their poverty, and deemed malingerers. Privileges to worthy poor were reflected in the fabric of the ward and personal deserving extras like issued tobacco rations et cetera.'

What were the specific criteria for *Classification*, and non-clinical treatment guidelines - *within* the closed poor-law institutions? Visiting then current Danish system of poor-law institutions as a member of a Royal Commission the Rev. F.R. Broomfield of Cardiff headed his designated good poor law notes as follows, viz:

> 'The poor and destitute are divided into three classes; (a) the friendly afflicted of any age, and those over sixty years of age who are workless, (b) those whose poverty is a calamity neither associated with crime or laziness,

together with the children who are innocent sufferers or (c) those whose poverty is a crime, being the result of drunkenness, sloth, improvidence, immorality or some related sin.'

Monday, 25th September 1967

Afternoon.- Mr Watkinson continued our guided tour of male and female Graylingwell hospital wards. ... Once again the sheer size of it all causes me embarrassment at the degree of my ignorance - and to-date incompetence - in offering practical mental health care - and, after-care. We concluded with a visit to The mortuary where a pathologist explained his work and we were shown a now yellow tanned aged male cadaver ...

Tuesday, 26th September 1967

Regular dosage of biology and physiology. During the afternoon a further tour of the Male Wards ...

Wednesday, 27th September 1967

Morning we concluded Freud, Piaget, Soddy - *Mental Development of the Child.* And greater depth on the digestive system. Afternoon a lecture by the Hospital Secretary on finances and how they are accounted for. We started aspects of practical nursing care with an introduction on bed-making.... vital in our daily duty of care.

Ah! ... Beds ... at the age of seven years, back in the orphanage in 1944, I had, *had* to learn to make-up my own bed (or else - I was in trouble) ; I soon learnt how to fold back corners to a right angle - and, to tuck the folds under the mattress, deemed Hospital Corners. I had learnt how to change my own bed-linen, top-sheet to the bottom, and new clean sheet as then current top-sheet.

And, as to *quality* of hospital beds. W.H. Ainsworth's doleful Jack Shepherd cartoon, looking down, full of remorse, at his demented, chained mother detained in London's Bedlam Hospital in the eighteenth century. [51] His mother's bed scant rushes or straw on bare wooden floor: ... Later years. Actual bed-clothing - assuming *a bed* - from dry-rushes - later mattress and pillows in stiff palliasses, as wartime and peacetime troops in barracks, extant many decades. To cotton sheets and snug woollen blankets - especially, if fortunate, in winter-time to have use of the blessed thick, all-wool pillar-box-red, top-blankets. In the late 1940s (even as a young child), I knew them as Red Cross blankets.

On top was a thin embroidered counterpane with a visible institution' logo (owned by). A Proper Institution Name - laid on *the* top of the bed, Asylum, *Hospital,* Orphanage; or other - giving secure warmth to the occupier. ... But twenty years earlier. I heard of, read about, many homeless, unemployed, and often *sick* ex-servicemen (aka Rogues & Vagabonds & Tramps), during the bleak 1920s and 1930s travelling to under-financed parish workhouse casuals and receiving wards, where they were lucky to have loan of a single thin worn blanket and an overnight allocated, cold floor space. [52]

But ... erm this in no-way implies I would subsequently *always* make my own bed up properly - I often (ahem!) just, sort of, well - tided it up. ... Grateful of having a bed. In the evening we attended an illustrated slide lecture, introduced by a guest psychiatrist, a senior lecturer from St. Bartholomews, on asthenic and pyknic - *Thin and Fat People* , and Psychology.

Thursday, 28th September 1967

Morning, the stomach studied in detail. A short cartoon film on *Flies and Food Hygiene* followed, with the inevitable discussion. Afternoon, a lecture by the Secretary to the J.J.C. on *Nursing and Management* . We talked of wage complaints and similar fundamentals, on practical nursing - and on beds. I enjoyed hamming the role of patient, and was duly shuffled around playfully by my student peers whilst the bed was repeatedly made on and around me.

Friday, 29th September 1967

Well, first month is up. Two short weeks and we will be on *active duty* on the wards. ...

Morning, and we continued physiology and theoretical psychiatry. Explored past and present use of the psychiatric lexicon. Mr Ilford reminded us and quoted authority on this aspect. 'Despite all that is said and written psychiatry does *not* possess a body of exact and established knowledge on which all can agree comparable with medicine.' He looked up and across at us to stress a point. 'Rather it consists of attitudes, concepts, theories and therapies from which each doctor selects what accords best with his predilections, so that one is tempted to say there is *not* one body of psychiatry but many psychiatrists.' 53

Obvious first source for preliminary exploration, of the language, used in Psychiatry - and common parlance - was use of our mandatory text book

Ackner's 1964 *Handbook for Psychiatric Nurses*. Its Contents and rear index, and Glossary to the contents of the work. [54]

The Preface and *Introduction* explained its History (origins and topical meanings) was written on a need-to-know basis only; (presumably Exam orientated): Amongst the list of its Contributors there was only one qualified psychiatric nurse - a Superintendent of Nursing, SRN, RMN, STD, of the Bethlem Royal and Maudsley Hospitals. In the not so far off future qualified, RMN Nurses *per se* would produce their own textbooks. [55] As we perused Chapter headings of Ackner's 1964 textbook, lexicon words in common language, in use long before learned Dr. Johnson, like asylum idiot lunacy mad - were found absent in Ackner's mandatory work - but still found in a modern English dictionary in the 1960s. Old terms were erased (as clinical terms) from Medical and Nursing textbooks since Nineteen-thirty and subsequent decades; being made clinically and *legally* redundant , as each new Mental Health Act came onto the Statute books and new terminology came into use - for awhile.

In diagnosis and treatment there were patients for whom it was difficult to admit to what was *chronic* - and *what* was not ; the former was always debateable if it inferred no-known-cure as *incurable* in one era, as for so many past condemned insane for centuries : But since *The Great War* and the rank horrors recognised in Myers and Rivers designated metaphor 'Shell-shock' - an awareness of war-neuroses, battle fatigue, neurasthenia, nervous 'breakdown' - discovered 'treatable' by talking-out therapies like psychoanalysis aided by mechanical aids. A new labelling terminology came from this hard won recognition for previous *NYD shell shocked* patients; survivors whose memories were fragmented with disturbed nostalgia, identified, *as* Anxiety Nervous Disorders, [56] as distinct from immutable Lunacy per se ; and labelled 'Psychosis and Neurosis' - two mental illness headings which definitions, existed in 1960s and 1970s. ... *not* damned as wilful malingerers; or even felons.

'There's often but a thin divide between them.' RAMC Mr Ilford reminded us - we green recruits. 'But sad, to this day it is often muted by some academic and media authorities that *any* generic *Mental Illness*, especially Hysteria and Nervous disorders, is a veiled cover for *malingerers* - at least sign of latent inept physical weakness and moral cowardice.'

I had no idea whatsoever how much of a controversy - a minefield, that this area of enquiry would lead in the future. And insight thanks to Admin Baz, Veteran Les, Doc Joyce, Graylingwell colleagues - and numerous personal observations. About the nature of shell shock treatment, neurasthenia,' aftercare for war veterans and families - war-pensions - as anxiety nervous disorders. And my own (to be) belief that *any* real hysterical behaviour is often a *real* symptomatic form of *not* coping distress. ... But certainly not malingering.

Watershed 1946

War Malingering *per se* was a reference to *wilfully* acting for gain. During *The Great War* Germany and Austrian military authorities, officially, had little sympathy, with their shell shocked troops, branding them as malingerers. In one footnote, to this introductory 'intake' chapter, I chanced upon the following postwar 1946 insightful remark, which complimented a serving officer's own personal experiences on shell shock and war neuroses. Despite a formal end to four centuries of Poor Law (what-to-do-with-the-poor!). As 1948 proved to be an immense watershed: birth, and rightly so, born in the introduction of the National Health Service (health care guaranteed for all British subjects - whatever their fiscal status quo); a philosophy of care born out of the recent, (albeit despite near bankruptsy) of our nation caused by the recent war years. ... But this was at the end of WW2 not the Great War!

> 'It is abundantly clear that we have not yet learnt the lessons of 1914-18 as regards the effects of stress on the less well integrated nervous system. True we have discarded the term 'shell shock' and substituted the word 'neurosis' but there still exists crass and unpardonable ignorance of the nature of psychological illness.' [57]

Author Doctor Beccle had, had wide experience, during the war as a psychiatrist in the Royal Air Force, and in his book described 'shell shock', war neuroses, and its symptoms. 'From an early date I became aware, in my training, (quoting RAF Dr. Beccle), of this often unjust mantle of war *malingering*. A term sometimes abused by a trenchant media (bred on heroic imagery), of not being really-ill, when a diagnosis of *hysteria*, war-neuroses, or other *nervous disorder* trauma, maybe first indicated.' A matter of attrition - and consequence. Any serviceman attempting to *Work His Ticket*, pretending, to be mentally ill with a view to being discharged from the armed forces; [58] such real life malingering in all H.M. Forces was taken *very* seriously - and, if diagnosed as wilful was treated as a criminal offence. ... The Royal Navy was most specific about this possibility in the 1940s:

> ‘ The malingerer deliberately feigns, or more often exaggerates, a disability in order to deceive others and gain some advantage for himself. ... In the last connection difficulty often arises over the distinction between malingering and hysteria . ... it is equally important to remember that no one is less of a malingerer than the genuine psychiatric patient, and no one needs more urgently, or repays more fully, correct and adequent treatment.’ [59]

But, ten years on, during the postwar 1950s (when I did my time serving in the armed forces), little had changed in attitudes, towards an accused *malingerer* in the armed services - *and in civvie street.* Psychiatrist Dr. Ronald Laing was not known by anyone of my acquaintance at the hospital in 1967 (though in later years I met people who had worked with him). [60] Laing did National Service in the Royal Army Medical Corps, serving from October 1951 until September 1953. At the time of the Korean War. He worked at *Netley* for a year, and later at Glasgow’s *Gartnavel* long-term Psychiatric Hospital, and much disaffected with his experience during the early 1950s. One of Laing’s early tasks was to assess a soldier’s capacities for service and in particular to ‘downgrade’ a genuine disabled person - and also, to learn to distinguish a certain skiver and ‘malingerer’ from a diagnosed disabled serviceman; Laing often had problems in this area, and he admitted he had:

> ‘developed an intense desire to ferret out the differences between deception, malingering, self-deception (hysterical), neurosis and psychosis, functional and organic.’ [61]

I have of course already well researched this mindset, as it was in 1914-1918 and afterwards - between the wars. To recap. In the early days of the First World War, *before* pessimistic more realistic appraisals of *The Somme*. Barbusse’ and his trench *poilus* idly differentiated between grades of Front Line ‘dodgers and shirkers’; those soldiers, not *really* wanting to die (for nothing). And reflecting non-combatant’s open opinions, especially civvies, often lauded mantra. Of civilians and of intellectuals reverence, as non-combatants ‘*respect for those that got killed.*’ [62]. I found no yet direct reference to the translated word ‘hysteria’ in Barbusse ; but ample on grades of capacities, in wartime madness; limits to personal boundaries, their capacity for survival. And attrition.

Before starting as an adult student RMN, I had, had a certain belief that *all* and *any* form of generic hysteria - degrees of stress - was symptomatic of *some* malady or other. And was *not* an attempt at deliberate ‘*malingering*’.

And this applied in aspects, of so-called peacetime attrition experiences - *not* just in war-zone activities. Both were individual reactions to coping, or not coping capacities. And a million miles away from what a few years later would be termed 'Political Correctness', such falsity, based more on socio-economic opinion - than cultural-denial, and classification (qualifications for any eligible disabled *War Pensions* or peacetime entitlement).

The original 1894 ground plans of the Wards of Graylingwell Hospital, and Classification and distribution of its accepted inmates, patients, was reflecting the class-based poor laws (what to do with ... where to place ...): but, twenty years *after* the introduction of the NHS., ... as I discovered, the old workhouse ward system (with compassion), is essentially, as yet unchanged. But, *that* aspect will concern me more in the years ahead - working in the community as an advocate for disabled men and women. As yet, *still*, it seems, our so called ruling establishment, *appear* to separate really diagnosed insane - from shell shock, neurotics (who are it seems), those with nervous disorders, not really ill but alternatively, often branded, weak or worse, as but work shy malingerers (to be punished) - a view in the past Drs Kidd, Freud, Jung, Myers, Rivers, Grafton Smith, Nicholl, Beccles, Laing, et al, protested against so much. But *first* I had to qualify in the next three years as a professional Registered Mental Nurse, an RMN.

To The Wards

Friday, 29th September 1967

Afternoon, practical nursing in First Aid. Now well under way. In wry amusement, I was again asked to volunteer as a patient for bed-making. And we covered more aspects of primary-care. Today, we concentrated on *body-lifts* into and out of bed. It reminded me - sort of - briefly of Boy Scout, and Army days! This day I received my first month's salary cheque as a first-year student psychiatric nurse for September 1967; the princely sum of £33.14s 0d...

Monday, 2nd October 1967

Morning film *On Obesity*. Afternoon, practical First Aid theory and bandaging.

Tuesday, 3rd October 1967

Morning, lower extremities of the digestive system. General psychology. Afternoon, bandaging and First Aid, types of bandage, use of figure of eight, reverse spiral, spica.

Wednesday, 4th October 1967

Several films shown on *Faces of Depression*. One film was prefaced by a still from Hogarth's Bedlam Scene in *Rakes Progress* : One an American made film on Psychiatry. ... Afternoon, some academic exercises. Definitions: The patient this-that-the-other. The nurse this-that-the-other. ...

Thursday, 5th October 1967

We began work on the cardio-vascular system - the heart first. Saw a film on the same. Afternoon, and more paper definitions. We had an hour's lecture from the hospital's Roman Catholic Priest, interesting but in no way revealing anything new.

Friday, 6th October 1967

More on blood and the arteries. Afternoon, basic on temperature, pulse and respiration, and syringes for injections. ... discussed little used tourniquets. Then we five students sat a two-and-a-half-hour Examination. ... In the afternoon I was informed by Mr Ilford, that I was to start work on MA1 the Male Amberley admission (aka receiving) ward, on Monday 15th October 1967.

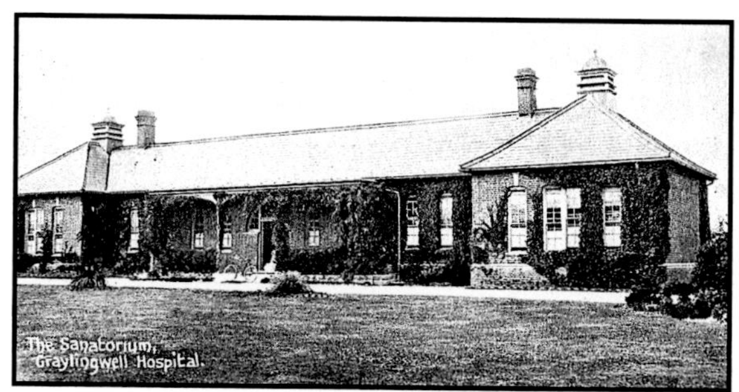

Sandown House, 1909.

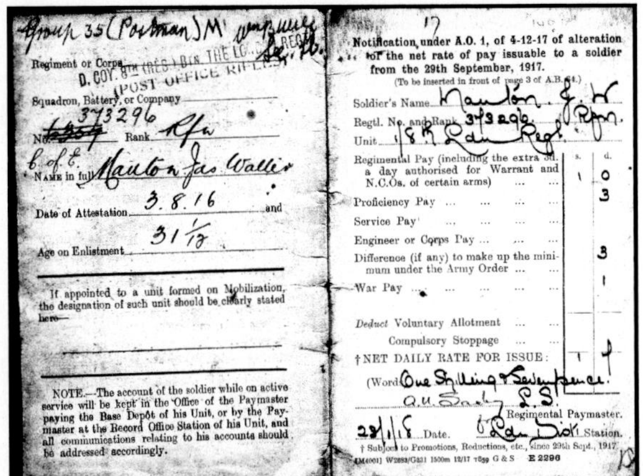

Group 35 (Postman) M'

Regiment or Corps D. COY. 8th (RES.) Bn. THE LO... REGT. (POST OFFICE RIFLES)

Squadron, Battery, or Company

No. 373296 Rank Rfn

Name in full Manton Jas Walter

Date of Attestation 3.8.16 and

Age on Enlistment 31 1/12

If appointed to a unit formed on Mobilization, the designation of such unit should be clearly stated here—

NOTE.—The account of the soldier while on active service will be kept in the Office of the Paymaster paying the Base Depôt of his Unit, or by the Paymaster at the Record Office Station of his Unit, and all communications relating to his accounts should be addressed accordingly.

17

Notification under A.O. 1, of 4-12-17 of alteration of the net rate of pay issuable to a soldier from the 29th September, 1917.

(To be inserted in front of page 3 of A.B. 64.)

Soldier's Name Manton. J. W.

Regtl. No. and Rank 373296. Rfn.

Unit 1/8th Ldn Regt.

	s.	d.
Regimental Pay (including the extra 3d. a day authorised for Warrant and N.C.Os. of certain arms)	1	0
Proficiency Pay		3
Service Pay		
Engineer or Corps Pay		
Difference (if any) to make up the minimum under the Army Order		3
War Pay		1
Deduct Voluntary Allotment		
Compulsory Stoppage		
† NET DAILY RATE FOR ISSUE:	1	7

(Words) One Shilling & Sevenpence.

Regimental Paymaster.

28/1/18 Date. Ldn Dist. Station.

† Subject to Promotions, Reductions, etc., since 29th Sept., 1917.

(M4001) W2883/G331 1500m 12/17 G & S E 2296

The Somme

1916. First World War. Above. A leaf from my maternal grandfather's Tommy Atkins AB 64 paybook on Active Service (1916-1918), in the Somme trenches : 373296 Rifleman James Walter Manton.1/8th London Regt (Post Office Rifles) 47th London Division. **War Pay** bonus, *allowance of* **One Penny per day** for fighting, wounded, shell shock - or dying, in World War One. **Siegfried Sassoon** said in his, *The Effect.*, *'Don't count' em ; they're too many. Who'll buy my nice fresh corpses, two a penny?'*

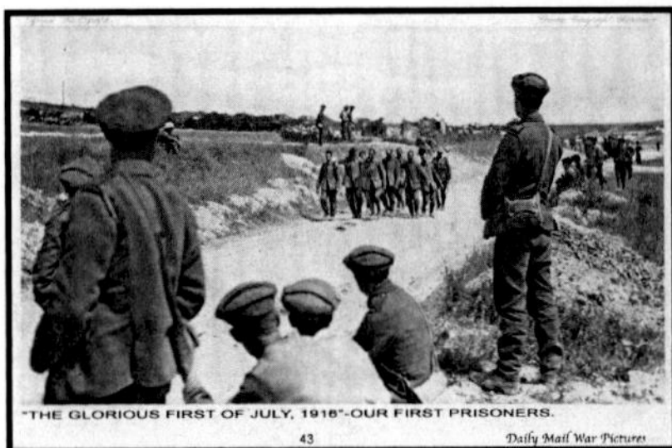

"THE GLORIOUS FIRST OF JULY, 1916"-OUR FIRST PRISONERS. 43 Daily Mail War Pictures

Left. The first day of *The Battle of the Somme* in 1916. The optimistic Daily Mail photo postcard's caption read: '*The glorious First of July, 1916. Our First Prisoners.*' Soon numerous NotYetDiagnosed shell shocked casualties arrived at Netley Southampton - a number transferred to Chichester's **Graylingwell War Hospital.** But. ...

It was *not* glorious. The first *Battle of the Somme* would last 141 days. Combined (with German) military trench, casualties exceeded a million persons. Statistics could not, in attrition, anticipate numerous survivors, yet-to-be hospitalised by shell-shocked, war-neuroses - with uncounted civilian casualties.This was but one awesome battle in The Great War.

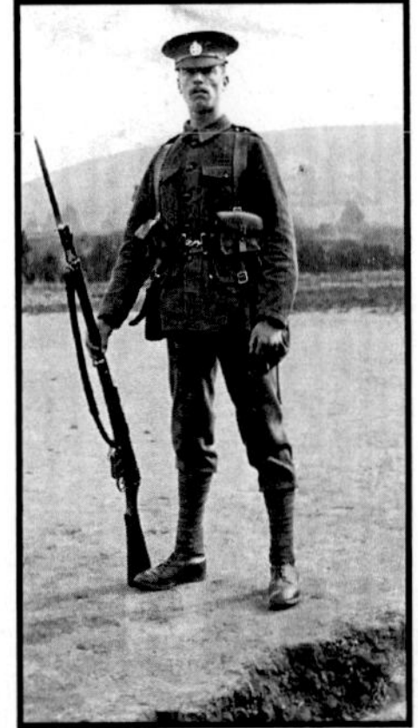

Left. 1916 replacement rifleman pic of *my* maternal grandfather, James.Walter Manton, posted to The Somme. *His father* James Leigh Manton (1849-1914), was an ex-regular of the 59th Foot (East Lancs): *Ahmed Khel (1880)* 2nd Afghan War;- retired on a minute out relief Chelsea pension as a regular Sgt. Rifleman Instructor.

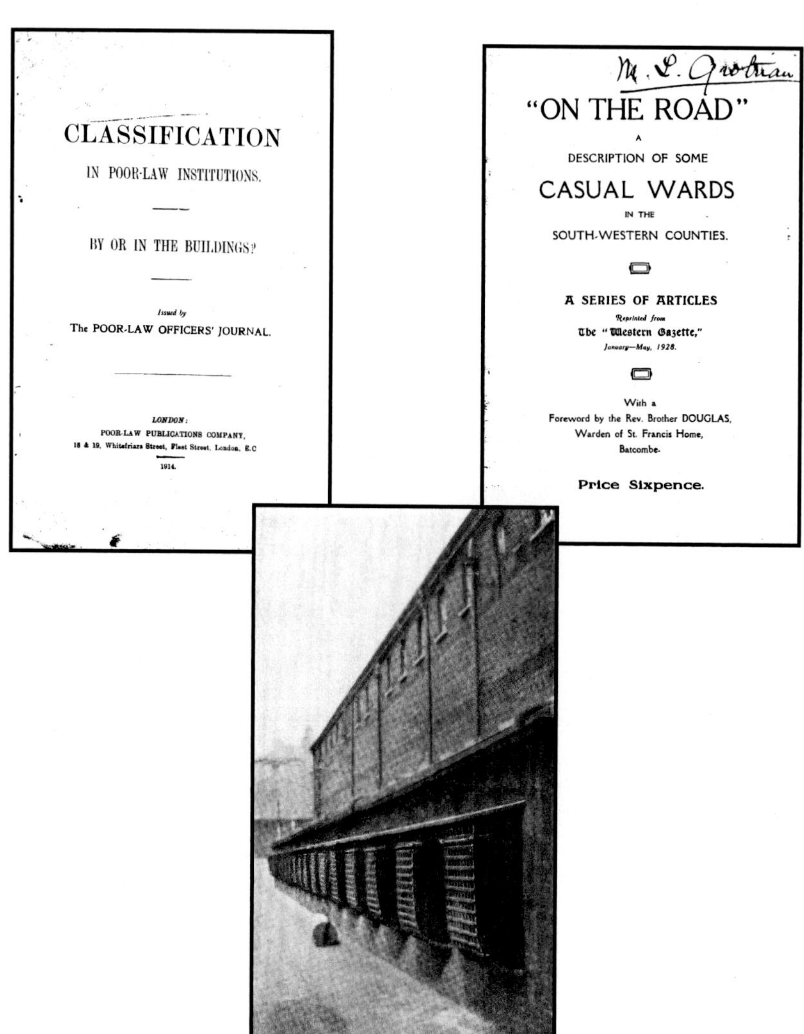

CLASSIFICATION

IN POOR-LAW INSTITUTIONS.

BY OR IN THE BUILDINGS?

Issued by

The POOR-LAW OFFICERS' JOURNAL.

LONDON:

POOR-LAW PUBLICATIONS COMPANY,

18 & 19, Whitefriars Street, Fleet Street, London, E.C

1914.

"ON THE ROAD"

A

DESCRIPTION OF SOME

CASUAL WARDS

IN THE

SOUTH-WESTERN COUNTIES.

A SERIES OF ARTICLES

Reprinted from

The "Western Gazette,"

January—May, 1928.

With a

Foreword by the Rev. Brother DOUGLAS,

Warden of St. Francis Home,

Batcombe.

Price Sixpence.

A view of stone-breaking cells in an old London workhouse reception ward yard where temporary inmates had to labour, in order to be lodged and fed. Note the grids through which the casuals had to push the required size of stone. The Poor Law existed till 1948 until the coming of the National Health Service. Graylingwell did NOT employ stonebreaking for its sick patients (see C.4. Vagrant Joe) : but, nearby Chichester Workhouse (as ALL workhouses) did have its casuals so employed in its back yard - to complete this task under the watchful eyes of a parish overseer. (Source of pic; *The Monasticism of the Casual Poor*, by J.R. Battley; F.R.S.A. Westminster. 1940.)

Chapter Three
Amberley One Ward

' The human body consists of about 60 trillion cells, and each cell has about 10,000 times as many molecules as the Milky Way has stars. ... Every person has nearly 400, 000 radioactive atoms disintegrating into other atoms in his or her body each second . But there's no need to worry about falling apart. Each body cell contains an average of 90 trillion atoms - 225 million times that 400,000.' [1]
Isaac Asimov. Facts & Trivia. 1979.

15th October 1967 to 11th February 1968

Amberley One Ward—Initiation—Regulations 1897—Meet the Patients—Staff—The Night Nurse—Reception Ward—Nausea—The Drug Round—Staff Breakfast—The Beds—Act of Attainer—The Mental Welfare Officer—New Admission—Essential Reference—Duty of Care—Felo de se—Efficacy of Care & Treatment—Detoxification, Antibuse & Aversion Therapy—Steve Antibuse—Flower Power—International Times & Playboy 1967—Spider—Methadone—Khalid—Incident—Irish—Shaun—Domestic—Blind Spot—The Blanket—Pad—Routine

Monday, October 15th 1967
Initiation

At a quarter-to-seven, on a cold Monday morning I reported to The Charge Nurse in the office of Amberley One (MA1) ground-floor male Admission (Reception) Ward; the large long-stay ward overhead was called Amberley Two. The patients' breakfasts were delivered for eight o'clock; before this time all patients were expected to be up dressed and washed - ready seated for the meal and early medication. Amberley's dormitories and sideroom occupants were roused at seven o'clock but, before this time, between six-forty and seven o'clock, the duty Night Nurse would formally hand over the ward to the morning duty Charge Nurse and his day staff, reporting on the night's events and any new situations.

After duly accounting for each bed and each patient, the night ward report was signed by the Night Nurse and the Day Charge nurse, and the report was then taken to the General Nursing Office. This ritual was repeated twice daily,

Night Report and Day Report (at the end of the day shifts), and produced each day of the year, every year - to date. Many thousands of old Notes and Reports were stored in the attic above Patients' Affairs - Medical and Nursing Records shelved on ground level - behind the Clerks front *Enquiries* office.

From all reports, medical, nursing and legions of administrative ephemera, the Hospital had audited and constructed an Annual Report. Copies of its *FIRST ANNUAL REPORT,* [2] dated for the year ending 31st March 1898, were still held in the attic over Medical Records. Regular reports have continued ever since, recording the day to day events of the hospital's staff and their dependent patient charges. Reports due - today.

As customary I was placed with one Charge Nurse and his shift to generally work with his opposite on days off, or be transferred to another ward during an emergency or staff sickness. Essentially there were three working shifts in 1967; two day shifts and one night shift, consisting of staff hours of day duty - Morning duty Six-forty am - to Two pm (twenty minutes for breakfast break) for six days a week. The Afternoon duty rota was One-forty-five pm to Five-past-nine (twenty minutes tea break) - for Six days a week. And Night duty; 9pm to 7am - three nights one week and four nights the following week.

There was seldom enough staff to back-up shifts covering all holidays and sickness and so from Charge Nurse to Student, one was contracted to work *both* shifts on that one day per week, known as *The Long Day* for it meant you worked, a minimum, from morning Six-forty am - to Five-past Nine at night (odd times to allow the shifts to overlap at The Handover), and our Time-sheets recorded this duty.

As a first year student I was off the ward one day each week, which was known as the study or School Day, when I would join up with my intake at the nursing school. At the Ward Handover staff arrived from within and without the hospital grounds. Within the life-time working memories of both Charge Nurses, staff formerly slept on their wards (off duty) and, ate, washed and dressed on the same wards with their patients during very long shifts. As an admission and observation ward Amberley One received a wide canvas of referrals whose patients initial diagnosis would invariably include somatic and psychiatric symptoms. On investigation an outcome could lead to a transfer to a local General Hospital, a Neurological Unit, or other Specialist treatment — outside the remit of a deemed Psychiatric Hospital *per se.*, or to an early discharge.

Dr. M. a long serving Graylingwell Consultant Psychiatrist said to Admin Baz: 'It is not unusual for relatives with a cantankerous relative (patient) to expect 'Recovered' to mean a much nicer person.' The doctor would then quietly explain that with treatment he could only overcome the episode problem and return them to their former self — whatever that was. (What was their normal pre-morbid self, might actually have been unpleasant rather than affable or sanguine. Can't make a silk purse out of a sow's ear!)

Regulations 1897

The hospital's Social History (albeit all social history) was of interest to me; and a salutary reminder how long and hard our predecessors worked. Hospital staff *Asylum Regulations*[3] were kept in the Admin Office and available for all staff and visitors to see on request. From the mandatory regs I read that, in 1897, as a rule the following leave will be granted:

(1.) Daily	-	from 8pm to 10pm (except when on Reserve Duty).
(2.) Weekly	-	Half a day, from 2pm to 10pm.
(3.) Monthly	-	One whole day, from 6am to 10pm.

All nursing *staff* had, *had* to be in bed, in those late Victorian and Edwardian days, with lights out at 10.30 pm (or else?), and up again, on duty at 6 am till 10 pm. Although official meal breaks were detailed it was *not* a matter of *How Many Hours* you worked, rather, when you were ever *Not On Duty*. And, given that you slept on your ward, too ...

Clearly, this could easily compare to employees of most past Institutions, Armed Forces, Abbeys and Monasteries, yes, even Hospitals, and at another level as house domestic servants. All were *'In Service'*, to Masters who were the employers, and servants as employees.

The point was you were *not,* in those Asylum days, allowed away from your place of employment *at all,* even when not working and off-duty, unless on official business. And, *no way,* could you anticipate matrimony, for married staff could not both be employed in the same institution: and, as customary, if a person *did* wish to get married, in any employment, you *had* to gain official permission or it was a no-no — and this meant you or your spouse had to leave your occupation if, of course, able to do so. I would meet numerous retired and present staff who confirmed this rigid mandate.

I was informed that this formal requirement for all employees. To obtain permission to get married applied to *all* staff as late as post-war 1945 and into the 1950s as in HM Forces and the Civil Service. As Baz of *Patients Affairs* confirmed, he too had had to ask permission in this Hospital. Indeed, as pre-war records show, most public institutions had this absolute requirement of employment — masters and servants in common law.

In retrospect, the foregoing description of day-to-day life in the asylum and its austere regime sounded quite depressing. But I found it useful to realise patients-and-staff were effectively 'all in the same boat' creating a warm community family relationship, removed from the outside demands of society — what we now call a therapeutic community — despite the relative harsh times they lived in before the war.

Doctor Joyce (not his real name) was an icon of integrity, a Consultant Psychiatrist for Horsham, later Worthing and District area. He was also years later to be a close colleague of mine working in The Community and Hospital. Dr. Joyce recalled to me, that back in the early 1950s it greatly increased your chance of entering employment if you were able to say you played a musical instrument, or played a sport of any sort. He chuckled when he recalled his first interviewer, a Dr. Rice, who was oiling a cricket bat whilst he was being interviewed. Dr. Joyce, then a young physician, ex-Major of Burma and recently demobbed from the RAMC service (he said), 'told a fib, that he enjoyed playing cricket, and Dr. Rice' face lit up,because he was a keen sportsman. Nineteen-sixties folk singer Bob Dylan sang, in the ballad *Gotta Serve Somebody;* 'Everyone has got to serve' (even surrender to) 'somebody', abstract anthropomorphic. To rightly submit to God - and shaped man or woman, which probably included any new employer.

Meet the patients

Initially, what struck me, coming on that first duty, was the homely air of normality about the ward. There were no media described screaming idiots or stereotyped aspects of lunacy, nor any 'stand to attention' militant staff to greet me behind a white coat.

As I entered the Amberley ward passage, I met a patient carrying a tray with teapot, milk and sugar, and walking behind him apace was the white gowned Night Nurse, who was carrying several large clean white mugs. The patient delivering tea was, I learnt, an often vied for, self-appointed duty that, if it worked, allowed him to continue for their duration in the hospital — or at least whilst resident on the one ward. On several of the long-stay wards the same nurse-and-patient had been resident for years. A safe factor for transient occupants; some dependency was essential, to acutely depressed, hallucinated, paranoid or deluded residents, patients in their own inner-worlds of sometime chaos, who experienced their ward as a warm haven.

To show *how* to survive was an expected first-aid function of all caring psychiatric staff. To rehabilitate sick patients, where possible; and to always, give old-fashioned altruistic care — whatever prescribed clinical treatment. I realised that many working relationships between staff and patients in this long-stay hospital had evolved over many years and built-up trust and dependency.

Gently, I knocked on sideroom doors before putting the lights on. And our patients, called by their Christian name, one-or-two by Mr, known to be more appropriate. Most patients were roused quite cheerily but several irritated, not surprisingly, at being disturbed from their sleep, though they accepted this inevitability.

Staff

The Admission (Reception) Ward's day-time staff were supervised by two Charge Nurses. Charge Nurse Bob, and his opposite, Charge Nurse Norman (both staff ex-RAMC). Two truly gentle giants with the latter's sometimes gruff tones often veiling true genteel emotions. Both Charges' wives were serving Ward Sisters in this hospital.

Two regular Staff Nurses covered the two day shifts. On Bob's shift was Tom, medium height, small moustache, athletic build, very humorous, intelligent and, dependable. And, his opposite number, on Norman's shift, was Harold, taller less athletic, more intense. As a number of other RMNs both Tom and Harold were double-qualified, with an SRN (State Registered Nurse) qualification.

There were two posted RMN students. I was one student on duty with Bob and Tom, and my opposite colleague, was Jacques, a tall, lean, lively tanned Mauritian; a third year student RMN who played the guitar. Sam was our witty cheerful brown-coated ward orderly. He always accompanied the morning shift. And last, but absolutely not least, was our ward's worldly, white-coated evening, volunteer, Astro Tony (his daughter practised astrology readings). He was a Chichester day-time shoe salesman - who would briefly, be-friend Sara and I. Astro Tony completed the daytime staff compliment.

Not forgetting the lone, staff - Night Nurse.

The Night Nurse

To the North of the E shaped MA1 ward the observatory dormitory accommodated sixteen acute beds; at the end of this long-room three single side-rooms. Two patients presently occupied two rooms. In the right-hand corner one converted side-room housed Gerald the duty Night Nurse; a Staff Nurse who kept a watchful eye on all new admission cases. Within Gerald's minute white-painted room were locked side cupboards with medical equipment, and a table and chair, with a green-cloth shaded sidelight. Just outside, against the wall, located between the two side rooms and nurse's corner-room, were other locked white cupboards with red warning lights which switched on automatically when opened. These cupboards held some drugs and stored clinical apparatus.

Each bed-space had a ceiling supported steel curtain-rung around its bed area, with dark-green moveable curtains against the wall (ward curtains funded by the charitable hospital's *League of Friends*). These curtains could be drawn by the patient during the night for privacy, if desired. The opposite, South-end of the observatory dormitory looked out onto the ward-gardens, and one early morning I saw a deer close to the window which had during the night strayed from the nearby hills. This turned out to be a rare event but also an early reminder of how close the northern perimeter of the hospital's estate was to the verdant South Down hills, woodland, and scattered copses.

Reception Ward

The long narrow dayroom had a variety of furniture, scattered rugs but no carpet, and included old long-back bamboo-cane chairs, around its periphery. At one end, the west-end, was a full-size billiard-table room. And at the entrance before the billiards room, outside a single room in one corner stood a black-and-white 17" television set, which sat on a low wooden table. Charge Bob told me that television was permanently introduced into the wards at the time of the Queen's Coronation in 1953. And television, tannoy radio, and weekly cinema shows in the Main Hall popular in the 1950s and 1960s (at the turn of the century there were occasional Biograph slide-shows and silent movies) were regular facilities.

In front of the television were three well-worn armchairs, which suggested late occupants of the night before. Close by the wall on another table was a much used portable record player, and a disorderly pile of gramophone records, long-playing 33 rpm vinyls, seven-inch 45 rpm's, and brittle 78 rpm's including, Elvis Presley soul; rock-'n'- roll Bill Haley; and lively Scot Jimmy Shand and his accordion band. Several battered paper-backed books accompanied the records. One book was open and placed face-down on an indented arm-chair and a partially filled mug of what looked like stale tea sat next to a white plastic portable radio — both items on top of the television set. Evidence perhaps of one patient who could not sleep and wanted to sit up during the night, in company with a cuppa from Gerald, the sympathetic night nurse.

On the south-side, off the ward's dayroom and adjacent to it, were two spaced doors and a wooden partition which led into a separate, outside enclosed verandah, which dated back to pre world war one days when open-air treatment was mandatory for certain types of illness such as consumption; and for patients in need of convalescence - and it had once housed a number of beds. The verandah had a ramp and steps giving easy access to the gardens it overlooked.

During the first world war, when Graylingwell was a designated war hospital, a number of photographs were taken showing recovering soldiers on this verandah but now, fifty years later in 1967, it was used by the ward as a dining-room area with tubular steel tables and chairs within the verandah space.

Early every morning around six o'clock a patient was woken up by the night-nurse and the kitchen opened up (it was locked late in the evening) so that he could lay the tables ready for breakfast — it was presently the same gentleman who brought us morning tea into the handover. I later learnt that Bill was, for various reasons, unable to reside in the community and normally as a long stay patient should have been placed on a more appropriate long-stay ward, but at his own request he had asked to stay (at least for a while) on Amberley One. A few months later, bureaucracy prevailed and our friend, to his consternation, was moved to a more 'appropriate' long-stay ward, because it was an Admission ward bed he had occupied. But, until then, Amberley Bill resided in one of the much sought after side-rooms, with its own door to close - and which provided a measure of privacy - and security.

Ward Residents

Our patients were slow to get up, which was hardly surprising, since many were suffering from depression, *deep* depression, a dark-black personal swamp that I had yet to learn about. This clinical state which had at some point made some of them attempt suicide or self-mutilation on at least one occasion in the recent past. Thus our entering with a purely cheery appearance was not sufficient a social posture - but it helped. And jokingly punching cracks with individuals, who were known by us, to create response, we worked our way around the two dormitories and every side room.

Most ward patients were ambulatory, but one man was bedridden in the observatory room, his legs bandaged around the calves due to severe ulceration. He was in his early forties a married man suffering from acute depression. I was duly detailed to every morning henceforth change his dressings and assist Depressed John with his breakfast and toilet ablutions; a student nurse using recently taught knowledge. I enjoyed this basic task, and he was content to talk about himself and his life.

The age range of patients on the Reception ward was between seventeen years and mid-60s — this a topical problem. At The Handover the Night Nurse related how one drug addict had jokingly threatened one of the older patients on an issue, and then challenged the night nurse that one night he would unite the d.a.'s (drug addicts) to raid the drug cupboards at the end of the observatory ward and close by the night-nurse station. Charge nodded his head and said that for some weeks he and Norman, his opposite, had strongly recommended that all drug addicts and alcoholics being *dried out* (both, off their supplies) should be separated from the other older patients, who often felt frightened, intimidated by specific individuals — but insisted they were *not* all of this disposition.

On my entry to the ward as first year student there were six drug addicts resident on the admission ward and before my three months would be up there would be a total of nine, a high proportion, too high. The Magistrate courts asked probation for medical and social reports, and thus numbers of drug offenders would be either in hospital pending a Crown court hearing for their particular offence or, offered a Section 26 1959 Mental Health Act section (being at risk) and required to stay in hospital for treatment of up to a maximum (subject to a possible Mental Health Review Tribunal) one year's duration — of which *no* d.a. to my knowledge, ever remained on a Section for that time. This was by most d.a.'s seen as a soft option, a placement of an open-ward — as opposed to the alternative, a more bleak formal locked-in stay in prison, probably Lewes. There were in residence both users and the dealers — the 'pushers' who made new uses of cocaine, heroin and its derivatives, cocktails (a mixture of drugs) and barbiturates.

A number of Section 26 addicts were in due to an overdose, including LSD cocktail offences. Several suffered dangerous after effects, including episodic flash backs, which often triggered a spell of psychotic behaviour; and less exaggerated physical symptoms as hallucinations, nausea, and other unpleasant experiences. They called these episodes 'bad trips' — which led for some, who were hell bent on self-destruction, to sudden death.

Nausea

From the outset, Kafkan and Sartrean *Nausea* displayed itself as a dominant symptom, for many of our psychiatrically ill patients. Nausea with or without actual sickness, for those with acute depression, paranoia, phobic complaints, alcohol or drug abuse poisoning — or, an extreme negative state of mind - a diagnosed affective disorder. A much lesser degree of nausea I had myself experienced, as physical *per se* sickness and nausea — but, surely never as these sufferers.

Another range of psychiatric illnesses found amongst our angst, young and old alike patients, were those experiencing one of the diagnosed schizophrenic (aka dementia praecox) illnesses. This disorder proved much more difficult for me to learn to nurse and understand, for whilst depression was not uncommon to my knowledge, schizophrenia was new to my world of experience.

And, finally, a third arbitrary class of new patient resided on our reception ward. These were aged persons who, *in addition* to diagnosed psychiatric symptoms, also displayed symptoms of senile-dementia, pre-dementia, or brain-damaged trauma — which needed observation and a differential diagnosis. On admission in the 1970s, most patients had some (or all) prescribed drugs suspended — surprisingly a number showed improvement.

The Drug Round

From that first morning I assisted in essential chores. At breakfast time the small medicine trolley was unlocked and wheeled out of the clinic into the dayroom verandah space by the Staff nurse and, as per regulation, with-one-nurse-to-check-in-attendance, prescribed medication was handed out to those who queued at the trolley. Initially, I found the prospect of handling with exaction over two dozen and more patients drug prescriptions at each meal-time rather daunting. A knowing patient would say helpfully; 'I-know-what-I-have-two-big-white-ones-and-a-small-blue-one' (two largactil and one stelazine in his case) or; 'one-large-white-pill-and-a-little-yellow-one,' (largactil and orphenadrine aka disipal).

This was but one vital routine, The Drug Round. Numbers of patients would be reluctant to take their medication; and needed gentle persuasion. The right dosage was of paramount importance at all times, and I learnt to not only identify *all* the current drugs and name all the patients but, like a milkman, memorise each persons medication and *always* to check, according to the written prescription sheets, and witness each signature by the qualified nurse as each patient received their medication. In time, my own signature would be witnessed when *I* came to measure out the medication.

After breakfast was served and early medication completed, the trolley was wheeled back to the main Clinic room off the ward corridor. It was then chained up, and the clinic door was kept locked when it was not in use. Then, there was clearing up, both by patients and staff. A daily duty washing-up roster was posted up weekly by the charge nurse, when two patients would be expected to clear up and wash up the dirty crockery. The list was always staggered throughout the week to keep it fair and reasonable, patients could swop names around as long as it was achieved. Always, I experienced in human institutions, there were slackers and skivers with the pressure from peers to effect results. And, of course, there were those who were genuinely too ill or depressed to execute any ward duty.

Whilst washing-up was being done, a number of the patients prepared to go to the hospital shop, occupational therapy, social therapy, or one of the industrial therapy workshops. Individual patients would be asked 'to remain on the ward' so that their Consultant Psychiatrist, or (if he had one) his Senior Registrar, could examine them, in the ward clinic and interview them, with the Charge Nurse present in the nursing office.

Staff Breakfast

The ward nursing staff prepared for their own breakfast. If a staff member wished to go to the staff restaurant for their twenty minutes, they could do so. Most staff members remained on the ward for a bowl of cereal, boiled eggs, and toast and marmalade, with a pot of tea — supplies bought in by the nursing staff (and they were!). It was another ward routine, the Staff Breakfast.

Amberley Ward's Staff breakfast location was in the corner night staff station off the large observatory dormitory, where there was a phone extension. A precautionary ritual was allocated to the junior nurse. It was mandatory to count up all the knives, forks and spoons, particularly the knives, *after every meal*, and after the rota patients had completed their washing up. This routine had been executed for many years, Charge Bob informed me, because of occasional depressed patients stealing the articles with intent to use them for attempts at suicide. Sure enough, on several occasions in the months ahead knives or forks were found missing, and such attempts at suicide were feared.

In addition, each article of crockery to be used by the staff for breakfast was re-washed and sterilized as it was placed under the scalding hot water from the urn jet. This habit originated from an awareness that occasional patients had, in the past, exercised some rather unusual uses for the crockery, and cutlery, and earlier vivid recollections of contagious diseases — therefore, no risks were to be taken. It was left to my imagination as what such uses there could be... It was probably, I concluded, just to confirm they were clean; a matter of common sense really, not a superstition.

Each day, for *The Staff Breakfast,* a pristine white table-cloth was used. During their 'formal break' staff were able to be available to patients still about the ward, whilst having their own meal and, sure enough, were frequently interrupted by anxious patients. The breakfast also provided an informal discussion of the expected day's work ahead, any anticipated problems, and the personal anecdotes with peppered topical conversation gleaned table talk from the daily press or TV shows of the night before. After I washed and cleaned up the crockery of our staff breakfast I joined the charge and staff nurse in the ward nursing office off the ward corridor.

Close by the office, off the ward corridor was a larder and clothing cupboard; several doctors' consulting rooms; the ward clinic; and a minute room with patients clothing and suitcases stored for the patients duration stay in hospital. At the other end of the ward corridor, the kitchen with its two doors at a right-angle, one into this corridor and the other into the dayroom. Another door linked the ward-corridor with the male admission dayroom and it was this door, and the kitchen doors, that was locked each night and unlocked when the day staff arrived, and left open during the day. It was as an open ward; thus the layout of the reception ward facilities.

During breakfasts our male brown-coated ward orderly arrived, and after first joining us for a cup of tea, began his domestic duties — with segregated wards, female staff rarely worked on male wards, and vice-versa. Although the ward orderly naturally exchanged amicable conversation with staff and patients; his specific duties were cleaning and polishing about the ward, but this was *not* cast in concrete and he could help out when common sense prevailed as well as when any ward crisis came about. (Not long before this time, and the coming of hospital orderlies — ward maids on the female side — all cleaning had remained the duty of the nursing staff.) Each ward was generally inspected *daily* by a Charge nurse and the hospital cleaning Supervisor. Admin Baz recalled that in one hospital an orderly / cleaner *formally* joined the Therapeutic Team, as their availability to converse with the patients was recognised.

The Beds

Unless a particular patient or situation required attention, the next routine, after breakfasts were completed and cleared away and patients directed to their various groups or occupational therapies, was The Beds. Although there was no longer a formal hospital wards daily inspectorate, in earlier times the Charge Nurse (under a rigid inspection by the Medical Superintendent, the Head Male Nurse (Matron, on the female side) and entourage) expected his ward to be clean and smart in appearance, and with no obnoxious odours — at least those that could be cancelled out.

Few patients bothered to re-make their beds and most were restless, although night sedation secured a reasonable nights rest, and bed clothing was found all over the place in the morning. Smoking in bed was actively discouraged as a severe fire risk, as well as risk of self-injury if suddenly dropping off to sleep, but I regularly found a number of beds were heavily soiled with tobacco ash, one or two holes and even crushed cigarettes located amongst tangled sheets and blankets. Several beds were also usually saturated with urine, and faecal stains.

One bed remained occupied at ten o'clock in the morning, in the Non-observatory dormitory adjacent to the billiard room. Ron was in the depth of a black depression (melancholia in an earlier diagnosis), had refused his breakfast, only wanting his medication, and said he wanted to be left alone. For a while this asylum would be granted, before we slowly talked him up and out of it.

Unless a bed in being remade was found soiled, when bedding was of course changed for clean linen, *both* sheets were changed minimally once a week, as in most homes or institutions. Not many years past, it would have been regular changes of straw and dry rushes.... I recall being issued an empty cloth-sack palliasse and straw in peacetime 1950s army huts and, as a teenager, I daily changed straw in the chicken-shed back in our home backyard.... What about the obvious, legions who had only hard dark dank earth, sand, or gathered leaves and bracken to lay down on ...

Twice a week on Amberley, Tuesday and Friday mornings, the treatment of ECT - Electro Convulsion Therapy (previously known as Electro Shock Therapy) was conducted for selected patients. Beds were specially made up with rubberised under sheets to receive anaesthetized and then recovering patients. The ward observatory dormitory was, during this treatment, closed off to other patients and staff, not involved in the event. And, contrary to public opinion, ECT was popular to many patients, as a form of physical treatment for depressed, who found it really did improve their morale even though memory was for a short time inhibited after recovery.

When a patient vacated a bed returning to the community, or transferred to another ward, or deceased (rare on this ward) a new admission bed would be made up, with the top sheet turned over at its bottom. This meant that the bed was made ready to receive a, possibly unconscious, patient.

A New Admission was another hospital routine to be quickly learned, as I would admit hundreds of patients (and assist in discharge) in months and years ahead. At face value, resident patients would be in old-fashioned terms, certified or uncertified, unwilling or willing, following a primary diagnosis which was presently either compulsorily into hospital by a Section of the *1959 Mental Health Act*, or informally under its Section 5 arrangements with no compulsory papers required. This procedure depended on the degree of *insight* and control an individual had over their *diagnosed* psychiatric illness, or disorder. If a patient was clearly *at risk*, a danger to themselves or to others in the community, *and* they were considered mentally ill then a hospital admission, a Place Of Safety, was deemed the appropriate place for immediate treatment and care. But to a patient wilfully moved against their will... Well, *their* feelings on the matter can only be imagined....

Act of Attainer

In an 1815 'Law Dictionary' by Thomas Potts, Gent; a work Charles Dickens would certainly have been acquainted with twenty years on in his early writings; Potts defines:

> 'Attainer, is property where sentence is pronounced against a person convicted of treason or felony: he is then tainted or stained, whereby his blood

is so much corrupted, that by the common law his children or other kindred cannot inherit his estate, nor his wife claim her dower, and the same cannot be restored or saved but by act of parliament'.

Quoting Potts again, in looking up *Lunacy* 'lunatic', he refers directly to his entry, 'See Idiot':

> 'Idiots, an idiot is a fool or madman from his nativity, and one who never has any lucid intervals; therefore the King has the protection of him and his estate, during his life, without rendering any account; because it cannot be presumed that he will ever be capable of taking care of himself or his affairs...'

I found Dickens, always sympathetic to disabled and elderly people throughout his lengthy novels. So it was Mr Dick (Mr Richard Babley), who 'was a little mad',was cared for by Betsey Trotwood, David Copperfield's great Aunt, in his wonderful novel *David Copperfield.*

Statutes, in some form or other, have been in operation in Courts and public life, at least, since the Thirteenth century, for *idiots*[4] and deemed *lunatics.* Inherited *property* of idiots and lunatics was put in trust to a Monarch, or other notable. Post-diagnosis a lunatic body was put in the care of a named individual or imprisoned, or hospitalised, through common law, written law, or even private mandate — as shown by King Henry the Eighth (1491-1547) who instigated a *private bill* to escape interference with his judgement on the young Queen Katherine Howard and deemed conspirators. King Henry's' private bill read:

> 'AD 1541 - Cap. XX - *How Treason committed by a Lunatick shall be punished, and in what Manner he shall be tried.'*[5]

I queried in what *original* writing, this bill had first used the word *lunatick,* when first drafted as a formal *legal* document was it in Latin or English, and was it an early *social* use in Tudor Law of the word *Lunatick*?

In retrospect, an act was passed in 1540 which reflected the *duties of care*, as it were, of the *Royal Prerogative*[6], which laconically read as:

> 'Cap. XLV. The Erection of The Court of Wards, and Names and several Duties of the Officers thereof, in the Governance of the King's Wards, and their Estates .'[7]

I wondered at what age a Ward ceased to be so. Was it laid down or variable? Erm! If a person was under 21 or 18 or 16 years old and married at that age did you owe, technically, a duty of care to them as both a Ward and as a Spouse and, when applicable. as a Sick individual? Perhaps I am being fatuous. This beneficial *Court of Wards Bill* was on Statute until the reign of Charles the Second[8], when the office of the *Royal Prerogative* over idiots and lunatics was transferred from the *Court of King's Ward* to the *Lord Chancellor.* (In the 1960s this was known as Chancery Lane, *Court of Protection.*)

King Henry was able to *legally* dispose of his Queen, and Lady Rochford (who was examined and declared *compos mentis*, at the time of her treason, conspiring as Lady in Waiting on behalf of the Queen) by invoking, in 1542, An *Act of Attainer* [9] in which Parliament bypassed the need for a public (democratic?) *Trial for Treason* by judge and jury, using the Bill and 'supplanting' a judicial verdict. This *Act of Attainer* had been in use at least since the 14th century when King Edward Second's parliament deposed the DeSpencers, who were executed when Queen consort Isabella, who in turn was usurped by son Edward Third in 1330, and her lover Roger De Mortimer overthrew Edward II. This *automatic* use of a Statute was used when a monarch or standing parliamentary body wished to defeat a foe *without a trial* and be able to dispose of their properties and titles if the accused were *compos mentis*, and even after the offender's execution. If they were deemed idiot or lunatic then any property, et cetera, was held in trust while in life, and after death any residue passed to entitled family descendents.

The above research presented a *so-what* question I shared with tutor Mr Ilford from our first lectures; when did a *clinical* judgement differ from a *social* view on being a lunatic? I pursued this historical conundrum, specific use (or abuse) of the word *Lunatick* as integrated in Dr. Johnson's English from Latin origins. This was a reliance on the work of scholars (whatever profession), from early Greek (i.e. Galen) and subsequent Roman and Arabic, or more latterly in legal French translations. The *somatic* origins of *diagnosed* insanity, a madness believed, caused by internal humoral imbalances manifested in a patient's behaviour as a '*frenzy, mania, melancholy and or fatuity*' (from the Latin). What caused insanity? Ideocy (*fatuitas a nativitate*) was seen as more obvious, and deemed clinically untreatable, as well as in need of care and compassion;

but to be insane. Why? Why historical interest in this term of *Lunatick*. Because of its implications, and being guilty ... but of what?

Katherine Howard (born 1521, Nineteen-year old fifth Queen of Forty-nine year old, and ailing King Henry the Eighth) within one year of marriage was accused, and found guilty of treason, in that she was *not* 'pure' before her nuptials (married 28th of July 1540) and unwisely been in the company of young Thomas Culpepper *since* the marriage. Her lady in waiting, Lady Rocheford, acted as a go-between for the Queen with Thomas Culpepper, and was found guilty of treason for her complicity but 'she went mad on the third day of her imprisonment, recovering her reason now and then ...'

This questionable fact, was she *malingering,* in '*feyning madness or not*', initially proved a legal problem for Henry who was determined to put Lady Rocheford, sane or insane, on the scaffold with her mistress, for she had already confessed her guilt *before* at the King's Council and found proven of High Treason:

> 'but, happened to "fall to madness or lunacye" (and) should be the subject of a special Commission of Oyer and determiner of Treasons.' [10]

King Henry's - self-appointed Head of Church and State - answer was the 1541 Act; and Lady Rocheford was subsequently executed on the green of the Tower Of London - after her Queen - on February 13, 1542.

It's one thing to observe, diagnose and treat a natural (medical) body phenomena, such as ideocy, or a 'decayed' person in organic dementia (non compos mentis) no longer, as previously, being in control of his or her mind and subsequent actions, and quite another for a human in authority to designate a socio-political cause (reason?) as being insane (unreasonable) - and removal of an other to an asylum, prison, hospital - or destroy for hearsay or worse an culpable act of treason. Being deemed 'insane' itself appeared at times to be a crime (in society) and in need of a trial or tribunal whether or not *and* be guilty - yet innocent of wilful intent - but still be placed in care or charge of an institution or designated responsible (for the idiot's actions).

On entrance in 1967 into Graylingwell Hospital, I accepted that many patients were in the long stay hospital (in its medieval use as a sanctuary) for not fitting (alienated) in the community and most in need of care and comfort as sheltered accommodation. If there was a vacancy on Amberley admission ward, it was unusual for it to remain so for more than one day as the hospital *always* had a waiting list, especially for informal patients.

With out-patients visiting the hospital to maintain a course of electro convulsive therapy (aka ECT), there was no question of non-sectioned patients being forced to have treatment. A Form had to be signed by either the patient, or nearest relative (for a sectioned patient). In the years ahead I would learn of possible side-effects.

Ward nursing staff would receive a telephone call from one of the Consultant Psychiatrists or their Senior Registrar, the delegated Duty Medical Officer for that day. Each doctor formally attached to one of the three designated areas in West Sussex; Chichester District, Worthing District, and Horsham District. Within two years Horsham patients would be transferred to Mid-Sussex at Roffey Park - or on to Haywards Heath at St. Francis Hospital.

"Have-you-got-a-bed?" was the most loaded question relevant to whether or not appropriate acute psychiatric care could be given *when it was most wanted.* If the answer was 'Yes' then a booking was made and a set of Admission Papers were made to receive the patient. A little known fact to the public was that getting *into* a psychiatric hospital could be harder than getting discharged back into their community of origin.

A Sectioned patient usually arrived accompanied by two ambulance men and a local-authority *qualified* Mental Welfare Officer. Sometimes, relatives came with compulsory patients, but *not* very often. Voluntary patients, on the other hand, usually came to the ward with a close friend or relative, sometimes even on their own if they had been admitted before.

As a new patient was safely received on the ward, any legal section papers would have to be formally checked as being in order. If the papers did *not* check out then it would be illegal detention and have led to a purported wrongful incarceration, traditionally the most feared and media sensationalised experience imagined. There is considerable literature on this abuse.[11] Victorian novels reflected ongoing fear of illegal incarceration. In the twentieth-century global, media records are replete with people wrongfully 'locked up' or 'imprisoned' in state mental hospitals and prison wings, as in the USSR - and other foreign locations. [12]

The Mental Welfare Officer

To be detained in an hospital (as a Place of Safety) against one's will was a sad inevitability with a number of patients whose psychotic or gross suicidal behaviour was loudly denied by the patient (unless mute - for whatever reason), whilst being visibly self-evident. A formal admission was arranged by the local authority duty MWO; The Mental Welfare Officer, a *duly authorised officer*, a local authority health man or woman employee based in the parish, the community. These previous beadle officers were re-named after The 1959 Mental Health Act. In earlier times such authorised Officers were also called Steward, Assistant Overseer, Relieving Officer and, more recently, re-named as Social Worker. Admitting officers worked in tandem (usually) with police, duty magistrates and two qualified physicians. Legally, one doctor's signature had, *had* to be an Alienist or at least an experienced Psychiatrist. If not a qualified physician, the section would be illegal, at least questionable.

Fortunately, for the majority of patients, admission proceeded without any particular problem. I learnt that *specific* written data on The Section papers had to be properly worded, *and* likewise the doctors and MWO's information, on their respected papers should be *identical,* or else *The Section* was deemed not legal (I was well aware it took away a person's Freedom - and, there *must* be a legal way back.)

In hospital, patients affairs would refer back to source if an irregular paper was realised. Serious errors were referred back to the MO, and informed the patient was not detained. The patient could then be discharged or agree and convert to a Voluntary (informal) admission (under Section Five of The 1959 act), if a compulsory admission could *not* be made at the time. (Years later I would sanction many Sections as a qualified MWO and, as an experienced Mental Welfare Officer, I found myself in such isolated situations on numerous occasions, a number in quite dramatic difficult scenarios, with a patient in dire need, to properly find and move them into a *legal* Place-of-Safety, as well as to resolve an emergency.)

It was also expected, but not always found possible in practice, that the MWO provide some basic written information about the patient's domestic circumstances. The doctor would be expected to provide Summary clinical data on the patient for the admission. I noted Charge nurses Bob and Norman, or other Senior nurse in-charge, *always* checked the admission papers, and these were referred to Patients Affairs if not correct, with the admission refused. If the patient was already known to the hospital then previous clinical notes (if it was in daytime and not weekend) would be brought to the ward from Medical Records. After section papers were sanctioned and the MWO departed, the papers would be taken off the ward (copy into ward case notes) and deposited with the duty Nursing Officer to be *again* checked by The Office - then again onto Patients Affairs to be formally checked. It was at the point of accepted exchange between the MWO *and the ward staff* that the admission became legal, if the paperwork wording was complete, and correct.

Paperwork completed and, after accepted admission, the admitting nurse would attempt to gain any updates to add to the patient's case notes, if the new patient (mostly unknown) was able to communicate. If he was too sick and unable to give specific information, then he was taken directly into the ward, curtains drawn around his bed and then requested to change into pyjamas, or get ready for a bath; if he wanted, and of course if safe to do so. Later on the duty Medical Officer would interview the admission.

The hospital Clothing-and-Property Card itemised all personal articles which the patient wanted to be listed, if they were competent to acknowledge this event, and the items were then temporarily removed, not including the articles to be kept, at his own risk, in or on his bedside locker. When completed, the *Clothing Card* [13] required two ward signatures as a check with valuables, and on delivery to Patients Affairs signed by patient-and-nurse (plus another member of staff if patient unable) overseeing this routine duty.

Any prescribed pills brought into the hospital on admission were left in the nursing office to await the duty medical officer's appearance on the ward, when the customary admission physical examination produced the human map details to join the other admission paperwork in the patients hospital file notes. At the conclusion of the formal admission clinical examination a new written prescription, and the in-patient, medical certificate would be issued. Recommended physical tests required separate *Forms* (aka chits) in the paperwork[14], also sometime after admission the path lab representative came onto the ward to obtain the usual pinprick blood sample.

All hospital *Admission* procedures had *had* to be learnt — *Stat....*

The personal touch would invariably be determined by the timing of the admission. So, if the meal time was some way off, the admission would be offered a cup of tea or coffee, and a sandwich, if he was hungry. It was the personal re-assurance that the patient needed, and deserved; it confirmed he was here to be helped, and *not* placed in harm's way.

New Admission

The New Admission sometimes provoked a crisis situation as the patient arrived on the ward. Initially, before admission, the patient might have been sedated, but on coming to, became confused and disturbed to such a degree that it was deemed inappropriate to remain on the reception ward. They were then subsequently escorted up the corridor to Bramber Two - a secure ward.

At a severe crisis situation, and they did occur at any time, a green-rubber cork-padded side-room at the rear of the main dormitory on Bramber Two Ward would (in 1967) be used for a time. If that was inaccessible, a pad on Chilgrove One (very unusual), or Eastergate would be used. It was a sensitive operation.

If our new patient had made a recent 'Suicide' attempt, and was still at risk, then a nurse was allocated on a one-to-one basis to keep a special eye on him. Over and above this *specialising,* however, it was normal to observe *all* patients behaviour following admission, and as long as real risks were apparent a formal duty-of- care remained in place.

All existent long-stay psychiatric hospitals during their living history as Asylums and Licensed Houses, reflected previous eighteenth century Madhouse Acts, and latterly the thick 1890-1 Lunacy Acts, valid until the coming of the 1946 National Health legislation and *1959 Mental Health Act,* which existed in the 1960s and seventies. The acts had explicit and *mandatory* instructions how to treat (or not treat) their vulnerable inmates. From the hospital's inception in 1897, 'The West Sussex County Asylum. Chichester. *Regulations'*[15] - marked on page twelve paragraph 36[16], in respect of the suicidal patient, a legal and moral code, which to this day remained enshrined in the robust duty of care of its patients - applying to all outpatients and residents. As such the duty of care was ignored at both patient and carer's peril.

But in the 1960s, with few staff, and on a full ward upwards of thirty patients to observe and carry out ward routines, to be *only* able to special one patient itself became a logistical, management problem; and at such times another nurse might be drafted in for the duration of the crisis period, if available.

The 1897 Hospital Regulations list [17] had 'inked' markers against *mandatory* rules of conduct, and to wantonly abuse any of these instructions any staff offender risked prosecution *as acts of felony*. If the hospital administrators and their employed staff neglected legal care duties in facilitating current law, especially if a fatality was a direct result of neglect, the authority otherwise risked a case-law prosecution. [18]

Lists like form filling will often draw a low groan when confronted with a task, and *what a bore* when references invoke labels, numerous laws, names and sundry forensic caselaw incidents. Yet, for thousands of years, ancient and recent manuscript written forms, stone tablets, papyri in need of decoding, disclosing fragments from someone's civic military or religious text enshrined as part of a recorded tedious list revealed a way of life in the distanced past. And investigating the day-to-day running of the hospital found numerous similar lists, especially a number of reference books from past Medical Superintendents' and general Administration Offices that were used since the 1890s and *still* on the Patients' Affairs shelves, in frequent use during the 1960s.

Essential Reference

I realised a revealing chronological list which was deemed *essential* reading in past Asylum hospital administration, by past and recent hospital administrators (including Superintendent Dr. Harold Kidd and his successors); Law Books, Journals and other necessary reference works for students, and professionally qualified Doctors, Nurses, and Admin staff, in their owed need of a due, duty of care to patients and junior colleagues. Without doubt first on the list was *The Law And Practice in Lunacy*, by A. Wood Renton. 1896.[19] valid and in use until the 1946 National Health Service Act and 1959 Mental Health Act. A supplement to Renton was *Law Aspects of Mental Illness Procedure* by William Gattie. 1933.[20]

And, from pre-war, *The Poor Law Code And The Law of Unemployed Assistance* by W. Ivor Jennings. 1936.[21]; and still in use in the 1960s was *Chalmers' Sale of Goods Act, 1893 including The Factors Acts 1889 & 1890* by Ralph Sutton. 1945 [22] ; *Law Relating To Hospitals And Kindred Institutions.* by S.R. Spelling 1947. [23]; valid until the 1959 M.H. Acts was the much used *Mental Health Services. A Handbook on Lunacy And Mental Treatment And Mental Deficiency* by F.B. Matthews 1950.[24] A Bible of Reference to nationwide hospital facilities, since Burdett in the 1890s was its successor; *The Hospitals Year Book. An Annual Record of the Hospitals of Great Britain and Northern Ireland.'* 1967. [25]

Last, in addition our *Patients Affairs* held a collection of published *Graylingwell Hospital Annual Reports* (copies for public perusal - on request, held in local public libraries). In another length of the library shelves - all past relevant *HMSO Mental Health Acts* and numerous slim *Poor Law* paperback commentaries, and supplcments to date.

Our United Kingdom government (in theory) guarantees its public, in its democratic society, that despite tight censorship and propaganda (encouraged by it) *any* controversial topics can be presented, at least debated, or acted in comedy, drama, documentary or by lampoon and satire, with libel not withstanding and free speech (not at all wanton aggression) without summary execution of politic dissenters - as in certain global dictatorships. Not so in U.K. legal contracts, and specialist textbooks, which reflect, in the small print, that instant resources *seldom* meet with new legislation. (Sociological jargon aka cultural lag.) Such ambiguity exists in exchanged Contracts and New legislation, and White and Green Papers, in the field of human care. Specifically in contracts paying for the care and wellbeing of others, mostly unable to care for themselves, and owed a duty of care. As I learnt.

Duty of Care

I do *not* recall in the 1960s and seventies ever hearing, or seen in writing, the term *duty of care,* which was to be mantra after 1980s towards *Community Care*[26]. Duty of care is deemed *implicit* in tenets of deemed 'qualified' professional memberships in Accountancy Education, Law, Medicine, Nursing, Social Work et cetera. The term *later* to become almost prolific in Nineteen-nineties and early 21st century in fictional Law scenarios, and Case-law courtroom dramas [27], suggesting all Organisations have legal responsibility for their own and members wilful actions.

Not till 2007, forty years on from my questions put to Admin Baz in Graylingwell in 1967-71 on *whose responsibility* is a duty of care?, would I see reference to a *National Health* administrative corporate body as *possible* perpetrators of *Corporate Manslaughter.* [28] On one National newspaper's Front Page, its Main Heading stated that:

> *'Hospital bosses could face charges after outbreak kills 90. MANSLAUGHTER BY SUPERBUG?* ' [29]

A later report *officially* vindicated that named hospital Primary Care Trust of wilful irresponsible neglect.

Government State institutions *and* their Managers are subject to rigours of The Law; a Senior empowered person from government down to local body, on retro enquiry deemed liable *if proven*, to be wilful abusing of their politic powers, for wilful read neglect, leading to predictable avoidable abuse, death, inflicted suffering, or wanton rank disorder, resultant from their written mandate? Junior staff not sacrificed as scapegoats; subsequently found guilty in neglecting a *Duty Of Care* of its public charges patients and caring staff.

One needed to differentiate between retro unwise but not wilful, human action, and deliberate advocated policy, whilst being well aware of its implications and responsibility. Case law in the 1990s specified that to prove such 'negligence' key elements had to be established, in a Court of law, to prove such *in extremis* negligence. A duty of care must be *owed* to the so-called victim (or victims); there must be a breach of that duty-of-care causing death or unwarranted suffering; and be proven, the breach sufficiently serious, to constitute actual damage by gross negligence. [30]

In the Twenty-first century it would not be uncommon to find the term Duty-Of-Care appearing in daily media; any assumption in neglect of DOC of any sick and vulnerable whatever their age or condition *may be* taken to task. For example:

> 'All schools have a 'duty of care' to safeguard pupils' welfare. Based on the "in loco parentis" principle.' [31]

But, the term duty-of-care was *not* found in 1960s initial enquiries. I noted the metaphor *shell-shock* was absent in Clinical Textbooks from early 1920s, but retained in existent *Dictionaries*, reflected in common language. Shell-shock resurrected as concept in Medicine *after* the second world war in 1980, as post traumatic stress disorder, aka PTSD. I found no *named* Statute headed 'Duty Of Care' (enshrined in the *Royal Prerogative*) in the Sixties.

Whilst I was not able to find in random searches any *early* direct references to abuse by gross negligence (worded) in a duty of care, I did find an old article in a Victorian 'Legal Guide' compendium dated 1839, a report on *Spring Assizes* held on the 'Norfolk Circuit at Bury St. Edmunds, April 2. Before Mr Baron Vaughan.' (Case) 'Mary Gleddall, By Her Next Friend v. Steggall.' (Abstract subheaded) '*Medical Men. - Their liability for negligence and want of skill.*' The action was presented in proxy, by a surgeon of the parish of Gedding, as the 'next friend' of the plaintiff, Mary Gleddall, who was too poor and unable to bring the action herself, and was only ten years old. It transpired that a doctor had maltreated a 'diseased' leg, and by proven negligence had led to a later surgeon having to amputate the limb when it could easily have been saved by more prompt and pertinent treatment. The young plaintiff won the case. [32]

But, again, in the Nineteen sixties I would *not* find duty of care or PTSD listed in any textbook '*Table of Contents*', or in any 1960 textbook's rear *'Index'*, yet it had been around for decades in small print and as legal (forensic and tort) case law footnotes. I asked Admin Baz to search his memories, and ask his retired senior hospital admin colleagues if they could recollect use of the term *in situ,* among our own hospital records.

Baz spoke with a former colleague, previously employed in the Supplies and Financial side of Graylingwell Hospital, who told me: 'Like me Roy M. does not recall the term of duty of care before the *Occupiers Liability Act* 1957[33] but there were standards below which no one could drop without reprimand or dismissal. These standards reflected the general expectancy of the local catchment area, hence they were often not so high in inner city areas.'

Following up these *bon mots,* Admin Baz suggested that an edition of Spellar might locate the term in use. He was right. I found a ref. in Spellar 1947 p87 [34] under the subheading: '*Liability of Hospital or Nursing Home For Acts Of Its Servants.*' Spellar quoted *proven* cases of negligence dating back to 1867 - and numerous other examples in the chapter:- 'A hospital or nursing home owes a duty of care to all patients ...'

I was puzzled. If the Law was so ambiguous about duties of care it owed to hospital's vulnerable charges, in writing, then apart from a proved individual's specific *neglect* of a patient or hospital staff member (or visitor on the premises) were The Laws to provide accommodation and sustenance for the afflicted enough. I pressed Admin Baz as to what source best provided such guidance; a law student would know immediately wouldn't he, or she? But I was a budding professional carer concerned about day-to-day-care of hospital residents and outpatients, not a barrister. Baz got my meaning. Straight off his loquacious tongue; 'No doubt. None at all. Most useful in Patients Affairs was *Chalmers. Sale of Goods Acts* .'[35] I looked bewildered. We were talking about people, patients. But of course, that was his point. Baz enlarged on the subject of *Contract law,* especially what was 'owed'; wordy but very useful:

> 'Briefly but simply it is a legally binding agreement made between two or more persons', by which the rights of patients (or whatever) are acquired, by one or more to acts or forbearance on the part of the other or others (Anson).

There must be offer and acceptance, capacity to contract, consideration (or deed), must be possible and legal genuineness of consent. In absence of one or more of above renders contract void or voidable. Contracts under seal had to be authorised formally by the HMC. Health authority et cetera. And Company seal must be kept under lock and key. Most hospital contracts related to purchase of goods (not overlooking contracts of employment).'

'I am *not* aware of any NHS hospital contract relating to patient care but there were contractual beds in Nursing Homes with formal nurse inspections to check that standards were maintained . Professional standards relating to standards are obvious to us , however, patient care involves all other staff as well as the hotel services, i.e. food, laundry, cleaning, et cetera. To monitor these services lay members of the governing body are required to make regular visits and to report back in writing. Adverse reports were acted upon by main body with remedial action taken subject to financial constraints. I realise we have *not* raised the subject of the law of negligence - as to how it applies to people *in care*. It involves a breach of a duty to take care owed to the person (plaintiff) by the carer (defendant).'

'Should a case reach court by a person claiming a lack of due care it will be decided by the ' law of reasonableness ' as seen by the foresight and caution of the ordinary person. To take this further - I found a reference to 'duty of care' back in 1932. This arose when Lord Atkin and Lord MacMillan discussed Donaghue v. Stevenson, 1932. This was a case of a woman suing the manufacturer for injuries suffered from drinking their ginger beer but it is a matter of tort' (private or civil case law) 'common also to care expected by patients which it is claimed was lacking.' [36]

Felo de se

Felo de se is a term of Anglo-latin origin, 'from Latin *felo*, felon plus *de*, of and *se,* oneself: formerly a Statute used in Criminal Law till a very late date, identifying 'a person who attempts - or succeeds - suicide'. Felon a now obsolete legal term indicating 'a wicked person'. In common law a person, a cruel evil one, who 'committed a felony' from old French; *villain* of medieval Latin origin of uncertain conjecture. [37]

Until 1961 any attempt at suicide as self-murder was formally treated as a statutory crime. How did police authority treat a *successful* suicide? Answer; possibly fault relatives or others, inferring neglect (by default) - in *complicity.* This to be proven in a court action? Any person deemed to assist in a suicide (whatever their motives) - after the 1961 Act, was and is still indictable. An accused *unsuccessful* suicide would have been formally charged with (attempted murder of self) as an act of felony pre-1961. And the unhappy criminal then arraigned before a Magistrate in Court (accompanied by a policeman), and placed on probation for committing this offencc. And...crm... probably instructed to receive formal care and therapeutic treatment for their affliction perhaps, even, deemed a *temporary act of insanity* and placed in a psychiatric hospital.

With no detail, an 1656 *Upper Bench Roll* of the Cromwellian Commonwealth protectorate, dated *before* the Great Plague and The Great Fire Of London[38] recorded deaths by suicide as acts of felony (in the absence of earlier complete Coroner's rolls) numbered fifty-males and twenty-six females, and one other of whom the sex was not identified. The Bench decided under the harsh criminal law of *felo de se* that of the seventy-seven prosecuted dead, it was said, they were: 'Indicted for that they did wilfully and feloniously kill and murder themselves.' And of the total only three bodies were named to be true 'cases of insanity'. The result under the law was not only every body was ignominiously buried, but that representatives of the deceased lost all claim to any property, which was forfeited, just as if an act of High Treason and consequent Act of Attainer was applied.[39] Why, I asked, the ignominious unchristian burial. It was deigned a crime against man, and God; a statute passed down into Twentieth Century psychiatric hospitals, and prisons until 1961. To name the infamy.... what happened to compassion?

Our so-called Christian Brotherhood (and *any* fundamental human sect which declares an un-believer was, or is ,not one of us, and criminalised) did not give consideration to a poor human-being who, *no threat to others*, felt *so* wretched and unhappy that life was not worth living and needed human charity. Instead, the *felo de se* sufferer was legally punished as being a heretic, committing a crime *against* an icon of *God* and image of The Family. And, if the poor imperfect soul succeeded in taking their own life, *then* burial inside any Christian churchyard was forbidden, with *only* unhallowed burial ground allotted to the corpse. It was customary to bury an *unholy* suicide at the centre of a crossroad where the Dracula devil (sum of all imperfection) could claim its own. And, although social changes occurred over the centuries relating to suicide - as I discovered for myself in the years ahead, on the surface few people expressed sympathy for the para-suicide (unsuccessful attempt). Mostly, it was short shrift for them as *malingerers,* taking a bed up, etc. etc. I suspected this attitude more likely to reflect an unconscious atavistic *fear* in most people - rather than a deliberate, derisive and unfeeling callousness.

This attitude to suicide, by any confused individual, or worse, lost soul, thus prevailed in our culture. If Suicide was no longer condemned by Statute as Self-murder and, *worse,* a moral sin against mankind, a sin *against* a legal God, surely such profound suffering was enough without criminalising it as an illegal act. *Felo-de-Se* (self-murder) in origin, I believed, the act derived from an adopted culture of the ancient Germanic Teutons. The Teutons set up altars at crossroads, a place where *criminals* sentenced to be sacrificed to their gods were executed. After Christian politics became established and heretics were criminalised, malefactors and suicides, along with innocent unbaptised children, heretics, and other victims of a fear-ridden and unsympathetic community were demonised and, of old, were buried during the night, to emphasise a heathen burial of the devil's own at a crossroads.

In our twentieth-century English psychiatric hospital, until 1961, specialising a deemed suicidal patient meant the need for a one-to-one staff and patient ratio, and formally signing of a hospital printed red SPECIAL CAUTION card.[40] The card was a mandatory receipt, used to monitor an *at-risk* (suicidal) patient's well being.

Efficacy of Care and Treatment

As with the majority of psychiatric admissions, what was required was unlimited patience and ability to talk, and listen, for hours at a time. Hours and hours of sitting or standing and talking, talking listening and listening, and feeling. This then was the backbone care and treatment of psychiatry. Other treatments, medication ECT or whatever, were but supportive and not intended to be curative in themselves.

On admission there were few incoming patients, however sick or disturbed, that did not respond to a treatment. Manic, hallucinated, paranoid, and deluded patients needed a different approach in psychiatric nursing on the ward, and I learnt to handle each case, to learn the gut action reaction which constituted professionalism.

A new admission in the 1960s was placed in pyjamas, and dressing gown (DGO - Dressing Gown Order); personal belongings temporarily removed to avoid a premature discharge. Confused patients sometimes wandered off the ward, outside into the hospital corridors, and even, into the grounds and gardens. Some patients reached the outskirts of town before being detected. Their pyjama-clad distressed bodies invariably advertising their condition and returned to hospital care.

Most new admissions were only too pleased to collapse into a chair or stay in bed and, let go ... accepting a necessary asylum, before beginning the long haul back to so-called normality and the pressures and pleasures of our community at large. After three days or so it was expected that the new admission could be given their clothes and be able to consider one of the Therapies — or other suggested course of treatment authorised by the Consultant, and the Charge nurse of his ward.

Patients on the road to recovery, would go for half-a-day or a single day's excursion out of hospital, before returning to the safety of the ward. The next stage was weekends; from Friday afternoon until eight pm Sunday evening; and then anticipate a planned hospital discharge. Sometimes long weekends were advised from Wednesday or Thursday through to the Sunday night or Monday morning. Finally, a week or two *On Leave* would be advised and, if found successful, a date for formal discharge arranged.

On Monday mornings, staff and other patients on the ward would experience the results of patients returning from home leave. Most patients who departed on leave, took medication with them. Leave medication constituted another basic ward routine, known as the TTOs, indicating medication *To-Take-Off* the ward on leave. TTOs were prepared by the nursing staff during Friday mornings, but anticipated the Monday or Tuesday before, to allow time for medication to be obtained from *The Pharmacy.* Another ward routine, 'Doing The Drugs', restocking the ward clinic supplies of medicine for the patients needs.

One morning each week the drug trolley stock was examined for empties to be refilled. In addition other clinical stock would be examined in the Cupboards, and deficiencies to be indented for from, the CSSD. (Central Sterilized Supplies Department), hospital dispensary and pharmacy. A large reinforced thick-cardboard locked box (one to each ward throughout the hospital) was collected by a porter with the wanted list, and duly taken for recharge to be returned filled later in the day.

Similarly, all laundry stock and other domestic ward supplies had a specified day when the nursing staff would organize replenishment of supplies. And surprise, there were *chits for everything*, all to be properly signed.

More routine work.

Detoxification, Antibuse, and Aversion Therapy

The Admission Ward accepted a limited amount of Alcoholic patients and Drug Abuse dependants who needed *Drying Out*, before being discharged or transferred to another ward. In the 1960s an experimental scheme encouraged a group of young DAs (there were no old addicts) to liaise with mature Alcoholics, often world-worn ex-professionals and long-service Naval and ex-RAF personnel from Tangmere, Portsmouth or Southampton, who were based at the *Therapeutic Community* of Sandown.

As a new student, I was soon acquainted with both groups of patients.

On the admission ward one programme selected patients (this was not compulsory) for conditioning behaviour under the direction of the Clinical Psychology Department. Treatment involved the prescribed *Antibuse,* using *scoline*, a neuromuscular paralysant drug, (similar to curare), whilst offering the subject a real heroin fix, or a measure of alcohol. As a Student, I was invited to help out at one of these traumatic experimental sessions.

The patient signed appropriate forms for treatment and, at a pre-arranged time, was met in The Clinic off the ward corridor. I remained with the patient throughout the experience. The Consultant (or his Senior Registrar - as I recall), entered with the Charge Nurse. On a table, adjoining a leather couch, was a CSSD clinical tray with two syringes, ampoules, cotton-wall-balls, and cleansing fluid. The doctor informed our patient *exactly* what to expect, and explained *before* he signed an agreement to the treatment. He again clarified whether he still wanted to undergo the antibuse test.

The drug-addict I first attended was a teenager, an 'old' Seventeen year old, hooked on heroin, currently on a methadrine preparation whilst being taken off the stuff. As with most of our drug addicts he had also tried acid (LSD) but was not specifically dependent on that mind-bending preparation - Heroin was a greater concern.

Aversion Therapy was a fashionable treatment offered to help him off his drug dependency. He did *not* have to undergo antibuse treatment but, it would help his case at Court when it was noted he had co-operated in a Treatment Programme. I call him Steve for this description.

Steve

Steve lay down on the ward clinic couch, and was encouraged to fill an empty CSSD syringe with a pellet of heroin and distilled water (as I recollect); but at this stage only allowed to contemplate its use. ...Then the doctor drew up a second syringe with a measure of scoline, a drug that would, for a brief time, paralyse all muscle tone including his chest muscles, and thus oppress his breathing. (I stood close by with a face-mask off an oxygen cylinder to give instant first-aid if needed.)

Steve's right elbow was bent, and for some reason (not known to me), a piece of cardboard placed upright on his arm, to shield the injection of the scoline from his view as he lay on his back. Then, the scoline was given by the doctor. Steve had full consciousness throughout the experience. As an observer, I thought it might have been terrifying for him but, *compared* to horrors from drug addiction, probably not as I imagined the experiment. He was told he could then inject the *'Fix'* if he wanted to, but was inhibited and found it physically impossible. Subsequently, the idea was that each time he later craved a fix, he would associate the antibuse and scoline experience with his wish for a heroin dose, and suffer an inhibiting *nausea*. That was the theory anyway. (I believe *this* treatment was *not* adapted as a norm.)

Antibuse

Alcoholic patients, too, were offered behavioural aversion therapy as an emetic with their dependent beverage. I learnt that oft to-be quoted mantra, if an alcoholic hates their dependency, they hate life *more*, and loathed themselves most of all. Drink, an answer to forget and to be in denial of not coping and hide in a shroud, all obnoxious causes of their despair. Other Sixties fashionable aversions were designed for phobias; sex offenders; and, a variety of clinical disorders and anti-social criminalised behaviour, this latter group also overseered by The Hospital's Clinical Psychology Head of Department, Dr. Harrod.

This Pavlovian aversion as a topical subject was not new to me. I read in *The Sunday Times* [41] aversion therapy treatment programme was intended as a therapeutic clinical measure to improve the person's quality of life, *not* to be an addict, dependent on drugs or alcohol or on *any* anti-social, illegal activity. Working with drug-addicts on the admission ward opened-up other areas of insight to me. In observing our addicts after-effects of drug abuse and of aversion therapy, and revealed a horror, for me, that such dependencies were *no way* an escape.

Flower Power

I had no personal experience, or desire for taking unprescribed drugs. In Spring 1966, *The Sunday Mirror* front-paged '*Teenagers make hallucination snuff.*

Drugs. A Ban on Seed Sales'.[42] People of all ages, in an open consensus, admired the Peter Pan imagery of 'Flower Power'. To *Make Love Not War* . I bought a graphic Soho Carnaby Row red and black poster of a Cat & Mouse making love - not war. Other Flower Power posters and T shirts said 'Talk talk not War war.' Another '*Jaw not Wa*r' displayed on one's chest, thus over the heart. Believers displayed *real* flowers, instead of metal bayonets. I admired genuine sixties Beautiful People, despite feelings that disciples were but naive Wellsian eloi, grazing on Establishment fields. Gentleness, naive or not, was experienced as a virtue when found to be genuine; a good happening.

But, with the public advent of the unprescribed, and manufactured, hallucinatory drugs, that image of peace and gentleness became for me, and others, a falsehood unreal in its surreality. Many illegal drugs consumers appeared *not* to offer peace to all men and women, but became aggressive, insular and anti-society; in a word, hostile, to any *real* practice of a brother sisterhood of mankind. The pure, icon folk like imagery of the flower people was becoming tarnished; fortunately, much of the music remained, and a number of true believers continued to attempt to work for '*A Good Life'* without the will to stamp on others to gain their narcotic supplies.

International Times and Playboy, 1967

It was customary for our ward drug addicts, sent by The Courts, to be regularly sent free copies of the so-called underground newspaper *International Times*. And, several of our ward patients regularly obtained copies of the American produced *Playboy* magazine. Both of these, IT and *Playboy*, often published letters and articles on psychiatry, or rather anti-psychiatry or subjects related to it. On my being given, by ward patients, 'spare' copies of the *IT* and *Playboy*, I noted these articles and letters, frequently evoked comment, especially on Aversion Therapies and ECT. Is cannabis harmless or a socially dangerous drug? At least illegal, at worst it tempted its consumers onto harder drugs, for greater kick; escapism into becoming a *pretentious* seeker; into their own heaven and hell. Inevitably, involvement as a student with our addicts accented my need-to-know *which* drugs were listed as forensic dangerous class A drugs, and to which a doctors prescription alone would allow legal consumption.

Under the *Dangerous Drugs Act,* opium morphine and their derivatives as pain killers were banned presently from public prescription, and used as recreation drugs. A few years ago, any dispensary could sell opium laudanum and *mixtures* as easily as porter and wine were prescribed by the parish doctor and local hostelry.

Also listed as dangerous drugs were cocaine; pethidine, amidone (physeptone) and The Analgesics; as dromaron, dilandil, proladone; all drugs for which access meant authorised signatures in the DDA book. *The Poisons Acts* also included most of the alkaloids and barbiturates which similarly needed medical authorization to consume.

I realised it was important to recognise side-effects coming from listed drugs.

The major and minor tranquillizers were invaluable helping many of our chronic patients back into the community. But, the Tranquillizers could cumulatively of themselves give great distress; if they were not treated, controlled. Chlorpromazine (or Largactil its other name) was a powerful example, a great reducer of symptoms of stress, but with a number of side-effects as penalty, such as the shakes which affected motor regions of the brain — Parkinson's syndrome; rigidity, tremors; excessive salivation; mask-like faces; loss-of-power in walking gait; drowsiness — dyskinetic, dystonic reactions; epileptiform fits; disturbances in metabolic activities, increasing weight; affecting thirst, retention of micturation and constipation, jaundice, photo sensitivity and skin rashes.

Medicines were dispensed in pill form, liquid form or by injection from the medicines trolley on the ward; Largactil was given in either pill form or by liquid. After several weeks of dispensing medication on the admission ward I developed a strange (to me) rash on my hands and arms. Years ago, serving in HM. Forces on Christmas Island in the Pacific as a sapper in a transport troop, I developed a nasty rash from contact with diesel oil and from then afterwards kept away from direct handling of this fuel.

A visit to our staff doctor Dr. T. quickly diagnosed the probable cause as contact with liquid Largactil. For a short period, I wore white linen gloves to off-set contact with all liquid medication, but it was only a few days before the need for gloves ceased and this skin rash never reappeared.

Spider

Spider was the colloquial of one outspoken sixteen-year-old Amberley' patient, a tall dark-haired arm-tattooed broad-shouldered youth. He usually dressed in a black-singlet and worn torn blue-jeans, often in bare feet. Strong and cocky in Sussex speech, a resigned d.a. in hospital on Section 26 of The *1959 Mental Health Act*. I liked Spider.

Why Spider? Not, perhaps, because he was tall and gangly, but, more likely due to the blotches and ugly blue-black-track-marks on his arms and legs and face and torso, marked by unattractive spots and acne. What I remember was his cheerful resilience. Spider was elected by his peers as ward-leader and spokesman of the nine drug addicts on Amberley during my three months stay on the ward. And, in fairness, he was pleasantness at all times towards myself, not at all to all other staff. One may say cynically it was to get round me, possibly true, but he had far more to gain by befriending other staff.

Gregarious Spider stayed the course, despite numerous hiccups and inevitable confrontations — with the community, courts, family, peers, and in Groups in therapy. In my recollection, he did not have the Aversion Therapy course of treatment; he may have declined the offer. Pre-section, he was first acquainted with cannabis reefers at school when 14 years old, tried LSD, and became dependent on cocktails of heroin-and-cocaine mixtures which, pre-admission, had almost killed him. Spider knew he was courting death with dependency.

Methadone

Methadone was a derivative given in hospital, in an attempt at breaking off illegal drugs dependency: In time, methadone, perhaps, was no less addictive as a DDA drug than other banned drugs. However well supported, going 'cold turkey', like Frank Sinatra in the 1956 film *The Man With The Golden Arm,* completely cut off from all drugs and nurturing back to good health, was the only way for many DAs. But, as I learnt, hard, so *much* depended on motivation. Addicts *must* want to get off drugs, and not *only* go into rehab through motions steered by courts, relatives or others.

Both Spider, and Kevin (who was a short-bum-fluff-beaded philosopher and intellectual 17 year old) chatted daily with me on the ward discussing various subjects including *New Age* exponents Gurdjieff,[43] Nicholl, Orage and Ouspensky, Indian music, Bob Dylan, psychedelia, artwork, buddhism, and other writings, as well as fragments of their personal domestic life. The patients openly admitted that cannabis supplies were delivered by friends and sometimes buried supplies in the hospital grounds for collection, as Cannabis to them in no-way represented any harm; cliche ridden 'just like your tea or coffee' (and of course, alcohol, a more loaded comparison).

The hospital was fortunate in having excellent medical staff, and one Consultant in particular was incredible. He developed rapport with all (or most) of the d.a.'s. I was privileged to sit in on a number of sessions when 'the issues' and specific patients were discussed with Dr. R. at ward meetings.

Khalid

Every ward had its characters; young, middle-aged and elderly; colourful and manic; bland and depressed; passive and defiant; single, isolated, married, divorced, separated and estranged. Local dialects and foreign accents peppered the ward population, with patients from distant counties of England, Scotland, Wales and Ireland. And, a small number of patients whose homes were one time abroad, including Polish, Italian and German, a few from the war years. Most European nations were represented among the hospital residents. Throughout most U.K. institutions, a similar spectrum of hospital residents were likely to be realised.

One quiet young man was Khalid, a common name like Smith, a lonely young man diagnosed suffering from florid schizophrenia. He was from Pakistan, and something of a mystery since we had so little information about his background. Due to the apparent severity of his symptoms; hearing voices, hallucinated and generally withdrawn, he communicated only with occasional monosyllables. About five-feet-four in height, usually clad in hospital pyjamas, he had broad shoulders and a round face. His eyes were dark, and to me reflected a hidden inner, and unknown man, rather than the seeming docile person he compared to other ward residents. But, how much was his behaviour cultural, and an obvious lack of English vocabulary, and how much stark illness. With physiological evidence it was difficult to diagnose.

Khalid was generally left alone by other ward patients and not placed in the role of buffoon, as some loners were, in the sub-culture of ward domestic day-to-day life. He had a habit of eating without utensils and piling lots and lots of food on his plate at every meal; eating as if he had starved in the past (or feared to in the immediate future) or, who knows, if these rituals were symptomatic of illness; or reflective of habits abroad and more so. Of what were his dietary habits at home, and where is, was, home?

What of his religious faith, Islam? *How* did he come to be in the hospital in the first place? I developed a particular soft spot for lonely Khalid whilst he was with us.

Some months later I learnt, through enquiries, that with the help of a Refugee Association Khalid had returned to Pakistan and I heard no more of him. Throughout my ward stay, as student, Khalid remained identified largely through the daily deliveries of prescribed drugs; Imipramine 50mg, Stelazine 3 mg, and Largactil 50 tds.

Incident

It was shortly after the patients had finished their mid-day lunch. Staff and Charge were in the nursing office. Two ward-patients were on rota turn for washing up and, as usual, the rest of the ward residents were yet to be dispersed about the hospital, prior to afternoon Industrial Therapy Occupation or other treatment programme. I had just gone off to the canteen and was in the queue waiting to order my meal.

'Quick, quick, return to the ward Barry. Trouble!'

Jack my opposite student colleague, due on the afternoon shift, had arrived, puffing and out of breath, on the ward as sounds of an on-going aggressive fracas in the billiard room became obvious.

Jacques had been sent by the Charge Nurse for my assistance.

On arrival at the ward billiard-room we were stopped at the door by Tom, our Staff, and cautioned. There, standing up on the middle of the billiard table, was an angry Alan, one of our recovering manic-depressives. He had been playing snooker with Dusty, a young d.a, when a contentious point led to an explosion of temper by Alan.

He had smashed the cue against the wall, and started throwing the hard coloured balls at random about the room. Two patients and our Charge had already been hurt by the ball missiles. Alan was *now* threatening to throw two remaining billiard balls, red and white, one clasped in each hand like hand grenades, staring down at the onlookers, bemused, and surrounding *his* island — the billiard table. What?

I assisted in ushering patients out of the room, Charge Bob directing traffic, and in sight of an angry, distressed and perplexed offender, Alan. His hurt victim Dusty, clasped his left elbow. Dusty, piqued and somewhat perplexed, also departed the billiard room, albeit reluctantly, and threatened to get his own back.

'It's okay Alan. All over now', said in-charge Bob, matter-of-factly.

We began picking the balls up off the floor. Bob limped from a leg injury where a green coloured missile had bounded off the wall, shattered a mirror and struck his thigh as it fast descended to the floor. His tone was reassuring, and certainly not threatening or reprimanding. Rather nervously, Jack and myself smiled and nodded agreement up at Alan following our Charge's example. Staff Tom sentinel at the doorway kept other patients away and outside and out of sight of Alan, beyond the doorway.

'Eh! Eh!' Alan was clearly puzzled. It was obviously *not* what he expected from the ward staff. In his surprise, and probably relief, the two balls dropped from his hands onto the now feet bruised green baize of the billiard-table.

The incident, my first, was over. I replaced the balls in the corner pockets. Not on the table, just in case! And, cautiously, we begun to pick up large pieces of broken mirror glass. I swallowed balls of saliva called up to wet my dry throat.

Suddenly, Alan jumped down off the table, and mumbled sheepishly, 'Sorry Nurse' - to Bob, on the way out, as he turned away and strode off into the toilets area.

Yes. It was over.

As Bob began walking away, he called me over and suggested I accompany him back to the ward office. As we sat down, he reached into a drawer and, from a collection of forms, pulled one out and placed it on the office desk before us.

'Right Barry. After any unusual event, whether it's an accident on the ward or an outbreak of fire causing damage to property, patients or staff, whatever it is, you will be required to write up a report as soon after the incident as possible and get a copy off to Patients Affairs and to the Duty Nursing Officer.'

He had my full attention. After all, surely most establishments and corporate institutions have a similar procedure, think of Case Law, Insurance and liability where there is severe damage, especially where the origin was *not* wilful but caused by an 'Act Of God', as some wits would have it. But this is, was, here! And Charge added, 'In this case I shall be writing up the incident. Fortunately, it sorted okay,' compassionate Bob concluded.

I noted Bob's slight limp from the hard billiard ball missile that had hit his right leg, but that was on a rebound and not thrown directly at him. Indeed, no-one had been hurt, except one or two bruised egos. And the other two patients who had received glancing blows from the thrown, hard, billiard balls had fortunately retained but minor bruises. And, yes of course, it might have easily had another outcome; other past recorded 'incidents' certainly resulted in more serious repercussions.

As I watched Charge Nurse Bob fill in the relevant *Graylingwell Hospital* report (*Incident form*) in 1967, I was unaware of how many such reports on a patient's (clients) behalf I would myself write up, or witness, in the many years ahead as a student, RMN, and Psychiatric Social Worker, as well as, not much later, as a qualified *Approved Social Worker,* working thirty plus years outside in the community.

Apart from the Incident Form, numerous other hospital forms were stored in the office drawers, including an elastic bound supply of 'chits' for the various Engineering and other Trade departments — Stores, Upholstery, Painters, Plumbers, Electricians and other sundry departments *not* directly connected with the needs of the ward patients; and naturally each tradesman had in his office whatever reference textbooks to assist them in their labour.

But, most important, I had to learn and locate the variety of forms *essential* in the diagnosis care and on going treatment of all our ward patients. And well thumbed in use were a number of reference Legal Medical and Nursing books and pamphlets which adorned one shelf with several on the office desktop.

Sometime later, following, a number of late Nineteen sixties media reported severe fires in old Mentally Handicapped hospital institutions about the country — and one or two minor ward incidents when our own fire alarms had sounded. I asked learned Baz, in my student innocence, about possible outcomes to such incidents, both to people and property?

It was *not* a question of someone's guilt or purported felony, but a matter of State damage liability. Given that the Royal, rather Sovereign state *Prerogative* prevailed, I thought, this question addressed two aspects, about repair or replacement to property and about subsequent damage to people, staff patients and whoever. Ultimately, it demonstrated how this long stay psychiatric hospital was run as a *living* entity, an organic institution, the fabric and its occupiers, on a day to day basis.

I was amazed, when I was informed that State Hospitals were *not* insured. Indeed, no state hospitals, institutions, schools, prisons, in fact no government buildings were (was this true?). A matter of logistics, pure weight of numbers. And, of course, why the need; surely being of our elected and trusted Government (whatever the nuances of individual elected members, its formal representatives);

being of the government was *the* insurance backup; it shouldn't need belts *and* braces in support. This should bc cvidence of a true elected living democracy: ;duties of care safeguarded.

Well, it ought to be; whatever the use of the legal, nebulous *Prerogative* web-like powers of Management by The Ministry of Health.

As I read and learnt, from both casework and day to day exchanges with colleagues, systems can always be abused, exploited in default or worse, through wanton misuse by people in positions of authority; *in extremis* even in a Democracy. In the robust memories of many staff and patients in the hospital, a number of postwar refugees that existed in the populace, on record, had been seduced (shackled) by obscene misuse, lies and propaganda, in prewar and wartime experience in Europe and elsewhere.

In Truth! *What is said,* and *what actually happens,* is often different to many survivors, in their subtle experience; as the following press statement directed at an aghast international press, with a subheading, 'Democracy As Camouflage:

> " The lie goes forth again that Germany tomorrow or the day after will fall upon Austria or Czechoslovakia. I ask myself always: Who can these elements be who will have no peace, who incite continually, who must so distrust and want no understanding? Who are they? ..." Hitler, Berlin, May 1, 1936.'[44]

Reality. So much suffering.

Irish

From that first day, on the Admission ward in autumn 1967, I could not miss the sight of sad figures sunk deep into worn-armchairs in furthest corners of the ward or, seeming to be endlessly asleep, sprawled on their beds or, hung in tortured states over the arms, seat, and back of corner ward-chairs. These were patient' postures of the depressed. Not relaxed, not passive. Not submissive. But, apathetic, alienated and lost - catatonic in their misery.

'Irish' was one of our newly admitted depressed. In early middle-age, grey-hairs amongst an untidy hay of brown hair, lean face unshaven and, today, unwashed (without staff persuasion). The dirt off of several past meals mapped out, stained, about his once white-shirt — now, grey. And, dressed in shabby black-creased trousers met at his feet in an old pair of ward-slippers long-ago left by a ward predecessor, no socks on unwashed feet. He was admitted one week ago, accompanied by a taut straight faced wife in a neat, dark, suit, a surfeit of tears long dried-up in their shared sorrow. But Kate had held the family together, as she loved both of them.

Kate suffered in silence, when Irish was given early retirement due to ill health. His long reactive depression dated back to the loss of their second child in an accident. And, exacerbated by his due promotion passed over, to a younger less qualified man. And, finally, the break-up of their sexual life. They slept in separate beds for at least two years prior to admission. But, still she cared and treasured her man, her husband, and father to Eric, their fifteen-year-old son, who too recollected his previously so capable, so confident dad.

And most of all, worst of all, was Irish's loss of dignity and self-respect. This led to self-neglect, and ultimately led to a suicide attempt with an overdose of prescribed medication and a filled up bath. Kate found him just in time. Irish was fortunate in receiving regular visits from Kate and Eric, and would recover and be discharged back home, during my ward placement of three months.

Shaun

One of our more active residents was a colourful, slim young patient named Shaun. Aged twenty-five, his father was a local Managing Director and owner of a large cannery, casing imported fruits. On admission, Shaun was given one of the two single side-rooms in the main observation ward, not because he was a private patient, but due essentially to his manic, religious behaviour. He was too often rushing excitingly in every direction, and verbally gushing out either expletives wanting to gain someone's attention or, too often, on his way to make unnecessary urgent purchases at the hospital shop.

One of his last manic actions, before being sectioned, was to sign half-a-dozen large personal cheques, including the purchase of a new car (he couldn't drive) and to give a donation of £500, in a Saturday afternoon collecting box, to a passing by amazed representative of a national charity.

I had, on a number of occasions, been led by Shaun to his room, where several well thumbed books on comparative religion and sheaves of hand written notes were used to lecture anyone, on a pet religious theory of his. But, of most concern, was the regularity with which he upset other patients in his manic behaviour, often interfering with men who wished to be left alone, at least by Shaun. He frequently changed his clothes. It was a wonder he retained any layers of skin, so often did he wash himself in the kitchen and bathroom sinks, or by soaking in numerous hot baths.

On the surface, harmless, and of a kind gentle disposition but, sadly, an enormous risk both to himself and to others during his manic phases. And worse, in his low cycles of depression, he was a self-mutilator and had attempted suicide on at least half a dozen occasions. Shaun was heavily dosed with Lithium Carbonate, which helped to reduce his energy output — the serum-level in his blood had to be checked regularly or else it led to toxicity, and even more confusion. He was another patient I came to know well during his stay on the Admission ward. Like Irish, Sean would recover from this acute episode, and be discharged back home.

Domestic

After several weeks of house and flat searching I remained unlucky, and was travelling by bicycle from Chichester to Lancing on days off in order to visit my wife Sara and the children. But eventually, luck dawned, and a sympathetic local Farm Manager, married to a nurse on The Edward James Estate out at Singleton, North of Chichester, offered to rent us a small tithe-cottage at the hamlet of Chilgrove, called Hoggs Back; a much neglected small two-bedroomed building with a large lightning gutted-tree outside its broken front gate. It proved unsuitable on internal examination but, a second offer by the same gentleman turned up trumps.

One of two *Stonerock Cottages,* it answered our prayer. Small two-bedroomed with a solid-fuel kitchen-burner, the internal structure recently renovated and a covered cesspit at the rear of the cottage; itself in front of a small wood inhabited by deer, pheasants and other wildlife; all for the princely sum of £2.50 per week plus running costs. It was also *very* isolated, and reached by a long unlit unpaved earthen lane, between a network of fields, and woodland, up from the Main Road which passed through Chilgrove. At the beginning, it was relative heaven; and I had my bicycle.

And so, just before Christmas 1967, we descended off a once-a-day, single-decker bus, my wife and I, holding a pushchair with infant Kit within, and young Paul, his two-years older big brother, who stumbled along holding the chair's metal arm. It was in a cold dark mid-winter afternoon with only a small hand torch to search out our new abode. Due to the fact that the cottage was unfurnished, and would remain so until the early new year of 1968, we made a quick visit, then caught the last return bus back to Chichester.

Sara and the children returned to my in-laws at Lancing, and I to the hospital and to duty, on Christmas Day.

Blind Spot

Adam Mitre, aged forty-eight-years, had been admitted to the admission ward a day before, direct from the Chichester Magistrates Court. He was a broad bull of a man, six foot four inches tall, heavy thick set shoulders with well developed muscles, 'Ugly though,' I thought, not unkindly, merely matter-of-fact, as I passed him.

Mr Mitre sat up fully dressed on his bed, both hands clasped to his stomach, an opened magazine face down on the bedding in front of him.

'Nurse! Nurse!', he looked straight at me. 'Can I see you for a moment please?' His voice was strained and demanding.

'Yes, Mr Mitre. What can I do for you?'

'Could you get a doctor, please, I'm in pain. It's me insides. They 'urt somefing dreadful,'. He clasped his trunk tightly, as if to retain certain organs within, attempting to escape his form.

'How long have you had these pains?' I enquired. I might be only a first year student; but it was an obvious question.

'Oh, erm, sometime now. They come and go you know ...'

'All right, Mr Mitre, I'll have a word with the Charge for you.' I walked off to see Bob, who was busy seeing someone's relatives in company of a visiting Nursing Officer.

I had to knock loudly to interrupt the talking behind the closed office door. It stopped, and Bob opened the door.

'Yes, Barry. Anything wrong?', he guessed straight-away from the look on my face.

'Sorry, Bob. Just in case, I thought I'd better come and see you. It's about Mr Mitre. He's says he has severe pain, stomach, I think. And, as Tom is off the ward, I thought I'd better come and see you. Just in case...'

'Quite right! Barry.'

'I'll be out in about three minutes and I'll talk to you about our Mr Mitre.', and Bob, of necessity, returned to wind up the heated conversation in his office.

A few minutes later, Charge Bob met me by Mr Mitre's bedside. I drew the green bed-curtain around the bed, to give some privacy from the growing audience of other ward patients.

'Wotsa matter wiv 'im?' lisped young Ted, himself a recent new d.a. admission.

'That's what *we* are going to find out, I hope.', as I closed the curtain behind me.

'Right, Mr Mitre,' Bob in sympathy. 'Where does it hurt?'

'Here!' Mr Mitre pointed to his lower abdomen, and looked up into Bob's face as he reached forward and lightly touched the spot with his right hand.

'There?'

'Ouch. Yes, that's it. Its been coming and going for some months now.'

'Hmm,' mused Bob, and lowered his voice to a whisper so that only Mr Mitre and I could overhear hear his question.

'Mr Mitre. It's on a Court Report asking for your remand. That *you* have been complaining of *not* being well for sometime but, *you* did not specify to the probation or police officers of a pain in your abdomen... in fact,' Bob paused, in posed question rather than remark.

'One of the reasons you are in our hospital, and not in Lewes Prison on remand, is because of your clinical depression and *not* feeling well.'

There was a momentary silence while Mr Mitre framed his reply.

'Well, erm, you know about my case then. I'm not admitting to anything. I love my wife, and daughters. Ask 'em, any time?'

And, in afterthought, 'This pain is still real you know.' He clenched his stomach. 'Even if the police and probation think I'm only trying to get sympathy.'

Bob paused, and indicated I could draw back the curtains.

'I will ask our doctor to have a look at you on his next ward visit.'

'When's that?' Mr Mitre challenged, vindictively; doubting that anyone would come onto the ward to examine him.

'About one hour's time actually, Mr Mitre.'

Charge Bob walked back towards the office, beckoning me to follow.

The curiosity of the other patients abated and left the vicinity of Mr Mitre, who had returned to the magazine he had been reading.

At the office Bob launched into an explanation, after closing the door behind us.

'I'll be as quick as I can Barry as I want you back on the ward. I'm sorry I haven't told you anything about our passing through resident.'

'Oh?' I looked puzzled by his turn of phrase and lack of patient reference.

'Mr Mitre is an unusual patient for this ward. He has apparently been committing incest with all four of his daughters for over ten years. Several weeks ago his eldest girl broke down, more out of consideration for her youngest sister who is only twelve now, than her own damaged feelings; and those of her other two sisters.'

'Christ' I spluttered, wondering, what next....

'And', Bob continued, 'since being taken into custody he has complained of one thing and another so that, as I read it anyway, no one is inclined to believe his pleas of occasional pain. A question of crying wolf I guess.'

'And what do you think, Bob?' I enquired, not sure what to make of this set of information.

'Well, Dr. Crampton will be here shortly to take a look at Mr Mitre. Remember, Barry,', he added sagely with a nod of his head, 'we are *not* a Court but a hospital, and should behave like it. Hmm! He's not on a Section, he knew what he was doing in his incest during all those years. We don't, yet, know the forensic psychiatrist in liaison between Mr Mitre and the court, though we know the mental welfare officer who brought him in. I suspect it won't be long before he's transferred out of here.'

True to Bob's word, Mr Mitre was shortly afterward escorted up to the ward clinic room where duty doctor Dr. Crampton gave him a full examination.

'Well I don't know if he is pretending or not, as the officers say in their report, but I think you'll agree, Bob, we ought to get an x-ray at least?' Dr. Crampton concluded, as Mr Mitre was directed back to the ward in my company.

Several days later it was confirmed; Mr Mitre had a duodenal ulcer and two days later received medical treatment at the West Sussex County Hospital, in Broyle Road. Ten weeks or so on, and an item in the *Evening Argus* reported his conviction for multiple incest, and his removal to Lewes Prison to serve out a custodial sentence.

We concluded that his ulcer was a 'blind spot' for earlier examiners who understandably, if not in justification in view of the enormity of his offences, believed he was telling one lie after another to escape the inevitable track of justice underway since his daughters' accusation.

The Blanket

Breakfasts over, beds completed, medicines new orders boxed, patients were 'out' to their respective treatments at Occupation or Industrial Therapy, Social Therapy, or to the Dentist, and only two patients left on the ward, Jim Howes and Fred Jackson.

I was in conversation with Jim, a depressed patient who had stayed back from IT, to see the Duty Doctor to ask for Electro Convulsive Therapy, which he had had some months previous. The ward staff did not feel that he needed ECT but Jim insisted he wanted to see the doctor and persuade him otherwise. He was looking for a shortcut, rather than commence *talking* out numerous problems, which had led to his recent overdose of prescribed drugs. He was about ready now.

I was engrossed, with Jim, in a corner by the billiard room entrance.

'Can I see you for a moment?' Bob said to me and, aside, politely remarked to Jim that 'Barry will be off the ward for a few minutes but he'll be back to you afterwards.'

I excused myself, and left the Day Room to join the Charge in the ward-corridor.

'Barry. Office rang. They have a bit of a flap on up on Bramber Two. Would you go up and give them a hand. It'll be good experience for you?'

In some haste, I strode up the main hospital corridor and ascended the concrete stairs up to the locked ward of Bramber Two. As I inserted the jig-saw key in the lock, I could not avoid hearing shouting and singular threats from somebody. And, just as I opened the door, another nurse, also called upon to assist as back-up, caught up behind me. Panting, it was Mauritian Jack, our third-year student.

We entered the ward together, and I locked the door behind me. Normally, in the day time, this ward was left unlocked, as with most wards in the hospital.

Jack and I marched into the Dining-Room area, where the noise was coming from, and there was Dick the Ward Charge talking, or trying to talk, to a man dressed in pyjamas and brandishing a knife, screaming out... 'I will, I will, I'll kill myself, don't you DARE stop me, or else.'. Distress blazed in the patient's eyes, who was unknown to me, but apparently well-known to Jack who echoed, 'Hi Dick.' to the Charge nurse. To the distressed patient, he cautiously added at a whisper... 'Hello Vic, can we help?'

'Vic's rather upset, as you can see?' the Charge Nurse quietly said to Jack and I, across Vic's vision. 'But he's not ready yet to tell us what's upsetting him. Are you Vic?'

I noticed several other patients, sat quietly over by the television watching the ward's drama. -They were used to ward incidents of one sort or another. Charge Dick looked across to Jack and I, and asked, 'Could one of you fetch a blanket off a bed in the ward dorm for me, and fetch it here.'

Jack moved to the side of the Charge, and I, most curious, turned round and walked back through the short ward corridor, down into the dormitory. I took the first blanket I could see off one of the beds and returned to the ward dayroom.

I was bewildered. What did he want a blanket for, the patient?

Vic, in a then frozen posture, had a raised knife, and at that moment appeared not responsive to soft re-assuring words, but at least his shouting stopped. He too was wondering, as I was, what happens now?

'Thanks.', Charge replied as he took the blanket from me and, folding it in half lengthways, then asked of me, 'right, lad, take the other end.' I thought, we are going to fold-it-up, (whatever for?). No, he had something else in mind.

'Stand back a moment please, Jack.' Dick, to our colleague, and Vic, who was frozen now in a sculpture, both still puzzled as I was, looked on; the kitchen knife still a threat; speechless during this activity...

'Right lad, now walk around Vic, that way round please,' gesticulating as he proceeded to walk in the opposite direction, around the distressed patient, Vic holding his *felo-de-Se* weapon aloft.

The blanket went taut and, as we moved on circling Vic, it became obvious what Charge wanted and within two-seconds the blanket was effectively bound tightly around the distressed patient; and he was disarmed. Charge deftly removed the knife from Vic's perpendicular, up-stretched arm and clasped hand, just outside the blanket's perimeter.

Jack and I moved in, but there was no need. Instead of more aggressive movements, Vic collapsed in tears: 'All right Vic ole' son.' Charge Dick tenderly put an arm around him and, together, they started for the ward office. Turning for a moment, he remarked to Jack and I, 'Thanks lads, could one of you stay a while until my Staff Nurse arrives back from the Pharmacy.' Jack remained and I returned to Charge Bob, patient Jim, and the Admission Ward.

Back on my ward, and after relating the event to Bob, he recalled ; 'Ah, yes; that would be Dick; one of our old school of Charge Nurse Attendants.' He then added, 'The *Blanket Method* is very effective in certain situations. It's safe, and avoids heavier methods when talking-down isn't working, but still possible for innovation and non-restraint in defusing your situation.'

Bob continued, clearly thinking of past years, 'Not so long ago, we had few drugs to work with, and more patients could be acting out with few resources to deal with any explosive situation. Remember, *At All Times*, you never, ever use *any* restraint which can harm the patient. If *you* cannot handle the situation, leave it, and either do what you can *or,* go for more effective help. We no longer have a Heavy Group of staff to call upon.'

'Blow ups are few. Most are confused, frightened people, who lose control. Wilful violence is rare, but does happen. Remember, a patient's rights ought to be protected, and *not* have a violent as well as a psychiatric label to follow them on after discharge, if you can help it. A Heavy Group, sometime existed pre-war. This was a number of well built hospital staff, called upon if a nasty situation needed defusing. Since our modern drugs, few patients display such a range of florid symptoms, hence staff being called on from other wards with staff shortages...'

Jack and I, no-way being 'a heavy mob.'

This was the first, and *only,* time I ever saw this *Blanket Method* for arresting a potential violent situation. But, the safeness of this action, combined with the personality of the member of staff was just right. Vic recovered and was discharged several weeks later.

Pad

Eleven years before, in 1956, I had been a member of HM Forces embarking as a squaddie in *Operation Grapple* [45] for the H bomb tests off Christmas Island, one of the Line Islands. I was a thin immature institutionalised youngster, doing his duty for Queen & Country; a member of a Sappers' stores group. We were assisting in loading a small battered troopship, *The Charlton Sta*r. Nearby, we had the immense company of the giant liner *Queen Elizabeth* (not as our escort, no honestly) at Southampton Docks.

Sent down, into the bowels of our elderly, smelly vessel, several of us stumbled into a minute dark, odd-smelling black rubber padded room — walls floor and thick door all well padded. A ship's crew member informed us it was a room for crew who went *off their heads* by excessive drink, or whatever, and who became insane. Surely, all ships did not enjoy this facility. I thought of Bogart as the insane Captain Queeg in the 1954 film of Herman Wouk's naval novel, *The Caine Mutiny*. A lone episode, as part of an Royal Engineers stores troop, this incident soon forgotten — but brain stored in the trunk of my mind.

A few weeks after the incident, involving the blanket up on Bramber Two ward, one of our new patients, a rather burly gentleman, went berserk; and could not be managed on the admission ward — I was not aware of all the details, but I was asked to assist his temporary transfer. The patient was subdued, after an injection, placed in a wheelchair, and taken up the corridor to one of the pads on Eastergate One ward, at the other end of the hospital. It was an emergency treatment, *already* on the way out in the hospital but, as we entered the dark, green-dyed, cork padded side-room in 1967, I was instantly reminded of that prison-like cell in the 1956 troopship's belly.

The full extent of new post-war controlling drugs was still underway, to pave the way for Community psychiatry. *No* member of staff, past or present, in *our* hospital's records of seventy years, remembered use of the extra-long sleeved strait-waistcoat or, better known, strait-Jacket in Graylingwell. In the United States and in Europe this straight-Jacket, I understood, was still used, I was informed, in some State hospitals but, not thankfully in the United Kingdom.

Years later, my mother gave me an anecdote of my father, an Australian Vaudeville artiste and Stage designer, of whom I have no personal memories of at all. Anyway, she said he had worked very closely with American Vaudeville (burlesque) comedians Olsen & Johnson for some 13 years or so in the States. Came the 1929 Wall Street crash and subsequent Depression, and the movie Talkies in America, he came over to work in showbiz in London in the 1930s, then met my mother and married her in Jan 5th 1935. He would be in the theatre foyer, as customers arrived, and be seen tied-up in a straight-jacket in the foyer. Shortly afterwards, he would be seen as a straight man on stage with the comedy pair, and in his own acts, whatever they were. Then, as the show concluded, he would again be seen, still apparently bound in the straight-jacket, by exiting theatre goers as they passed through the foyer and out onto the street.

Critics, in the 1960s, were already referring to powerful new tranquillizing drugs (merits and demerits) as chemical strait jackets but, sadly, seemed to miss the point, either or what legitimate alternative treatments were available; viable, when a person was very 'ill' and, talking down unhelpful, to control *in extremis* disturbed behaviour towards themselves, and towards others. These new drugs, despite cumulative side-effects, in the main really did arrest many of the causes of disturbed symptoms, and allowed acute and chronic patients more 'freedom' from adverse *biological* chains. And more people discharged from the long-stay hospital back into The Community.

Routine

Christmas 1967 arrived, and I was on duty throughout the holiday week of Christmas and New Year festivities. On Amberley, most patients were quite vocal, including the depressed, and mobile. A number were well enough to go home to relatives or friends, but for those who remained, within their clinical boundaries, all appeared to enjoy themselves.

Staff, and the better patients, were brilliant in putting up and making up Christmas decorations; being no exception, because it was a psychiatric and not a general hospital. The huge Christmas fare and wonderful *bonhomie* of all institution staff and patients was rewarding for me to witness as a first year student nurse.

Of special interest on Christmas Day, was a visit of the Chichester Mayor and his followers, accompanied by Senior medical and nursing staff. The corporate visit was brief, after all they had all the occupied wards to visit, but it was pleasant.

I was already identifying myself, with the patients and staff, as *us* when meeting outside visitors. A children's choir, from a local church group, accompanied the notables. It was their honest acceptance; no signs whatever of stigma or fear of the children, and their escorts, as they sung their Christmas carols to our gathering on the admission ward.

And there were the ward office parties across the hospital. At breaktime Bob sent me off for a half-hour tour of the wards; but not to accept drink: 'Because you are still on duty.' But, the odd sherry was accepted with the offered sausage rolls and ward fare. There was no untoward event to mar the Christmas festivities though it was quite exhausting at the finish.

Drug rounds, meal time distributions, medicine collections, new admissions, TTO. distributions, occasional incidents, callouts to other wards, and especially, patients being discharged home, for good. And, hospital schooldays once per week, every week (except Christmas). And beds to make up; ECT. sessions, talks with relatives, and lots, lots of overtime on offer. All soon became routine to me on the Admission Ward. And, it was a cold wet mid-winter day on February 11th 1968 when I finished my Amberley One duties and briefed by the Nursing Office for my next ward block, called *Chilgrove One* Ward.

Time to move.

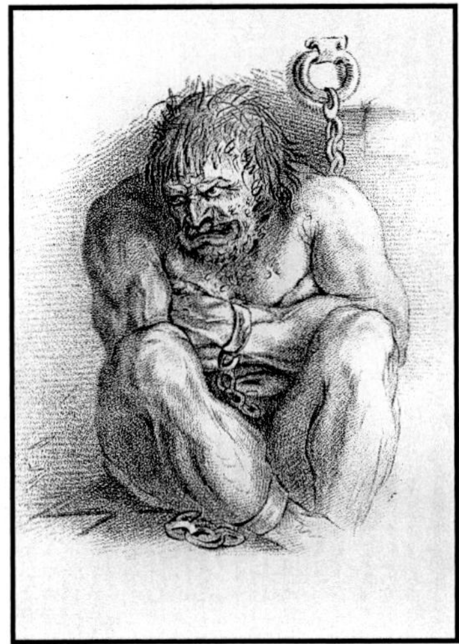

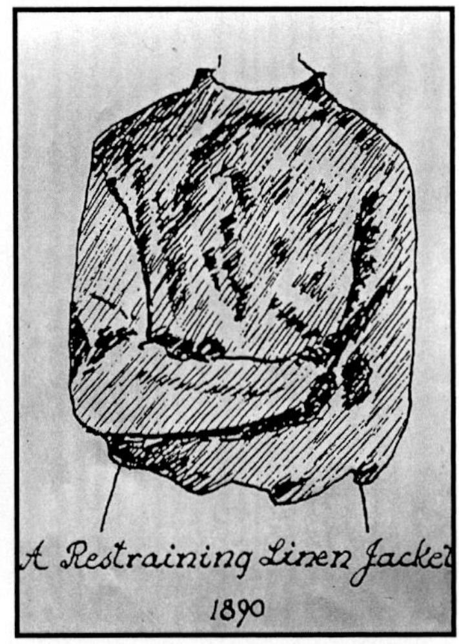

Left, Published mid-19th century drawing of a chained sufferer in Madness. A human being in absolute despair and resignation, seen 'in solitary confinement' - as *envisaged in 18th century* : caption read 'You see him in his cell regardless of everything, with a death-like settled gloom upon his countenance. ' (Source. The Anatomy And Philosophy of Expression. By Sir Charles Bell.(1806), Publ. Bell London 1877 ed. see pp 160-1). **Right**, a contemporary print of a late 19thc. linen strait waistcoat. Fortunately such treatment in 20th century U.K. Britain, with due compassion and better resources, such restraint, given as a duty of care in a hospital long redundant — but, perhaps not so in other countries.

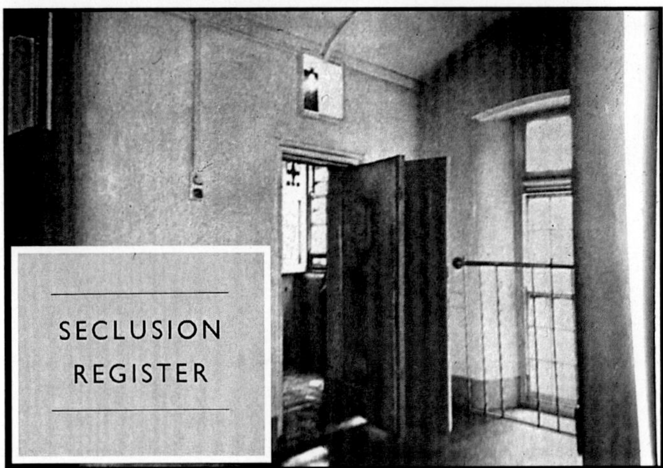

Single room 'Pads' were a fixture in all asylums to control and contain episodes of violence and self-mutilation when talking-down or other pacific means was ineffective. In Graylingwell Hospital and UK they were closed down in the late 1960s.

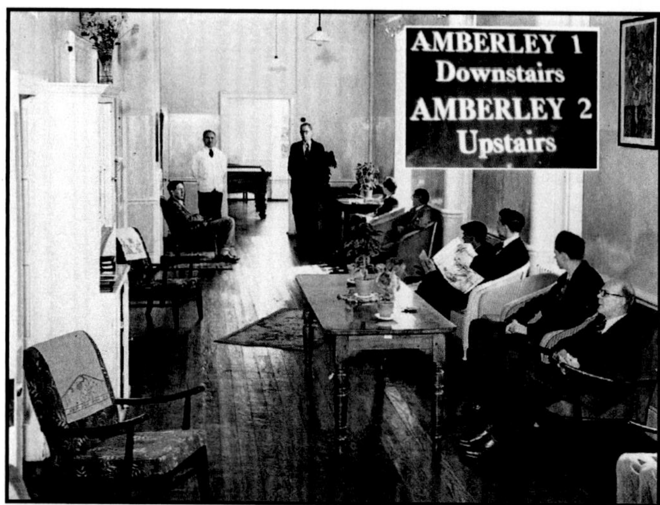

Amberley One admission (reception) ward, in early 1960s. Staff standing. **Left** Nurse Mr.J. Morris. **Right** (in civvies) Deputy Chief Male Nurse Henry George Clinch, a WW1 veteran, who qualified 21st May 1924. Dr H.A.Kidd was his Examining Superintendent.

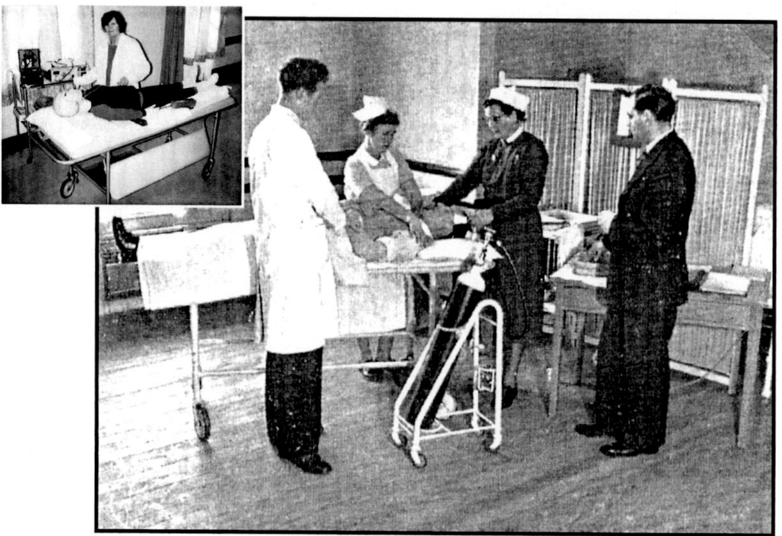

1958. ECT existed in WW1 as faradism: 1934, Meduna introduced Electro Shock Therapy, unsafe, until post-war Electro Convulsive Treatment — with Scoline. It did not cure Schizophrenia but, in low doses for short courses, was effective for clinical depression. But, heavy doses and prolonged courses — abuse! (Main picture from Park Prewitt Hospital, Hampshire, Exhibition Brochure, 29th April 1958.) **Inset**: Brenda Wild, RMN, Graylingwell ECT Suite, 1997.

Chapter Four
Chilgrove One Ward

' When memory begins to decay, proper names are what go first, and at all times proper names are harder to recollect than those of general properties and classes of things. '[1]
William James. Principles of Psychology. 1890.

12th February 1968 to 11th May 1968

Chilgrove One Ward—Boo and Kipper—Alzheimer's—Hospital food—Pharaoh Ants—Vagrant Joe—Staff Ahmed—Captain Jones—Incident on Barnet Two—Barney and No Names—Mensa Charles—Prancer and Mr Smithers—Domestic—School—Harrow—Outpost, Acres

February 12th 1968
Chilgrove One

The gaunt Chilgrove Block, located close to a brick tubular passage, formerly led to Medical Superintendent Dr. Harold Kidd's house, which was now a Male Nurses' home, situated off an elbow bend of the west Main Corridor. I entered the downstairs ward through an unlocked dark-green door; a spiral flight of grey concrete steps immediately to the right led up to the rehab ward Chilgrove Two. Moving on, along the ground floor, I passed, on the right, two low small closed doors; rooms dark in shadow, situated under-the-stairs. One space hid a still used ward store-cupboard, the other was a small locked disused pad.

Forward, a few yards on, there was a locked door; using the heavy male key I entered another short passage into the open-area of Chilgrove One ward. The ward office on the left, and a small square kitchen to the right, on a corner. A right-angled extension housed a narrow central corridor, enclosing a dining-room space and separate ward ablutions — toilets, sinks and bathrooms. At the end of this horizontal passage, on the right of the H frame structure on its vertical, was a second, long-stay dormitory; this arm extended down, and back into the Main hospital corridor by another access door.

Ahead was a seating-area, on its left a separate built-on 1950s Conservatory annexe with the ward-garden (airing court) outside. North, straight ahead, was the main acute-and-bedded-dormitory, with two small side-rooms, one to each side, at the end of this ward.

An obnoxious smell impressed itself upon me; a strong odour of urine, excreta and a sweet-smelling citrus cocktail of mixed chemicals. This was a common feature of a number of long-stay wards; mostly elder (white flowered trees with much *pith*) despite ongoing effort on the part of patients and staff to keep it clean and to arrest any noxious smells at floor and bed levels, as well as help abstain from a spread of infection.

Initially, I felt nauseous and occasionally retched, and surreptitiously sniffed an old empty perfume bottle of Sara's, that I'd brought along on the second day, to offset the ill effects; but a week or so on duty and I became used to this resident odour. It was an inevitable feature, of caring for elderly-demented and acutely ill (sans dignity) that 'have you been' was a fatuous statement rather than a polite question, with so much evidence of incontinence needs continuously meant cleaning up; off uncomfortable, demented helpless patients, and off the floor, and frequently to change sheets, pyjamas, underwear and trousers; so self-evident, and essential in our duty of care.

The traditional imagery of nursing angels chirpily offering bottles to patients who ask to go is a truism, but so are the products of the severely-ill and dementing-souls who then, just, let go... (and, in large numbers, frequently did so throughout the day).

On this ward, I learnt about *ward gardening*; joking, but not mocking, a colleague commented as I was about to mop up Boo or some other busy resident; the patient's fingers of one hand, a thick-crusted brown, that was dried-up and thickly sandwiched behind their nails (which acted like forks to 'dig' into their back-garden, insidiously, throughout the day).

Ways of coping!

For many hours during the day, bedridden Chilgrove patients and those others unmoving sat in fixed-chairs, or longbacks, and were seen with their eyes glazed and seemingly unseeing, looking around them. Residents, remembering fragments of times long past; confabulating, inventing memories they had wished for and, now, but mythologised icons. I observed patients tracing fingers filigree lightly through the air, tracing unseen willed shapes upon their bedding...

Bruce, a lean man with small moustache, thin thatch of white-hair and such piercing blue-eyes, wore blue-stripe pyjamas and would every few minutes through the day, call-out 'Nurse', to come over to him to ask for 'a fag', and for an opportunity to eulogize over his wife, and children who had recently visited him with all sorts of goodies. He said he eagerly awaited her next visit that very afternoon. The warmth of his voice, and twinkle in his eyes, completely belied the reality that we knew only too well and (thankfully) he could not register. The truth was that it was not 1946 as he believed it to be, it was 1968; and sadly his wife had died over ten years ago and nothing was presently known about his children, as no-one ever came to visit dear old Bruce. He was only in his late forties.

The forty plus patients on this ward had few regular visitors, but those few that did visit were invariably devoted, visiting a relative year-in-year-out with, probably, no hope, in this instance, of any likely recovery. Boxer and Kipper had regular visitors who displayed affection and concern for their kin at all times, until they eventually died. (I would later be present at Kipper's departure, on another ward.)

Proportionally, few patients expired in this hospital, though a small number stayed many years and even then, could either be rehabilitated, with new social skills, or discharged back into someone's care; somewhere. Better off In bed-sitters, in the community.

On the Admission Ward, patients came and went with relative rapidity; many left after a few days, or a maximum of six weeks; an experience I only came to appreciate when serving on a Long-Stay Ward for the first time.

At most times a sick (in the physical sense) patient was transferred to Lister, the sick ward, down the corridor or, if worse, transferred down-the-road, to the Royal West Sussex Hospital in Broyle Road. Sometimes, a sudden bout of pneumonia or stroke brought on a man's demise during the night, and I assisted in drawing a screen around the patient, laid out for departure to the morgue.

Boo and Kipper

There were a number of endearing characters on Chilgrove One in 1968. Two were fondly named as 'Boo boo' and 'Kipper'. These two long-stay patients lived in open single-rooms at the end of the observatory ward. Another notable was Boxer, who was a professional boxer in his youth and now bedridden at the end of the left row in the main ward observatory dormitory.

Boo had been admitted into a hospital, not this one, at the age of eleven years of age over twenty-years ago, in the post-war period, having survived a serious heart condition as a blue baby which left him severely mentally handicapped. At birth it was predicted he would have but a short time to live, and yet he still existed...

My introduction to Boo, by Charge Nurse Big Jim , was in retrospect quite a humbling.... I was being shown around the ward for the first time and, having toured the length of the observatory dormitory amidst considerable noise emanating from confused demented, elderly and late middle-aged patients, on their beds, some in long-backs, with one or two in locked in chairs with their swing-in circular wood-tables, we reached a single room with a closed to not locked door. The door was ajar....

'And here, my lad, is Boo, who needs *special* care and attention', Big Jim said, as he nudged the unlocked door wide open.

A bare grey mattress was on the floor, with clean and soiled crumpled up bed-linen balled at the foot of this bed. In one corner a battered aluminium-pot for toilet had recently been used. Sat on his haunches crouched in the corner was Boo, diminutive, well-fed and naked; his discarded pyjamas remained clean and screwed up in a ball before him. There were no murals about the lower walls; clean and spotless, it all reflected a well-cared-for room and patient. There was *no* faecal smell apparent in this room, which surprised me.

Big Jim spoke slowly, gently, almost cooing, indicating we were going to give him a wash, exchange clean bed linen, and maintain the tidiness of both room and Boo. Boo's grey eyes glinted and tightening his crouch, he looked up at Big Jim with clear affection, his eyes showing that which his poor white-body otherwise lacked in animation.

It was on this occasion that I first met Big Jim, the ward Charge Nurse, a tall lean-man with uneven dark hair, sunken cheeks, and harsh gravelled voice that, when called for, bellowed to students and staff alike, reminding me of an Regimental Sergeant Major, but *always* incredibly firm and kind. Sussurated in his slow patient speech, even with the harshest of his dependent charges. His white ward-coat always appeared as if it was too short at hem and arms, and billowed around his lean agile torso.

In the three months placement, I often went into Boo, but remained reserved and, honestly, a bit scared at times. I was too ignorant, however well intended, to establish any rapport with him. But, I had considerable respect for Boo, as an unfortunate deprived of ability to function in the so-called normal world outside. Oh yes, he had dignity too. Boo-Boo (I did learn his proper name, he died in the early 1980s) was *definitely* an exception in this hospital in the degree of his infirmity, whereas Kipper, his close neighbour, had a lived pre-morbid past and considerable, concrete personality. Sometime later I met a micro-encephalic; but that's another story — for later.

Kipper's single-room was opposite Boo, only five feet away and, whereas it was seldom that Boo emerged from his safe station, Kipper often came out into the dormitory with something to say; in his lone mono-syllabic way. One sentence he frequently uttered, in fact I recall he could say nothing else, was 'I've only got one lung!'

Indeed, he had *only* one functioning lung; a result I believe of pre-hospital caught tuberculosis. His kipper-like wraith shape and visible concave rib-cage, where no inflated lung matched its peer, was self evident. Tattooed down his arms and indented on his frail body was evidence of his youth in the army of the 1920s serving in Singapore and in the Far East, before life dealt its fateful card and led Kipper into this hospital, about eight years ago.

I did wonder, regarding Boo and Kipper; with no prospect of any conversation, what *conscious* memories did they experience?

Alzheimer's

In the first bed, on the left side of the non-ambulent part of the observatory ward, was a young man with black hair, lean-face and thin-body; scar-thin and sat-up, propped-up against four pillows for comfort. Alec seemed out of place with the rest of this wards' residents, though he made movements in the air with outstretched hands and pointed fingers, tracing deliberate shapes upon the counterpane.

Alec had a pre-senile dementia, it was irreversible and terminal. He had been hospitalized for over a year, with his condition insidiously deteriorating. The clinical diagnosis was *Alzheimer's disease*, the brain's tissues breaking down, the body's intellectual functions affected and, accordingly his willpower, consciousness, control (call it what you may) was slow, shredded and disappearing.

But, and what a notable but, Alec's dignity, what was his pre-morbid persona, seemed to permeate, even in this demented state. His eyes and mannerisms were confused and anxious but apologetic for his behaviour, in the fleeting moments his brain allowed a painful emotional comprehension.

These insightful moments were most noticeable when his family came to visit. There was a wife and children, two young girls and an older boy, all school age; tender and often tearful. They visited him *every* visiting period and almost every other day. Alec had been a successful insurance broker in the City of London, but three years before.

In a matter of weeks his emotional communication too had diminished, and one morning, a few weeks later, Alec. who was only 43 years old, was dead... and, already, a new admission was accepted for his bed, that very morning, such was the continuous pressure for beds in the hospital.

A sad maudlin true story which could have easily been an anecdote for a Nineteenth century religious tract (SPCK). However, the majority of the residents on this medium and long-stay ward did not stay long, bedridden or terminal. A number of the more ambulant would be transferred onto a Rehabilitation Unit, and discharged out of the hospital back into the community.

Hospital Food

Contrary to media jokes, which insisted all public-institutions' food, like the proverbial British Railways' sandwiches, was awful, our hospital produced good cooked food which was rarely sparse in quantity or bland in choice. The hospital was well on record as good housekeeper and monitored its budget accordingly. Quality of food was good to excellent and, again to further surprise, nearly always 'More' if patients requested it. Staff (or patient) would journey back to the kitchen, or phone through for more, if the meal trolley had run out of any particular item.

At ward breakfast, there were bed-patients, and ambulant patients from the other end-dormitory to be fed. There were three staff in attendance; Charge, Staff-nurse, and student, with between thirty-five and forty-five patients to be served from the two dormitories and medicated. Helpfully, there were at least three capable rehab ward patients, who regularly assisted in pouring tea or refilled the large metal pots from the steam-urn in the kitchen, who received a small remuneration for their assistance. Mostly, it was good teamwork. Staff and patients working well together.

One particular patient, John, was an epileptic *compos mentis* resident, who (his wish) assisted on selected domestic duties, and wore a half-white coat overall to emphasise his *special* status. The media was vigilant that patients should *not* be exploited as supplementary labour, even if they wanted to help out, but humane commonsense fortunately differentiated from such extremes. And epileptic John was a great help, and paid an allowance each week, thanks to Big Jim's insistence for payment.

Breakfast, chosen from fried eggs, sausages, bacon, baked beans, boiled eggs, poached eggs, scrambled eggs, haddock (bones removed), tomatoes, and grapefruit was all regularly offered in daily combinations, along with customary special diets and, as with all hospitals and homes worldwide, the most helpless were spoon-fed (e.p. John is marvellous in this gentle task). Liquid was given in the long spout vessels designed for this purpose.

Pharaoh Ants

Most days, I remained on Chilgrove for my breakfast twenty minutes and, on one rare occasion, at breakfast we watched a wee mouse emerge from behind the kitchen skirting board, whilst we sat for our meal break within the small square kitchen space.

And, despite an half-hearted humorous chase by myself and auxiliary John, it escaped back behind the boards and into safety. But, it was a one-off, for such intrusions were rare, though during the Summer-nights cockroaches could sometimes be seen scampering across the kitchen floor. Yet, the floor and surrounds were always kept immaculate as hygiene was kept to a high standard, as staff were always vigilant against any evidence of infestation.

When I later spoke to Admin Baz of this brief encounter with the mouse, I also mentioned the parade of marauding cockroaches, usually when heat of the kitchen and, more so, Summertime propagation brought them out from under linoleum, and up from the cracks between tiles, floorboards and wainscot boards, in evenings and night-time. Baz, who had been employed in admin and finance since 1950, related the following anecdote of a time when the hospital still had its own functioning operating theatre.

'Do you know about Pharaoh ants?' Baffled, I looked at Baz, and thought, what on earth has Egyptology to do with hospital infestation?

'No Baz. Never heard of them.'

He then recalled several incidents from pre-war and post-war years.

'Infestation in old heated buildings was a common problem, world wide, and was difficult to control, especially cockroaches. However, ants do not readily come to mind under this heading, especially Pharaoh ants. They were light yellowish coloured, and were more of a nuisance than a health risk.' (But not so, we were wrong. The ants were in fact a common infestation throughout most institutions and required continuous vigilance on the part of the administration to keep such vermin nests at bay.)

Baz recalled first hearing of these ants, who are attracted by blood, and had read in hospital documentation about forty years ago, (the 1920s?) of a surgeon in the middle of an operation finding a Pharaoh ant on his sleeve. After checking, it was noticed that they had started to form a trail up on his trouser leg. It was assumed they were trying to reach the blood on the operating table. To the best of Admin Baz' knowledge, the only such ants recorded in Graylingwell appeared on the female geriatric wards, and logical argument gave support to their appearances elsewhere in the hospital. He was advised, more than once, of ants gathering near the bed of a patient in the last hours of his or her life.

A new Catering Officer had recently been appointed, and generous changes in the menus were in the making, in addition to social changes. On my arrival in 1967 there were two distinct catering facilities; the Staff Restaurant (my room was over it) which was largely used by nursing staff and junior medical staff, other employees and visitors; and the Doctors' Restaurant, (though its days were numbered) which was a second Staff restaurant, called *The Blue Lagoon*[2]. *The Blue Lagoon* restaurant was located off the eastern link corridor, close by The Main Office and Admin rooms, and was initially taboo to all employees, *except* Senior hospital staff and administrators. Four separate tables rigidly divided the hospital hierarchy; Medical, Senior Nursing, Paramedical & MRC Technicians, and Administration.

Fifty years before, both areas served the needs of all junior hospital staff, including (pre-war) servants, and nursing attendants. The few Asylum alienists and Senior doctors had their own private messes, set apart, located close to The Front Entrance, and The Medical Superintendent had his own supreme detached facilities.

Baz recalled the *Blue Lagoon* restrictions in early post-war years; within the Officers' restaurant facilities strict convention was *demanded,* with penalties, I don't know what, for offenders. The Restaurant Manager rigidly ensuring Medical Officers were *not* polluted by the nearness of other ranks.

On one occasion related by Baz, a visiting admin clerk had cause to approach a Consultant's table and, intent on delivering the message, put his hand on the corner of the table. He was immediately rebuked; '*Are you aware you are resting on the doctors' table*?', said the horrified Doctor. The humbled clerk was again, further castigated by the Head Waiter, who reminded him to 'Please keep your place in the future'.

Up until the Nineteenth century, *safe* drinking water was always a major problem in family households and all institutions and, therefore, it was customary for an asylum, workhouse or poor house, to have their own on safe tap beer brewery (gin was safer? Low alcohol). Cholera and typhoid was otherwise all too common - as Norman Longmate's excellent written social histories liberally illustrate.[3] And, there is a local Sussex example; a watercolour, held in the Chichester County Archives, dated 1856, of the East Preston (Worthing and District) Poor House clearly shows its brewery, included in the drawing.

Graylingwell from 1897 was most fortunate with its distilled Lavant waters down from the chalky South Downs. Tea and coffee was previously mostly for the middle-classes and nobility, being too expensive a luxury for the labouring classes and poor law institutions. The hospital rightly took pride in its own Farm Produce and closely monitored the quality of its own Supplies Department. And this fact extended to patients and staff enjoying the best possible (despite inevitable austerity) quality tea. Graylingwell employed its own professional Taster of Tea.

Baz recalled, in the 1950s: 'Tenders were invited to supply tea leaves by the tea-chest (lined plywood boxes approx. 18" x 18" x 24" high; empties in demand for storage, house moving; another form of recycling). Firms had to submit samples of their product and costs. These samples were laid out on the long wooden counter in the Supplies Dept. A Mr Ibbitson was contracted as official tea-taster and sampled each leaf. Based on his professional opinion, the best taste (quality), at the best price, was selected. This system lasted until the 1950s; possibly into the '60s. It was estimated that over 2,000 cups of tea a day were drunk in the hospital in the 1950s. Persons permitted entry into the Supply Stores, until the late 1950s, would have seen long-slatted shelves, full of cut blocks of cheese in their cotton cloth wrapping. Not unusual was to see the liquid dripping slowly from each cheese. This practice continued until they were considered fit, dry enough, to uncloth; and cut with the aid of a wire before issue to the Catering Department, and the wards.

And times, again, were a' changing in the late 1960s for our fifteen hundred plus total patients and staff. A new catering officer, on following his arrival, had recently been one of our lecturers at the nursing school behind the Summersdale Villa wards and explained in detail his new improved budget proposals for all hospital staff and patients.

One of the nursing staff's early morning duties was to go around the ward with a clipped board list of all its residents, new in 1968, and, where possible, show every patient a prepared kitchen Menu offering a choice out of three possible choices per meal *per day* for the following day's deliveries in the heated ward food trolley. And thus, the kitchen staff, knowing the collective quantity of each item, would only prepare what was ordered, cutting back a quantity of kitchen waste and *not* over filling the ward pig buckets. Admin Baz told me the hospital steward presently had a contract with local farmers, since Graylingwell no longer retained its own farm and livestock, to have and supply from the hospital's daily pigswill; a profit to duty of care of its patients. Although inevitable changes ensued in the decades ahead I noticed this clean disposal of organic waste was kept on for many years.

Breakfast on Chilgrove was the best time to catch rehab patients on the ward, as the men in the end-dormitory would afterwards depart to OT, IT, or other appointed hospital duties. The following days requested menu needed to be returned to the kitchen manager before 11 am and I was pleased as ward student to be assigned this, *then,* new duty.

As to the staff. Momentous change, end of a long-era; *The Blue Lagoon* was to be formally closed-down as an exclusive Officers' Restaurant, modernised and refurbished as an all-staff democratic, self-serving *Grill Room,* with individual orders for whatever ordered at a hatch; a number slip allocated. Then, also new, access to a vegetable and salad bar, before sitting down, anywhere; *with anyone* in the room. For a short time, par excellence. Beef steak and even salmon steaks were available on order but, I noticed, the budget soon removed those (then) luxury items a few months on, though the self service Grill Room and waiter service Staff Restaurant remained for some years as alternative choices for all visitors and staff. There was always the small hospital shop, or the outside in-the-grounds Naunton Pavilion run by volunteers aided by the worthy *Friends Of Graylingwell* charity organisation.

Vagrant Joe

'Cleanliness is next to Godliness' was a saying engraved on my generations earliest memories. And, coupled with the truisms that to be warm, to have a hot bath, to be washed and have dressed hair, clean clothes (better still though rarely so, new clothes), a shave and a means to relax, at least partially from the dirt and grime of life, both real and metaphorical, was a personal experience I acknowledged all too easily and perhaps took somewhat for granted; a physical chore at times, but always beneficial.

And I looked to others...

It was wintertime when I began working on Chilgrove One, and though the recent 1967 Christmas festivities were already history, several 'vagrants' were being admitted after our so-called Winter holidays were finished. Till recent times, the local Union parish Workhouse 'Casual Ward' had catered for many indigent travellers. I noticed some of our discharged moved on (as next address) to the *Brighton General* Hospital's Casual Ward, then located conveniently adjacent to the main road on Elm Grove hill's summit and adjacent to the open main road. I recall visiting this excellent provision for the homeless, and could find only praise for its range of facilities. There were also a few welcome charitable Salvation Army hostels.

I learnt each year a number of admissions of tramps, casuals, were made into Graylingwell, to nurture and protect those vulnerable souls for a few days, or weeks, needed recuperation during the harsh winter holidays. Vagrant Joe was one of them, probably a tramp, in his mid-Sixties, though looking presently much older.

I was on a morning shift when Big Jim asked me to help out with a new admission. Joe, a vagrant, had been discovered attempting to sleep under a road-side hedge, North of Chichester; he was found half-frozen and in an de-hydrated state by two sympathetic police patrolmen in a panda car. Initially, when the police found an unprotesting Joe, they wrapped him in blankets then, having radioed, transferred him into an ambulance and rewrapped him in what appeared to me as thick silver paper, used as thermal protection. His confusion and mild aggression on admission, in beginning to come around, meant he was diverted in transit from the Royal West Sussex to our Chilgrove ward in Graylingwell, by the kind policemen.

Vagrant Joe had a tangled dark beard with a strong smell, thick mould patched in growth about his not so ragged clothes. But, it was the length of his nails which first grabbed my attention; they were long and hooked over, with black grime packed into and painted onto his fingers and toenails. As he protested, he clawed, at first, whoever was in his reach, before collapsing with obvious relief in the realisation that no harm was intended; the opposite in fact.

Behind the closed round bathroom curtains, on a drawsheet placed on a wooden chair, sat Joe; and another chair for a folded drawsheet to assemble his filthy few belongings as they were onion peeled off of him; one reluctant thickness after another. His skin was blotched and patchy, with islets of permeated filth (how long for this to happen, I wondered), but he was *not* emaciated, which suggested he had been eating, aiding his, to date, wintry survival. Joe had no money about his person. Before being admitted to Workhouse or Public Infirmaries casual wards it was customary to bury any monies outside, as you had to be destitute, before being admitted and signed in for a bed and meals bath and disinfestation in a House or Hospital ward.

Together, Big Jim and I attempted to gain conversation, any conversation, to gain a response from old Joe and, as we drew off his tired brown corduroys, a further surprise, but in no-way so for Big Jim, Joe's one time white underpants were heavy, thick, with stale and recent congealed faecal matter. Big Jim beamed good-naturedly, albeit in mutual awareness. 'Get rid of that Barry eh.' I gingerly dumped this evidence of neglected body into a bright-red cloth dirty laundry bag hung, suspended, in the wire frame on wheels, much used on all hospital wards (all clean clothes wanted) and a warm wash sponge down began. Not a bath yet, probably later; his thick hair a matted grey-skein slowly had a metal-comb through it catching any intruders amongst the general mix-morass. Joe was changing before our eyes.

'All right Joe. Fancy a cuppa *and* a bit of breakfast yet?' Big Jim matter-of-fact asked of Joe. We helped him into a striped hospital dressing gown; ready for the duty doctor to do his admission physical check and mark-up on his blue body geography sheet contribution chart, to be added to a set of then customary hospital admission papers; this would come a little later in all good time.

'Yus please, Big Jim.' (Yes! They did know one another.) And he opened up, looked to the affable Charge Nurse, and grinned. 'It'll do a treat'.

And they knew each other... rather-well, and for many past years, on occasional visits into the hospital, a Sanctuary had always been provided.

Care and charity in the community was not a modern innovation.

Only its form changed, sometimes.

Two large white pint-mugs (as typical *issue* supplied towards servicemen and public institutions for many decades) of tea, and a doorstep cheese sandwich later, old Joe sat still, in dressing gown, while together we awaited the duty-doctor and listened to the radio tannoy in the warm Conservatory day-room.

Out on the ward Ahmed had been busy preparing for the routine ward ablution round. And Pete, our brown coated orderly, had arrived and was chatting away to Auxiliary John, our ward-aide, as he poured a measure of disinfectant into the oval metal-can. The floppy white cloth-mop, with its brown stick-handle, was already soaking as he prepared to do a section of the ward-space floor.

On Staff's polished metal-trolley, two white enamel bowls of water were placed on the top with two white folded flannels; underneath were two square-neat, fluffy piles of white towels; and, a number of sets of various coloured pyjamas. Supplies, to be regularly restocked, as we travelled the ward and likewise refilled the water bowls. The small white plastic soap-bowl was set adjacent to the two larger bowls, on the top shelf.

For most bed patients, one of us did the washing, and another followed along to do the shaving, but a number of gentlemen were not passive and required immediate reassurance; one or two very truculent patients needed gentle restraint, and required two staff. If it was a matter of infirmity or general illness *per se*, even mild confusion or dementia, persons requiring hospitalised care would have been admitted elsewhere but, there was a need to remember why were they here and resident on *this* ward.

Need to know ...

There were, in the observatory ward, two bedridden men, diagnosed as Elderly Mentally Ill (aka EMI); in their early 80s, they appeared relatively fit, physically, but in an ongoing, obvious confusion; probably dementia. They were often at war, frequently punching and kicking out and, as for their language, it would have put any long-serving soldier to shame. Perhaps they were old soldiers.

Both gentlemen had formerly been admitted into their local general hospital following admission, after attacking their wives and smashing up their homes. Sidney, had set fire to his home lounge whilst leaving unlit gas on in the kitchen. His poor wife had had a stroke after that incident. William was sadly worse; he had suddenly attacked his wife with a kitchen knife, whilst accusing her of infidelity and deceit. Both incidents were wholly out of past pre-morbid character, the two elderly residents with otherwise normal histories. Both Sid and Bill quickly became unmanageable on a general hospital ward, and were transferred by ambulance to our psychiatric hospital. Although considerably quietened down (medication obviously helped) now, each time Bill's family visited him the sad aggressive episodes were triggered; fortunately this did not deter further hospital visitations. Most of the daytime Sid and Bill remained quiet, sleeping, but, they became truculent at any human contact, including ablutions.

Ways of coping with reality, theirs and ours.

Staff Ahmed

Chilgrove' Ward's Ahmed, recently qualified RMN, was one of a number of young men and women recruited as student nurses from the Island of Mauritius off the east coast of Africa. An evening soiree had been arranged, at our family rented lodgings, nearby the village of Chilgrove up in the South Downs. Sara played the guitar. I'd owned a bongo drum, but was no drummer. I'd been a Professional Dancing Teacher for *Arthur Murray Dance Inc.* in the early 1960s[4] but, though a dancer, I was *no* musician. Together, out at Chilgrove, we enjoyed the company of three of our lively Mauritian nurses in an hour or so music session. Staff nurse Ahmed was *not* present, he was on duty. One performer was a third-year student Jacques who had brought his own guitar, and was great on-the-strings and sang to all French lyrics. The event finished with a low limbo gymnastic dance, much to our two children's glee. An enjoyable Saturday evening out at our rented Chilgrove cottage.

Our morning ablution, round on the observation ward, was practised to the light company of voice-overs and popular music from a portable radio; or a tannoy box up on the wall of the conservatory annexe. This essential Nightingale routine had been carried out for centuries, wherever sick and fragile vulnerable persons were gathered together in need of care and attention. But, as a daily routine to do so for others, it was new to me. It was not, as alluded, *not* just a matter of going from bed-to-bed, and assisting patients at their level of competence in cleaning themselves; there were daily considerations to be included on *every* round.

Under one brief of daily ablutions; washing, shaving, dressing, change of bedding, bowel functioning, emptying and cleaning out of long-necked urine glass bottles (kept in wire baskets affixed under the bed frame, and easy within hand reach of competent patients), as well as temperature-pulse-and-respiration charts (aka TPR charts), that needed regular updating. We also had to take readings of *all* our bedded patients, passed faecal stools and colour of urine; basic observations of *any* new changes, blood, functional, indeed, *anything* that needed to be actioned upon, reported and recorded, as such all basic observations. And this was *not* the designated hospital Sick Ward...

At *all* times, I learned to be 'alert' to the ward as a whole; to notice any sudden or ongoing anticipated needs of our *dependent* patients, and of other colleagues in hailing distance; and to include the almighty phone-ringings. To our lay public audience and ever critics (if the media was its reflection) outside the hospital perimeter, such personal needs of our *psychiatric* patients were non-existent, and could only perhaps be stressed when in an association with a General Hospital; or when *Home Care* treatment was a consideration.

Captain Jones

Ten o'clock in the morning. Big Jim was in conference with our Ward Doctor M. in the nursing office; it included a discussion and further examination of old vagrant Joe. All mobile resident patients from the other dormitory of Chilgrove One were about their chores. Orderly Pete and auxiliary John were busy putting the chairs up on the square dining-room tables of the day-room, chatting away as they continued their daily clean-up ablutions.

Staff Ahmed and I attended our bedded patients in the smaller observatory ward. We had a total of twenty-two people in bed to attend to in the acute dormitory; this included, Sid, Bill, Boxer, Bruce, Boo-Boo and Kipper. As customary, affixed to each white painted iron-bed head, over the head level of each resident, was a name tag and birth date reminder — mostly for any visitors rather than regular ward staff.

As we approached each bed space, the curtain was pulled round for privacy and each patient was reminded of what we were about. We asked each patient for their own shaving preference (where they could answer); wet or dry shave? Behind each bedspace was a recently installed electrical plug fitting which allowed access for a two-pin-plug, and use of the ward electric shaver. The majority of our patients preferred the considered luxury of a wet-shave, though it was certainly more time consuming; its benefit was quickly self-evident and found to be therapeutic. Wet shaves? Moi? Me, as *barber,* and to others?

Now, that too was a new experience. And there was no learning time of shaving a balloon, or other such demonstration, as I had seen in some advertisement. It was to be done, executed, slowly and tenderly; now. I did it, in the expected ward experience, albeit with some hidden trepidation. But, thank God, there were no accidents. Halfway along, we came to a giant of a man, sat-up and with a clear confident posture, complete dignity, his blue eyes reflected a great sense of presence. Mr Jones had experienced the use of considerable authority, as Mr Arthur Jones, aged 76 years, had been a long professional sailor in his past, pre-morbid, working life.

Ahmed paused and gave me a cue as we drew his bed-curtain round with a cheerful, 'Good Morning, Mr Jones. Is it all right if we do your ablution?'

He did not answer; for like Sid and Bill, although he became truculent in his body language, he otherwise remained mute, for he too was sadly dementing but remained confused in any attempt at communication. Mr Jones was given to sudden bouts of physical aggression in this probable total confusion. His valid frustration in not being right and able to be his pre-morbid previous normal, so earlier otherwise competent self.

But, together, we always assumed dignity.

Mr Arthur Jones had been a sea Captain for most of his life; a war-time sailor in both world wars as a member of the Royal Navy, rising to the status of Captain and, after an early retirement, transferring to the Merchant Navy and, lastly, as a Captain for a major tourist line travelling the world, responsible for all passengers and crew aboard a sea going liner. How on earth did he end up here, was my first inward response?

After his wife died, and his children being too distanced overseas, dementia led to his eventually being admitted into our psychiatric hospital, as the private nursing homes concluded they could, unfortunately, no longer cope with his needs; a euphemism for his bouts of aggressive behaviour (but fair comment). Captain Jones weighed about fifteen stone and was, largely, inert. So, Ahmed and I gently, firmly, cleaned him and trimmed his Players grey beard, washed him; and changed his pyjamas; finally (with some difficulty) putting his own black silk dressing gown around him (one of his few remaining personal belongings to hand), and lifted him into a longback padded armchair by the side of the bed, with a clean drawsheet on the seat and propped pillows to lay back against. We then made up a clean bed ready to receive him later in the day, and gave him his hot morning drink.

But, unfortunately, Captain Jones soon became restless (the moves probably triggered him), and he fell out of the armchair onto the floor. And, reluctantly, we transferred him into one of the wheelchairs with the screwed-in, half-round, crescent wooden-table, which enabled him to safely receive his drink without accident and risk during a fall. He would not remain in this chair for long and, after finishing his drink, he would be re-seated in the longback, where we could again put a pillow behind him as he appeared to settle down.

The Captain would again need our assistance before the end of the round, as he would need his bed-curtains drawn to complete an ablution. Such regular actions, made me feel rather humble. 'There but for the grace of....' It was an essential fact. Never, ever, leave anyone (let alone Captain Jones) on the toilet any longer than necessary. Dementia was irreversible. Matter of fact. It was all about loss of competence and, most important, about dignity, a loss of dignity.

Incident

Several weeks later, in the midst of a morning shift ablution, Ahmed and I were interrupted by a call from the office-end of the ward by Big Jim. 'Just had a call. Bit of a situation on Barnet Two. You won't mind going along to the female side will you, an' lend a hand?'. His tone suggested some urgency.

'Not at all Jim.'

'Thanks a lot Barry. Pop along then. I'm sure Pete'll be happy to give Ahmed any help he needs.' Now, Barnet Two was the female equivalent of Bramber Two ward, almost exactly so, like half of a Rorschach butterfly. Both were acute wards for the, mostly compulsory, Sectioned disturbed patients; with often locked wards for its younger mobile residents.

And I departed for the acute, female locked ward of Barnet Two.

Only Senior staff had master keys, which would open male and female doors; otherwise my key only opened male wards. But, on arrival at the top of the stairs, I met up with a Senior nursing colleague who waited at the door and ushered me through the doorway. Screaming and crashing noises greeted our entry, and suggested where the problem was as we stepped into the ward passage. Mrs. Vatson, the Senior Nursing Officer, a well dressed lady with a marvellous kind-but-firm demeanour, locked the door behind us, as we headed for the dormitory from where the shouting was coming from.

It was all too obvious where the upsets had taken place. Mrs. Vatson gave me the distressed patient's name, Jenny. Her footsteps were, as it were, seen everywhere; evidence of a human hurricane about the whole ward area. To our left we saw the dayroom with all the tables and chairs thrown about; torn books, broken glass and a huddle of patients sat silently looking down the corridor at us (hopefully) — as we turned right and passed the nursing office and into the dormitory.

A large lady with long dark hair, colourfully dressed, (but partially so, for it was torn, with one bare shoulder and ample breast exposed showing substantial scratched flesh), sat on the waxed wood floor, propped up against an overturned wardrobe. Exhausted.

'Hello Mrs. Vatson. Thank gawd your 'ere. And reinforcements too. You need 'em. Jenny's gone barmy again' Jean, an FB2 patient, looked up at Mrs. Vatson who she clearly knew and trusted.

'Thanks Jean. You *are* a bit bruised yourself. You all right now?'

'Yes, now.' Jean said, sad, subdued and resigned to poor Jenny's fate. 'And Jen a nurse 'erself, before 'er illness. Me, 'er friend...', Jean concluded.

Mrs. Vatson turned meaningfully to a third party, Alison, a Staff nurse off one of the other wards; who had preceded us. 'Look after Jean for us would you dear. While Barry and I go down to Jenny and, Sister ...'

And as we moved on, Alison promptly crouched down to tend Jean, who sadly had seen it all too often before, after all, she and Jenny were good mates. She had in all probability tried to calm her down, but Jenny's too loud tormenting inner voices were overwhelming, so Jen just struck out.

As we strode through the centre of the dormitory, stepping over considerable debris, we spotted Sister James at the end of the room trying to talk-down Jenny who, at first, was out of sight behind a surviving standing wardrobe and not overturned bed. Sister's blue uniform was torn and marked, where she had at sometime got too close to Jenny in an earlier attempt to placate her and Sister had been thrown to the floor.

'But, I tell you it's not true. The police are not coming to arrest you - for something *you* have not done Jen...' Part of an ongoing dialogue, Jenny was convinced, by numerous hostile voices and imagined phone calls received in her head, that she was guilty of some heinous crime. Her screams had covered the noise of our oncoming footfalls. Jenny was small, about twenty four years old, and presently naked, her discarded clothes thrown off about the dormitory.

As we came in to Jenny' and Sister James' view, our diversion interrupted their sad melody and appeared, momentarily, to stop the aggressive confrontation. I had no way of knowing (or time to think about it then) how disturbed Jenny was, and whether she was anyway influenced in that moment of diversion by my added intrusion, but no matter for within seconds she again began to sound off at Sister James; trying to ignore our new group presence. But, not for long, as Mrs. Vatson had peace and order to instrument and, matter of factly, said to Jenny, 'All right Jen. I want you, for a while, to rest in the side room. Now!'

Moving towards Jen, Mrs. Vatson indicated to me, with a sideways head movement, to assist her in persuading Jenny to step back into the already prepared single bedroom — but not before a final protest as she reached for a bed-side chair, and in one swift moment hurled it at a side window and succeeded in shattering one more window pane. Mrs. Vatson, Jenny and I moved as one body, and crowded into the small room and, backwards, I tripped over the made up bed and mattress, but quickly gained composure and avoided Jenny's flailing arms and legs as she collapsed onto the soft mattress below her. Dr. Trowel, a locum duty doctor, arrived with Sister James to give a PRN medication.

'Would you turn Jen over please.', Sister asked of Mrs. Vatson and I — we obliged.

I noticed, as we held Jenny for Sister to administer the injection, that although she had managed to effect considerable damage on the ward, as well as toward Jean and the ward sister (and who else?). Surprisingly, Jenny had few flesh marks, whatever, despite her nakedness, though how long she had been thus I had no way of knowing.

A strong pungent odour occurred, as Sister produced a filled syringe. It was a relatively popular, in long usage, hypnotic and anaesthetic, prescribed drug called *Paraldehyde*, a turgid thick brown-syrup-like liquid which I found, when giving, slightly more difficult in application than other prescribed injections (I had already given numerous injections, including Paraldehyde). I knew its quick effectiveness made it relatively safe in helping to bring down highly disturbed patients. It needed a glass syringe; rather than the new sterilised plastic CSSD syringes replacing the old 'glass' stock, as Largactil (Chlorpromazine) would soon totally replace the former Paraldehyde stock of medication.

Sister James kneeled down and gauze-wiped a place on Jenny's right-buttock (upper-outer-quadrant); we observed a little bruise on the left-side which suggested a possible not so long-ago similar incident. As Sister stood up, Mrs. Vatson put a clean nightdress over Jenny and I pulled the clean bedding out from under and over her already, now quiet, prostrate form. Dr. Trowel had remained just outside the door; no room, or need, for all of us in there. The door was left ajar on our departure, so Jenny could be observed from time to time until again out and about the ward and hospital grounds.

As we headed back towards the nursing office, Sister James to no doubt write up her required notes, Sister explained, for our benefit, how circumstance had left her alone on the ward, her own Staff-nurse off-sick, and her auxiliary off on an essential errand, when Jenny suddenly, went *up-the-stick*[5] and attacked her friend Jean, before going on the ward rampage.

Back on Chilgrove ward, Big Jim seemed a little surprised at my quick return from The Incident on Barnet Two. I had been away only twenty minutes or so. As I rejoined the ward-round ablutions, I thought of the enormity of such waste of a young life that Jenny's paranoid schizophrenia was creating for her. In the months and years ahead, I would get to know Jen quite well.

Barney and No Names

It was early afternoon, the second Handover completed and I was asked by Ahmed if Pete was still on the ward. Someone wanted to speak with him on the telephone; it sounded like it might be his wife. I had searched the whole ward, except the dormitory at the other end, which should be empty as its residents had returned to their chores after their dinner break. At first I thought, oh well, empty, no sign of Pete, must have left; when I spotted Barney a long-stay resident of the rehab section of Chilgrove ward. He was partially hidden, blending in a corner of the dormitory, behind the last bed and behind a closed door which lead into the main south corridor.

In his slight middle-aged frame, a fixed-smile ruddy-cheek full moon face, with a crown close-cropped haircut (obtained from a visit to Bill the optional part-time hairdresser) who improved his inadequate hospital income by working as a part-time ward auxiliary. Barney was dressed in typical, but soon to disappear, hospital uniform clothing; care of the incredibly overworked hospital laundry.

He wore a shrunken light brown jacket, its two-buttons tight across his growing corporation (and clean that morning); its pockets bulged with sweets and cigarette-papers and grubby handkerchiefs — innocent house-debris. Barney's grey, unpressed flannels were also clean that morning, and at half-mast his button flies invariably remained undone as he leisurely nondescript walked the long corridors, or the grounds in Summer, bothering no-one. Black shoes were clean; though his laces mostly remained untidy rather than undone. Below the tight much worn shrunken jacket, Barney displayed a brown woollen cardigan stained with evidence of this days breakfast and dinner menu choices; and food remains on a tartaned tie, properly done up against his off white shirt. For all of that Barney was, in sum, clean and tidy, like his bedspace and shared dormitory.

What drew my attention, from my twenty-feet away in the dormitory, *his room,* in my unavoidable, stumbled on, distanced observation, was the frenzied activity Barney was visibly indulged in. He was masturbating himself. So what;

it was quite natural, but ... 'Barney', I called out, across, *not cross*, but matter of fact nurse calling out.

'Please. Be more *private* if you relieved yourself in the toilet.'

And I left him alone, to finish his natural need for relief, in private; hoping no one would inadvertently again interrupt him, and perhaps more abruptly so. There was, after all, little enough privacy for the long-stay residents. The previous week, Big Jim had found Barney performing his understandable need for relief on the *other* side of the door, out in the public ward corridor, and persuaded him to, in future, relieve himself somewhere hopefully more private.

How many years had Barney been in the hospital? Ten, twenty, certainly a long time, and now, his previously florid (and often threatening to others) paranoid schizophrenia was almost burnt out. Though he rarely spoke to anyone, his lips were almost perpetually mumbling as he responded, whispered in reply to his voices. He regularly paraded the corridors, suddenly, to stop, turned to face a wall, touch it with both hands, then shout or argue something inaudible. He used to furiously mash his head against the wall, and threaten 'others' if they interfered, but this was now rare. Barney would continue his otherwise *free* meanderings within the grounds.

There were already fewer *visible* Barneys pacing the ward-corridors; secure in their custodial nurture-webs which allowed them as apparent damaged souls, to be *themselves* and otherwise anonymous, but still accepted individuals. Their dignity too, as much as possible, was respected in this their un-invaded, private world.

Big Jim knew the names and personalities of everyone of the forty two patient residents on this ward. The twenty two people on the observation-block; and twenty plus long stay rehab men resident at the other end dormitory in Barney's domain.

And if the twenty two acutes could not functionally identify others, many of the long-stay group of individuals certainly did; and when they talked with Big Jim (and other established staff), despite the obvious formal whitecoat boundaries, they appeared to interact with confidence and measured affection; certainly *not* in fear or even awe, as outsiders might imagine as truth. Auxiliary John, our helpful short-white-coat auxiliary was a long-stay resident on this part of the ward. And so was Mensa Charles....

Mensa Charles

Chilgrove Charles was, at one time, gauged with a functioning *savant* high Intelligence Quotient (IQ) of 163 plus (my own, a feeble 120, at one estimate) in the Mensa class; and, for a brief period before mental illness overtook him, could communicate on difficult textbooks on higher mathematics and logic; and sundry works on philosophy. In conversation with him, one abandoned item of his came to my attention; it was a book titled: *Introduction To Logic. And To The Methodology Of Deductive Sciences* [6] It was *not* a Lewis Carroll *Symbolic Logic.* [7] Charles' book by Tarski was *way* over my head, yet Charles, and the subject, the language, fascinated me, despite my gross ignorance.

Mensa Charles lost his balance, and developed a mental illness which left him so emotionally disabled he could no longer cope with *any* requests or demands, either real or imaginary, from anyone, without becoming disturbed, and this often led to him attacking others; or attempting suicide, with numerous recorded *Incidents* of self-injury. He tried real hard to overcome his problem, his emotional block. Admin Baz and I marvelled at the man; we knew he had a photographic memory (paradoxically 'like an autistic, or an *idiot-savant* at the other end of the IQ strata), a brilliant mathematician and an excellent pianist. Onetime, at his request, as part of his rehab, arrangements were made for him to attend a local college; but the tutors said Charles knew more than any of them, and put him straight into exams. He started to answer the questions then suddenly stopped, tore up his paper, and walked out. Obviously, he failed. Later, he said he had found the exam paper was insulting, as it was too easy for him. If an average person is said to be at about six o'clock, a brilliant person around mid-night but insane, perhaps, on this graph at five-past -twelve, Charles (at that time) was just beyond midnight.

Mensa Charles, diagnosed as schizophrenic, had 'autistic' [8] features in his behaviour. With Charles in mind, I found a relevant reference in Leo Kanner's 1943 paper on: 'Autistic disturbances of affective contact.' [9] Charles gross difficulty in containing his emotions, albeit dissociation from *any* social-reality in relating to other people, was identified with a form of Paranoid Schizophrenia. At another level he was viewed as an *idiot-savant.* [10] Presumably *savant* as 'a man of IQ rote learning' but *an idiot* with little to zero moral control of emotions.

In the near future, in 1970 during RMN Community Block, and afterwards, I was to have considerable first hand contact with children with Autism - earlier diagnosed as symptom of 'Child Psychosis'; and their needs to include a provided bespoke Special Education. And, in 1971, newly qualified would transfer to St James Hospital ' *Wessex Children and Parents Unit* in Hampshire; where I would work with autistic children and their parents for two years, and later be awarded the *Diploma in the Psychiatric Care of Children* by Portsmouth Polytechnic.

I recollect 'all' those long-term Graylingwell residents, who willingly attended rehabilitation tasks at Industrial and Occupational Therapies, or worked either with the gardening section or closely in tandem with one of the hospital tradesmen. Many of the older residents had, not so long ago, worked on the hospital farm at some time. I respected, and was even sometimes bemused, by Chilgrove's Mensa Charles, despite his aggressive anti-social tantrums. Charles worked in the hospital Printing Department (good with letters and numbers). Chilgrove Barney worked in the Tailors Department. Another patient worked with the boot-repairer. And, though small remunerations (due to government policy) these rehabs earnt the then maximum therapeutic earnings; and gained a portion of dignity and self-worth, as well as regular employment.

All wards were overseen by minimally qualified (RMN and SRN) Charge nurses like Big Jim; who also monitored and organised the clinical, cleaning and sundry support needs for his long-stay residents. There was no room, presently, for wardrobes for the twenty rehab men in the Chilgrove second dormitory. And so, bed lockers were somewhat full, with whatever few belongings they may have accumulated. A side room at the bottom of the rehab dormitory was, at one time, used by a sleeping in nurse-attendant. Big Jim said he knew a colleague who slept in there only a few years back. One adjacent locked side-room was presently used to store cases, coats and other personal belongings; this single room was formerly occupied by a patient.

Unlike the acute dormitory, this long-stay rehab dorm of Chilgrove One was untroubled by any noxious odour of soaked-in urine; instead, it smelt pleasantly of wax-polish rising from years of bumper polished and naked pine-wood planked floor. It was odd that the floor reminded me of, only a few years back, 'Pounding the pines'; as we dance teachers, of Arthur Murray Dance Inc. in Oxford Street London, called it in the early Nineteen-sixties. The thickened wax ward pine planks had been produced by decades of routine custodianship. No wonder there were fire-piquets at night.

There were several strips of carpet and one or two personal rugs; no curtains and no signs of the modernisation that other wards were beginning to receive as the size of the hospital population diminished. This dorm was home for the twenty-plus souls.

Home

In a short time, all of Chilgrove's long term would be moved out, moving home, to other more presentable quarters, as the hospital was re-furbished and up-dated. This long stay dormitory section in 1968 recalled for me childhood dormitories and early manhood — raw memories of immature orphanage and army days. Pre-fab floors with red asphalt, or grey concrete, or bare black earth, and overseas coral sand floors under sun brittled tented accommodation. Existence in Blighty under wartime built thin cold corrugated roofs, in long camp huts accommodation. Organisations to which in my brief thirty-one years, I had contributed many, many acres of red wax polish, and uncounted hours on my hands and knees, pushing heavy-metal bumpers, to 'pound the pines' and make wood or red asphalt floors shine. As norm, countless thousands of no-names around me.

Perhaps, it was because most Chilgrove rehab were off the ward all day long; out and about the grounds at most times, compared to the continuity of necessary, daily, ablutions with more acute-patients on the observation wards. Subsequently, I recall few faces, even fewer names, amongst the long-stay human community. Back on the receiving ward, recovering residents spent little of their time off the ward, but joined a substantial number who came and went out of the hospital in a relative rapid-turnover. I had little time to get to know them; but too, most patients were soon hidden in past anonymous algorithms and statistics, among files in hospital records — *sans* names.

Prancer and Mr Smithers

It was an accident. Poor Mr Smithers, after being still for such a long time, had suddenly moved with such a velocity he rolled off his bed and onto the floor, and injured himself. There were no cot sides to his bed; there were only four sets in use on Chilgrove One, which after all was *not* strictly a sick ward, and only borrowed a set of cot-sides when found necessary.

And as I filled in the Incident (accident) Form details, Big Jim was phoning for the Duty Doctor, whilst Ahmed tended Mr Smithers injury on the floor. With a blanket and pillow in placed position, he was not to be moved until the Duty Doctor said so.

'Ha!' I thought to myself. 'Where's that Prancer now?'

Two weeks before, a passing-through part-time auxiliary, who said he was a student something or other, was doing a back up. Ahmed and I were not on duty and Big Jim and Pete (out of goodwill) were on that mornings ward round ablutions.

His name given as Harold Prancer, he was initially received as grateful help, having been sent by The Nursing Office to 'help out' where he can on the ward.

But, within minutes, (Pete later recalled to me, as witness) Prancer, a 'Know-it-all', had begun to expound in a high-pitched tone on the 'Wanton cruelty in all these old Victorian asylums', with clearly fixed views. Pete described the incident. Prancer's spectacles dancing up-and-down on his large but narrow-boned nose, in their fine chrome-frame. As for Pete, his short van-dyke beard shook in embellished indignation in recalling the incident.

Prancer after all was criticising him, as well as Big Jim and, blanket wise, *all* staff working in this hospital, as well as *all* long-stay hospitals; a dire declaration.

As if to prove Prancer's much laboured point, on his having relieved Pete (humane ward orderly, musician, and lay philosopher we knew him by experience), he was directed back to clean the floor.

Prancer, small, tight-lipped, thin and spiteful, chip-on-shoulder, then assisted Big Jim on a routine ward-ablution; when Captain Jones promptly fell onto the floor, his well fat-padded frame protecting his body, if not his dignity....

And so the Captain was temporarily put-up into a wheelchair, placed in front of the then risky bedside chair, and, the protecting round-table adjusted by the purpose built screw fittings; Pete to settle him with a drink until comfortably reseated in a padded longback.

'Mumble, mumble, mumble, mumble', Prancer with curved shoulders sloped head downcast commented, as the necessary task was adroitly completed.

'Sorry, Mr Prancer', Big Jim politely asked of him. 'Did you say something. I couldn't hear you properly?'

Pete was but a few yards away, and the ward radio in the dayroom was hardly audible, so there was no barrier to hearing their discourse.

'I said, It's *cruel* for all patients to be locked-up on these wards, like this if you like', head still downcast as he pontificated.

A speech Pete thought he must have embellished in that dirge numerous times to ignoramuses who needed his spiritual guide of enlightenment.

'Oh', Big Jim gently rather than indignant (as he had every right to be, he was no cruel advocate). 'Do you think we are abusing our patients then, Mr Prancer?'

'Erm, erm!', Prancer paused and spluttered, not expecting any defence; as if it was necessary.

'How? Do you mean because we have lifted this poor heavy, defenceless (demented) gentleman into a chair, and locked him in it?' Looking to Captain Jones...

'W-ell ... Y-es', Prancer murmured.

'And, All! All patients *locked in*, in this hospital. Really ... is that what your own observations have told you...?'

Pete recalled the event with some sadness. For the next few minutes Prancer had tried to apologise for his known inaccuracies, as Jim explained point-for-point aspects of health and care, and what could happen if proper precautions were not made to safeguard against injury to a patient in our care.

About being responsible.

We stood in the conservatory; Pete with his mop and bucket and citrus sweetening compound, and me with a newly laid up clothing-trolley — and other 'stuff' for our residents' home comforts...

'God, Barry, you should have been there. Wotta-sour-puss, Prancer, eh!'

Pete in grim satire.

Raising up his right arm, crooked about 90 degrees, he then raised his palm and with arched fingers mimed a wave on water, dipping it up, and down, up, and down. Meaningfully, the wave turned into a fork tongued snake, as Pete hissed, 'Ssss..sss ... Steerforth ... Steerpike. ... Prancer.'

I too joined the movement, raised, then moved, my clasped hands in tandem with Pete's sentiment. I added in a low, sussurated tone, 'Sss...sss... Worm tongue.'

We later heard that Prancer had written a Formal Complaint against Big Jim and the practice of 'locking patients up against their will'.

Captain Jones. in his frailty and tendency to frequent falls afterwards, remained a silent witness to Prancer's accusations, since his vote had never been enquired of by that political advocate for freedom and fair play...

The last I heard about the Prancer 'crusader' was he had left a trail of written complaints before disappearing from the hospital; perhaps to scribe some learned PhD thesis on how Big Jim and others could better care for Captain Jones and Barney and Boo Boo, and all our Others, if they were asked, and could lucidly reply, as consumers. Disposing Eureka babies with his own murky acid bath-water. And as to Big Jim and Bob and Pete, and their peers as 'devils incarnate'; my senses could not deceive my own integrity in lying for some politically media-correct attitude.

Cooled down ... !

We did discuss the chairs' design and possible viable alternative ways of providing care for our demented many. The growing focus of Barney and others being asked, told, they will be re-settled back, somewhere, into a community which hitherto rejected them; and their ways. We wanted better care facilities for all of them.

But, we had not needed Prancer to act as catalyst in that debate. His cardinal offence was 'not cricket'; and essentially so. His proven evidence was given in bad faith; given in rejecting what is displayed in ward-routine, as good-nursing, and generally good-caring of others — whether or not it was custodial or community. In the here and now, carers and consumers alike are only able to use what resources are precisely made available, for patients and carers.

And so the duty physician, Doctor Crampton, arrived, and carefully examined an uncomplaining mute (though just audibly groaning) seventy-five year old Mr Smithers. He had a lean and fragile frame, with too large blue-striped pyjamas, stick-like chest and twig-like bent sprawled legs (he could only digest minute quantities of liquid food).

'Yes. Thought so,' he said to Jim, talking across Mr Smithers, that seeming lost personage (he was a one time school teacher, and father of five) with vacant blue-eyes and surrendered body. 'Fractured femur I think. Better transfer down the road for an X-Ray, and onto Lister sick ward when he returns from The Royal...'

Within minutes, Mr Smithers was slowly, carefully, manoeuvred onto a stretcher trolley (brought onto the ward by Jack, one of the few hospital porters) and he was taken up to the front entrance to await the ordered ambulance.

And, as Mr Smithers vanished off the ward, Big Jim saw Doctor Crampton off the ward, and proceeded to phone the nearest relative, the eldest son who lived in the West Country; Mrs. Smithers, his wife, had died some years ago.

And we resumed other duties...

Domestic

Thc long hours, the outside cold weather, my lean-frame, and a proneness to catching colds and stomach complaints, lead to frequent bouts of influenza; presumably from the centrally heated hospital milieu and, not so well heated cottage we lived in; out at the rural South Down isolated hamlet of Chilgrove.

So, collectively, a circle of petty ill health circulated amongst my family. And Sara, our two children, and myself appeared to either take it in turn, or sometimes in tandem, experience some fractious malady, but *not* enough to warrant staying off work. Indeed, I was increasing overtime duties and periods of study, to the consternation of my good lady. Sara had little time off work. But, otherwise, there was that reason for existence, our steel motives and purpose in all this already routine, of work, work, work.

We had no real time to dwell on ideals, or other more idyllic occupations. Most moments of domestic pleasure were occasioned by Paul and Kit, those innocent infant sons of ours. The price of work, work, work, would evolve a long time off, but remedial episodes, for myself, were sometimes provided in the stimulation provided at work, by hospital School days.

School

Mr Ilford informed us that until quite recently, General Nurse Training *and* Mental Nurse Training, until the *State Intermediate Exam* - had been identical (generic) in its substance. And this was reflected in our mandatory reading *Handbook for Psychiatric Nurses* (*The Red Handbook*). [11] Due to developments in Psychiatry and management of sufferers of mental illness, the latest *'Red Handbook'* during the 1960s was exclusive to Registered Mental Nurse students. The *first* year of the three year RMN syllabus generally remained much in common with our SRN general nursing colleagues.

Since our 1967 Autumn intake completed its six week induction programme and we had entered the wards, we had regular Study Days. Initially, one day per week for eight weeks, and two further series of Study Days for eight and twelve successive weeks.

On Chilgrove One Ward, I was well into the Eight-days sequence on the run up to obligatory Night Duty with the Inter-State Exam, which was due on the 1st October 1968. And, although we were well steeped in the physical states of mind body and its care and attention, the metaphysical was often presented in one guise or other by our tutors, especially, ex-RAMC warrior Mr Ilford's eye-witness accounts on the horrors of war.

Harrow

I recalled another RAMC instructor in 1966, when I was serving in part-time terriers in a Harrow, London based branch of the Territorial Army. Our Staff Sergeant gave a graphic description of active service during the war with the Desert Rats in North Africa.

One vivid anecdote in particular holds, about attitudes, and about oneself. He told us, that there had been a lot of casualties, following a bloody tank battle, and he was on duty in a tent with the bodies of recent fatalities laid out about him. Exhausted, he was taking a short break — alone. Due to the intense heat it was necessary to prepare recent dead bodies for burial as soon as practical; and he had been hard at it, due to the intensity of the desert campaign, for sometime. Our Staff described the incident to a hushed (male and female) audience during our, long-ago, evening lecture. He had had, at one time, enough... and knew so from self-observation — for there was no-one else present to witness.

'I took a break. In the middle of writing a letter to a relative, back home, with the heat of the tank-battle still about us, I realised, with horror, that I was using a man's still warm dead body as a table to rest upon, and had not previously realised *what* I was doing...', he paused. 'In short, I had become *too* used to it, and forgotten the deceased rights to dignity. And, of course, in the act; my own. I had *no* wish to be so brutalised...'

We did not know if this anecdote was apocryphal, though it sounded true enough. But, his message was clear. It was about dignity and self-respect, for one's self, but especially of vulnerable Others. And, our Mr Ilford, hospital tutor, was certainly of that brand, of that same experienced generation, who had served in the wartime RAMC.

Mr Ilford, RMN, SRN, had been captured in Singapore, and survived a long forced march, led by his Japanese captors. Throughout many lectures, at the Graylingwell School, he illustrated points to make with wartime anecdotes, and stressed that attrition of shell shock had its parallels in peacetime casualties; our patients. Talks always well received, and well remembered. Many of his anecdotes were about humanity, and not seeing all as black and white. As human beings, there were many of the enemy who hated war and its infamy, had to do their duty too, and strive to survive.

One talk, given to us early in 1968, was about human physiology. Basic, but easily missed, if one becomes involved in memorising the trees; but forgets the unified collective forest; and ignores all the 'outside' and inner dependence on the trace elements on which we continue to exist. 'Yes, you will learn much what you followed in your previous schooldays' biology and general science. About different body-systems and constituent parts. And, when things go wrong, what in diagnosis that wronged-condition was called, and how possibly to relieve and even cure that human failing....'

The foregoing was roughly an introduction, for I cannot recollect his exact rendition. And, he paused for effect, his high then balding head high. He was a tall man in his late fifties, his white coat informally undone with casual wear beneath. Again, the pith of the text: '*Remember....* all the body-systems are always *interdependent* on each other. And, if *one* system is affected, in some way, expect its action to effect other parts of the body; look always to the part, and to the whole ...' And, though most hospital School-days interrupted a week's ward-duties, we were sometimes presented with other opportunities, especially, in my case, by adding extra overtime for essential increased income.

Outpost, The Acres

Spring. 19th April 1968. I agreed to a morning overtime shift, to wherever The Office wanted me to go, then to resume my afternoon shift on Chilgrove One. And so, I found myself on an outing to Worthing, in West Sussex, by way of the Southern lip of the South Downs and the castled town of Arundel. A journey, I was informed, by Tom, staff nurse off Amberley One, who was also travelling in the hospital van, to *The Acres* in Boundary Road; a busy Early Treatment, Day Hospital and Outpatient Clinic.

I knew a little about this outpost part of the psychiatric services, for the Worthing Firm, from a talk given at the hospital school by one of its Consultants. A talk, headed; *'The Worthing Experiment*'. Ten years ago, it completed a successful two year *Community Care* project, led by the charismatic last Medical Superintendent, Dr. Joshua Carse. The Experiment ran from 'Jan. 1957 to Dec. 1958'. *The Acre* had been operating as a Day Hospital for *Worthing and District* out-patients, ever since.[12]

Before The Acre's inception as a Day Hospital, it had served well, since 1943, as a residential unit for recovering female patients; with Medical and Nursing staff, two hospital social workers, an Almoner and a Psychiatric Social Worker (Mental Health Social Worker) in situ. It was first used (after its purchase) as a convalescent and preventative unit for psychiatric patients whose homes were in easy local travelling distance, rather than the twenty plus miles, each way, between West Worthing and North Chichester.

Since my experience of psychiatric patients was limited to those residents back in the long stay parent hospital, I had no real expectations of *The Acre,* except the obvious; it was another Graylingwell Hospital Ward — but outposted twenty odd scenic miles away.

Spring was in evidence, as we journeyed through miles of glorious green countryside with long acres of woodland on both sides of the A27 high road. As we travelled, I enjoyed clear views of the sea, and Sussex downland. Below and seen to the South were islands; villages, rills and copses, amid town pocket patches scattered about this delightful map — all the way to Worthing.

Finally, we entered a short gravel driveway, to park in front of a detached house in its own extensive gardens, with numerous outbuildings and even a man made stream, alight with goldfish reflecting the Spring sunshine off golden scales. There were two front entrances, (there was a side entrance). The one on the left had a hand painted wooden board with an 'Entrance' sign posting the way in for unfamiliar newcomers; the other was for patients and staff into the Day Hospital rooms.

It was a charming property, originally built viewing the sea to the south and later converted from two previous pre-war houses, then in private ownership to an ex-Major and his large family, and had warm brown wall panels, as well as carvings about ceilings, bannisters and other decoration; and numerous rooms varying in size, converted for the use of the National Health Service but retaining the decor of bedrooms, two lounges, kitchen, studies, bathrooms and ablutions.

Outside, was the residue of the former well-to-do owner (who was believed to have had the first electric 'outside' lamp-post in Worthing?), with converted stables now, a Social Therapy hut; greenhouses, garden sheds and various outbuildings with well tendered green-lawns, fruit-trees and patterned flower-gardens. The landscape was cared for by a hospital paid gardener, himself an ex-patient. Our van-driver unloaded his other hospital deliveries of food, medicines, and various clerical ephemera, and departed through the main Front Entrance. The deliveries were checked in by The Secretary, who appeared to be a general factotum — head clerk, housekeeper, and one of the visiting Doctors' secretaries.

Staff Tom led us off through the other door, into the Clinical areas. On our immediate right was The Clinic and patients' Waiting Room. A number of out-patients were awaiting ECT (one of twice weekly for some, till their course was complete). This was why we were there that morning, to assist with the ECTs. Tom and I turned sharp left, but not before he pointed forward and indicated up a narrow, short spiral-flight of wooden-stairs; the back stairs, where the toilet (only one), and kitchen were to be found. A house indeed.

We entered a large area, of two adjacent rooms, linked by a single-step. Both rooms had Treatment beds ready and made-up to receive out-patients who hoped, no - expected, after a short memory-lapse as an after-effect to eventually be relieved of their angst — more so, if several sessions had already been completed.

The mystery of ECT. Much talked about, a physical treatment with a low-voltage controlled flow given to an already temporarily anaesthetized patient. Despite its debit critics, for some unknown reason it 'mechanically' actually lifts depression, though mostly endogenous (unspecified causes) not, necessarily so, in a reactive episode.

Several staff were putting finishing touches to preparations for the ECT session. Two Charge nurses, a broad-shouldered man, Acre John with fair hair, broad smiling face and hospital grey uniform suit, shining black-shoes and with customary white overall. He was chatting to a red haired nursing sister with a dark blue hospital dress, dark stockings and a broad belt with silver buckle. The name Sister Brigit and, yes, she was from Ireland, came across from John, as Tom and I approached them. I guessed both to be in their mid or late forties.

Acre John was lining up the filled syringes, on the top of the wheeled trolley, and Brigit was about, checking the fittings and glass measure on the top of the oxygen cylinder — its heavy weight set in an heavy two-wheeled iron-barrow, to move behind each bed in turn, as each patient receives their treatment. Seated on a chair, the other side of this small day ward, was a dapper, dressed Consultant Psychiatrist, who was busy checking through his list of private patients. His out patients were to be done first; and presently treated four private patients — not under the NHS.

Tom formally introduced me to John and Brigit, with a nod across to acknowledge Dr. Watson, the Worthing physician attending his own patients. John and Brigit normally covered different shifts, but on the two ECT days they both attended as there was no regular staff nurse; hence, our help, sent out from the parent hospital at Chichester.

After re-checking preparations, we adjourned to a back room called The Clinic, adjacent to the small back-kitchen. When there was no ECT, this whole area served the *Day Hospital*. The Out-patients Rooms and The Office were located over the other side of the building, this was the 'other' Acre House. One had a Cupola mounted on its South-west roof-corner. Below was a first floor Consultant's room and, below it, was the main Acres office, housing the Medical records, Secretary, Clerk, and telephone switchboard.

Brigit teamed up with Tom to attend last minute preparations, which included the Waiting Room, and ticked off an list those patients who had already arrived for ECT.

John took me under his wing and escorted me to the second of the prepared beds room, mentioning that two Doctors were expected, one of whom an Anaesthetist, which enabled The Session to begin; whereas our Consultant Psychiatrist had yet to arrive from Graylingwell for all the NHS out-patients; he would afterwards hold an afternoon Clinic from his upstairs office.

On this first visit to *The Acre*, I had little time for instruction by Acre John; though, fortunately, I had already attended a fair number of ECT sessions on Amberley One Ward. My present task was two-fold; to double check each patient had not had any food that morning and to enquire whether it was a First Visit, and to see whether any patient, or relative, was anxious in any way about the forthcoming treatment. There were no patients present who did *not* want to be here; no compulsory (Sectioned) patients, a possibility back at the parent hospital. And I assisted, after treatment, in helping to turn over unconscious patients onto their sides, and await their awakenings. Afterwards, I assisted in giving out the tea and biscuits. The whole treatment Session had taken about two hours.

And since I had to return, with Tom, to the Main Hospital for the afternoon shift, we had no time to chat with patients and staff; or to stay and eat lunch with the patients in the Acre dining room. Not all patients stayed to lunch, meals had to be booked in advance. But, Acre John managed to give me a lightning tour of the compact, *Acre* estate. I was impressed by the Social Therapy area; in a converted coach house. And, also, a separate, small loft-conversion overhead, of a previous Two horse stable; this premise, with a trapdoor into an attic overhead, was converted like a den, or inner sanctuary, as part of an Art

Studio. This studio was used for patients, by Beryl our Graylingwell part-time Art Therapist, who travelled out to this outpost several times a week. And so we returned to the main hospital, after a too brief overtime session; but with a promise of a return to work at the Acres, and hopefully on a day that ECT was not ongoing. Thereafter, I experienced the Acres as a preventative, Early Treatment Outpatient Clinic, as opposed to mostly Custodial Care. I was more aware of the breadth of psychiatric care in hospital, and outposted work – *In The Community...*

Before leaving Chilgrove One, I knew that my next ward placement was not going to be the same experience. I'd visited *Bramber Two,* the often locked acute-ward, sufficient times to be shakily uncertain of this new unknown.

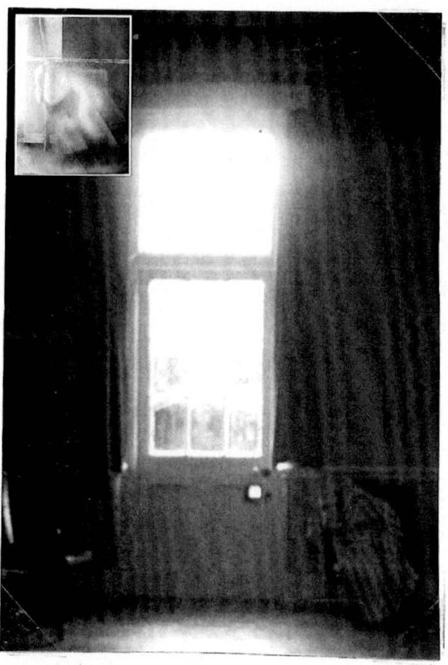

Boo, (aka John C.), four o'clock one summer Sunday morning, in 1980. No idiot savant, he died in 1982. Inset, 1983 painting by Reading artist Steve Bruce, based on the above photo.

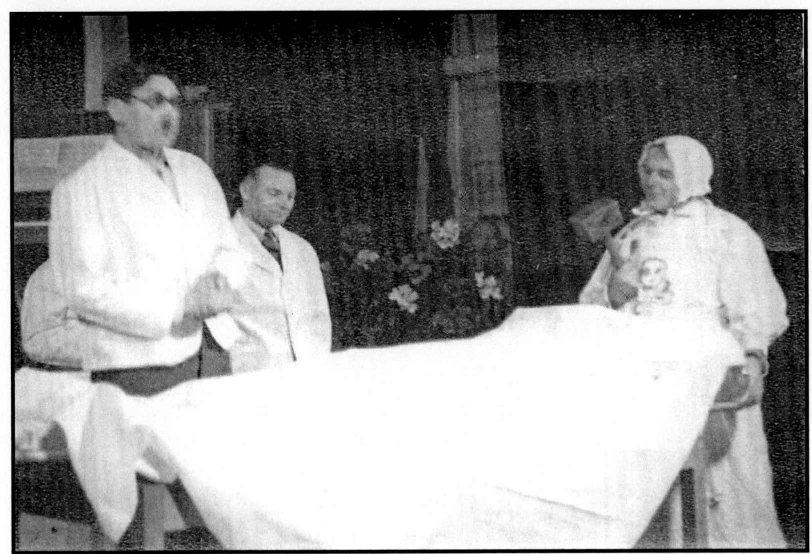

Christmas pantomime given by Chichester County Council staff at Northview PAI in early 1950s. Left to right : Mr Simcox Ass't County Treasurer's Dep't ; Mr. K.McFadyen County Treasurer's Dep't : and Mr George S. Pople (Relieving Officer for Bognor & District, Mental Welfare Officer attending Graylingwell Hospital in 1960s). Photo from George MWO.

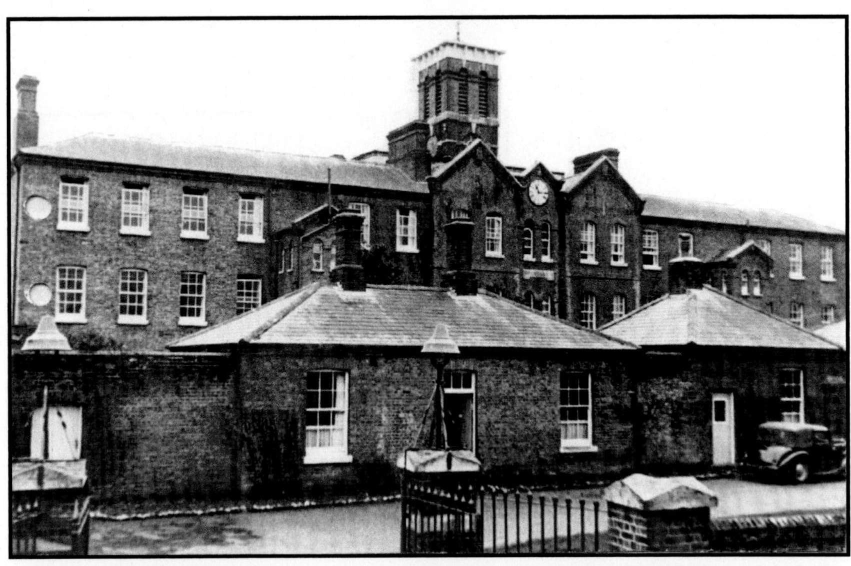

The East Preston (Worthing and District) Workhouse, known as 'The Spike' (after Spikes atop the Workhouse front gates). Front Entrance to Northview, East Preston Public Assistance (Poor Law) aka PAI Institution. Closed July 1968, demolished 1969 (Pic Source. WSCC Archives PH266)

The Interpretation of Dreams

Sigmund Freud

An Entirely New Translation by James Strachey

George Allen and Unwin Ltd

SIGMUND FREUD

AN OUTLINE OF PSYCHO-ANALYSIS

Freud's last major work
First publication
in book form in English

THE INTERNATIONAL PSYCHO-ANALYTICAL LIBRARY No. 35
EDITED BY ERNEST JONES, M.D.
THE HOGARTH PRESS AND THE INSTITUTE OF PSYCHO-ANALYSIS

1890s. Dreams, written about for millennia; but Freud's (et. al.) approach, in 1890s; introduced benign psychotherapy, used as compassionate treatment for casualties from WWI.

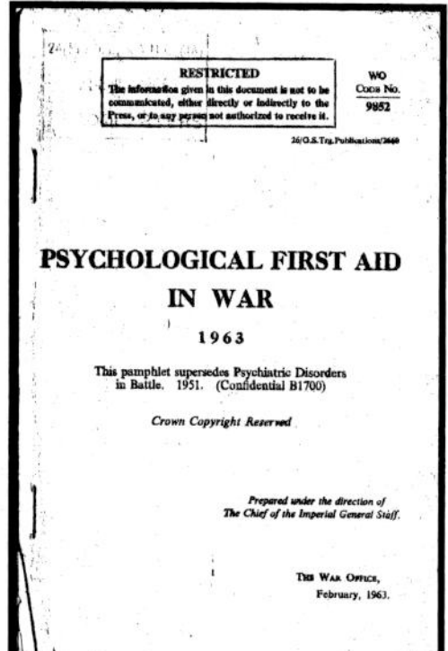

RESTRICTED
The information given in this document is not to be communicated, either directly or indirectly to the Press, or to any person not authorized to receive it.

WO Code No. 9852

26/G.S.Trg.Publications/2660

PSYCHOLOGICAL FIRST AID IN WAR

1963

This pamphlet supersedes Psychiatric Disorders in Battle. 1951. (Confidential B1700)

Crown Copyright Reserved

Prepared under the direction of The Chief of the Imperial General Staff.

The War Office,
February, 1963.

1963. But, often rationed, Psychological First Aid, in War (and Peace); restricted.

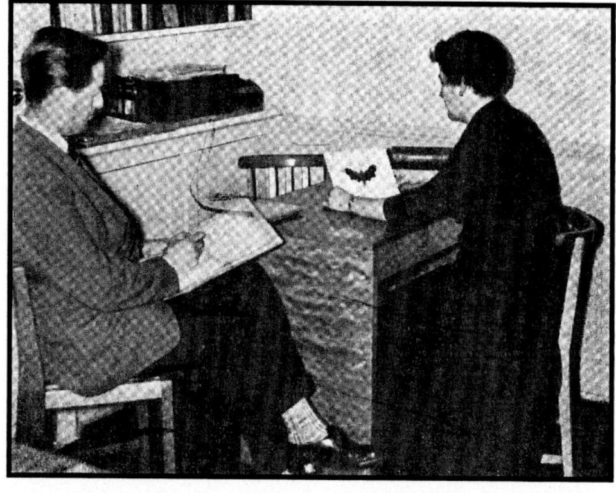

A talking out therapy. The Rorschach (after Hermann Rorschach 1884-1922) ink blot test - one of ten - used by Psychologists as a profiling technique, projecting aspects of a client's (patient's) personality and state of mind. ... 'Now what do you think this ink blot picture could represent?' Source: Park Prewitt Hospital Brochure, 1958.

Chapter Five
Bramber Two Ward

'To run a distinct line of division between sound and unsound mental functions, however much to be wished in theory, is impossible in fact, since there are intermediate states of development and disorder making an unbroken gradation from the sanest to the insanest thought and feeling.' [1]
Henry. Maudsley. MD 1939.

12th May 1968 to 3rd June 1968

Bramber Two Ward—Doug and The Twins—Ward personalities—Responsibility—Talking down Tiger—Bath time—Walkabout—Dougie—A Chat—Master—Voices—Other voices—Treatment—Reference—Handbook—Glossary—Schizophrenias—Relief—More on Treatment—Recreation Hall—George MWO—Temporary Insane—Rules of Freedom—Order—Heavy

May 12th 1968

I'd worked Bramber Two ward on a number of occasions, during staff shortages, and when a crisis called for additional manpower. In truth, it installed in me a prejudice that, on the male side, this was *the* ward where the most disturbed and most aggressive (real and potential) patients came to; to be nursed, cared for and, where necessary, contained.

It was often locked, *not* always, one of the Acute Wards, and I was more than a little afraid, but determined that in no way would I reveal my inner fear. Another term for the ward, supposed outmoded, was Refractory, to which the unit was often referred by experienced staff and seen in some documentation. *Refractory;* In a Collins 1968 New Gem pocket dictionary definition said:

> 'Unmanageable; difficult to treat or work; resistant to treatment; perverse; ungovernable.'

Those references could certainly have been given to numbers of our patients on their entrance into the hospital and, in the degree or nature of their infirmity, whilst resident on the ward, and could be improved.

As I recall, there was an average of 15-17 patients resident on Bramber Two ward at one time, bedded in one long dormitory or in one of the singular three adjacent side-rooms; one of which was a Pad. When the ward was *very* full, an extra side-room was in use situated off the day-room at the other end of the ward-corridor.

Bathrooms, toilets and a small treatment room were located off the dormitory; the dorm with its singular three-foot-wide beds, wardrobes and bedside cabinets. The wardrobe could be locked if the patient wished and a patient could hold onto a key, but because of possible illegal use of drugs etc., it was an *acute* ward, staff too possessed a key. It did provide a measure of privacy, against theft or intrusion, by other patients perhaps hunting for cigarettes or other valuables. For practical purposes, the dormitory was locked during the daytime, unless patients were given access to lie down, have a bath, or be transported to a side room for time out during periods of aggressive disturbance, when *talking* out had proved ineffective.

The Refractory ward was situated on the first floor, over Bramber One, an elderly, long-stay ward. On climbing the grey concrete steps, and using the large skeleton-like iron key to enter over the threshold, you stepped into a short narrow corridor which was effectively a nerve centre; given that it was located at the centre of the ward rooms and offices.

Opposite the entrance was a small kitchen, where I would in due time spend many hours. The kitchen door could be locked, but it was only secured for short periods to maintain cleanliness. Turning left into the corridor, a minute room on the corner was used as a storeroom, and next to it another small room which was the ward's nursing office. This room possessed a clear window looking out onto the Bramber Ward gardens, in those days — the mid-sixties — it was enclosed with iron palings and thick hedge. Not many years later, this barrier would be permanently removed and patients taking the air (the gardens were once called airing-courts) could walk about the extensive green parklands of the hospital or go out into nearby Chichester.

The Ward office was locked when unoccupied, otherwise the door was left open to allow patients continued access to staff. A few yards on, past the office, was a door to the dormitory, with a large iron radiator attached to the wall adjacent to it; this spot was often used by patients to stand and have a quiet smoke, or to have a relatively private conversation.

At the other end of the Ward, adjacent to the kitchen and on the right of the ward entrance, was the large Day Room. This rest room also served as the Dining Room, with its square tables and four chairs to each table. Long-back red plastic easy to clean covered lounge-chairs were around the periphery; and a black and white television was fixed in a corner on an overhead shelf, for all to see, with in arm reach of controls. The TV set was on much of the afternoon and evenings, but mostly off by eleven-thirty or so at night, with night medications having taken effect.

However, restless patients were allowed to stay up and, if patients wanted to see out a particular television programme, this was no problem. A large number of windows were on one side of the day room, and it became clear that these panes of glass were easy targets for angry or disturbed patients; most would take up a chair and use the legs to penetrate the small linked panes of glass. Only seldom would a patient use his hand to break glass.... fortunately, in my first week no windows were broken; whilst I was on duty.

Two other rooms were sited off the day room. One was a side-room for patient accommodation (it was believed that many years ago this was a second pad but there appeared no evidence of this conclusion) and the second room was relatively empty with a strip of carpet, a table and chair, and a large chair. The room was used as a patients quiet room, relatively, since its voluntary occupant could close the door behind them; alternatively, patients would entertain visitors in this room. Last, round the side of this quiet room, a narrow passage was linked to an out of sight storage space and the day room toilet.

Doug and The Twins

Doug was my new Charge Nurse; six-feet plus, broad and muscular; a full head of dark hair swept back in one thick wave, and with an accent I could not easily identify. Simon, small wiry Charge, was his opposite number. Both staff in their late forties . There was no regular Staff Nurse on duty with Doug, whose shift I was attached to, but Fred, a tall gentleman of substantial girth — he had a twin brother Harry — was our acting Staff. Fred and Harry were both retired Charge-nurses, staff who returned from war-service twenty years ago. It was an accepted practice; retired staff (retired at 55 years, if they had had thirty years service *minimum,* like Teachers, Police, Firemen etc.,.) could be re-employed as part-time Staff-nurses, greatly valued by staff and patients alike.

Fred had a marvellous sense of humour, and would entertain staff, and patients, with anecdotal stories taken from his thirty-plus years personal history of wartime RAMC, and long service at the hospital; which had begun as a probationer in the mid-1930s, and only interrupted by war service. Apart from Fred and Harry, known as The Twins, there were half-a-dozen other pensioned staff who, like Les, a retired Chief Male Nurse who first entered the Asylum as a boy member of staff in 1917, were re-employed by the hospital.

Young Geoffrey, twenty years old, a brown coated ward orderly (only on for morning shifts), completed our staff complement.

And, of course, there were *the patients.*

Ward Personalities

As with all our long stay wards, the patients one soon came to know were those characters who, like staff-twins Fred and Harry, had been resident in the hospital for many years; they were the chronic core who filled the long-stay psychiatric hospital's quotient *statistics* of occupied beds. It was all too easy to reinforce media myths in stereotyped beliefs of wanton neglect cruelty and ongoing abuse of patients on the long-stay and refractory wards; but the private agony and suffering, where so, was in the degree of patients' diagnosed mental illness; their inner torments, whatever made that judgement, *not* at all in the quality of care and often affection demonstrated by ward staff, and fellow patients.

Routines were duplicated on every hospital ward, so I quickly absorbed its catalogue of basic duties. On that first Sunday morning on B2, most patients stayed in bed and avoided breakfast, for there was no OT, or IT, over the weekends. And during The Drugs Round (the trolley was kept in the Clinic Room off the dormitory), I assisted Fred in giving out the medication. There was no ward orderly on that Sunday, and dinner delivered for one o'clock had only a slightly higher ratio of patients — laying in bed was still preferable. A few residents expected visitors after two pm, but I noticed there were very few visitors to this ward.

And, by the time I left the ward hand over and finished my morning shift, I concluded it had been a quiet introduction to this refractory ward. I had been introduced to our patients' names and identified the core residents, as well as those men who, though in an acute stage of their illness, would be expected to improve sufficiently for either transfer to another ward (from which they might have originated) or who were expected to, hopefully, be discharged. A dozen or so, two-thirds of the residents, had already been on this ward for some years and knew each others foibles, and their caretaking staff and the ward milieu so well they were relatively secure and did not want to transfer (even if offered) — a discharge would have been a different chalice.

The core of ward patients' personalities, included two Harrys; one Harry H., 60 years old and quite rotund who was an Oliver Hardy comic to his duo

Stanley side-kick — Manny, in his fifties. The other H. was little but lively Harry A. (he had a sister on the female side) who often appeared to be seen chuckling to himself, he seldom spoke, though he could, and constantly wrung his hands in some eagerness or other. He appeared to furiously pace about as if he had a bus to catch, but would rarely offer any conversation, yet he remained quite friendly. Harry A. had a reputation for disappearing off the ward. One day, written into his case notes, 'Harry. A. missing for the whole day. Eventually, he was found in the dank underground service corridor maze, which runs under the main corridor.' Underground, this eerie dark subway would have been experienced like ghost Great War sapped trenches and earthy tunnels, yet '*Somehow he had got past the security*'. An engineer's key was used to keep this area locked, unless egress was required. Admin Baz recalled ward nursing staff ringing him after Harry's return to Bramber Two as a found 'missing person'. Harry, on emerging from the low subterranean stygian darkness, most observant, laconic, said to staff (in his notes) on return to the ward, that he had seen '*Rats, as big as bloody cats*'.

There were three Bramber Two Johns, and one Johnny, and there was a silent Ted. Ted serious, and potentially deemed dangerous. He presently had one girlfriend, who had been admitted from Broadmoor having previously attacked her husband in a fit of pique with an axe. Ted was agile and vigilant and, notably, always took great pride in his appearance. In the future years I knew him, I always stopped to comment on his smartness; he would stop, pause, glow, and give me a thin smile (rarely did he speak), and walk on.

Cecil C. always wanted to sit down and be engrossed in his schizophrenic daydreams — but did enjoy the television. Counting, 1- 2- 3 ... William was tall, like Fitz, but Will enjoyed conversation and, like a character out of '*Hard Times*', insisted on *only* hearing about *The Facts* about whatever; 'Tell me the facts please.... what's the weather like?' He liked data on the weather, geography, and mathematics. Obsessional William, not a savant, would often repeat himself, and double query your replies. He could often be seen, head down and loudly counting lino tiles or paving stones, when out on walkabout; a likeable character. Will was one of the few patients, on the locked ward, who enjoyed regular visits, but he could do very little for himself.

Ex-Merchant seaman, paranoid schizophrenic Jim, in his late twenties, enjoyed playing board games — I played many a game of chess, and draughts with Jim. Notably like debonair Ted — he too enjoyed the company of the ladies. Jim would talk to Ted, but Ted would seldom initiate any greeting or conversation with anyone — except privately with his lady friends. But for some reason, based on his past, an angst and schizoid Jim was terrified of any dark African or West Indian, and would suddenly launch an attack on some poor innocent, unsuspecting stranger, even if the unknown man was just walking down the corridor.

Fitzwilliams, also known as Fitz; a tall, wispy haired man who always seemed to move in stops and spurts and would stop, and then slow march; ever occupied with his eyes glazed; he was one of two previous professional painters, and loners on the ward. The other was André (not his real name) a one-time Surrealist painter, who was always a mystery to me. He was small, a stocky pyknic build, in thick brown corduroys and hacking jacket, singlet (no shirt) , and thick soled leather sandals (no socks). André enjoyed his food, was often seen munching something he had purchased from the Naunton, and was a recluse.

Tall John was then the youngest, at twenty three years old (more of *this* John later). Rotund Harry was the eldest, just over sixty years old. Will P. (DOM), was a young schizophrenic who stayed a few days whilst I was on the ward and who, after I briefly became acquainted, presented me with an esoteric pic of the goddess Isis, which he painted for OT on the ward. A few of Bramber's residents.

Only three of Bramber Two's patients received regular visitors, all three Johns, others had occasional relatives or visitors. These details were relayed to me, matter of factly, prior to Sunday afternoon's visiting time, and to ensure they would be up and decently dressed to receive their guests. On arrival, it was probable that they would be out of the ward for the afternoon.

Responsibility

Sundays were generally quiet days, in the suspension of off-ward activities treatments and investigations. The ward, in theory, could sustain fewer on site nursing staff as escorts on off-ward duties would be minimal; but since a shortage of staff (at least qualified) was a basic norm then I found myself 'acting up' from an early date. Acting up meant that even as a student RMN, I was senior to auxiliaries, pupil nurses (for State Enrolled Nurse — SEN) with any untrained support staff, and so, if there was no charge nurse or staff nurse on duty at any time, the senior student would be expected to cope with all ward duties — and to only phone out for help if an emergency situation occurred.

The foregoing was common sense, and probably general throughout all institutional settings. But what could it mean for me — or any student suddenly placed in such a position of trust. Staff to be trusted with all ward patients, continuously *dependent* on you in authority.

On the general receiving Admission Ward on Amberley One, the patients were more easily organized and approachable than here on Bramber Two Ward, where the more acutely ill and disturbed could less easily cope with demands made upon them by staff or other patients and visiting relatives. It was abundantly clear, as a first year student, my own frailties could easily, so suddenly, be put to the test in any reality confrontations. If Doug, or Fred, were called off the ward, or not turn-in for whatever reason, then I assumed my professional mantle of responsibility. It was never to be treated as an ego trip or fatuously, but in this ascribed role — very cautiously.

Most of our patients, however seriously ill, could read the staff's moods and integrity crystal clearly. Your measure of competence was quickly tried and tested, from '*Can I have a cigarette?*', or '*Open the kitchen up...*', or other I wants, to potential aggressive episodes, due to a patient's own disturbed inner world (needing external expression), or in confronting other people in verbal threats or physical attack. You had to cope, or bear the consequences. In effect, you were always having to confront yourself and *not* be able to hide behind a white coat, or wear masks of indifference, or await in time and hide behind other persons authority or competence. Reality.

During one energetic fracas, with Dougie and I having to break up a vicious encounter between Can Terry, small, sure footed and wiry, and Tall John, clumsy, heavy and a bulldozer, my watch glass cover was smashed, and my necktie, with its tight neat Oxford knot and shirt top-button properly fastened, was grabbed by Tall John who, using the tie (it could be long hair) pulled my head down into the floor, before Doug prised us apart. This wasn't the first time my tie had been tugged in such a fracas.

At last, I realised why most experienced staff often removed their watch and hospital grey tie, before breaking up any ward battles. It was following one of these not uncommon B2 fractions, that I decided to never again wear my watch with the face normally on the top of my left forearm — henceforth I always wore the glass-face on the inside of my wrist (I still do); strap only, exposed on the outside arm — and generally took the watch off altogether, when appropriate. I took to wearing a loose silk cravat, which easily just fell off if grabbed by a disturbed patient — fortunately quite rare an event, so under an open-necked shirt, finding this was not objected to, I continued in this garb on duty on Bramber Two.

At first, with set ward routines for all persons, I too only needed to do what I was told, and expected to do by staff and properly — as our patients expected of me. And in such set routines was a measure of security, which meant I was one of a number, mechanical and not a threat - and I performed in good-faith.

There was no nausea in such basic ward routines; of feeding, ward prescriptions, counselling, making-tea, giving out cigarettes or chocolate bars, obtaining or discussing possible goodies for patients; tending first aid on cuts and bruises; such actions were as much custodial-care as acts of a responsible parent caring within their home and family. And with continuous numbers of residents to care and watch-for, there was too little time for any intense therapeutic work with individual encounters, in this reality: but exceptions did exist twixt staff and residents.

Talking down Tiger

It was one of the Johns — Tall John, who went *up-the-stick* early one evening when I was left in charge. Doug was on his day off, Simon on leave, and the duty Staff had had to leave the ward. There was, at that moment, only Geof (on overtime), our young ward orderly, and myself, in the day-room, chatting with patients after supper washing up had just been completed. And the twins were off...

Suddenly, we heard a lot of shouting, coming from the dormitory, which had been opened up a short time ago. Quickly checking it was safe to leave the vicinity; the television was on, and a group of patients were enjoying a popular weekly comedy show, Geof and I swiftly made for the dormitory. As we entered the room, we could see Tall John holding a chair up in the air and threatening another patient. It was Manny, who lay prostrate on his bed beneath him. Two other patients were rooted to the floor beside them, uncertain what to do with themselves.

Tall John was strong and volatile. He was on an incredible amount of prescribed medication, mostly largactil. His system, it appeared, was becoming more immune to prescribed tranquillizers, perhaps biologically too used to it, over a period of time; but this was pure presumption on my part, and *not* an informed clinical opinion. John could be a handful.

I had chatted to him a few times, whilst on overtime at the ward, and played various table games with him in the day room. As I approached him, I took stock of the situation as it was presented to me. Several panes of glass were broken behind the bed, and he appeared to be frozen like a statue, with upraised chair and staring eyes fixed downwards onto Manny, who was looking up, terrified, at looming Tall John. I had a lone situation in hand.

First things first... unfazed, I asked, 'What's up John. What's the problem?'

Only yards away, over the mantle of the no longer in use fireplace (the hospital no longer had iron coal stoves or any open fires as these were replaced by cast-iron radiators), there was a one-time early warning bell, marked *Emergency.* It had a black electric press nipple, which connected to the ward office up here on B2. As a precaution (this being the at risk refractory ward), this wire also connected to the office of B1 *downstairs.* But — this alarm was *disconnected.* Perhaps, it'd been deliberately disconnected, having been abused by residents too often sounding this dormitory alarm. Much as unfortunately, too often, a patient would break the glass of the red fire alarm outside the ward office when there was no fire.

I was reminded, in good humour, the first time I had experienced a similar 'So what, *Get on with it'* situation as a squaddie soldier back in 1955, when detailed on a routine sentry fire-piquet patrol at Saighton barracks in Chester; there had been a number of armoury break-ins by the IRA, and our patrol was issued with wooden pick handles, *and* an WD whistle *which had no pea in it.* This was mentioned to the NCO in-charge, who giggled and said matter of factly, something about '*Are you taking the piss* ?' (knowing I wasn't). But, erm, so what? All I discovered, in a torch beam, which *did* have batteries in it, and needed no whistle, was an outraged energetic copulating couple, seen in a Rabelaisian half-naked embrace and quickly, I back-tracked out of sight.

The 1968 ward emergency buzzer was *not* on, and was in effect useless. I gestured to Geof to take the two bystanders away from the scene, back towards the day room. John appeared, frozen, still, threatening — and indifferent. I got to the bedside, and Manny, and looked up at Tall John. Full of concern, I asked him to: 'Tell me about it. Come on John, all right?' I smiled up at our disturbed, fractious patient, and reached down to Manny's arms, gently lifted him off the bed, and directed him off towards the day room to join Geof, still looking directly up at Tall John.

Psychiatric First Aid. Training instantly came in to play. Isolate the incident, remove all unnecessary onlookers and, if possible, remove any potentially dangerous objects which at that time, could be used (like the chair) as weapons.

I had watched colleagues on Amberley One, and here on Bramber Two, still such situations, and given me excellent models by example. Only seconds had passed since my arrival, and the other patients departure from the scene; and Geof knew to ring for help from The Office. I realised I was alone, with Tall John, who transferred his threatening gesture from Manny, to me.

He answered petulantly, 'Manny wouldn't give me a fag'.

And, I caught myself in the act, what I was doing ...

Me... me who hates violence. Loathes bullies.

And after what seemed hours, but was only a few moments silence, 'Would you like *me* to give *you* a cigarette from the office, John?'

'Yes please Barry. I'd have been all right, if Manny had given me one'.

Tall John lowered the chair, mumbled incoherently, and heavily followed me in line down the polished pineboards of the ward dormitory, for his fag. As we approached the office, Geof came out of the dayroom and opened the entrance door to two white coat staff coming up to help out.

Bath time

A ward resident could ask for a bath any time he wanted, but Health & Safety house rules determined when this was viable; especially, if there was a need of 'specialising' a patient. And laid down in stone, as it were, there were mandatory instructions to ensure this practice.

Carers as well as facilitators, we were responsible for all the ward's residents health and welfare; and this included cleanliness. It would in later years be called *A Duty Of Care*; in past years it came under *Moral Treatment*. It was certainly addressed in the written mandatory 1897 Bath Rules, and if *any* wanton neglect was recorded, the hospital and its deemed responsible carers would be sued. In past Annual Reports such incidents had occasioned and the accused member of staff subsequently dismissed. [2]

On the Admission Ward of Amberley, all patients were shown the bathroom facilities, and then left to use them, as they wished; except again for *specialising* (suicidal risks, epileptics or others with specific levels of disabilities). And on Chilgrove long-stay, the bedded patients would be helped to wash, with curtains drawn around bedspace and assisted or bed bathed as needed. But, Bramber Two specified a different routine. There were very real risks with those younger more agile residents, on that acute ward.

Bath time occurred once per week when patients who needed to be 'reminded' were organized and coaxed to have a bath and a change of clothes.

This weekly ritual (mid-week afternoon when possible) was monitored on the list of all ward residents tucked onto a clipboard. This list of names was appended on graph paper, its squares tabled from Sunday to Saturday. As a resident had a bath, his name was crossed in the appropriate square. Of the sixteen to twenty patients probably resident at a peak period, perhaps, half a dozen would have needed to be regularly organised during a bath time. Now, in a home-setting, parents with a large family would (I presume relatively) have little trouble in administering its members bath time, given available facilities of course.

I personally had very vivid memories, of Numbers of boys needing to be bathed in a set time, when I was in an orphanage home institution. Due to the time element, and dearth of facilities (quantity of possible hot water, numbers of baths, et cetera) we often had to share, two bodies at a time, in often already well used bath water. Not always but at most times. And, consequently, most bath times were seldom relaxing, or fun-times, but a chore of necessity, Like Now. No choice; doing as I'm told by my senior colleagues. Another duty of care.

As much as possible, dignity and privacy were built-in to our week's routines. There were four baths; two in one room and two in an adjacent room, with green surrounding bath curtains. Very few patients needed to have all stages of their bathing watched — even from across the room. Ample fresh hot water and large dry clean white towels were taken from a ready made pile, specific to these occasions, which were made available.

Clean clothes would be asked for, as required, by those Bramber Two residents who did not own their own private stock (so named), which they generally had laundered and pressed awaiting in their wardrobes — or piled in the clothing store cupboard. But the number of our patients who needed 'reminders' included those who would quickly 'lose' any stock of clean clothing if it was left till required in their wardrobe or on top of their lockers. And so, for this small group of patients, clean clothing was produced as it was needed, by the staff, as at bath times.

Now all the foregoing, though necessary, could have been tedious, but problems could, and often did, arise at bath times with some of our patients, who experienced regular thought disorders, hallucinations, and worse, devious paranoid delusions as well as other florid symptoms of their illness (whatever their causation). They often related them to anybody outside their own body-space including us, myself no exception. Thus, for Bath time, it was safe and sensible to have at least two experienced staff to organize the facilities and be ready to deal with any problem situations. In fact so vivid were the 1897 *Rules and Regulations* of the Bath times, there were several printed notices on the walls for staff and residents to read and be reminded of — especially staff.

Staff had no excuse for not observing *The Bath time Regulations.* [3] The relevant paragraphs covered all possible eventualities and was equally valid in 1968, under the administration of our ward staff. Bath Rule. No. 9 said:

> '*The Bath Key* is never to remain on the tap, and must *never* be trusted to a Patient. When *not* in use it is to be kept locked up.'

And, before that, No 8 suggested:

> '*Before the Patient enters the Bath the temperature is to be ascertained by the thermometer. The temperature must not exceed 98 degrees (Fahrenheit), or be less than 88 degrees.*'

Indeed, although some terms of reference may have changed in the past seventy-five years or so, these good practices were still very much in use, and I observed them!

I observed the large printed-up, wall mounted poster copy of these *Regulations,* fixed to one of Bramber Two's bathroom walls. There was also a separate, smaller notice which referred to the necessity of checking that bath temperatures were correct — *At All Times.* A large iron steam water radiator on one wall, ensured room temperature would be comfortable for bathers.

The baths were of large deep iron construction, with white enamelled surface and with a large hot-cold mixing tap, which had an hexagonal female socket fitting on top. This required an independent separate metal male key, with a moulded twist handle, to insert down and into this tap fitting, before any water could be dropped into the bath. This metal key, as required, was kept in the nursing office of the ward. Common sense prevailed and, whilst at most times rules were applied by the nursing staff, there were patients who were allowed to ask for use of this key without the normal supervision. This privilege was certainly recognised by any patient, trusted not to misuse its property. History, and the media, will likely produce examples of insufficient supervision and patients being scalded, even drowned, in a hospital bathroom. And it is more than probable that an acutely disturbed patient might wilfully drown themselves, or others.

First Bath time routine on the ward, I was on duty with Doug and Fred; Twin Fred and I supervised the bath time. Tall John was on the list, and he did not want a bath, neither did Ted, Jim and Terry, though Jim usually enjoyed his baths; all four were young and lively, diagnosed paranoid schizophrenics — exhibiting florid symptoms. The wooden duck-boards were down to raise above any bath water overflows, and to avoid slipping on otherwise a too wet floor. And two chairs for the lads to use, if they liked for clothing towels whatever.

Ted came into the bathroom. Small and physically quite fit, he was chuckling to himself, grinning as he entered the room. It was evident, to Fred and I, Ted was enjoying whatever dialogue he had with his hidden voices. But Tall John too heard the chuckling, and saw Ted's face lined by his grinning, and instantly became convinced that Ted was laughing *at him.*

Tall John suddenly screamed across at Ted and, reaching down, begun to pick up one of the duck-boards and threatened to hit him; '*if he doesn't stop laughing at me*'. Fortunately, Ted was quickly diverted by Fred into the adjacent bathroom and I reassured Tall John, who then became more easily managed as he concentrated on wanting things to wash his hair; and I obliged. The rest of the afternoon session passed without incident, as The Names were ticked off the list. In subsequent weeks, I was better prepared for such incidents at ward bath times, and numerous minor events did ensue during the then necessary weekly rituals of Bath time.

Walkabout

The structure of all ward work, night-and-day, was similar to most wards. After all, our patients needed to be clean, clothed, fed and given prescribed drugs. Contrary to media opinion, 'all' patients did not need prescriptions, though chemotherapy was a major prop, and, appropriately, patients needed to be occupied and therapeutically treated during the course of each lived day.

But, *not* every patient adhered to every laid down routine, however well intended, and despite expectations of others; due to the identity of this ward as refractory (even if not admitted), and occasionally locked. We did *not* really expect our patients, to behave like robots and recognised individual idiosyncrasies; at times having to bail our patients out of trouble; either within the hospital, or on their occasional walkabouts out in the community at large.

The ward elder, Harry, aged sixty-years, small and barrel rotund, round-faced and mischievous, was also rather irascible. Why was he on this acute ward, I asked? Well, one of the reasons, was one or two of his anti-social habits were deemed not normal or acceptable, by good folk in the nearby community. He had a ward friend and kindred spirit in Manny, who was not so rotund but of similar age and height and also deemed anti-social.

One day, the telephone rang in the nursing office, and our Chichester policemen, helpful colleagues at the other end, reported that they had two gentlemen in custody at their station, benignly held, like Laurel and Hardy, but, having committed lewd offences, those two loveable film comedians would never have performed in public.

Harry and Manny, on occasions, voluntarily assisted the police by standing at a Chichester crossroad to help out, in directing the city traffic and, spontaneously, during these outings, *might* have decided to wash lucky citizens motor vehicles; by urinating over a citizen's car body-works, whilst rendering song in colourful most musical ditties...

And, being so sociable to passers-by, they would let *some* privileged ladies know they were seen and admired, by calling out to them in cheerful language, whilst they then executed their whatever well-intended *good* deeds; but never ever intending harm.

Although, over the years, one or two anxious 'phone calls were taken about Harry and Manny, there was no proven evidence of any hostile act, *but*, The Community had its *Rules and Regulations*. Community and Society, of course, also had its stygian fears of the unacceptable. Removal of any unwarranted pollution was mandatory. And we could not prove, or guarantee, that our two residents could or would not stop their occasional anti-social acts; and *not* in the future frighten horses and proper norm folk, by their Rabelaisian behaviour. But neither, in practice, did we feel the right to lock them up for ever *and throw away the key,* as some offended critics proposed to the hospital management, after one or two recaptures from a walkabout; as they escaped off the ward or from OT.

In 1968, there were about one thousand in-patients resident within the hospital milieu, plus numerous visiting out-patients day-patients and a considerable amount of attending staff; a considerable quantity of people, a definite community on its own account. And our patients were part of it, and walked about within the hospital estate.

And sometimes outside its perimeters.

Most patients on the ward, if at a reasonable level when the door was locked, might have asked if they could be let out — and were. But, as the foregoing anecdote recalled, a number, deemed anti-social or specialised, required escorts if they wanted to go walkabout; but another small group would have preferred to take root, like proverbial lounge-seat cabbages, and *never* leave the ward unless made to do so. And so, organised walks and outing excursions were frequently encouraged, by visitors and hospital staff.

The sheer depth and unremitting quality of care and concern for our patients, by the majority of my colleagues, could only have been acknowledged by those who experienced its daily occurrence. It was especially noticeable during my days of employment on the most disturbed wards — warts included. On weekends and early in summer evenings, those patients who were unable to go out of their own accord were asked if they would like to go out for a walk with the staff.

A number of the most popular long-walks were up around Summersdale, up towards Goodwood, Lavant and the lower slopes of the Southdown hills, meandering through country lanes and over sunken brooks. They were pleasurable walks for all of us staff, and patients, who usually managed to stop off at a local country shop and pick up some goodies to devour en route. We would have had to keep an eye on Harry and Manny, if they accompanied us, in case they sloped off or spotted ladies underwear hanging out to dry as fair pickings.

Douglas

Our Charge Nurse was, without doubt, the hub on which our ward-shift revolved; safe and secured for all our dependent male residents and to all junior staff colleagues. Doug was one of a breed apart, late forties, a tower of strength over six feet high, thatched with thick dark hair draped over a wide high brow, broad cheeks and, more often then not, a real warm knowing sparkling eyes smile. He displayed a sense of guffaw humour, and range of intellect which often appeared to charm us even in the thick of ward crisis and able to demonstrate what he was — *Integrity*. But, Dougie knew wrath, and when the occasion demanded it his constant integrity would have his accented deep boom of voice, tell you (patient or staff) *what* was right and *how* to make it so. Thankfully, this constant approach worked well on our refractory ward and reflected as ward policy in its found duty of care to all its dependants.

Bramber Two's charge nurse Doug, not his real name, was, I believed, of Russian birth, of Tartar or Cossack, and had in pre-war childhood lived in the Ukraine. He saddened in talking about his past, and remained faithful to his home origins. Well educated and an intellectual, he was no fan of Josef Stalin (or of the Nazis) and the regime of censorship, deprivation, terror and secret police. One of Stalin's purges caused the death of millions of Doug's countrymen in the 1930s, by starvation and mass re-settlement programs; whatever exact, his past life sounded colourful to me, in a description given during a ward tea break.

Doug had experienced considerable suffering and privation, during his war service as a one time officer; and, I recollect, for a period as a prisoner of war. I felt the circumstances of his past sufferings were not to be pursued, unless he introduced them; only about his survival, and the humane philosophy he demonstrated in his character — a bonus to the hospital, patients, and myself as a student. But there were occasions when his views on life became self-evident.

In retrospect, Georgian Doug roled to me at this time a cross between affable elder brother, mentor and father figure; much admired by others, as well as myself. But, no rose-coloured spectacles or sycophancy, he had his feet of clay; he was a widower, with a young son to bring up, and was courting one of our nursing staff over the female side of this hospital. Why I, as student, acknowledged emigre Doug, as a ward mentor, was *not* because of special medical knowledge or psychiatric insight, *but* a strong personality in the way he behaved, which was clearly for real whoever, whatever you were; and our patients warmed to this capability. His integrity was constant. A good rock professional.

Bob and Norman, my previous Charges in Amberley, were very English, tall, broad, the quiet gentle giants I have described, but rocks with a different softer timbre; ageless carers and good professional role models. In no way would all colleagues encountered in work be, as such, rich and deserving in commentary as I found Bob and Doug; but *many* were and they demonstrated for me the essence of living Gentle men, (and Women).

Not hyped up, invented, media designated images, in political masters of our majority, those in perpetuity, of negative value, meanly based on owning money and abusing power ... but in truer culture. What they were 'inside'; tall and, always, all so human for others. Such Charge Nurses (and Sisters) were of that breed apart, gentlemen who were among the uncounted staff of benign institutions, unsung heroes who cared and nurtured in turn, their too uncounted historical millions over the centuries; and to our nowadays. Not, not ever, those wrong fruit or rotten apples, those models for instruction so well depicted by Charles Dickens; the exploiters, the abusers, greedy crass, gross, self servers, who are never true gentlemen in the foregoing context. But, the rank and file, to which I aspired, who otherwise quietly, diligently, dependably just did their jobs, in good-faith, often for their whole working, duty-of-care, life-times; in caring for others. Almost Saints *but* with mortal achilles heels.

American author Harper Lee might have based such a role male model Atticus Finch in her novel *To Kill a Mockingbird.* [4] The lawyer as truly such a caring person. I'd found Amberley Bob and, Bramber Two Dougie - examples of that special breed of man, (and- woman). Those gentlefolk - as Miss Maudie said (of Atticus) in her book:

> *'I simply want to tell you that there are some men in this world who were born to do our unpleasant jobs for us...'*

A Chat

We had just finished our breakfast of cereal, tea, toast and two eggs, sat in a corner of the day room, when John R. approached Doug and I and asked if he could have a chat in the office. He was lean, some five feet eight inches tall, dressed in grey trousers, bare feet and black sweater; body mounted with a long stern face, his dark eyes hooded with long eye-lashes and concave sunken cheeks. We could've touched his taut drawn anxiety in the lines of one possessed. Day and night, he lived with an inner permanent terror.

'Of course John', Doug said kindly, as he rose and beckoned me to follow them into the office. Doug sat behind the office desk, John R. in a chair facing him and I to the side; it was a small room, so we closed the office door for privacy. Anticipating, encouraging his conversation, Doug said objectively, 'Had another bad night did you, John. Bad dreams?'

'Yes Doug. They came down again last night, and I'm frightened of them.'

John then gave a graphic picture, of a fiery chariot with angels or devils descending to lay their claims on him. He was clearly very much afraid. To John R, they were not divorced dreams, unthreatening half-awake hypnagogic images, but very vivid figures, that were real and unexplained, subjective experiences.

Charge had obviously been through this dream of John R.'s and other nightmares in previous requested chats and, slowly, John R. was believed and comforted and reassured of our being depended upon to defend him, as the needs arise. John believed Doug and, as suddenly as he had approached us, he stood up with arms straight and rigid against his body; his face straight lacking animation - but his eyes, momentarily blinking, seemed to relax, just a trifle, alleviating his tormented soul.

And John. R. walked away and off into the dormitory, with a departing, *'Thanks, Doug'*. There was also an affable sideways nod as his eyes looked directly into mine, as he acknowledged me as Doug's aide. This brief encounter was about *fear*, naked fear, that appeared to always be hovering over *him*, haunting, persecuting and seldom ever leaving him alone, night and day. In the daytime inner voices would, with varying frequency, frighten and cajole him to do ugly sometimes violent things towards himself, and others, against his will. But John R. continued to deny their ascendency and, on occasions, wanted to talk about these voices and attendant hallucinations. The ward was a safe haven for John R., who only wanted to leave its arbour if someone safe would accompany him out and back.

Master
May 15th 1968

It was a quiet, long, day on the ward. I had already completed a mid-morning crocodile walk out to Lavant, with Harry and Manny and a number of other satisfied residents and, lunchtime over, Jim and I had completed the washing up an hour or so ago. Tall John and I had enjoyed, in a fashion, a board game of draughts and, minutes later, I managed an uneventful short chat listening to Can Terry.

I always applied our tutor Mr Ilford's axiom, to treat our disturbed patients as if they were normal, *but* to anticipate a five-per-cent possible nonsensical response. Charge Doug was again busy in the office with John R. and his concerned visiting father, who was planning to have his son home for the next weekend. Staff was on his day off, and our orderly had finished his shift and gone home.

Nondescript William Pace, in his thirties, arrived on a Section brought in by an MWO (not George) and two of his work colleagues, two days ago. He was suffering from an awful paranoia, which left him out of touch with reality; and quite vulnerable. Will was a civil service Clerical Officer who spent most of his working days (according to the brief case note assembled on his admission) filling in forms, checking up data, using the telephone and conducting authorised visits anywhere in the community, in pursuance of certain truths, in formal 'checking' out numerous, albeit mysterious (to us nebulous, even secret; what was fact and what fiction was impossible to gauge of his real working life; of his relatives we had no information) investigations.

Amongst his private possessions, locked in his bedside wardrobe, Will closely guarded a dossier of writings and drawings, rather good ones, which he insisted provided evidence of abuse by Aliens, the American CIA, rival Russian KGB *and* the British Secret Service — about black art & science technology goings on. Will was visibly, mortally, afraid of dire retribution by his enemies; '*And* so-called friends...', added sub-rosa. Clearly, Will felt safe, he said so, on our Bramber Two ward, in the *real* sanctuary of an English Psychiatric Hospital, here in Chichester.

'Honestly Barry... it's really going on... *I know...*'

In the not so distant past, when I was employed in the armed forces as a squaddie, and, more recently, but a year or so ago, working as a civvie Clerk at New Scotland Yard in The Press & Information Department, I had routinely, no idea why, been required to sign a copy of the Official Secrets Act — just in case, I supposed. So, I took Will's ramblings with a pinch of salt, yet his underlying fear was all too real and visible.

Will, like Charge Doug and myself, staff and colleagues and our nation's populace had, for sometime, been reading in the media of Russian spies, of defectors and politic dissidents, et cetera, as well as, lately, of protesting Alexander Solzhenitsyn's writings, that were censored in the 60's USSR, and of rogue, to the KGB, Doctors, Scientists and Engineers currently being illegally, amorally, detained through *misuse* of State secure Russian Psychiatric Hospitals.[5] Hadn't Doug and I, only the other day, had a long chat about this very issue; and compared it to the Sectioning of our own patients, and proper use of Mental Health Review Tribunals under the 1959 Mental Health Act. Of proper use, and abuse of legislation.

During a number of Confidential, he requested, exchanges with Will I learnt, with some surprise on my part, that he was an accomplished poet and amateur artist with a font of information on Ancient Greek, and especially Egyptology. Following a friendly, intense discussion, Will asked me for some paper and painting materials, which Beryl, our visiting hospital Occupational Art Therapist, was pleased to give, for Will, and with a promise for any further materials, if requested by our ward. Two hours later, he presented me with a small, definitive esoteric theme, a multi-coloured painting of the Egyptian goddess *Isis,* which he insisted on signing and dating on the reverse with his-real-name. But, at the foot of the picture, down in the bottom right hand corner he signed his work 'DOM'; which, from my school day Latin, was an abbreviation for Dominus — Master. Or an alternative *nom-de-plume,* as Dominic. Ward based Occupational Therapy certainly must have helped.

But our temporary resident disappeared, several days later. It was my weekend off and, on my return to work on Monday morning, I heard that someone had called for Will Pace during Saturday evening and his Section rescinded. And Will, I presumed, returned to home, work and whatever. I never saw or heard of him again.

Voices

John R., Tall John and Can Terry were diagnosed schizophrenics, who suffered from a cluster of symptoms which suggested this label.

In my personal experience, ongoing thoughts in my head, mind whatever, were of a singular nature that I always identified as me. This was the only voice, if it could be called such, resident in my own head. To a limited extent I could control the flow of these thoughts; if I wasn't expressing thoughts as words within my skull I remained very much aware of 'me', even though not expressing thoughts or forming words through the passage of my mouth. Words out of sight.

In my life experience, the media of printed words, film recordings, and listening to other people were vehicles of expression which reflected thoughts to graphic pictures in story forms or lined visual illustration. Such expressions of thought, as disembodied (not mine) forms were not, in themselves, hostile but benign, visual communication which recorded others thoughts (as voices), and could include my own contribution. Agreed normality.

Names such as St. Joan of Arc, artist and poet William Blake [6] and religious prophets were regularly paraded in the media, as people who had experienced voices that were supposed not of their own thoughts. But, no matter what art form we, at least I regularly, had paraded before us it remained, in experience, not real; *not* within the province of my own conscious thoughts and physical experience and, as such, remained the sum of personal knowledge, in experience of others' voices and recorded by others' art forms.

On Amberley Ward were several young simple (hebephrenic) schizophrenics. They were simple *not* in lack of IQ function, but exhibited symptoms of bizarre behaviour and expressed words and emotions which in normal parlance were deemed incongruous (i.e. didn't make sense to others) and often displayed emotionless (flattened affect) behaviour. They would appear to laugh, or cry out, for no apparent reason, as if responding involuntarily to specific stimuli. Although I had observed several patients experiencing involuntary incongruent self-expressions, I remained distanced from their inner private worlds of experience; distanced initially much as familiar art forms in my own framework of experience.

These were *real* alive people, not statistics, not others' images; and on Bramber Two ward I was more aware of fellow humans who experienced voices mostly hostile to their me's and which voices were sometimes in their heads or outside outpouring through various mediums; like the television set, radio, read meaningfully (to them) by words spoken by others or words coming out of walls pictures or other outside phenomena. John R. had talked about his voices out of fear; Tall John's voices were more paranoid; they communicated to him that he was being talked about by others, a lot of the time.

Terry's inner voices were sometimes given a form or name by him; one name being a God from the Sun he called *Can,* who often spoke from the television set. I speculated that Terry's voices' receptacle, *Can*, was partly a concrete truism (i.e. it was the television set, but *much* more so) and this identity, for me, gave him the nickname of Can Terry. In an effort to try and comprehend the origins of our patients' voices, rather than what they were saying; and their different effects on them as individuals; I pondered on the lines of science-fiction as one possible (occasional) biological mechanism. It seemed *their* rational internal bio-chemicals which contained memories, words and conjured imagination (explanatory) were not under 'normal' controls; whatever normal was and is. I found many questions — but few answers.

Other Voices

It was a physical fact that *I* could *not* see, or feel, the electromagnetic wave vibrations which carried voices and images into the television receivers, or voices for the boxed radio. But, as an act of faith, I believed that it was the scientific inventions of man which could identify and harness these means to record and display these communications. They were thus 'under control' and wholly independent of me and my bodily mechanisms. I could well imagine individuals who experienced them; experienced this aggregate as a matrix of unseen uncontrolled incoming wavelengths, differently, from me. In an effort to understand those physical differences, I mentally researched a variety of other worldly interpretations of their, causes and effects, their mechanical, biological reality. Was it so different from my being?

Essentially, the volume of sounds of all people outside me *and* their various mediums of television, radio, or other recordings were separate and self-contained, and could be turned off by me, or at least by others outside me. My imagination, perhapsed, that as my *normal,* conscious, brain controlled and diffused all sounds and images, so I was *not* overwhelmed and otherwise confused by a babble of invading foreign voices. After all, I cannot consciously translate, otherwise identify, or separate, like different musical and human instruments, the abnormal Identity of *other* sounds, as possible beings, transmitted through my mind and body; *not* necessarily wilfully, but because the left side brain controls were out of gear (or brain in gear with?) with its right side as it were, and passes through our bodies. Such possible recipients might be diagnosed as mental patients, morons, human mutants, shell-shocked and traumatised. A consequence of being *ill,* or innate a norm *savant* gift given at birth. Pure fantasy of course.

I'd always been sceptical of mediums, and some diagnosed schizophrenics, and, past identified oxymoron, *idiot-savants* — as proven Science-fact; as well as concepts expressed by creative writers in Science-fiction, who declare they are the vehicles of others, by telepathy, live entities, or recipients of messages from dead personages who happen to be famous - or infamous, and beings from other worlds' dimensions, who just *happen* to speak our own native tongue, or identifiable Latin, Greek, whatever. But, exploring possibilities, integrity insists the rather obvious. Just because I am not a theoretical physicist, or chemistry professor, and profess I am ignorant and cannot converse in other known languages, or achieve going to the Moon or planet Mars or, like Hillary and Tensing (with or without technology), climb Mount Everest and other human achievements, doesn't invalidate or preclude the knowledge of, how what when or whys, of the concept, the capability, of a possibility leading to a probability.

Normal biology; is it *resistant* to sub-sonic, super-sonic vibrations and, I did wonder, as an ex-soldier on the Grapple Tests during these years, especially of nuclear radiation? Can any exposure cause *mental aberration,* in tandem with possible physical deformities and genetic mutation. Impossible? I recall discussing this subject several times with tutor Mr Ilford. If human guinea pigs are wilfully exposed, to physical and psychological Pavlovian trauma. At all times a human, as all things, is a matrix point of all and everything *in* and *about* us. Clearly (erm!), in nature this 'noise' exists for interpretation, in perpetuity. Beyond... x-rays, ultraviolet exposure, et cetera... and if there is *too much* exposure to radiation?

I was fortunate, being but one army sapper ('847. Sir!), a peace time nuclear veteran statistic, who attended the U.K.'s *Operation Grapple* on H-bomb tests off Christmas Island in the mid-Pacific in 1956-7. Fortunately I did *not* actually witness an explosion. [7] One Sapper of the Royal Engineers had worked in the Refrigeration Unit on Christmas Island in the late 1950s. (I'd visited a refrigeration plant a number of times, in a Bedford three tonner, delivering Petrol Oil and Lubricants (POL) as a member of 71 Transport Troop in 1957.) Sometime after I left the island, a Lance Corporal of this refrigeration plant *witnessed* H bomb explosions without any protection and, in 1966, developed a blood cancer and severe skin condition due to (claimed reckless) exposure to radiation.[8] In his Judgement, Mr Justice Caulfield ruled that the authority's rights, liabilities and obligations were transferred directly to the Defence Secretary and not to the Crown itself. The Secretary of State was (not) "the Crown itself" rather than an officer of the Crown, and could therefore not be sued.' [9] The soldier is still, '*owed a duty of Care*.'

I was to lose a childhood movie icon, John Wayne, one statistic, who suffered and later died as a possible contributory result of 1950s American dirty nuclear 'tests' aftermath in the Nevada Desert. Only 140 miles from the sites in Utah, named Snow Canyon (how ironic), during 1955, The Duke later developed lung cancer after he starred in an ill-fated film called *The Conqueror.* There were also other eminent actors, at the film location, who may have died as a consequence of the nuclear fallout, among two hundred or so actors and crew, including actors Thomas Gomez, Susan Hayward, John Hoyt, Agnes Moorhead, and Dick Powell.[10] Within thirty years or so, at least half of the nearby Nevada town population of St. George had died of exposure to slow burning toxic refuse from the infected elements about them. Hiroshima it wasn't, but exposure to down wind *dirty* radiation, it was, Ugh!, relevant; knowledge of others and my own, of those post-war days. I acquired information about colleagues, ex-servicemen, and civilians, about *genetic* offspring, affected by long-term ingested toxic nuclear radiation; and / or other traumatic shell-shock (PTSD) physical and psychiatric maladies from such unresolved trauma. Though I was then innocent of such dire existential knowledge, in the late 1960s and 70s.

After marriage and two children in the 1960s; and much, much later grandchildren, I feared, privately, would I, or my offspring, endure some post-nuclear fallout defects or malformation? (*We didn't.*) It was no longer but stuff of 1950s John Wyndham science-fiction stories; or of Official Secrets Acts, no matter how world governments denied any uncomfortable casualties, or to repeat Great War denials. NYD's (Not Yet Diagnosed) or, as the media might interpret, denial, in propaganda; not yet admitted (NYAs), a duty of care for pensionable disabled. Of after effects by exposure to toxic gas, radiation, or Agent Orange.

Imagine being a traumatised psychiatric patient, *just imagine*, absolute horror of your conscious brain; like a centrifuge which through a process of osmosis is unable to prevent, unlimited incoming forms of other *communications* — with *no* norm sorting-out control. Uncountable trillions of fine invisible thematic vibrations, sounds seen within you as variations of colour. Perhaps *some* human beings (out of trillions) have the *capacity* to actually 'hear' and 'interpret ' *some* of those extra foreign noises as inner voices, spontaneously mystic seen as graphic numbers or wavering abstract dream shapes. Such could blow your mind (erm, kill you, make you insane or *savant*). It's the stuff of A.C. Clarke, science-fiction fantasy.[11] How, I pondered, to recognise coded *interference* in the brain? And invasion of other human cells.

It's developed technology, not psychiatry, which allows mankind to morally, assimilate, more and more to tap into the mass wavelengths (whatever) *in-and-about-us*; and there is eternity to tap into. But, my hearing alone does *not* amplify and assemble those abnormal (in experience) unknown voices and sounds; I think. Already a then truism, it seems, I my senses perceived, read varying thicknesses of specific wavelength spectra as colours, angstroms threads; each sense reads such and such as what we hear, see, taste, smell and feel. And the unified me interprets such a range of recorded knowledge - through its fragmented memories and experience.

But ... if, for whatever reasons, the fine range of what was normally, perceived (viz by balanced internal bio-chemicals, whatever) is unbalanced; then the brain is inevitably going to be confounded and most confused, for its norm range (library of memories) knows *not* the pitch of sounds, images etc., presented out of the norm teleological (meaningful) framework, within the framework nexus of the brain and skull.

It's inevitable, that in order to make a personal sense of any added *new* sensory data, in aggregate, anything and everything ever recorded and dormant with previous memories, may be unconsciously called into play (called logic) to rationalise and make some sense, a declared truth — in a context, related to an (to norm) insensible. Words and images, as poetic metaphors, meaningful symbols, codes, artistic line images, glyphs and cellular trace memories, all, could be used and subconsciously called up from Karmic unconscious to make a *new* or old identification. (Where is love in all this?)

What is biological a norm, and what is diagnosed as an abnormality?

It was at this stage I observed (no, not visualized, but believed as such) that a person's behaviour might perform bizarrely, or irrationally, as *not* appropriate by my norms and mores. For example, if disturbed Terry insisted he had just received personal instructions from the Prime Minister or The God Can, or one of the prophets via the television — *what* mental mechanism was absent or impaired, (chemical - an aneurism) that would inform my 'me' that it was not real but imagery on the television, and was mis-translated in Terry's own brain-box (that was scrambled, to use one popular term) as his existential reality?

A different mental process was clearly, I thought, at work for most, if not all, schizophrenic, thought disordered residents, including John R, Tall John and Paranoid Terry.

Too often, in schizophrenic communication, the metaphorical was used as concrete; that was not consciously interpreting any symbolism or key words — as such ?

And, quite often, if words were used metaphorically by our ward patients John R. and paranoid Terry, they were clearly *not* conscious that it was the use *they* were putting the metaphors to, i.e. people in glass houses should not throw stones because the glass in their own houses could be broken — true in concrete terms, but more meaningful as metaphor. How could I help and treat our residents whose thought disorders and other symptoms were the cause of continuing distress to themselves, and often towards others? I further researched, at face, my own present limitations by self-observation.

Treatment

The word 'treatment' was emotive, as much as objective, to patients and staff. Clinically, it suggested medication, or one of the physical applications such as ECT or, more drastically (and rarely), leucotomy. Additional methods of treatment included some semi-skills taught weekdays at occupational and industrial therapy, all available facilities, and Psychotherapy if deemed appropriate and fiscally possible.

In the above definitions of treatment, the inference was to improve and in some way benefit the patient. Whatever nit-pickers could aspire to, those range of hospital treatments were benign in their intentions. Primary Investigations were definitively *not* treatments in the former descriptions, whether they were pathological (physical), psychological or other diagnostic means to further exploring a person's unmet needs; but, in a broader context, anything and everything pertaining to contact, with or on behalf of an individual was, in my view, a treatment (or about) intended to generally, ultimately, even temporarily be of some benefit for them.

The staff's attitudes, my attitudes towards John R, Harry, Manny, Jim, Terry et cetera, and staff colleague relationships were, in effect, equally valid as how I behaved was, too, a treatment of them; in early Victorian parlance this interpretation included Moral Treatment (loosely put, being kind to, instead of punitive). I felt it went potentially much, much further than the foregoing common sense approach; potentially, it was (and remains) infinite, given that to learn everything about anyone or anything, I would in that potential gain a key to eternity, which had to be an absurdity, as I had neither the brain-power or stamina, or indeed the arrogance to pretend such a summary of someone; not least about myself.

Yet, to retain an open mind on acquired knowledge became essential to me, however specific the *glossary* of psychiatric diagnostic terms of reference, hospital rules and regulations, medical and nursing terminology and common law and statutory, laid-down, *legal* framework systems, which were available to me to help get to know how to treat whoever, for whatever purpose.

Although I had not, then, any other professional rubber-stamp of credibility, (viz I was not a qualified physician, philosopher, psychologist, or other discipline; as yet) it did not prevent any eclectic conclusions on my own part, when combined with my own personal experience in reading (sensing) phenomena presented to me; whether it was something I saw or heard or, most important, what a patient might say to me, or in my presence; signs, symptoms, any criteria, I formed opinions.

And, of utmost importance, although frequently bewildered by what I saw and heard especially from our chronic schizophrenic residents, I accepted at once the real experiences to them as phenomenological facts, very matter of fact real enough experiences to them, and for them as persons. True, the reasons of what and why they experienced such and such was then judged on a normality from given systems, and then related to what I personally could understand.

Much depended on what my senses and memory *could* interpret (and retain), or had dismissed, no, more, *missed altogether,* because there might have been no nostalgic framework, no professional or other unconscious symbol, grammar for me to explain, cross-reference, interpret, and recognise *any* new strange phenomena — about The Unknown. Perhaps, it was easier to always dismiss the sounding impossible presented facts, than challenge the existing (told) systems of interpretation. But, mostly I, we, were safe in *Good Faith,* making proper use of present structures and glossaries provided to understand *all* our patients needs and our ways of caring, treating their presented needs.

Reference

Each profession, every skill, had its foundation body of knowledge which was invariably presented by words and graphics. And every work was in a sense a time capsule, as its date of publication would have reflected a then summary *introduction* to that calling trade and profession. Ackner[12] was one of my standard authorities of that time, essential for basic training as an RMN. Another useful book recommended to us as a source of reference was *Textbook of Medical Treatment.*[13]

There were countless other helpful, but past dated, Rosetta Stone handbooks in my lexicon, with iconic introductions, and rear glossaries, becoming new *specific* grammars of information. But *all* were just that, after all, *books of words* that were *not* previously in my head (let alone of *owned* experience). And, if I wanted specific information, I would, if possible, ask an *experienced* qualified person to *explain* something to me, which would remain *their* interpretation, received on *their* credibility ... and always assumed *fact* , superior to my range of ignorance, as an introduction. Key words as symbols and metaphors, offered for use in translation, placed in a context and *used*, or abused.

All the foregoing became essential in learning, to cope and treat our patients. Especially to better assist in learning more about myself, and others, and of *the voices* (not to confuse with thoughts). Kraepelin[14] described the inner voices in schizophrenic disorders, and paranoid states, as symptoms of *Dementia Praecox*, and textbooks until the post-war (1945) reflected this fact. A Swiss psychiatrist, E. Bleuler,[15] introduced the new term of *Schizophrenia* referring to a group of symptoms, suggesting one form of a mental disorder. And though often taken out of context by the media, 'schizophrenia' (a cluster term) remained an introductory word, which suggested sufferers with symptoms of this mental disorder.

Handbook

The Handbook for Psychiatric Nurses[16] instructed me that schizophrenic disorders often began to show in early childhood; and collectively there are more chronic unfortunates with this mental illness than all of the other mental disorders put together — illness as an inability to cope. As with other human ailments, there were varying degrees of this illness. A considerable number did recover from acute attack, though it's probable certain schizophrenic patients are subsequently, emotionally handicapped (obsessional, *spontaneous* thought control, and thought blocking), with a functional deficit — as a result of their previous trauma, slowed or impaired thinking, becoming too passive — or too aggressive; odd or eccentric behaviour by social mores; and disinhibited or too inhibited, perceptions occasionally disturbed, with a contracted or protracted sense of time and or other possible resultant out-of-tune disabilities....

Most of our resident patients, with acute or chronic conditions, had systems suffering a loss of integration of their various normal mental functions, in particular of mood and feelings (Affect) and their thought processes (Thinking). Patients, who appeared to experience *per se* delusions and hallucinations, were not necessarily schizophrenics, as other physical abnormal states may have produced these phenomena, but, combined specifically with a marked loss of this integration of mood and thought processes, indicated a schizophrenia as a possibility.

But the symptom of flattened affect, straight faced no tears was one interpretation, the reaction of, say, not appearing to demonstrate grief or loss internally, and just not able to demonstrate to others, this could have been an initial normal symptom of bereavement. Yet, to infer schizophrenics do *not* feel loss too, was wholly unjust; though how this was experienced and demonstrated to self and others may easily have been claimed as, at times, at least anti-social and at other times putting themselves or others very much at risk to life limb and property in not caring (or able) to demonstrate through norm *'integrated'* means.

Because of the foregoing, too numerous thoughts, words and other voices caused considerable distress to our patients — if they remained unchecked and uncontrolled: to arrest this stress, the type of schizophrenia needed to be identified and specified relief recommended to alleviate their suffering and normalised, as much as was possible. But, how to comprehend them? I sometimes found, in trying to hold a conversation with a patient suffering from one of the schizophrenias in an acute phase, was like playing a game of verbal chess — with your opponent winning all the moves. Knight's move thinking was one applicable term in the schizophrenic diagnostic glossary.

Glossary

Schizophrenia language was thus, to me, often of other worlds; angst identities, encapsulated within seeming passive skulls, or semi-wild screaming entities, emitting sparks, discharging uncontrolled energy, creative and destructive, out of turn. And I wanted, desired, needed a key; a gateway into, at least to look and, if possible, please, communicate rather than but custodial commands as need. I needed a schizophrenic vocabulary in translation. A number of words in the vocabulary of schizophrenia in Ackner's *Handbook'* [17] were introduced at the Graylingwell School, issued in a general psychiatric Glossary handout. As layman and student, I had long been perusing lists of *Contents* and *Indexes* of numerous handbooks, to better obtain an idea of the author's attitude or importance on a subject I was interested in. And most works, which included a *Glossary,* were, of course, itemised in alphabetical order; a useful model. A synopsis of content within the work.

Affect (emotion, mood); affective change, this suggested a definite alteration in a person's emotional state which might also refer to their possible withdrawal into an out of touch inner-world; a flattening of affect would have indicated, a false, or shallow surface mood with little sustained depth; incongruity of affect suggested a lack of communication between their mood and thought — viz laughed at a sad subject or bad experience.

Autism; an apparent withdrawal from an interest in other persons, or disengagement from life outside them which demonstrated unawareness of anything of potential or direct danger towards them — as changing traffic lights, speeding cars, intense heat or cold, electricity gas et cetera; a person might walkabout aimlessly any time of night or day stopping to look at a mirror smiling to themselves (or talking to it) for long periods of time and or be uncommunicative to any observer.

Delusion; more than any other word 'delusion' might have been experienced as most used in the language of psychiatry (this is a personal view); — it was used as a symptom in acute confusional states (functional), in depressive illness, in mania, in senile dementia, *and* in schizophrenia.

Ackner defined 'delusion' as a false belief, which in the face of contrary evidence, was held with conviction and was unmodifiable by appeals to reason or logic, that would be acceptable to other persons of the same religious or cultural background. The *content* of a delusion, can be a symptom which indicated a break with reality, and was described as an aspect of someone's psychosis; — a '*primary* delusion' would have appeared suddenly, fully developed, and without warning, as a dire revelation at meal time with crossed knives, and an upturned glass as proof of a conspiracy against them or a secret warning of a disaster or unfaithful wife, confirmed by a blood-red sky and the red-polish being used on the floor by the ward orderly (a CIA spy), et-cetera.

A *secondary delusion* (interpreting) was a response to other presented phenomena, symptoms, such as delusions of persecution - resultant from original primary delusions; paranoid delusions, which were all too common, using ideas of reference to people talking about them especially in a malevolent way, watching others in the distance watching them and whispering about them. The *evil* things, being conveyed about them, also broadcast on radio and television and even radiated from the distant sun and stars (like Can Terry). And in delusions of influence, the schizophrenic patients' florid systems included false beliefs that they were adversely affected by all electronic apparatus (especially the television), radar, the wind and rain, ultraviolet waves. Other people reading their mind or taking possession of them and alien forces controlling them. But all (though many persecutions might be real enough) delusions were *not* dire symptoms of fear, despair and of evil origins.

I was introduced to a surprising number of patients who declared they were mediators of God, and individuals, apparently, deluded as being immortal (not human) gods and unreal named prophets. And quite numerous re-incarnated Jesus Christs, who resided as Privileged, or cursed, as patients, resident in the hospital. I recall in 1968 at least three separate male patients who had insisted *they* only were the true Christ; yet, not one appeared to be aware of any other's existence.

But, patients who believed they were in the form of the Devil, or possessed by that negative evil configuration as source of all their wrongs, were much more apparent than others' delusions of grandeur and benign phenomena; *not* a wishing to be an important (dead or alive) personality, but deluded into actually *being* that entity, with all signs and portents provided as proof of identity. And, as *that* being, they owned whatever hidden or secret powers sufficient to change everything and everyone to whatever — *except*, sadly, themselves into being of good health, mentally well and able to leave the hospital. In later years, I became acquainted with several patients whose disturbed minds and bodies produced somatic delusions, changelings who believed their bodies were really known incarnate living or dead, film, stage or musician icons or other notables; one patient, a sad amateur musician, castrated himself in his anguish — fortunately this was a rare extreme.

Hallucinations; to a layman and general public, hallucination was *the* one word which they might have associated with psychosis (or mysticism) as an introductory term, rather than delusion. *Ackner* defined 'Hallucination' as:

> '*A false sensory perception which arises on its own, in the absence of a corresponding objective stimulus.*'[18]

Sensory perception, the glossary suggested, was demonstrated by use of any of the five senses of visual, seeing; auditory, hearing; olfactory, smelling; gustatory tasting, or tactile, feeling. Something, which is *not* then actually present, but probably produced by internal disturbed perceptions and named, conjured up and shaped from memories. A hallucination, as with all sensory phenomena, might have been experienced separately (identified), or in conjunction with other norm or abnormal bodily experiences. Such unified unbidden existential moments would too often be nauseous, awesome, and quite threatening and fearsome.

Small wonder, that delusions to account for happenings could have been initiated by a sufferer (or acolyte?). And I am attempting to comprehend the *false* sensory hallucination. Not at all, the possible real existential extra-sensory experiences, *not* of my *yet*, owned experience. Hallucinations can be experienced within *normal* dream-like states, as just before going off to sleep as *hypnagogic* images - or just before - an awakening. Or in other, abnormal mind and body conditions such as with fevers and toxic confusional states; images produced would have been familiar or fantastical, animals people or suggested from graphic pictures, any phenomena as visual projection.

Abnormal sensory phenomena could be found in conditions other than the schizophrenias, but the auditory hallucinations of hearing, the voices, appeared most typical and representative of the schizophrenic sufferers; they might have had another voice, or plural voices, saying they are evil and living a sinful life and should suffer for their guilt and subsequently punish themselves, in a response to them. Sometimes, such intruding voices would forcefully instruct a sufferer that somebody was evil and threatening to them and the world, and needed curing or eliminating.

Auditory hallucinations included anything from strange noises to unbidden thoughts, familiar and unfamiliar voices, tic or commentar. It, or they, might be a one off experience, occasional in acute crisis episodes — or unfortunately long-term chronic phenomena of their everyday normal life experience; the latter for our Johns, Harry, Jim and Terry then on Bramber Two ward in 1968.

Olfactory hallucination referred to an internal smell, identified as gas or strange odours, suggesting someone was trying to kill them; this experience might have been complimented by gustatory hallucinations, evoking strange or unwanted tastes, which often suggested experience that someone was trying to poison them.

Tactile hallucinations of touch were sometimes experienced as a symptom of drug abuse as, for example, with cocaine psychosis, which Ackner described as a sub acute, delirious, state due to prolonged exposure to the drug. Further, tactile hallucinations, drug addiction and alcoholic delirium tremors produced complaints that their skin was crawling, believing there were small animals or snakes whatever about them (aided by perhaps visual hallucinations to confirm their experience). These tactile sensations would be identified as 'strange feelings', sometimes localized (night or day) in the genitals suggesting someone or something was interfering with them in a sexual manner.

And all these 'descriptions' were sadly listened to, by me, as sufferers described accusations, voices and alien experiences, and wanted out. Illusion; if I felt nostalgic, or depressed, I could easily see a tree shape or wallpaper pattern or cartoon image, which reminded me of someone or something. But, an illusion was a false perception (or false belief), due to a distortion of a real sensory perception so that a sufferer would not see a tree shape or wallpaper pattern or cartoon image, but real (to them) other conjured images, that were illusory. *In practice*, it was sometimes difficult to gauge whether a patient, in a description of what they believed they saw and experienced, was experiencing hallucination or illusion (with a delusion as explanation for its appearance) in an altered state of consciousness. With sensitive discussion *other* symptoms might have confirmed or concluded otherwise.

Neologism; my red handbook noted in cases of chronic schizophrenia that the association of thought disorder and autism often resulted in the sufferers speech becoming odd and stilted; their words (and presumably thoughts) took on a private meaning for them, and were misused (to us) and may have been telescoped together to form new words — these were *neologisms*. Nonsense, to others; helpful towards a code interpreting fragments of symbolic schizophrenic communication (viz nonsense to others but meaningful to them).

I was introduced to a brilliant 1968 work entitled; *Pragmatics of Human Communication.*[19] A Study of interactional patterns, pathologies and paradoxes. A book about pragmatic (behavioural) effects of human communication, with special attention to behavioural disorders (see Intro). This work complimented Gregory Bateson, David Cooper, Esterton, Goodman, R.D. Laing, et al of those years. All these contemporary authors *explored* verbal, and non verbal communication (NVC) of florid schizophrenics. And included use of the following terms:

Neologisms, which, to a listener, might end as verbalised meaningless jargon, divorced from their owners precise inner-feelings origins, and could not always be decoded by Others, however well intended.

Paranoia; this was another word, much used outside medical parlance, but with a particular meaning in the psychiatric glossary; a patient suffering from paranoia — or a paranoid state, owned symptoms characterized by delusions of persecution and a lack of logical thought. It was very common in schizophrenia which symptoms included delusions of being persecuted, when all evidence indicated this was not so.

Sad, fascinating, one of our new Bramber's patients, Will P. produced a thick notebook with numerous sketches (by him) which proved the Special Branch, CIA, KGB (esp. KGB), and space aliens, were all after him, and forever whispering and scheming against him. But, as with many patients experiencing *paranoia,* their evidence could be most persuasive. This diagnosis excluded all persons who, in some-way, were, are, being persecuted and pursued, by others, and *could be* confirmed.

Psychosis (psychotic); in past literature the generic term of lunacy, madness, and insanity mostly referred to an acute or chronic (incurable in previous parlance) psychiatric condition, which suggested the patient lacked any insight; and a denial they were ill, though all contrary symptoms demonstrated what, to others, *appeared* self-evident. In a differential diagnosis, the patient could be psychotic and then, in time, improve and still be 'ill', but no longer in psychosis; and this included our schizophrenias. A matter of *knowing* you were ill — or not.

The Schizophrenias

Ackner described schizophrenic disorders and paranoid states in one section[20] (see Chapter 16). In the 1960s, the Schizophrenias (note plural), were differentiated into five, principal symptom clinical cluster types:

Simple, Hebephrenic , Paranoid , Catatonic and Paraphrenia.

However, as Dr. Ackner in 1964 reminded, these lexicon terms of reference were *not* absolute, separate conditions, but a matter of degree; mixed symptoms indicating considerable overlap. And patients did, *do* gain relief *and* recover from *acute* conditions. The *Simple* Schizophrenias (aka schizoid like) onset was usually met during early adulthood (though some adolescents experienced symptoms); they did not display gross behavioural disorders, or florid hallucinations or delusions.

Odd behaviour inertia and emotional impoverishment, were the first observed symptoms; at home. Perhaps, in inertia, staying in bed too much of the time, only getting up during the night (not to be confused with active adolescent sleep patterns). Then, slowly, with personality changes towards autism and bizarre, to severely neglect themselves, become vagrants and eventually to need others to watch over and care for them in the community.

Hebephrenia was most observed in the young, but would have added the more obvious florid schizoid symptoms of hallucinations and bizarre, delusions, preoccupied and observed giggling to themselves (unable to hear someone talking to them closeby, perhaps), this 'oddness' increasing insidiously as their condition deteriorated — but not inevitably. I recollect one young man, answering the above description, who was convinced his knee had its own brain, and waves were coming in through the roof and taking him over — and that was in the community; he was not hospitalised.

The fourth 60's definition of *Catatonic* schizophrenia, arrived later than the first two types; it usually attacked (invaded) in early adulthood. The patient stuporised, unmoving, having to be fed and mopped up and generally totally cared for in their frozen seemed paralysed posture. *Suddenly,* one might become animated, and move, having heard noise about them (previously unable to respond) and accidentally injure self or others, before retreating back into their catatonia (conversion-hysteria).

Ackner said they responded to electro-convulsive therapy. In their inner-world, an outsider would wrongly conclude catatonic sufferer's senses were not registering the goings on around them, but the person could hear and see, and would certainly later recall, much said about them, or done to them, during their acute illness. Due to the success of treatments in the hospital, I met no-one in this acute state, though a number had been so stuporised in the past by a form of shell-shock, or a side effect of an infectious malady.

I recall one female Summersdale patient, discharged in the care of her mother; she had been *catatonic* for some months. It afterwards left her *emotionally* handicapped with other deficits, as residue from her trauma. She described *to me* that, after recovery, her memory returned, nostalgia of an adolescent sexual rejection in her *only* romance; which had immediately preceded her catatonic withdrawal.

I observed some of our schizophrenic patients who experienced an unresolved depression, coupled with their shutting off of any emotional depths. In contrast with the former descriptive states symptomatic of schizophrenia, *Paraphrenia* appears to have evolved in later years of middle-age or older, with full blown paranoid delusions and often florid hallucinations. Such sufferers had experienced sufficient normal life to construct so called *normal* personalities, and thus, in their paraphrenia, their personalities were preserved and encapsulated but, due to their disorder and their attendant *morbid* beliefs, the police would often be called out to deal with alleged persecutors (i.e. neighbours).

A number of late middle-age sufferers were admitted, with this complaint of paraphrenia, whilst I was on Bramber Two ward; several others were visited by me, with a Psychiatric Social Worker, as out patients in Midhurst.

Two other words, associated with schizophrenias. *Schizoid* generally referred to a patient expressing odd anti-social and introspective behaviour, and similarly a *Schizo-affective* personality, suggesting someone whose illness leaned towards schizophrenia.

Ackner quoted the patient, leaving a ward with a suitcase and, when asked why, replied 'there is something strange about my case and I am taking it to a doctor to look into it'; an example of concrete thinking. In flow of speech, a schizophrenic sufferer could suddenly stop mid-flow, and explain that other thoughts had compelled him to stop, and so he was compelled to think certain other thoughts or follow certain voices; this thought-blocking, the patient insisted, was due to the *telepathy* intrusion by Others.

Another thought-blocker was demonstrated in a conversation (usually one sided them talking you listening) in full flow when suddenly, with you still earnestly attempting to relate, they stopped and walked off. I believed, often, it was because an emotion came into play, or rather it would not function. Any emotional demand, however minute, was non-functional at this acute level.

I had no personal experience of a mute patient *living* zombie like in a schizoid withdrawal 'catatonia' state in hospital, i.e. schizophrenic catatonia, *(not* of Edgar Alan Poe and buried alive by Voodoo use of the Zombie inducing drug powder *Tetrodotoxin,* through osmosis into the skin, to freeze all mobility for at least 12 hours; or induced by a dose of curare, aka scoline), but I found the foregoing *glossary* useful into current 1960s psychiatric vocabulary. And, apart from a strong suggestion of hereditary origins, the amnesia *whys* seemed often debatable. In one example, this was described by Emil Kraepelin[20] early in the Twentieth century as *Dementia Praecox*. There was:

> 'an attempt to describe symptoms of intellectual impairment observed in disturbed young patients; in fact it wasn't dementia (as such), but a loss of integration of the mental functions, especially of affect and thinking, descriptive of *Schizophrenias*.' [21]

Relief

To *diminish* pain in physical and mental distress, was to administer relief. And, at ward level, if a cure was not possible, then to offer any treatment which alleviated some suffering was relief (to do no harm). Causes of distress were varied, and depended externally on so many points of contact that a resident was able to experience. Illustrated books, magazines, newspapers, television, radio, music, other people's opinion, *all* provided audio and visual communications, as stimuli. Stimuli would have been therapeutic or intrusive and threatening, much dependent on a person's frame of mind. To the one impoverished, an item gave relief, to another it added further pain.

The hospital Estate, with its many acres, was large, with numerous green hideaways and ha-has a patient seeking temporary relief might find, to isolate for a time. And the main hospital block itself, with its numerous long corridors and myriad rooms and spaces, too would have been a warm rabbit warren which provided real asylum and comfort from a possibly felt cruel and much threatening world — out there. To some sectioned patients, the hospital was an alternative prison, to a disordered and distressed mind, which already provided an inner prison of free will, it colluded.

Malcolm, an eighteen-year old recently admitted into Amberley, frequently passed me on his perambulations about the corridors, loudly playing his portable radio, the sound vibrations which he deliberately blasted into his ear drums. He carried the weighty box on his shoulders, a seeming permanent attachment — to onlookers, it was seldom absent. His was a normal adolescent act of behaviour to play music loud and furious, often to the great irritation of other persons in earshot. But Malcolm played his vibrations for more practical reasons; it deafened the otherwise loud persecuting inner voices in his head, and in out shouting them the radio offered him temporary relief.

To Terry, God *Can* was *in* the television set which he found too frequently turned on, for Others, when, if given a choice, *he,* Terry, would have destroyed this offensive item (all that noise). The radio and television gave out regular news items on the war in Vietnam (horror, in use of toxic Agent Orange), and anti-war clashes at USA University campuses; and of conflicts, murder and mayhem across the globe — offering continuous assaults on patients, persons already suffering, victims from a surfeit of global persecution and despair.

Temporary relief to Malcolm was the noise of his transistor — at his control. To Terry, temporary relief was the television off — also at his control. And removal of conflict... in theory, perhaps, that was an easy part of relief, the reduction of stress by a direct removal of a cause, with evidence of these acts self evident. More of the immense therapeutic relief value of music later.

Relief from anxieties and stress was varied, and began with the realization of just how important 'ablutions' were and, in an upward scale, satiating first physical needs, to metaphysical and spiritual values, as self-worth and nebulous values as contentment. I later read of Abraham Maslows's pyramid of needs, which compliments the above descriptions, I think. The supporting value of measured, prescribed drugs, was always self evident. *Chemotherapy* — prescribed drugs, had developed enormously in the decade preceding my entrance into the hospital in the 1960s. So, too, had earlier decades produced treatments, which very significantly reduced the psychiatric hospital's population.

Hospital *Annual Reports* for pre-war years reflected, in their statistics, patients suffering from Tuberculosis; and others from Venereal diseases — especially the latter, with progressive syphilis and the phases of psychosis which accompanied this awful condition. And, too, Epilepsy was a major problem before the advent of the new stabilizing prescribed drugs which reduced needs for hospitalization.

Before the second world war, Isolation Blocks and long stay, Back Wards were sadly replete with chronic patients resident in the large psychiatric hospital; mostly as terminal cases. Yet within two decades those I*solation* Hospitals (Fever Hospitals, which historically replaced medieval Lazar Leper Hospitals), and numerous recent VD and TB Sanatoriums, built for recovering tuberculosis residents, were no-longer needed, for not just that relief was obtainable, but cure and preventative treatment was greatly reducing bed statistics.

And so, too, were the advent of these almost wonder drugs also used for Fevers, which were reducing that bulk need for hospital beds. My colleagues, then, were still producing a variety of post-qualification nursing certification, which anticipated such special needs; e.g. the *Fever Certificate*, in addition to the main RMN, SRN and RNMH certificates — each discipline of which took three years independent study to complete qualification.

In the Nineteen Sixties, considerable optimism existed that Relief could (at last) be given to sufferers with florid symptoms then indicating one of the schizophrenias; and other mental illnesses. This relief was possible, like Aldous Huxley's Soma pills, to give instant relief — but Huxley was then, in the 1930s, writing in a vein of futuristic *Science-fiction.* But, as with many good-things which brought wholesale relief, they had a collective price, initially perhaps unknown, i.e. *Side Effects.* It was a calculated risk, as many treatments on-balance were, with wisdom of hindsight and possible litigation... billed against good-faith carers.

In past centuries, scant knowledge of treatment meant that Doctor and Dame risked being indicted for Witchcraft, if a tonic gave a wondrous relief from madness without a full religious exorcism as its prelude. But the latter charges meant the accuser had to prove *'the imploying of wicked spirits to any intent whatsoeve*r' and this was, '*Felony within the statute.'* (See Law; 9 Geo.2 c5; Witchcraft Acts;1541-2, 1604, 1735, 1944.)

Today, in 1968, a persecuted (paranoid) patient, with somatic hallucinations and florid delusions of being poisoned, may still accuse their carers of involving the devil or evil spirits; but the accused would not, in the United Kingdom, be tried for Witchcraft or Sorcery in performing diabolical arts. But, if treatment was given in *wilful bad-faith*, individuals could be later indicted for malpractice... and proven gross negligence. About acts of relief.... I wondered, and compared Past and present given treatments for mental illness.

More on Treatment

Treatment fashionable in one era, becomes unfashionable at a later time; its definition is, inevitably, dependent on prevailing attitudes (law) as well as any possible later admitted cost in undesirable side-effects. On this note Dr. Jonathan Swift:[22]

> '... from a Redundancy of Vapours ... that the main Point of Skill and Address, is to furnish Employment for this Redundancy of Vapour. Thus one man chusing a proper Juncture, leaps into a Gulph, from whence proceeds a Hero, and is called the Saver of his Country ... another achieves the same Enterprise, but, unluckily timing it, has the Brand of Madness, fixed as a Reproach upon his Memory Leave to inspect into Bedlam, and the Parts adjacent.'

A century later, medications (tonics) in use for the different Swiftian symptoms of madness could certainly be listed in our own Hospital *Poisons Book*. General all purpose tonics, were available in the Nineteenth and Early Twentieth century, for rich and poor population; from tar-water to laudanum or port-wine, advised by the parish doctor — and a treatment ticket allocated by their parish *Relieving Officer* (Social Worker), to be taken to any nearby Dispensary.

A Victorian 1883 '*Book of Prescriptions'*, for example, recommended for the mentally disturbed and those with a *Nervous Disposition*: 'Cold douche.- Shower-bath.- Quiet.- Purgatives.- Opium.- Chloral Hydrosyamine. And Bromide of Potassium ... which was prescribed for someone with *Mania* .' (*Note use of Opium*). And for treatment of '*Melancholia* '(Depression), *was given*: 'Tonics. Purgatives. Wine. Pil. Hydrarg. Aloes'. Many were generic names, given that Tonics, purgatives and wine, suggested numerous brands and concoctions; not least, the Tonics with laudanum (an opiate derivative) which were in considerable use in the Nineteenth and into the early Twentieth century hospital prescriptions.

Renowned artists and writers of the 19th century including Thomas de Quincy and John Ruskin were, using current colloquial, sensitive workaholics who were properly prescribed Tonics which contained liberal amounts of Opium, recommended and prescribed in good-faith by qualified Physicians for their patients' relief. Treatments in use, during the course of the Twentieth century at this hospital, came-in and went-out of fashion, from enthusiasm at their entry, to distain in wise retrospect — as Dr. Swift had satirised so well in his literature.

A perusal of many psychiatric hospitals patients' folios and dispensary records held in the *Archives,* or illustrative literature on public sale (as I have demonstrated), reveal a past worth of varied ablution treatments, douches (baths) warm hot or cold, *all* to have been given at gauged temperatures in proper water containers — or, in the form of swathed hot-towels cold-towels, hot-sheets cold-sheets aka wet packs. And, till recent years, prescribed agitated therapeutic baths with wooden (or other) boards on top to ensure manic (disturbed) patients would stay in their baths (even given food and drink while under the dutiful eyes of their ward attendants) for prescribed periods. *Comfort, not pain ...* given in definite *Relief.*

A variety of physical treatments had lately been tried, tested, and then fallen out-of-fashion; Malaria therapy treatment, for General Paralysis of the Insane from terminal Syphilis; and, for violent patients (an example), a one-time tranquillizing cocktail of paraldehyde and sulphonal (the latter discontinued when its side effects were found toxic to the renal system) — both treatments used and disused by the outbreak of the second world war.

During 1939-45 and early post-war years, there was *Insulin Therapy* (later, Modified Insulin Therapy), and *Leucotomy*. Of course sixties ECT, still practised— derived from 18th century erratic static electricity, and later, WW1 Faradism. Now better *and safer,* known as *ECT* (Electro Chemical Therapy; also EST; Electric Shock Therapy, or Electroplexy) and lesser known *Narcotherapy*, a protracted sleep treatment.

Then, there was an allied *psychotherapy* stable of treatments; the use of *abreactive* medication as the minutely, homeopathic sized, prescribed doses of the active hallucinogenic from specific plants, *LSD* — already under threat, as unsupervised abuse and synthesised patents devalued earlier, believed, prospects. I heard, *and saw*, abundant evidence of debited and credited commentaries of all of these physical treatments; at the hospital. During the

1960s, many staff and patients (as consumers) experienced a variety of physical treatments; viewed at inception as cure-alls, unreal *Elixirs,* a Holy Grail of ultimate relief for all mentally-ill sufferers.

Certainly, they were treatments prescribed and given, in all good-faith; though their inventive Heroes would as customary fall by association into popular media disdain, for not coming up to Second Coming expectations. By the mid-twentieth-century, biochemists researching into improved elixirs produced more and more better pills, as food to relieve mental illnesses, and had as specialists replaced herbalists, alchemists, and philosophers of the dispensary forebears.

Opium, now in the 1960s a legally, Class A only, forbidden drug — though specific derivatives (e.g. Morphine) were obtainable by signed medical authorization, and, a must-be-done, duly entered in the Dangerous Drugs Book (aka DDA book). Arsenic is, too, a well recognised poison, though often, in *minute* quantities, was prescribed in the past for certain maladies. MIMS, our hospital pharmacist's bible, contained hundreds of prescribed drug entries and, as our local expert, would be available to the medical staff to prescribe medication. This bible defined a catalogue of side-effects from taking prescriptions.

Tall John and John R and Ex-seaman schizophrenic Jim were prescribed chlorpromazine (largactil); and trifluoperazine (stelazine), which reduced their over-the-top manic behaviour; and subdued unwanted inner voices — and reduced episodes of aggression. Relief... One recognized side-effect was a patient's eyes upturned to the ceiling, but then easily cancelled by the additional drug of orphenadrine (disipal), a small yellow pill. And so, combinations of prescribed drugs gave Relief to the sufferers, and also, in a knock-on effect, relief for other patients and carers.

If any person (patient or staff), was found to be taking illegal drugs; amphetamines, cannabis, cocaine, opium, or others which were banned by law, then cancellation of this source was equally deemed appropriate treatment. Numbers of our patients, were often confused about what *they* felt were safe treatments — as opposed to what the hospital staff prescribed for their relief. Connolly, Hill Tuke and other doctors (*alienists* — psychiatrists), of the early 19th century, well recognized the immense value of occupation, self-worth, dignity, and the moral-treatment of patients' owned finer-feelings, being always due consideration when administrating what-ever care and treatment was then viable...

Our hospital based Occupation Therapy (OT); Industrial Therapy (IT); and Social Therapy facilities, were well developed amenities in the hospital, since

1952 — and expanded, after the formal closure of the Hospital Farm in 1957, to this aim. And, everyday except Sunday, a member of the nursing staff would accompany a group of the ward's patients to the Industrial Therapy Unit (ITU) yard and stay with them until meal times — then returning with the patients to their ward. Bramber Two patients were regular attenders at these therapies — most, with escorts.

Recreation Hall

Between two short south connecting corridors — the right, off which the Grill Room, Restaurant, Nursing Offices, and Patients Affairs were housed and the upper left-leg, where the Patients Shop and adjacent Barbers were located — was a short connecting corridor forming an H shape, this linked across, on both sides, with the kitchens, north and south. On the lower part of this H was the large Recreation Hall. The north-and-south Main corridors, at each end, then boxed the H into two enclosed areas.

The Recreation Hall was very substantial in size; completed in 1897 at the hospital's opening, it was also the year of Queen Victoria's Diamond Jubilee. To commemorate that august event, a variety of social activities were organized for the new *West Sussex Asylum* residents. At the hospital's inception, a lantern slide show with 'animated photos' of the Jubilee celebrations was shown to patients in the Hall.

A wide variety of athletics, sports and other organized social activities, were subsequently held open to *all* staff and capable patients. And from the opening of the Asylum to the 1960s (and afterwards), very regular social activities were held for the benefit of residents. Radio was introduced to the hospital wards in the 1930s, and black-and-white televisions placed on selected wards from the date of the 1953 Coronation — about the same time of the renaming of the hospital wards by the (then) Chief Male Nurse (no doubt aided by the suggestions of his colleagues).

In 1968, regular film shows were held at least once per week, sometimes twice on Tuesday and Saturday evenings, from 5.30 pm or thereabouts. The projector, operated from a small balcony, at the rear of the recreation hall with some seating space. Advanced notice, of the new programmes, was posted about the hospital perimeter, including a substantial peg board notice propped up, placed outside one of the doors of the recreation hall, almost opposite the grill room restaurant, and nursing office.

Most entertainment, on offer, was free to all staff and patients, though for special 'Dances' and fund-raising activities, entrance fees were welcomed. Charity Fetes had long been a feature involving the local community population, who regularly supported those annual activities. I heard that, in the past, the Chichester City Guildhall in Priory Park (I'd seen, in evidence, a photo dated early possibly WW1 years) had produced numbers of past hospital fund-raising events; but most large activities were, are, staged within this hospital's own large grounds.

To the advantage of all past hospital's patients, these ephemeral social activities were an obtuse form of the local community's acceptance of the psychiatric hospital; very much a source of relief, and a supplier of employment. Much was dependent, on the staffing levels on the wards, as to whether 'specialed' residents would be accompanied to the film shows (or whatever), but, on most occasions, staff would phone another ward (via the nursing office) and ask for an escort, so as to not deprive a wanting patient; but most residents made their own ways to events and their suppers were kept hot for their return.

Stress and anxiety exacerbated more voices, deeper depressions, triggered by (or about) other people in and out of hospital, including relatives, or with other 'outside' connections; and, in order to sort-out and render relief, the aid of a PSW (Psychiatric Social Worker), or the then small, but invaluable, hospital *Patients' Affairs* office would have assisted in helping to resolve such issues. Referrals for such assistance were given by a doctor, nurse or the patient himself walking down to those hospital based offices.

On entry to the hospital, following admission, or prior to and after discharge back into the community, one key figure in those days was the local health authority, benign official — the Mental Welfare Officer. The MWO's job was to ensure that, in a welfare context, the law and the patient's rights (whatever) are properly administered in gaining their resources to Relief. And about Law.

George MWO

During the first year of training, our intake had little need of reference to the Chapter *Legal and Administrative Aspects*[23], except to witness an admission, on a section, by the ward charge nurse and the community duty Mental Welfare Officer (MWO) who usually accompanied the ambulance crew.

We were expecting an urgent section, one afternoon in May sixty-eight, and he arrived just as we had completed the after-dinner washing up and the IT group had been escorted off the ward — *not* due back till tea-time. Loud echoes, sound of the door being unlocked, and wheels and shoes heavy against the top concrete steps. Geof had gone off duty, Doug was at the door, and Fred and I were in the kitchen chatting away to several of the patients when we noticed the loud human activity, suggestive of our new admission — since it was taking place only yards away from us. Two ambulance men were helping a semi-conscious (clearly under some sedation) young man over the threshold. Behind them were two cautious uniformed policemen, and to their rear was George Pople, one of West Sussex MWOs, who accompanied admissions onto the wards.

'Hmm', we thought, must have been a bit of bother, some aggravated At Risk situation and suggested a probable disturbed and frightened patient. He was broad, muscular, though not very tall, and had several tattoos on his arms, as we could see from his flailing arms and limbs overhanging the metal and canvas wheelchair.

'Fred, Barry', Doug hush called out as he said goodbye and 'Thank you' to the ambulance men and police escort. MWO George stayed back, to deliver the section papers, and give some background information on the admission; and probably a chat. Our new patient, Rodney, an ex-paratrooper, appeared to be still hallucinated as he monosyllabled, lisped out 'Devils', 'Holy Cross', and other religious orientated words. At one point, from his sitting position, he was looking up at the ceiling and crossing himself in a prayer or protective oration, but mostly he was half-conscious.

Fred went off to turn-back a prepared bed at the end of the dormitory, and close by a side room — just in case. George had already introduced a summary of the events, which brought the two policeman out. Rod had attacked a number of people (mostly unknown to him - it was believed), and put several in hospital for examination. Details, Social History, would come later; and the full medical examination by the duty-ward-doctor, when it was sensible to interview the patient. Doug and George, chatted in the office, as I attempted to speak with Rodney (who sat in the wheelchair with a blanket around him) outside the office.

'This is a hospital... You *are safe now*... in hospital', I tried to convey to him, despite his 'hands-off' gesticulations attempting to strike off his devils, whatever. He was still quite disorientated. In Rodney's anguished disturbed state of mind and hallucinated experience, heaven knew what our looming bodies over him, and this new 'hostile' environs must have translated for him. It was hoped the applied pre-admission medication (given at the police station by the duty police surgeon to quell his violence and hopefully sedate his persecuting inner-voices), would eventually allow him to be more settled and effect some better insight, out of his illness.

'Better take him into the dormitory Barry. It's clear he'll be too disturbed and unsettled for a while. See if he'll doze off, eh?', Doug called out. And so I (with slight difficulty) wheeled our new patient down the dormitory, and Fred and I, we thought prudently, merely removed his shoes and jacket, and laid him on top of the bed covering him with a blanket and counterpane — till later. To my surprise, almost as his black-hair hit the soft white pillows, he contracted like a punctured balloon and went off to sleep. And we returned to the office, ensuring no other residents were about the dormitory. They were in the dayroom.

'He's asleep, Doug' I reported. He nodded and returned, 'Time for tea I think — eh George?', looking to our MWO, sat in the office corner, having safely delivered his papers and had them checked by Doug for later dispatch to the Patients Affairs Department. I'd met George briefly before, whilst admitting on Amberley One (no policeman necessary then). Though I had heard much of George, the MWO (and of his colleagues), I previously had not had the pleasure of listening to him at any length; this time I was not to be disappointed.

Apart from contact with occasional hospital visitors and relatives the MWOs (as social workers) were then our *only* formal *outside* community connection. A senior colleague of George's, had given us a talk at the hospital school during our induction last year and impressed us of their role in administering the Mental Health Act and Welfare duties, in liaison with Nursing Homes in the community. We heard of MWOs visiting relatives and out- patients in their homes (in common with the PSWs). But, with so much introductory details given out, a deal of knowledge was already forgotten.

The introduction of the '*Mental Welfare Officer*' (per se) was a recent title, which followed instrumentation of the 1959 MHA in the early 1960s. George illustrated many a tale, from his crop of professional anecdotes, including his mental welfare officer work as a local government 'parish' relieving officer since 1930 — with a provenance dated before Charles Dickens was born in 1812. The officious beadle (relieving officer) Bumble (lovely name), was depicted in Dickens' *Oliver Twist.*[24] In his day, Dickens, a journalist in his youth, attended criminal courts like Bow Street — and local workhouses, and home visiting in his local parish. His first published work, *Sketches of Boz*[25] emphasised:

'The parish beadle is one of the most, perhaps *the* most important member of the local administration.'

Pre-Nineteen-sixties statutory admissions into hospitals and public institutions was one of the duties of the 'District Welfare Officers'. *Before* 1948 and the NHS, officers were still known as '*Relieving Officers.*' Their many public duties, as social workers, working with other appointed parish officers... in-the-front-line... administering often harsh (by default lack of resources) poor-law. Welfare Laws extending back to the Elizabethan Poor Law of 1603... and, before that date, overseered by a medieval *Steward,* or by other names.

In 1960, there were three Mental Welfare Officers for West Sussex; one based at County Hall Chichester; one at Horsham; and one based at Worthing—but initially their duties *only* related to the deemed *Mentally Subnormal.*[26] Our George had been in the business of caring for forty years and more, a pre-war and wartime *Relieving Officer* working out of Bognor Regis, which was about seven miles south of Chichester and the Hospital, and worked with the Mentally ill. In fact, as I would learn from George, he had been employed by the County as a Relieving Officer for West Sussex since 1935: a long professional pedigree — and as a parish officer since 1930.

From the 31st March 1961, District Welfare Officers ceased admitting patients into the psychiatric hospitals; those duties formally transferred, full-time, to the new Mental Welfare Officers. George then, to his pleasure, as he enjoyed his mental health work and was clearly good at it, became full-time in Mental Health (Social) work, as a new *Mental Welfare Officer*; and here he was, on Bramber Two ward.

George was not tall, or particularly well-built, but he was well into middle-age and close to retirement, when I met him in the Nineteen-Sixties. At sometime in the past, he had had a car accident and lost the use of one eye, and consequently wore a black eye-patch. But, oh how that pirate-eye twinkled so... His voice was soft and mellow, with speech unhurried; and his knowledge (of all and anything) seemed limitless; more, he was not brutalised. There was no arrogance or holier than thou utterances, and no whatever hints of a shell of seemed indifference, brought on by long exposure to life's harsher realities in altruistic, long working for others, over almost forty years — close working with the sick and needy, as a parish employee; and all that *before* our hospital meeting.

Perhaps most notable, George's often philosophical quips were always interlaced with humorous anecdotes, many in laughing at his own past behaviour in his professional duties — out there!

Staff Fred agreed to keep an eye on the ward, including our new patient, allowing time for me with Doug and George, to discuss the Section 29 '*Emergency Application for Admission for Observation*' [27] papers for certification: and to have an in-depth discussion on *Law and Order*; Mad or Bad, Hospital or Prison — and other such highly emotive, but herein (new to me) vital aspects of care and treatment alternatives. The MWOs needed to know aspects of The Law and Mental Health, and now, so did I.

Temporary insane

A few days later (pure coincidence), not long after meeting with Mental Welfare Officer George on the ward, I received a phone call from The Office, asking me to meet up with a patient on Amberley One, and act as an escort (only as a formality, they insisted as there was no risk) with a sectioned *patient*, to attend a *Mental Health Review Tribunal* hearing in a room close to Patients' Affairs. It was only a short journey — from the ward to the *Tribunal* (what a term, politic rather than clinical). I didn't know the patient, a young registered drug addict on an customary 26 of the 1959 Act but, *he* acknowledged he knew of me from Spider C. and clearly a proxy faith was already in place at my arrival on Amberley. I sat alone outside the room, whilst the hearing was taking place but, at its favourable conclusion, it was the patient's advocate, MWO George (not surprised at my brief appearance) who came out of the room, with a clearly satisfied client — off the Section, formally discharged, but to continue attending the hospital for after-care rehab and therapeutic treatment at his own request.

I had, in past experience, worked as a civilian clerk in *The Press and Information Bureau* (and briefly with General Orders) for the Metropolitan Police at *New Scotland Yard* in the mid-1960s. There had, at no time, been cause for me to relate to such vital *legal* issues; I had always been able to keep at complete arms-length, any notion of in-depth personal experience of law, let alone called on judgements of Mad-or-Bad, or, Mad-And-Bad society ascribed issues, as well as about innocent victims of circumstance, wilful acts in law breaking, or in being mentally ill or so disordered.

On Amberley, my acquaintance with law-breakers, the drug abusers and one-off incest case, had not then led to any particular digression on my part about Law and Freedom, since it was the 'other' aspects of those patients; the philosophical, the social, the personal details, but 'not' of the Law itself. I was having to examine, in honesty, numerous aspects of the Law and Freedom, and in the making and breaking of Rules and the subsequent possible (even life threatening) penalties.

MWO George might have been involved in one case, relating to a patient already in Graylingwell, which indicated that the prescribed 1959 MHA did not (couldn't anticipate) answer all potential crisis situations, and left it to the integrity and experience of the involved professionals to resolve any unique life or death situations. Admin Baz recalled one such case, a caselaw in which he was personally involved in during these years:

Dr. Joyce, Consultant Psychiatrist, had had a medical / legal problem in that the patient he had been treating in the community had been brought to the hospital, by the emergency ambulance service, suffering from a diabetic coma. He consulted with Baz (who told me about it) and the admin head of the hospital, explaining that his patient who had been earlier, refusing admission, did *not* meet the criteria to be compulsorily admitted for treatment; but *she would otherwise certainly die* if her wishes were respected. And, she was in his care as his patient. She had threatened to sue through the courts, if she was admitted against her will. After going into *a duty of care,* detailed discussion, it was agreed that the situation was *not* covered by the Mental Health Act 1959. However, *the patient's health came first,* and the hospital would opt for the latter if it was a case of appearing before a later Coroner's Court, or The High Court. This agreed, the patient was admitted for treatment and recovered. True to her word, she took legal action, which had led to the case of *A Patient v. Rex,* which was heard in the Royal Courts of Justice before Lord Chief Justice Widgery. [28]

For the informed observer, the foregoing was a most interesting case with the M.H. Act. being analysed, word by word, with extended discussion on the ambiguity of the words 'may' and 'might'. This led to reference to the Royal Commission Report, to seek the thinking in Parliament at the time of drafting and passing the previous 1959 Act. 'Rex ' was found at fault in law, but with a rider, that the legislature should look further into this shortcoming. This contributed to the passing of a later 1970s Mental Health (Amendment) Act.'

Rules of Freedom

Rules, boundaries, freedom, will-power and choice. In experience anybody, every-body, is bound by its minute, time-capsule, their own time sense, their own unique physical state. A Being contained and maintained within specific quantitative, and exactly qualitatively, structured forms, components, and physical temperatures. Such is biological science. So for all our patients, myself, staff colleagues, and others outside. Facts of life. More. On Bramber Two I'd experienced first hand new knowledge about a variety of laws - divine and mortal.

We are bound by established human-made rules in Law, and social mores which too if *not* maintained, evoke penalties - for patients and staff alike. This an cultural legal Establishment. The fact human-rules are *man-made* is just as much our being's real world, as its demanding physical dependent atomic components. Thus, the alchemic and metaphysical are in application, just as true.... all patients, all staff, are bound within — by rules, but often certain personal rules of a patient could no-way conform with the expectations of others; conflict often inevitable.

Order

Colliding worlds, physical and metaphysical parts alike, meant friction conflict and degrees of pleasure and pain. Whatever collisions were felt in an individual twixt their emotive I AM and its husk; or relative to their external worlds, was much about what concerned, and affected our diagnosed sick patients (in conflict — or in chaos), and of our efforts in trying to help our patients as a duty of care.

However we treated their, our situations, abnorms, conflict, whatever signs and symptoms detected and presented, it was to a harmony we aimed for as a primary goal. But this primary pacific goal was a generalisation. It was the minutes, life's details which were to be investigated and benignly treated, whenever however practicable and sensible.

Hospitalisation, in this context, was *my* becoming involved in ongoing situations with patients and colleagues, and in attempting to replace *abnormal* states with so-called normal states — as normalisation. About talking — *and* doing, and the consequence of *not* doing. Normalisation in patient care, and my own responsibility, as I had came to understand it, meant conforming to such rules as would render a peaceful, at least acceptable, state of being. But such conformity would, where quality-of-life was concerned, seem of questionable value, even if unavoidable, if it brought *more* pain with a reformed ability to cope, and be coped with, given day to day existences?

Ex-seaman patient, paranoid-schiz Jim, already an occasional chess partner (ironically able to have bouts of insight in his Knight's move thinking) and I were in the kitchen sharing the lunchtime washing up, and chatting abut 'girls'. Jim was eulogising about rainbow Jill up on Barnet Two. Out in the dayroom we could hear laughter from a group of three or more patients amongst a general cacophony, anticipating some real or imaginary event in the afternoon.

All other ward staff were engaged in a Handover in the office, with their door closed. ... And something was wrong.

Suddenly, it became church quiet in the adjacent dayroom; two seconds later zombie Tall John stood, on my right, framed in the kitchen doorway — but three feet away from me. And ignoring Jim, who was on my left, John, glaring directly at me, coldly demanded, in a threatening tone, '*I want one* now *or I'll knife you* !', (he wanted a fag). Sure enough, he had one of the kitchen knives in his right fist, waving it meaningfully towards me.... Initially, I felt more annoyance than fear, and said nothing, gathering bemused wits to respond, when to my astonishment, before I reacted to the possible, awful impending incident, Jim (himself a potentially dangerous paranoid schizophrenic) slowly lifted his head up from the filled sink, gently placed a soapy plate on the wooden sideboard to his left, and slowly swivelled his head to look directly into Tall John's snarling face. And in a low *deep* terrifying tone said to John, '*You leave him alone. Barry's all right.*'

Tall John seemed to shrink and, quickly putting the knife down on the floor, just inside the kitchen to admit compliance with Jim's warning, he fled towards the dormitory. Jim (and I) relaxed and carried on our conversation, and resumed the washing up.

Heavy

I found working on the *Refractory Ward*, despite the excellent guidance and support of Doug and colleagues, still had me feeling *very*, very heavy, and often inadequate — and tiny inside.... But perhaps it was a matter of growth, a growing awareness of changes taking place in my own personality; which was more than exposing my own achilles heels (in service, treating others) in becoming a professional.

Perhaps, it was one aspect of humility I had long recognised intellectually; or was it pathological, in feelings of insecurity and immaturity; even inferiority, perhaps, not withstanding any pomposity. I could honestly grant myself a *tiny* admission that this humility was a germ of robust compassion for fellow man, which transcended my well established ego-bound self-centre: and would it last, could it last, would *it* grow; or remain minute and so stone heavy within my self-centre.

There was still Fear.. rank fear *within* me, though there was I suspect more than a germ of real Charity, and a wavering glow in my darkness, even an occasional blip of Clarity; *but* still I felt within... closed and contained; *too* many fears — yet (please!) to be exorcised.

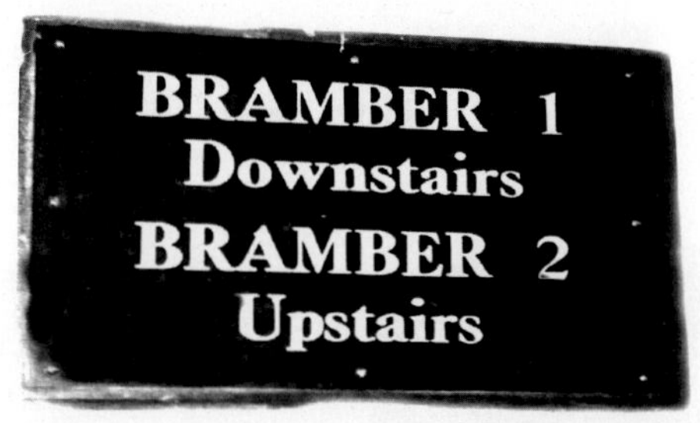

THE LISTENER, 26 *July* 1933

SYMPOSIUM ON MODERN ARCHITECTURE

The Listener

Published by the British Broadcasting Corporation

Vol. X. No. 237 26 JULY 1933 [REGISTERED AT THE G.P.O. AS A NEWSPAPER] THREEPENCE

Principal Contents

1933. The year Germany opened (misnomer) Dachau concentration camp - first of hundreds of NAZI camps to be. In the UK long term results of unresolved NYD NotYetDiagnosed, Battle Stress fatigued, twenty years *after* WW1 ended, *many* previous shell shocked veterans remained hospitalised - but *not* on military pension statistic lists, incurable and paupers - anonymous survivors - war veterans, housed in public assistance Institutions and U.K. County Asylums.

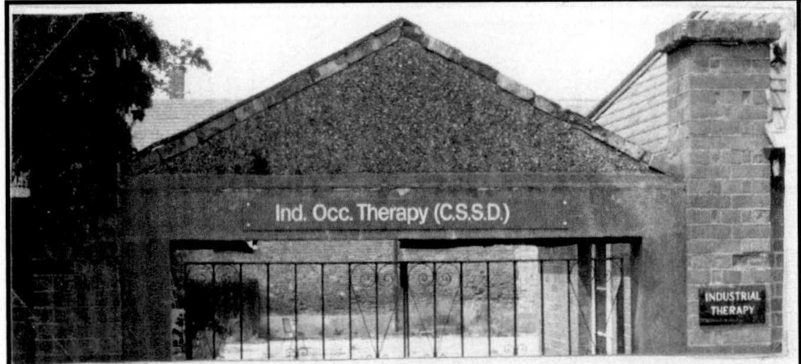

Entrance to **The Yard** in the 1970s. Photo by author.

Right. The author **(centre)** as 3rd year RMN student supervising assembly contract work in No 5 shed. Present are hospital resident patients *and,* out-patients. And (for the pic) in charge Mrs P. an SNO; and, student colleague Harry **(on R)**. *Photo by Chichester Photographic Service Limited* - taken Spring 1970.

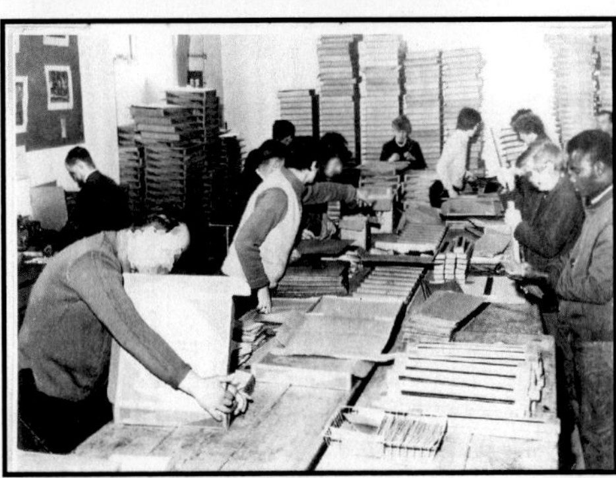

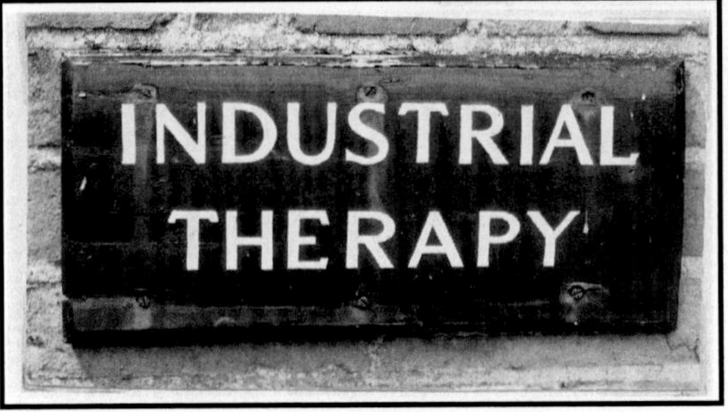

Left. IT sign attached to the right hand entrance pillar of **The Farm Yard in 1970s**. Photo by author.

Right. Nine Bramber Two patients attending O.T. - occupation therapy (disassembly work under supervision) in No 2 shed in The Yard. *Photo taken by Chichester Photographic Services Limited* - early 1970.

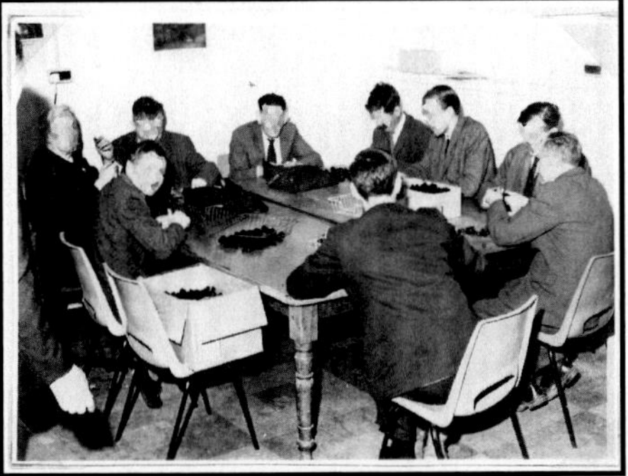

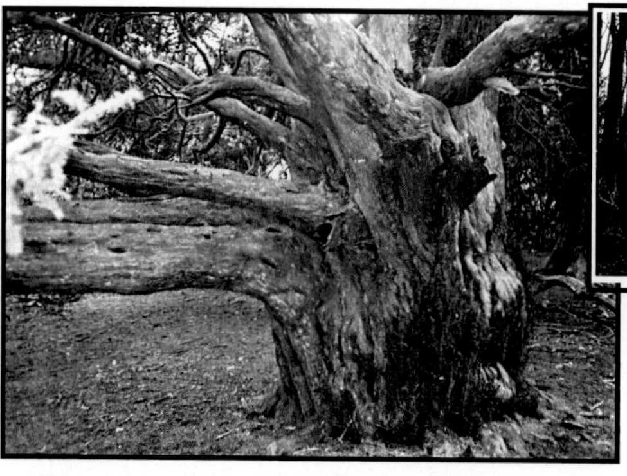

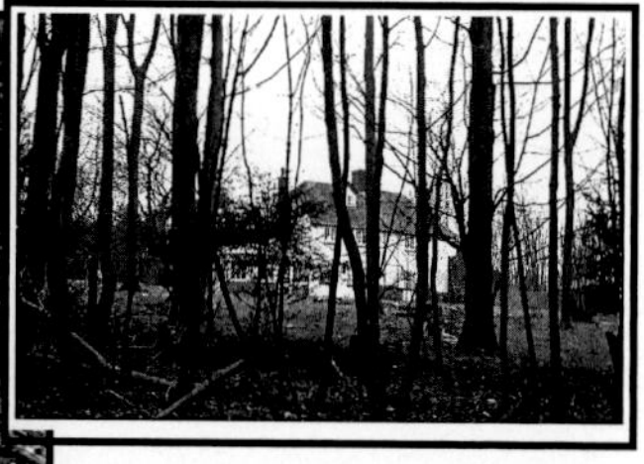

North of Chichester was hidden Kingley Vale, with its cluster of ancient yews rooted in a coombe (on my left), as I travelled home after work to minute Chilgrove — on my bicycle. The rank rural scene encouraged many surreal Sartrean thoughts and feelings about our patients, and about all human existence.

Each day in 1968, I was aware of up, above and beyond (out of sight) Kingley Vale, on dark South Down wooded hillside, the existence of a Binderton cottage, a former 18th century Pest House (Dr. Joyce informed me). And, nearby, stone remains of a hilltop on-guard phantom Roman camp. Nothing scary — just respectful.

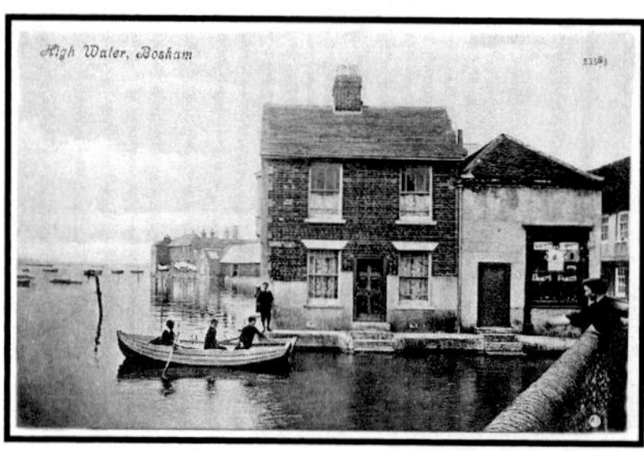

Bosham. (See C8. Summersdale, p355)

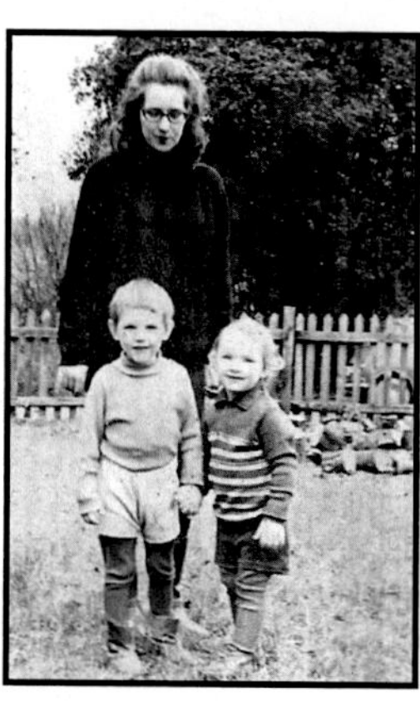

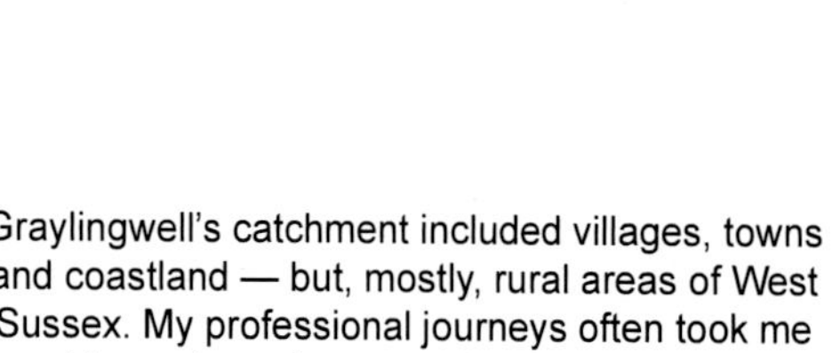

Graylingwell's catchment included villages, towns and coastland — but, mostly, rural areas of West Sussex. My professional journeys often took me out to such rural scenes, throughout Sussex.

Right. Home for a few months, 1968. Sara, 5 year old Philip (Pip, Paul) and 3 year old Chris (Kit), in the rear garden of Stonerock Cottage (owned by the Edward James estate) in the hamlet of Chilgrove, north of Chichester, situated by a farm and woodland, up amongst the South Down hills.

Chapter Six
Nausea

'Let me add that poets walk some distance above the ground on quickly melting snow, into which their footprints disappear. All this does not make the work of remembering and resuscitating ghosts any easier. '[1]
Jean Cocteau. 1956.

4th June 1968 to 9th June 1968

Nausea—Sartre—On Leave—Journal, The Grammar of Being with Others—Can Terry—Kafka—Philosophy—Depersonalisation—Chesterton and Superman

Nausea

Words, words, words: structured learning organised through the hospital school and its prescribed ward experiences; aided by compulsory, and suggested, reading matter, was mechanically working within me: juxtapositioning with all detritus of collective past-reading, learning and lived experience: a massive collection of words: Traces, threads, connections, *memories,* my own and of others; *never* of *the* experiences — per se. And, in order to better help myself digest so much new knowledge and new experiences, I commenced a brief *Journal,* which centred as a Commentary on current domestic and hospital routines. During this time, I would include appreciation of extra-curriculum studies in this Diary. I began by reading a paperback of Jean Paul Sartre's *Nausea.* [2]

I felt, in writing this mean little commentary on Sartre's work, a nemo, a nobody. In truth. I was addressing, quite frequently, invisible icons and signatures of Olympian gods. My trivia. But what I stamped onto the ground surface, who only knows. Only too briefly, as if in isolation, I read *translated* Ancient Greek writings of Homer (lead on by Bertrand Russell's *History of Western Philosophy* [3] and other tasty introductions and, of others, in aggregate; fragments of Hesiod, legions of Mythology and its myriad gods, heroes, villains. Introductions to Names; Archimedes, Aristotle, Empedocles, Epicteus, Heraclitus, Paracelsus, Parmenides, Plato, Plotinus, Socrates, other awesome commentaries on life.

Was I pretentious (*no* - but I was *very* curious) in just reading (*what* else!) about those illuminates? Greats always, *always* in others' translations (*how* else?). But, still, I adored Gilbert Murray's thin green paperback translations of Euripides, Dionysus and *The Bacchae*. Plato through a glimpse of Jarrold's translation. William Blake's art and poetry. Enjoyed Dante's trilogy, in Cary's translation of the *Divine Comedy*. Milton and Virgil. And, a little dipping into something tasty from great Philosophers like Plato and his tutor Socrates.

All these classic excitations — coupled with memories of adolescence. Through the keyhole, forbidden erotic 1950s Hank Janson and Mickey Spillane's lurid cheap paper-backs. Earlier still, as an infant, being read to in wartime, of Enid Blyton[4],Rudyard Kipling, Mark Twain. Hearings competed with vexed voices as, overhead, nearby 1944 doodle-bug and dog-fight droppings, explosions amid lightning flashes — whilst being read to by an anonymous lady-carer in *Spurgeon's Orphan Homes, Dingle* underground shelter. But, so what. All are now (and now and *now* — in time erased) minute memories. Information and experience, mingled within my own social history. No matter what my senses read, and record in chemical traces, already I knew, as yet ... *I know in experience* nothing. A being deaf, blind and lame, in this context. Intellectual, accrued, memorised and reasoned data, is not Being.

On Leave

In the early 1960s, I enjoyed reading Colin Wilson's book *The Outsider* [5] and the critic Edmund Wilson's essays, on Giant others. In the year before entering the hospital as an employee, I'd been engrossed in Henrik Ibsen, T.S. Eliot and Bernard Shaw's — *Plays and Prefaces*. Yet, *all* the foregoing meant very little, so much literary name-droppings — except as an introductory font with all comic-musings; memories mixed into a centrifuge of words, and imprinted icons; which unconscious, anticipated attempts to interpret my *nausea* in facing inner-fears, and ignorance, and more so, in the attempts to translate others. Rote learning is one thing; but Knowing is something else, eh! After Bramber Two ward initiation, I experienced a week's overtime on Chilgrove One ward (again); and proceeded on a week's home leave to our rented cottage, at Chilgrove hamlet seven miles away up in the Downs.

Tuesday, June 4th 1968
Journal, A Grammar of Being with Others

On one week's leave. Finished duty on Chilgrove Ward, a chronic male ward of forty-two mostly aged patients. Just concluded an introductory period on the disturbed patients *acute* ward of Bramber Two. I'm reading to relax; Jung's *Psychology of the Unconscious.* [6] I'm well into Jean-Paul Sartre's *Nausea,* aware of the latter's (misunderstood in media) influence on Sixties anti-psychiatry politics and later demise of Psychiatric Hospitals. And, by my past acquaintance, with writings of Ouspensky (via Colin Wilson's voluminous works). At *first* found a definite *frisson,* between these savants, an ongoing debate on *raison d'etre* about *All and Every-thing* (Ouspensky) and *Existence. Being from No-thing* (Sartre). How nihilism, post-war dialectic in the media, arrived, to eventually affect mental patients and policy care-planners. A trend among some politicians and philosophers, to *deny* insanity in any form. Ironically, it seemed, to *prefer* prisons to psychiatry, with disturbed behaviour.

Wednesday, June 5th 1968

Ten-fifteen pm. A few brief notes. I'm very tired... On Sara's return around mid-day, following a visit to the dentist and shopping, I learnt Paul our eldest had been a little naughty, over-tired... Around three pm, a new acquaintance Doug, a Charge Nurse colleague from Bramber Two, arrived along with his son. They collected us by car and relayed us to Chichester, where we were pleasantly entertained in their home. A problem arose around seven pm or so, when Kit our youngest fell into a fish-pond in Doug's back garden, much to our horror. I dashed out from the kitchen, scooped him out and, dangling him upside down, hastily drained the surplus water from him, aided by pats on his back from the palm of my right-hand. Paul, unaware of the implications, was laughing merrily at what he thought antics. We removed all his clothes, wrapped him cosily in a borrowed towel, and consoled his surprisingly quickly-cured tears. I, too, borrowed a pair of trousers and removed my wet jacket. On returning home, both Sara and I felt extremely weary. She retired as soon as the boys were laid down, around nine-fifteen pm, in order to unwind and after making us both a cup of tea, I finished a first reading of *Nausea* by Jean-Paul Sartre, but I'll comment on this when I read through my notations, on a deemed empty existence.

Thursday, 6th June 1968

Visit to mother and step-father, in their 35 Highland Road confectionery shop at Southsea.
I was thinking of Sartre's opinions. Started reading Franz Kafka's *Metamorphosis and Other Stories'* [7]

Friday, 7th June 1968

Kafka

Few hours sleep last night; much thought, much discomfort, little rest. If only one could record revelations of thought and digression as one enacted them well, sometimes, anyway. I concluded Kafka's *Metamorphosis,* late last night. An excellent insight to a state of hysteria, and the absolute animal-state it can reduce one to. As Sara, who too had read it, and I agreed — his self-inflicted condition, appears a direct escape from his ever-demanding family and 'Chief', and the debts and guilt of responsibility laid on his being. Kafka's style is uncanny, unlike any I've read before. Since beginning Sartre's *Nausea*, I've read an old *Playboy* magazine [8]... his philosophy and literature now constantly amid my thoughts. I should like to peruse, in depth, some references I have underlined. Most speak for themselves. From *Nausea* [9]:

> 'All these characters spend their time explaining themselves and happily recognizing that they hold the same opinions. Good God, how important they consider it to think the same things all together.'

Can Terry

Egotism. Adoring others, who agree with one's own superior opinions. Abhorring those who feign disagree. And worse, expound their own — ignorance... On reading Sartre's quote, I remembered an incident last week on Saturday night, a couple of hours before departing on leave. Terry, one young patient on our locked ward, is a very disturbed twenty-six year old schizophrenic. A week or two back, I had only just come on this locked-ward when in, what I thought sympathy, I struck a chord with him. At least I thought I had. For nearly two hours, Terry and I talked together. He talked, I listened. At the outcome, he made known to me his pleasure, that I *appeared* to understand his theories. The same deluded convictions that admitted him to Hospital seven years ago, amongst other anti-social actions. For two weeks afterward, I was on good terms with this often potentially aggressive young man. Beliefs superior-opinions, and his outrage at the idiocy of television nonsense. It was a television show, that sparked Terry off and made him *high.* Shortly after, I as 'someone-who-understands-me' (his words) was approached.

As the hours followed his behaviour worsened, and he got more and more frustrated. *Why* didn't *anyone* comprehend? After all, it's all *so-easy* – he lamented. I must admit, that I was really scared for a while. When he went *up-the-stick,* he smashed windows and attacked other people with flailed fists, legs and body. Thanks to the moral presence of Dougie, the Charge Nurse, things were *just* kept in check. Eventually, we managed to divert his aggressive thoughts by nodding agreement and gently leading him away from the presence of the other patients, who felt quite threatened by Can Terry's *physical* presence. It was a sad, frightening encounter. The anecdote vividly brought to mind Sartre's quote. True an extreme case. But still one based on the human tendency to want everyone to agree to one's own superiority:

> 'Objects ought not to touch, since they are not alive ... a sort of nausea in the hands.'

Said Sartre.[10]

Philosophy

Sartre experienced an opposite to conclusions of Gurdjieff and Ouspensky. The latter two advocated *all* named objects as individual by the state of their own existence — *but* remain, integrated as part of The Whole.... and identified by their Heideggar named uses; a place coded in a consensus language strata. But, this does *not* describe feelings of alienation (alienation — aka nausea). I agree with George Gurdjieff and Peter Ouspensky. For me, not *Nausea;* but pleasure! The wonder and pleasure of holding, and then concentrating on, an object in an unknown, in words, physical communion with its portion of divine universality.

Apathy, rank indifference, boredom, man's worst enemy from my limited experience. That is *after* striving to maintain existence; post Survival, much of Sartre's philosophy in *Nausea* on inanimate objects, I viewed as truisms. But only if one deliberately blinkered oneself, from that which is common to mankind. He *alienated*, or appeared at first reading to do so; isolated the human component as but an abstract idea; *not-real*; unreal; surreal. Thus, the body alone may become repulsive following this de-personalization.

> '... and the varnish melts, nothing is left but a pale streak on a piece of wood. And everything is like that, everything, even my hands.' [11]

Sans feelings. Sans humanity.

Roquentin, or rather Sartre, is of the opinion (in his novel) that if a future is predictable, fated - then it is worthless because of this fact. Always the gloom and shadow, seldom any gold or warmth. Exit, experience of both pain and pleasure - or is it. Why this attitude. When ' *... nothing is left but words ...*'[12]

Depersonalisation

De-personalisation complete; de-civilising; regressing. ... Sartre rightly, realised the dependence of, mankind - *on words* - and, decried those words ... or did he - my naïvetè, in retrospect shows up clearly in these early responses. Roquentin appears to have lost himself and was not prepared to enquire into his positive potentialities as a thinking being. ... Rather isolated himself in self-pity ... Later on in this marvellous short philosophical novel Sartre admits to that unit named happiness:

> 'I am happy as the hero of a novel ... you feel that time is passing, that each moment leads to another moment ... that each moment destroys itself and it's no use trying to hold back ...'[13]

Heraclitus' state of 'flux'; and, that hoary chestnut, 'time-waits-for-no-man'. For Sartre, again, it is fate. Man has little to say in the matter... back to Rollebon on whom Roquentin is composing a potted history. The human Saint, who dares to pass urine and faeces. The human Hero, that desires someone else's wife. A god (not God), that shows a human trait. The Professional Man, who momentarily loses his dignity. Mother, Father, Son, Daughter, Husband, Wife. Human history appears to prove, that in the eyes of the one of the the-other, no-one is allowed to 'err... an icon is an icon is...' T.S. Eliot, Neitzche and Koestler were three notables who sympathised with this fickleness of man. Later on, in *Nausea,* I found that Roquentin, too, finds things not up to his ideal 'Rollebon' and promptly decides to drop his history; clearly the historian did not feel comfortable — with a 'warts an' all' human being. It seemed odd to me, at first, through Sartre's *Age of Reason* and *Nausea* his so-called Heroes are anti-heroes — those for whom family life is repellent, all too binding. Not just different. Visited Chichester and cycled my way miles through the gorgeous evergreen. Lingered a while in the second-hand book shop, next to *Shippams*, the fish paste factory, and medieval raised city wall in East Street, Chichester; shop owned by one of the Meynell's.

Chesterton and Superman

I purchased a paperback, G.K. Chesterton *Essays on Orthodoxy,* which writings I found optimistic and most inspiring. An answer to gloomy pessimism, of a dead-end blinkered materialism, God Is Dead — e'en as a metaphor, as to our origin and destinations; and that there really is nothing else, (viz those deluded humans who know everything - *really* ?) being the be-all-and-end-all, ultimate, end of man's doctrines. From Chesterton [14]:

> '... *Even* the wildest poetry of insanity can only be enjoyed by the sane. To the insane man his insanity is quite prosaic, because it is quite true ... Oddities only strike ordinary people. Oddities do not strike odd people. This is why ordinary people have a much more exciting time; while odd people are always complaining of the dullness of life ...'

Saturday, 8th June 1968

I imagined Chesterton in an *imaginary* reply to Sartre about Heroes and Supermen:

> '... Who thought that men would get on if they believed in themselves, those seekers after the Superman who are always looking for him in the looking-glass, ... all those people have really only an inch between them and this awful emptiness, ...' [15]

Stating the obvious, I feel, that there is an *infinite* quantum of knowledge 'we-do-not-know' *albeit* ... 'will *never* know'... *as homo sapiens*. I am often confounded when a personality, in one of the Sciences, or politicians, makes a new discovery and then declares, at last, that *they* have realised *the* secret (previously unknown) of *the* universe. Such arrogance.

Sunday, 9th June 1968

A beautiful hot sunny day. One of those days, when only the continual harassment of 'four' hectic young contesting, demanding, fighting, screaming, crying, hurt; lovable children; could at times colour the air. I took the oldest two boys, our eldest Paul and his cousin Mark, into the woods with me, armed with my newly sharpened axe, to gather the daily collection of deadwood for our kitchen's Rayburn boiler. And, air... 'Mm'm!' delicious, it clears my head of all and any maladies, a treatment I often apply when in need of 'cleansing'. Wild life, too, is in much abundance. I have seen pheasants, rabbits, hares, rats, stoats and even a stray doe deer from the larger woods at West Dean. The country has many advantages, moving direct from London — but I still miss London.

Today, I avoided reading, thinking, writing or discussing any of the P's... Psychology, Philosophy, Psychiatry. Instead, my relaxed reading, when possible, was Len Deighton's *Billion Dollar Brain*[16]; a light-weight thriller with his usual two-sided view of Russia, America and Britain, that Deighton's literary force can relate so well. Deighton promoted the right sort of interest and sympathies, so much needed perhaps these days when nations *hopefully* strive to move closer together. I'm due, now, to start my mandatory minimum of three months *Night Duty*. I suspect this will be of mixed blessings, as I must also continue additional daytime overtime shifts, essential school days attendances. And, full night duty; how will it influence my domestic life.?

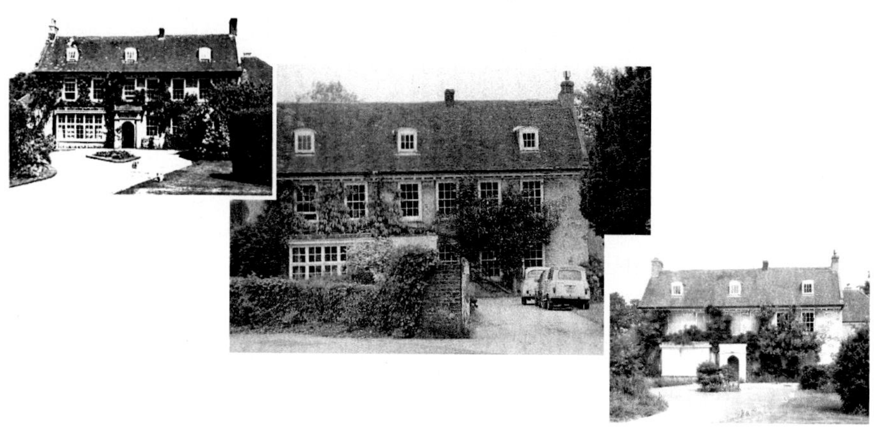

Graylingwell Farmhouse, home to the Sewell family, 1853 - 1857. **Top left**, private residence of farm bailiff, Mr Peacock, and family, in 1909; **centre**, as a day hospital, in the 1970s and early eighties; **bottom right**, closed down in late 1980s — now a listed building.

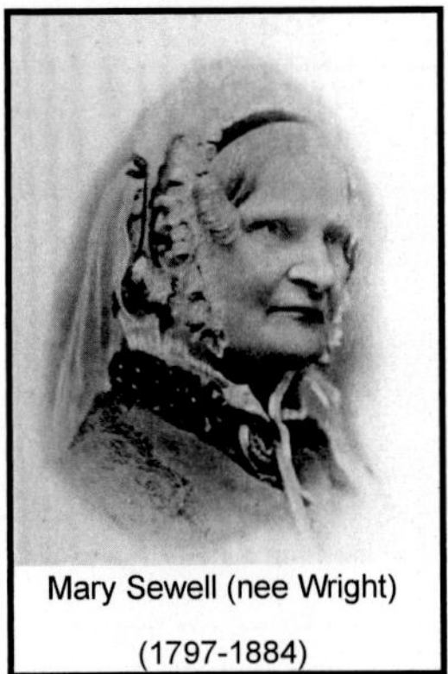

Mary Sewell (nee Wright)

(1797-1884)

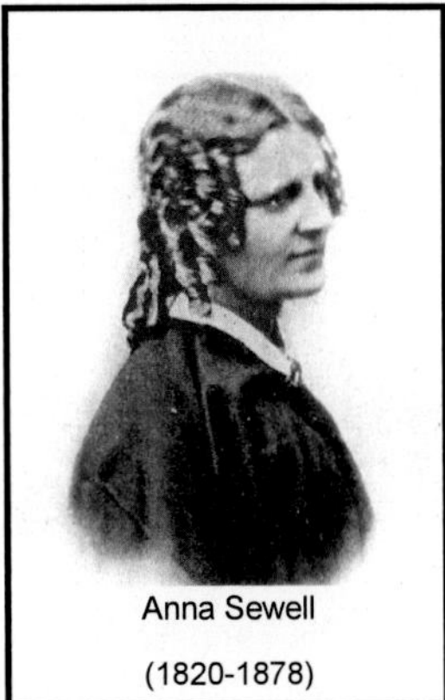

Anna Sewell

(1820-1878)

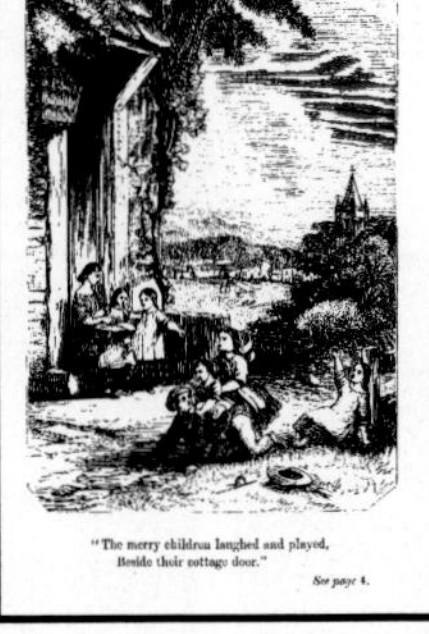

"The merry children laughed and played,
Beside their cottage door."

See page 4.

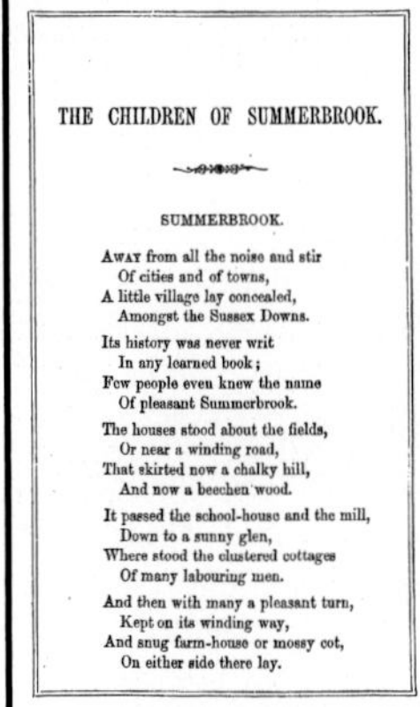

THE CHILDREN OF SUMMERBROOK.

SUMMERBROOK.

AWAY from all the noise and stir
Of cities and of towns,
A little village lay concealed,
Amongst the Sussex Downs.

Its history was never writ
In any learned book;
Few people even knew the name
Of pleasant Summerbrook.

The houses stood about the fields,
Or near a winding road,
That skirted now a chalky hill,
And now a beechen wood.

It passed the school-house and the mill,
Down to a sunny glen,
Where stood the clustered cottages
Of many labouring men.

And then with many a pleasant turn,
Kept on its winding way,
And snug farm-house or mossy cot,
On either side there lay.

First published 1859

Pictures from Bayly; Jarrold.

(1884 ed.)

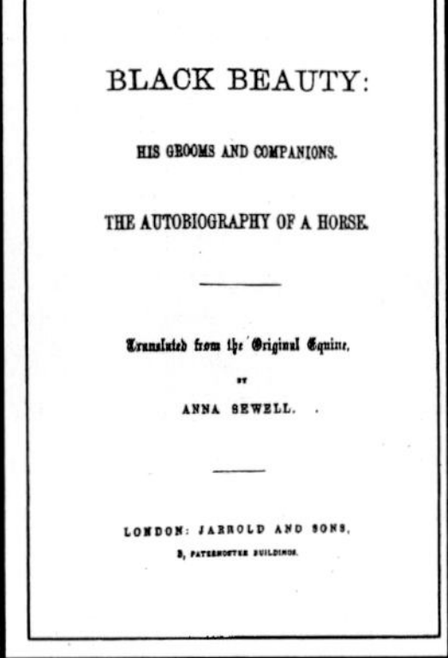

BLACK BEAUTY:

HIS GROOMS AND COMPANIONS.

THE AUTOBIOGRAPHY OF A HORSE.

Translated from the Original Equine,

BY

ANNA SEWELL.

LONDON: JARROLD AND SONS,
3, PATERNOSTER BUILDINGS.

First published 1878

Anna Sewell, borm 1820 in Yarmouth — The Sewells, afterward, moved down to London and, later, to Sussex — Brighton, Lancing, Haywards Heath and then to Grayling Wells, Chichester on October 1853, where they stayed until 1858 — hence, westward, to Bristol and Bath. Anna's mother, Mary Sewell, published, in 1859, a collection of verses, written for young persons, called Summerbrook. The first page, shown above, apparently describes Grayling Wells farmhouse, in rural, 1850s Summersdale (Near Chichester), in the river Lavant valley, near Binderton. Lavant village had a mill way back to Saxon times; this recorded in the Norman Domesday book.... Hospital staff regularly took groups of patients for walks about this same lovely countryside previously frequented by the Sewell family.

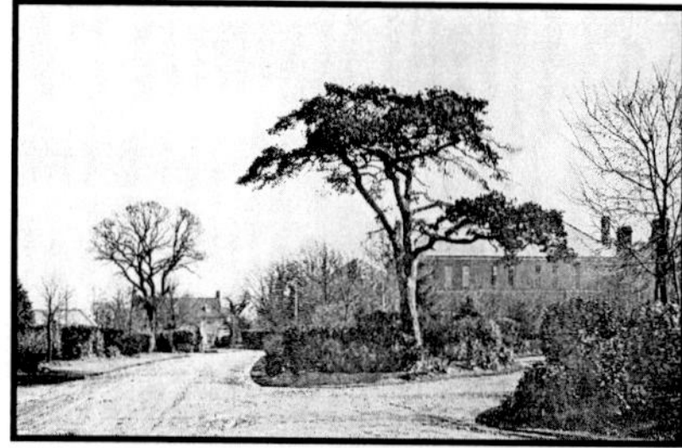

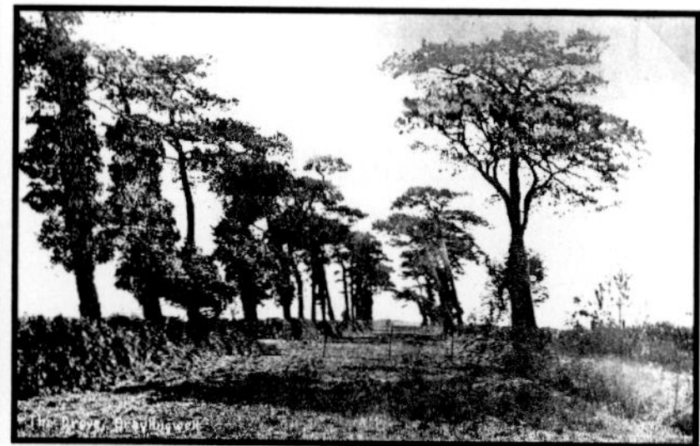

1909. The Farm Road. At left end is the farmhouse. Photo taken from a 1909 brochure.

1909. The Drove. Running from the Yard of the Farmhouse, to the south. Photo taken from a 1909 brochure

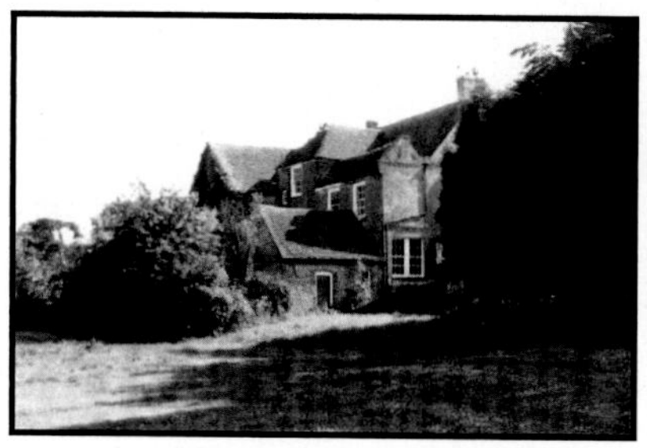

1980. Farmhouse rear. Showing how large the property is — or was. Photo by author.

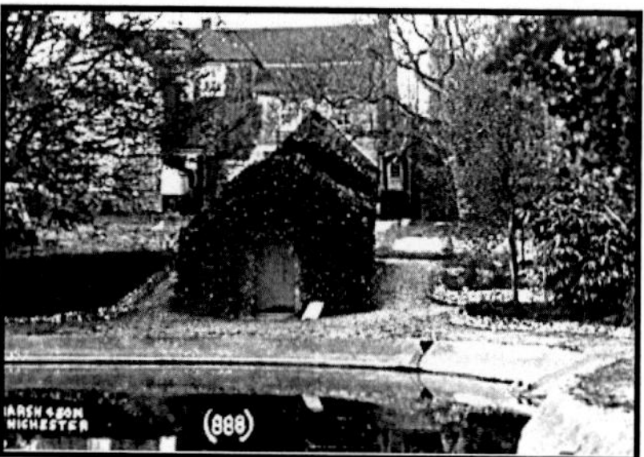

1915. The Grayling Well. Near the pond was a crab-apple tree; the pond filled in, during the 1960s.

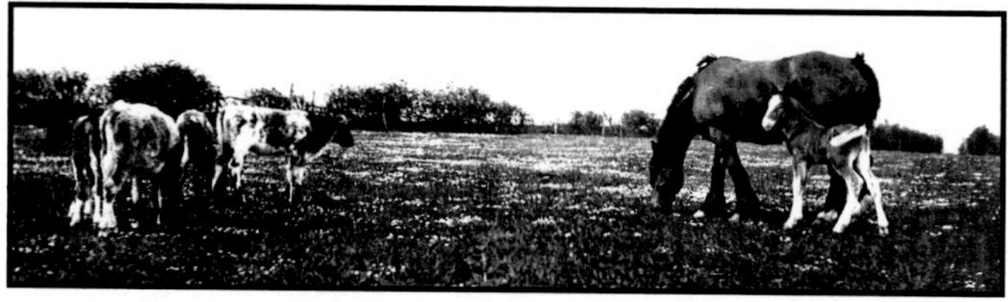

1950. One hundred years since the Sewells left; in a Graylingwell Farm meadow, cows and horses were kept. The farm was closed, and the stock sold, in 1957. Photo courtesy of the Green (Brown) family.

Chapter Seven
Night Duty

' Not the power to remember, but its very opposite, the power to forget, is a necessary condition of our existence. If the lore of the transmigration of souls is a true one, then these, between their exchange of bodies, must pass through the sea of forgetfulness.' [1]
Sholem Asch. 1939.

24th June 1968 to 1st October 1968
Night Duty—Night Thoughts—Mysticism—Gradgrind—Surreal—Rehab—Physicist John—On Patrol—Richmond Villa—Memories, The Time Paradox—Dreams—When is Real?—Can Terry—Experiment—Nothingness—Insidious Death—Fragile Beings, Robb & others—Commentaries—Faust—Refractory—Deja Vu—An Experience—Stress—Atavist—Admission—Ghost—NUPE Mike—Flies—Fechner—Existential Dave—Drug is a drug—Psychology

Night Thoughts
My maternal grandmother, *Beatrice Sarah Manton* (nee Ayres nee Wilson (1889-1968), *Beat),* was born in Eighteen-eighty-nine, as were, in that natal year, playwright and poet Jean Cocteau and stage and screen comedian Charles Chaplin; the latter both performers, geniuses of their art. By pure chance, Chaplin and Cocteau met between the two world-wars, half-way-round-the-world on May 11th 1936: 'on board the Japanese tramp steamer *Karoa* plying between Hong Kong and Shanghai, on the China seas.' Cocteau could speak no English... Chaplin could not converse in French. Fortunately, the latter had a secretary with enough French to be able to render translation. Afterwards, both artistes wrote of this meeting of the two Masters. Cocteau In an autobiographical account of his Jules Verne-like *Round The World Again In 80 Days.* [2] And. Almost thirty-years later. Written in comic genius Chaplin's *My Autobiography* [3], Chaplin recalled that their French interpreter, who spoke unemotionally, (had said to Chaplin) 'Mr Cocteau, he say, *You are a poet of zer sunshine,* and *he is a poet of zer night.'*

The Night is an oft used metaphor, in the language of art[4], by film-makers, musicians, poets and painters, to light-up insight into *dark,* mostly unrecognised, regions of the inner psyche (a generic term, like *ether,* for unseen and unknown content of an apparent vacuum — within inner and outer space). Cocteau, in an 1959 interview, which was later published in *The Paris Review* of 1967, [5] said: '*Art is a marriage of the conscious and the unconscious.*'

And so... in writings about Night Thoughts and any artistic compound, made out of Freudian Dreams, I believed all human beings, in addition to fulfilling innate complex instincts to eat and gratify bodily needs, also *experience* a plethora of *emotional* needs to 'think and feel' and, above all, the crucial need to be able to *think* and express freely for oneself, and not always be bound by others. And, if *not* free, there *might* well be problems. Three months compulsory Night Duty provided an abundance of *new* thoughts, and unexpected meetings, some confrontations, which in time I would translate and link up with threads of past of legion others; especially day and night thoughts among our patients.

Tuesday, 25th June 1968

In the hospital nine-months as first-year student, I was detailed *Night-Duty*. Initially, base on most nights was Lister Ward (The Sick Ward), with the Senior Staff Nurse on night-duty. Duties varied, most nights in set-routines; including essential fire-piquet patrols.

Each night, emphasis was on helping-out, in giving-out suppers and night-medication, helping patients to bed, assisting on any New Admission and being called-out to Emergencies. Routine was to assist other night-nurses on ward rounds — changing dressings and any wet and dirty patients, and opening up ward-kitchens for patients going out to work, or to lay breakfast tables on unstaffed night wards. Early morning included helping out in getting patients up, dressed, and beds changed and made-up, if possible, by the morning handover.

Last duty. each night early morning, was to visit every male ward and collect their night-reports, and deliver them to the Night Superintendent, or other Senior Nurse in charge at *The Office*. I was unused to night-duties and underestimated its effects on my domestic life, physiology and in timing on my mental development. To remain true to myself, I had to frequently examine what I was doing, the circumstances and surroundings I was working within; and to enlarge my reading (separate from formal study reading). Where possible, I decided to experiment (never, *never* with any drugs) when viable on myself; and write-up such self-observation. Unfortunately, my amateur literary style at times would show as a regrettable handicap.

Whilst the purpose in being a student Registered Mental Nurse was to study and practice grounding in psychiatric (and psychology) nursing, for me it also demanded an exploration of what (and whys) many of our patients express, in verbal and non-verbal communications... intangible subjectivity.... on sensing, seeing, hearing, feeling, and attempting to identify... ghosts, gods, demons and, aspects of joy and despair.... during *their* days and nights.

And, of encountering other beings, other *human* beings, in their *other* worlds, and of what physiological effects may (and do) do to the 'inner' and 'outer' worlds of patients when chemical norms are interfered with, by prescription or abuse? Also, topically, existential enquiries relating to others; myself, my inner-space, and worlds; out there? Sartre in 1947 [6], declared he was 'atheistic.' and said: 'It is impossible for man to transcend human subjectivity.' At this time, in 1968, I compared Sartre' with Wilson's[7] writings, which ask the kind of questions that were once regarded as Religious; questions about *The Meaning* of human existence (and), of God.

I found psychologist William James[8] had explored both belief systems, the atheist (Nothingness — '*the beyond*') and religious (God the creator and destroyer)... and combined them; observing, but frail portions, of porous skin contained inner-and-outer worlds of *living* creatures. Every creature is part of 'all and everything', known and unknown. Forty years on, collating my notes, at 70, I discovered Dr. Darold. A. Treffert's monumental book called *Extraordinary People* [9] which affected me, just as Professor Will James *Principles of Psychology* [10] had done in 1968. We are still but embryos. Yet to explore what is potentially human. All we seem to look at is our shell. I knew I was, at most, *only* scratching at the hollow surface *of things,* like a Darwin chimpanzee exploring its body for fleas. Just scratching at the surface; curiosity was already a permanent, *living* itch.

Monday, 24th June 1968
Mysticism

Last night commenced night-duty at the hospital; first shift was from eight-fifty-five pm to seven am the next morning; started on the Chilgrove block long-stay wards and moved on to Lister male sick ward.

For light-reading (home and time-out at work), I completed Rider Haggard's *The People of the Mist*[11], a pattern of Jung's archetypal mythological symbols; and finished *Orthodoxy* by G.K. Chesterton[12]. I was impressed with Chesterton's commentary on *Ethics, Morals and Paradoxes in Christianity*; his analysis applied to all world religions; which faiths seem based on written down *inflexible* human dogma. I was confounded that, on *forensic* evidence, most inflamed wars between humans and humans, were on behalf of their own particular 'brand name'; and evoke most vicious bloodletting, between sects and schisms, seem *within* their own designated faith edicts that were cast in stone. Surely contradicting the *real* goodness written, *within* their own Holy Books?

I began a work, helpful as a philosophical buffer, in the oft stress laden work of the years ahead. It was *A New Model of the Universe* by P.D. Ouspensky[13]. In 1966, only months before entering the hospital, I had been mesmerised by Russian Ouspensky's 1922 *Tertium Organum;* an update of Roger Bacon's 13th century *Opus Tertium.*[14]

The above writers indicated... 'Whatever we are' and 'wherever we come from', and in death, as spirits 'in flesh depart'. The Master! The Mistress!, we're not - Not! Are we not but global robots (or puppets) examining our allocated half-life molecules? Back, in the Night-time, to the moment when the first hypothetical man and woman, *Adam and Eve*, issued from whatever Laboratory appeared on Earth. Mankind made a mistake; according to Tradition. He thought, by himself, he could guide and direct his life without any help from 'the outside'. Ouspensky's early utterings, on *The Fall and Mysticism,* are about subjectivity; human emotion. He said [15]:

> 'Mysticism is entirely emotional, entirely made up of subtle, incommunicable sensations, which are even more incapable of verbal expression and logical definition than are such things as sound and colour and line.'

In between shifts.... back to concrete reality. Our portable Dansette record player was on; the small radio turned off, its batteries dead; no shillings-and-pence to replace them, and no television. Rachmaninov's vinyl *Concerto No. 2,* a favourite of mine, was being played. Upstairs, both boys were happily asleep. I returned for a while to study Ouspensky.... very tired.... Tomorrow *must* read up on Psychiatry! And work.

Mysticism and the Fall, of man's innocence and sin... who, what defines? Surely, such dialogue must always be subjective, and not scientific, according to a, seeming, blind Establishment. My head was full of raw dialogue, as I put the alchemical work aside and retired to bed. Up to bed, fifteen minutes of Arthur Koestler's *Spanish Testament* [16], and bliss of a fashion. Sara downstairs, typing contentedly away on a short story. Psychiatry is about healing sick minds, and I am learning about this field. Ouspensky, esoteric, exotic, and physick, continued to be, for me, a useful catalyst. A counter, amidst all hospital work. Mental and physical, living, working, midst zombie death, disorder; hope and resurrection....

Tuesday, 25th June 1968
Gradgrind

For the past few days there has been nothing but gales, and rain, rain, rain, rain! Last night was my first night at home, since beginning night duty. I have had little sleep and little rest. The boys, both of them, got us up during the night. Result; I am over-sensitive, over-tired and short-tempered. Presently, Sara and boys are out, dressed up; *out*, in all this stinking rain! I'm trying to catch up with some rest, but being blasted by noisy blue-bottle flies.

I curse the flies. Their Beelzebub loud buzzing assaults my searching temporary peace of mind, as they so often do. Curse them; The Flies. What can I do? Tired. And angry with myself for being tired and bad tempered. Yes, Yes, Yes, I know; subjective emotion is the key to human self-control, for and against. Nothing mystical about that. Family returns, the gates outside close.

Rain! The Strain remains but all else, this time, resolved. The boys, bless them, are laying down for a kip, much needed since they were awake so early. I Resume (consume) reading. Sartre's written answer to the Philosophy of Andre Gide[17], found in *Playboy* of May 1965[18], copy from a patient on Amberley; Spider. An article on Sartre and, topical, R.D. Laing; on anti-psychiatry. One Dickensian notion bubbles to mind, as Sartre quoted in the aforementioned magazine interview:

> 'I can wonder if it wouldn't be rewarding to act like Gide's character.' (Surrender to sensual joys - search for God in everything.) 'But advice of that sort is lost on a worker who does eight hours on an assembly line. He's tired out. How can one tell him to go out and ransack the universe for sensations when he has been stupefied by a day of brain deadening, brutalizing labour?'

Chesterton on complementing Sartre (I imagined) in his *Orthodoxy* [19] said, he felt that:

> '...true philosophy is concerned with the instant. '

I am too tired to continue any more Commentary on Sartre's seminal *Nausea*[20]; or anything else. This afternoon, shortly, I will again be up, and cycle through this monsoon rain to the hospital, for *another* overtime shift.

Surreal

Back. Night-time. Close to midnight at home. I recalled I'd been on an overtime shift, on a long-stay back ward. On return home, cycling back from Chichester, up through the so-green South Downs, to here at Stonerock Cottage in Chilgrove, surreal thoughts pass through my biological brain and its visceral vehicle. All inner visualised thoughts, perceptions, and concepts are active, *as I live,* in this earth molecular instance. Last evening, a young patient I helped on Amberley, four to five months ago, approached me. Dave was taken ill during his first year at Manchester University. I recall, when I first arrived on the Admission Ward, he was sat down deep down in depression, trying hard to concentrate on one of Kafka's works. We talked. I noticed all his readings were mostly on nihilistic, pessimistic philosophies. Dave was fascinated by Kafka and Sartre; and well read on Kierkegaard and Heideggar's works. He showed interest in Hesse, Ouspensky and Gurdjieff' and collective Universality; perhaps, more optimistic philosophies, a new Pandora's box?

Early evening, Dave appeared on the ward on which I was working. He was feeling depressed and wanted to lift his spirits. His object was to ask my opinion on some poetry he had written. 'Dave', I said, 'This is much better than a few months ago.' Eventually, he persuaded me to borrow two books off him, *Existentialism as Philosophy* by Fernando Molina[21], a study on Sartre, Neitzche, Kierkegaard, Heideggar and Husserl, and *Six Existentialist Thinkers,* by H.J. Blackham[22]. Both books were much scored and clearly well tattered in being, heavily read by him. I promised to read both books, before returning them. (Dave later, after his discharge, sent the books back to me, to keep as a gift; in thanks for my passing support.)

Treatises, of academy philosophers written works, run to many hundreds of pages; a collective, thick, jungle of *thousands* of pages, most of which are central to the examination of being; about nothing (yet everything), about human existence, relating to itself and everything, and Nothing-ness? There is no way I can presently (or near future) have time to read and digest all such demanding heavy tomes. I was, already, a compulsive bibliophile mostly dipping into 'whatever' out of raw curiosity and, long ago, recognised it was the *only* pathway for me to enjoy any communion with learned authors (it could only be one-sided; and my influency of any other language, except a number of French and Latin words internally fossilised from early grammar school days). And so, aided by Book Titles, Tables of Contents, Indexes and glossaries (especially with time locked First Editions; with annondations, and information in original context.)

And so, delighted, I later purchased two second-hand hardbacks. One, *Being and Nothingness* by Jean Paul Sartre [23] and the Second, *Being And Time* by Martin Heideggar.[24] The latter looked as if had been owned by a student in philosophy as the item was a little biro-scored and annondated by him (inscribed on flyleaf by a William ... in 1969); these scored additions would normally be commercially disastrous, thus cheaper, but for me they were a blessing, a bonus, as these helped initial (discuss) dippings, and provided several (discuss - argue) leads into foreign Heideggar's wordy labyrinth. And helped me to thread a labyrinth way, into non-sensual realities, that *must* exist as in the realms of science-fiction writers; about, eternal nothing-ness, paradoxically to imagine, formalise 'whatever' is presently out-of-bounds to mortal beings; in our time.

Cycling, mechanical pedalling away, I scanned the Sussex countryside in travelling home but, with a little *more* so than usual. I *added* a new Summary of thoughts in my transport. Looking across at a horizon of numerous anonymous trees (it was a clear but windy night — ouch!), waving well-decked branches from side-to-side like octopus tentacles. Gazing at the hill in which they were thickly rooted, I became *aware* that although I perceived the beautiful symmetrical greenery, as they faded and disappeared slowly dropping into the black shadow of the night, I thought....

'S' funny, they are all ... *its all'*, seen yet unseen, balanced, molecular whirling atoms, nuclei. But, built like live polyps, for they are; *it's all alive* - in some form or another; all around me... *Everything is alive...* mobile, as Ouspensky described so vividly.

More. And I withdrew into my egg-shaped shell (as then I envisaged my head).

All me, I, my body, is just like that, those same nuclei polyps...

I tried so hard to be *aware* of everything outside myself, and therefore isolate my seed of being from its tentacles, antennae of perception and sensations... *not to be.* I felt a physical pressure where, I believed, is my seat of emotions.... the frontal lobes of my brain. And I registered a definite holding back of emotional sensations. On realizing this attempt at a greater natural awareness (cycling mechanically all the while), an immense feeling of relief, momentary well-being, as if a headache was removed; and, once more, I in my body became but a traveller. It was unique, for me. Noise, without doubt, is the one sensation that singularly rapes my brain's awareness, when attempting peace or concentration in any form. I'm on double-shift (fourteen hours) tomorrow, I don't know on what wards. I'm continuing, where possible, a Pelican Original paperback *New Horizons in Psychiatry* by Peter Hays, for study. [25]

Wednesday, 26th June 1968
Rehab

It continued dark and cloudy; rained all the way to work, even harder on the way back. A long day, six-thirty in the morning to seven o'clock in the evening, all that day spent assisting a Charge Nurse on Cavell One, a new Rehabilitation Ward. Cavell was located on the still, otherwise, tabooed Female Side of the hospital. I'll not enlarge on first impressions, as they could only be first observations. I'll wait until experience allows me to comment. Suffice it to say that only 'one' Nurse would invariably be at the helm here, with forty-eight patients, I looked, listened and reassured.

I learnt of Assessment Tests (a fair number), which were to be used on this new Rehab ward, and how patients were to be coaxed towards being moved back into outside society, with self-assurance. This major move was certainly part of the de-institutionalisation (aka institutional neuroses) of our long-stay residents. This new rehab term was certainly influenced by Dr. Russell Barton's seminal 1959 *Institutional Neurosis,*[26] and the pioneer work of Graylingwell's own Dr. Joshua Carse's *Worthing Experiment.*[27]

The reason why I was asked to help, was that long stay patients were moving into a new ward, from the dormitory ward of what was part of Chilgrove One; they included burnt out Barney, Mensa Charles, and epileptic aide John. With these and other patients to assist me, we moved dozens of old tables, cupboards, case-note folios, baggage, clothes, kitchenware, etc. etc. I was introduced favourably to a number of no-name patients. But, as I was already acquainted with most of them, having worked on Chilgrove One and Two wards, the task felt like helping out friendly neighbours. All these new FC1 patients had moved into their, new home by the following day, and marked the end of an era.

On return home, Sara gaily informed me that she had been out in the potato fields, gathering new spuds into sacks. To my amazement, I learnt that here the rain held off till she had finished; seven hours, she worked. It appears that, early this morning, a local farmer called and asked if she would like to help in the fields; she jumped at the opportunity. The boys, it seemed, played happily around her and loved the mobile tractor turning up the earth. Too tired. Too late for any discourse. Well, another day over. Tomorrow another School study day at the hospital.

Thursday, 27th June 1968

Evening, and it was still raining. Rain, all the way to work, with a strong gale force wind; and, it rained again all the way back. Earlier that day, Sara had had to clear the front room up from falling soot. First impression, on arriving 'home', was the mess; flipping black, ugly black soot. Yet another solid fall, due to the rain... Sara's back ached. The boys had been very good. I played with them, briefly, before they went to sleep, a happy, quiet, sleep which soon overtook them. How my heart reached out to them, as they had giggled so chirpily, and again, a little later, when I had looked down at them, then fast asleep.

Nothing special, to record this day, with regard to private study, on which to comment. But... an interesting conversation on basic biology at work, with Harry from Ghana and our tutor. The talk originated just before tea break, when our tutor, Mr Ilford, sat down to chat to us. Something he said about *age,* started us off. 'Tell me, is it true, what some textbooks infer, that the 'entire' human body is totally changed over a period of seven years...?', I asked Mr Ilford. 'You mean the cellular structure?', he replied. 'Yes, all of it,' I said. 'Every bone, fibre, skin, and blood cell...?' Mr Ilford looked for a reference book; we three were seated in the Training School Library. 'Ah, here it is; let me see. Somewhere... here... there is a case....'

He had a little trouble in finding the reference, then pulled out one book off of the top library shelf and said, 'Ah, here we are. Well, anyway. If a man is deliberately held back from eating proteins for whatever reason or other...'. Mr Ilford then quoted clinical data, on Nephritis, or similar complaint and, in a gravitas tone, continued as a matter-of-fact: 'He wraps patient in a blanket to sweat it out of him...'. He read on. 'They found that, despite the fact that no proteins have been administered, protein waste products were *still* being excreted by the kidneys.'

I thought, is this what happens in starvation as the body begins to decay, as the brain and breath yet survive, while the will is sapped; blood drawn out like rubber tapped from a tree. Sort of implosion — mechanical eating of itself to stay alive... invisible to disappear like a Kekule snake up its own... and, in its spiral, is re-born as a phoenix. 'That the body is breaking itself down.... erosion....' Mr Ilford had our drift and completed the quotation.

But... Harry and I felt we had *not* really got The Answer. I commented, 'We were thinking of the ketone bodies?... Well, That... Yes, Mr Ilford, that's the sort of thing I mean... but *all* the body?' 'I'm not sure about the bones and tendons.' He said. 'But, it's basic biology, as you know, that all *living* bodies appear to be constantly creating, building up and, in keeping the bodies' status-quo, destroying older tissue by Anabolism and Katabolism.... the state in flux of the body...' Our tutor was called away, before we could complete our teatime exchange. Harry and I decided to continue the debate, asking questions of each other, more metaphysic and philosophical than somatic. And this was a tea-break, or smoke-break, for those who indulged (Harry and I did not).

Although Summer mid-afternoon, it was dark outside, (we had the lights on). Outside, a curtain of trees shook invisible, long-arms into the room and seemed to scratch like harpies upon the blackboard; as wind driven rain finger-tips dripped hieroglyphs upon our school window panes. Harry suggested a searching question. 'Barry, what do *you* think of Ghosts and the like?' Interesting, I thought. 'Ghosts?... Water shapes, that leak through brick walls, window panes and re-assemble, the other side?' 'Right!', he said. And, into it, I replied, 'Well. I like Leonardo da Vinci's introduction amongst his notes, Harry. If it's truly a Ghost, Spirit or Angel, then it's impossible for them to be seen *in their own shape* by us, unless interpreted by some terrestrial medium, and yes, yes; I believe a person can be possessed, in, erm, some way.', and I paused.

'Are you acquainted with Dr. Samuel Johnson, *the man* who put together the English Dictionary...?' 'Yes...' Harry's face wrinkled anticipation. 'Well, his friend Boswell asked Johnson *that* same question; he said: 'We talked of belief in Ghosts.' And Johnson replied (think I've got it right):

> '..."Sir, I make a distinction between what a man may experience by the mere strength of his imagination, and what imagination cannot possibly produce."...'[28]

'What do *you* think, Harry?' He looked at me as if at a mirror, and replied, *'I don't know;* books I've read don't discuss enough on neuroses and the electric, nervous system, since they only appear to define present and *physical* definition of *it,* the body... I am?' Still intense, my Ghanaian friend continued. 'Back home, most of us believe in a sort of holy ghost, whether we are Christian, Islam, or what. And, Barry, *I believe* in One spirit, as me, as a sort of ghost in my body. You know... What we, we were talking to Mr Ilford about, I don't think this is necessarily the invisible ghost, as a separate, *you know,* discarnate apparition?... Do you ?' Thinking about our patients, I hesitated. 'Well, yes, no, but...'

Earlier, we'd discussed in the classroom what some patients described as ghosts, angels, devils, even succubi that may have sexually assaulted them in the night time; David on Amberley was one acute patient. It was then diagnosed as but a hallucination, a dream within a dream, as I recalled... there was also the obvious, numerous, hallucinatory experiences, of countless others, to consider. What, again, is one to perceive as real, surreal, occult, or but a distortion of the senses...?

'Can we inhabit; can we, as a so-called ghost, or other spirit or, or other form be in, or be morphed from *Another World*?' I was trying to admit to my ignorance on the topic; and keep to our, implicit, integrity... (I had read a little on the philosophy of Physics and of other more esoteric works at this time.) 'Look across this room, and out of the window, *can you see the air*?' 'Well, no ...?', replied Harry in affirmation. And, I continued, questions *(not Answers)* we were then both affirming.

'Oh, you know it's there and you *breathe* it; but you had to *learn about it*, or *read it,* with perceptions?' I continued. 'And, metaphorically, allocate *it* a name. 'You seldom perceived or detected *it,* by your human I's senses. You had to deduce it or accept, believing it so, in integrity, in good faith. It's invisible. But can you deny its existence, just because you can't necessarily see, hear, feel, taste or touch it. *And what is breathing*?'

'Well of course not.', Harry agreed, well tuned in to our present thread. I continued, 'No, of course you don't! But is this not what most of us do. Unless their own senses can physically identify it, they will *not* recognize its existence; the air is but one example. There is much that we cannot sense; that we are unable to actually see, actually feel, actually smell, actually taste, sense and identify. The other day, I read something by Ouspensky; *emotion is a sense.*

We become *aware* by the emotions, of something, even though our other senses do not seem to detect it.'

'The emotions must be able to perceive,' I droned on, 'just as the eyes must be open to see: certain experiences are intelligible only in mystical states... viewed entirely by the emotions. Just as difficult to convey verbally, as *what* compound, colour really is; *in words*. Eh?' We paused. Harry blinked, as the wind noisily plucked the tip of a branch against the window. I said; 'Imagine our senses adjusted so that the air before us is rendered visible; *in its present state that is*. Then, naturally, this table, those chairs, yes, even you yourself, would be rendered invisible too (for others?), for you are in density as in 'air', remember.'

'Imagine, take this to infinity, to infinite dimensions, as worlds. Each one, a *scale* gauged by the capable, performance possible, by the human senses. Now I ask, on the same scale; *the same*...Why in its own state, shape or form, should not other live beings exist in their dimensions of sense equally as we are valid in ours? Just imagination?' [29]

'I'm not so sure, are you ...?'

There was another, meaningful, pause shared by us in a dyad. 'Could not so called djinns, spirits, angels, which after all are only agreed names, noises we make to designate and assign to the mostly un-knowable, Harry? Surely, such similar science fiction and factual entities exist in those worlds, *all in and about us at all times*? Artists and poets, using metaphors, appear to know of these threads, and revere more than fear; the unknown.'

'It's the inevitable lack of direct import that seems impossible to change: for us, me, to communicate, the *scale must* be changed — yes, new concepts, applied in chemistry and physics. But, once in transport, you have changed to view or communicate, you have killed or transformed the original... erm ... *or have you*? Is it only the observer and thus participant that changes, or, in a subtle way, both? You cannot be absolutely stationary and mobile at the same time, or can you? Can one penetrate, without destruction? I often imagine, visualise, Harry, our whole body as a matrix, potentially, expanding consciousness, into and transcending, even momentary, infinite dimensions. Sadly, we remain mostly only conscious in this *sensual* world, and indeed *only* of atomic Elements Table material, always buts...'

Round about this point, Mr Ilford returned, poked his head around the door, and hinted that our afternoon tea-break had rather over-run... and, our other colleagues had returned from their smoke-break, smoking outside the hut. About the time of talking of other worlds, I recall thinking it was *dogma* of many persons I knew, in an absolute dread denial (why?) of even the possibilities of unknown, other worlds. Here in the hospital, it seemed to be but a credible fiction, the province, only, of our disturbed patients....? We returned to the classroom to see an interesting film, called *Psychiatry and Art,* featuring children and creativity, its subject being Chaos; Base; Order....

Night work tomorrow. Detailed for the long-stay wards. Late shift. Ouspensky quoted [30] Mach's theory that:

> ' *a thing is only a complex of sensations.*'

Presumably, one-thing-leads-to-another. Philosopher John - Jean Paul Sartre's existential novel *Nausea* [31] seminal work was first published in French, between the wars, in 1938, entitled *La Nausee.* The first John Lehmann English translation, out in 1949, was titled *The Diary of Antoine Roquentin.*[32] But, it was the Penguin paperback, re-titled *Nausea* in 1965. This book was my personal *Rosetta Stone,* for introductory, existential, mental perambulations; and just why anti-psychiatry, as sanctuary, or imprisonment, was really *much* more than examining current methods of psychiatric treatment, in postwar Europe.

I realized that Ouspensky and Sartre appeared (to me) to be at one opposite pole to the other, in their philosophy; the former on a good life, the latter on angst and dread, and this belief would help to anchor me in my hospital day to day life. To legion Questions, but not, at all always, to answers. In good humour, I thought of Sartre's Roquentin, in his history, considering himself but *a thing;* and an unreal one at that. Was it, but yesterday or the day before, when cycling home, I *imagined*, or *really* perceived, everything I observed, in passing, as but nuclei atomic polyps; this the *so-called* limit of my so frail and narrow range of capabilities, my *reality*? We see, I see (understand in my mind's metaphoric eye) but the surface segments; even then, this and that surface is actually well gutted with holes (which we, I, don't see)!

This surface, being the lines, curves, colours, sounds, etc. etc. Ouspensky stated, rather well I think, that there is something perceived by us and our perceptive apparatus that sees, *in wonder*, the green of the trees, the blue of the skies and so on. Witness our *Ghost In the Machine* [33]... always, and in tandem, I pondered how many of my colleagues, and patients, experience *their* natural phenomena, on an every day to day existence?

To interpret Austrian physicist Mach literally, *man is but a thing,* would be but to deny *that they exist*, even though this existence needs far more definition. The colours (as Colin Wilson aptly described, the materialist measures colours as but, only, thicknesses in angstroms) are but seen, as *reflections* of the sun's rays. (We see what is lit up, but not what is a truer awareness, of what is behind the metaphoric sun — and I don't mean in norm distance) Ouspensky added that this is *much more* than a truism. In a way I am just starting to work on, Ouspensky suggested that *thought* itself is of the fourth dimension, since it passes all barriers by way of imagination; all walls of three dimensional time, and space, are bypassed... Just what *are* thoughts? What's that, as we prepare to go up to bed. *Man cannot live by thought alone?* Hmm! Food for thought; yuk, how juvenile.

Friday, 28th June 1968

Mid-morning. It's still raining hard, bloody hard; heavy wind blowing pounds of filthy black soot, down the chimney, into our Chilgrove front room. For a couple of hours before breakfast, the boys wouldn't eat (much to their mother's annoyance). I played with them. They had had far too many biscuits, as fillers since awakening... tut! tut! Shut in, kept in by the inclement weather, plenty of toning down and consoling needed, for infants Paul and Kit. The rain was not letting them out. They would quarrel over their toys. Inevitable, I guess. Roll on Summer sunshine. Before going on duty tonight, I must continue some substance on *Nausea*. Well, I've had breakfast. Now, with Paul, a toy lorry is broken; fixed it!

My recent studies on Sartre's philosophy, triggered a number of recent memories when, but two years ago, we'd lived in Teddington — opposite Bushey Park, nearby a Thames weir and King Henry the VIII's *Hampton Court Palace*, all places in walking distance from our rented home. Also, close by, was the National Physics Laboratory buildings and its staff; one of whom was our next door neighbour, a junior research scientist named John.

Physicist John

In 1966, before moving down into West Sussex from our short-time in Teddington, west of Central London, where I'd worked as a civvie at New Scotland Yard. Where Kit, our second son (who would study Physics at London University many years later), was born at 165 Park Road Teddington. Our next-door neighbour was John, a physicist, and his family. He worked at the local NP laboratory. I'd had a fascinating debate with John, who specialised in Laser and Maser rays. At the time, I made some notes in one of my numerous erratic red-notebooks (which I'd kept since, soon after being discharged from HM forces). My notes were on that debate, that was about words.... a debate on the value of Words.

(Words that Sartre had dismissed - but, used so well in *Nausea* - as unreal.)

I'd asked John to communicate, over the telephone, what a wooden chair was, to a person many miles away, without using The Word *chair*. Odd John was a devout believer in the absolute usage of Mathematics [34] as his language. That we talked, in the English language, appeared to have been bypassed by him. To me, it was an absurd *Alice in Wonderland* statement. He disowned the total value of words and all except, *per se,* mathematical symbols and any other use of metaphoric language. *Surely mathematics is a pure metaphorical language, on its own*? Now, in no way did I undervalue that wondrous world of maths; which certainly and sadly eludes me, and its kin, geometry. *But to eliminate words, well it was, to me, ridiculous...*

Lay boys down, for late morning rest. The rain was again descending in torrents, and the trees at the back of our small Chilgrove home leant as if, any moment, their backs would break. Trouble with this rain, was that it was difficult to gather fuel from the woods behind us, due to everything being so waterlogged. Oh well, it won't last forever... Memories. The debate continued... Physicist John insisted that *only* abstract metaphoric mathematics could describe any object *truthfully;* and not ambiguously to any stranger at any meeting; i.e. the *primary* communication to a lay individual, who is *not* mathematically minded. I challenged my neighbour, 'Imagine a man in Moscow you wished to talk to over the 'phone. You are to describe that object, that red seat, to your friend *without* ever using the meaningful words red, or seat?'. John attempted to describe it strictly in terms of dimensional space, symmetry and mathematical equations.

'All right!' my physicist neighbour declared, as the exchange began. Imagining sceptic myself, at the other end. So, after his description, given of course still in words, I concluded it was a cube, which exact size was first of all questionable, and any colour was impossible to diagnose. 'But your cube could be a dice, a television set, a box, anything; how do I know it's a seat for sitting on?' I challenged. 'That's my point', he replied, 'It's nothing but a cube.' Perplexed, I replied, 'Oh, I see.' I followed. 'You mean you *deliberately* discount all human words, shapes and analogies, because they are personal?'

'Of course, they're *not* real. This house is only a collection of bricks and mortar, etc.'

'But...', I was stunned. 'You mean you only accept, in finality, that the house is *no*t for human habitation at all; you deny its existence as such?' 'That's right!' he said, coldly confident. 'And your seat is but a cube ...?' 'That's right!' 'You insist, John, that this is your revolutionary universal language.... This mathematical breakdown?' 'Of course. It's better than millions of words.' 'But... but...?' I didn't really believe him. 'You must be totally *dependent* on the fact that, already, *all* your universal men and women are savants *well* versed in your common mathematical symbols. Your verbal equations. And, well *you, John,* can graphically draw those icons. How, *verbally,* do *you* communicate them to others...?'

I continued, 'What if you meet a primitive man, a man from outer space; an ordinary man like myself who does not comprehend your code? How do you *talk* to him, describe things, perhaps, way above his head?' John seemed dogmatic, rather than sure, of his answer on the value of words. And answered my plea, 'oh well; if you're going to bring the milkman into it. You can't expect everyone to be of the elite. It's a question of survival of the fittest.'

'Good God! I don't believe it,' I spluttered. This was out of his previous, unbiased, debate. Mortified, I asked for a precis. 'You believe *only* those who have already been schooled, primarily (and only) in maths, be addressed... no others...?'. John, a little subdued, answered, albeit reluctantly, 'Well if they're ignorant, as most of the masses are, they don't want to know about politics, economics, science and so on.'. Here, I thought of the over-specialisation that I had so often met, read, and heard of. He was not my Hero figure, of a survival by the futurist Supermen of technocrats! 'Well.' I concluded, disillusioned. 'I firmly believed that it was the common responsibility of so-called elite scientists and the like, like yourself, to communicate your scale to the populace in language; what is potentially with us....' It was about that time, as I recall, that the debate broke off for me to go back home. Next door, to Sara and some tea.

Friday, 28th June 1968

Here is a line from Judith Groch's fascinating work:[35]

> ' We use words and numbers' she says, ' to save ourselves the trouble of thinking about the objects and ideas they represent.'

I get one of our wooden chairs up to the kitchen table and join the boys for dinner. Damn this rain! Moments ago, I returned from collecting our milk from the churn, down at the end of our muddy farm road. Nice meal. Yell from kitchen, as I sat, reading, comfortably seated on the loo seat. 'Your sweet is ready....' Sartre [36] intrudes on my necessary task with words:

> *'... Words had disappeared, and with them the meaning of things, the methods of using them, the feeble landmarks which men have traced on their surface....'*

Roquentin, as Sartre, had found himself fast descending down into a realm of chaos. I thought, perhaps, like H.G. Wells's Mr Fotheringay in *The Man who could work Miracles* [37], believing, falsely, he had spontaneously (by wishing for the experience) found a route to The Source; he finds himself instead an unknown vacuous part of the flotsam, a mote being in no-where space, a blip in forever nothingness, alive yet dead, in absolute chaos...

Sara insisted, since the time was two-thirty pm (I had been on night duty), that I go upstairs for a rest. I was again on duty that night and, before Nightfall, must leave the cottage around seven-thirty pm. I would not arrive back home till around eight am the following day, at the earliest... Ha! Just managed to get up to the bedroom. Close the door, sit on the edge of the bed, and Kit came up the stairs in search of me; bless his little heart. Rest? I descended the stairs again, and carried him into the front room where Paul was engrossed, building towers with coloured toy bricks. I played for a few moments with the boys. My wife entered from the bathroom, where she'd been on her hands and knees cleaning the floor, and cleaned up around the fireside, where the carbon soot (how much the detritus of old past dead lives shredded therein) has again laid its engrained mementoes. I was gently shoved away, with a gesture, towards the boys. Paul the eldest encouraged me to, 'Have a nice rest, Daddy.' It was three o'clock in the afternoon and I was soon resting on my bed, scribbling these passing lines of commentary on mere existence. At that present moment in time, there was no-doubt it was a happy time. Historian (as Sartre) Roquentin had written:

> 'If anybody had asked me what existence was, I should have replied in good faith that it was nothing, just an empty form which added itself to external things, without changing anything in their nature .'

Why, why, why? Why, in commentary, should everything *always* be ugly and sordid in its not-known nothingness, its depersonified state; the veneer ignored (though just as true). I had to agree. that things shorn of their human utilities and sympathies were often at first *odd* but, good grief, to me they were often, also thrilling, wonderful, to just exist, as it did a minute atom, or a universe... To me, both were stark reminders of wonders that exist.

And what genius man has been gloriously endowed with, with clay, to shape and identify so much form and gracious beauty, from hitherto unidentified masses. Politics, filth, disease, destruction and barbaric ignorance are poles apart from bare existence, for although as real, to man, they are sordidness; never, but never, the things that existed, unknown, foreign perhaps; but hostile? Roquentin, Sartre [38] continued, true but, but - had he found his Rosetta Stone, his Holy Grail - the one Einstein unifying factor? I doubted it. But it was an observation. He said:

> 'I understood that I had found the key of Existence, the key to my Nausea, to my own life. In fact... Absurdity... the world of explanations and reasons is not that of existence.... Movements never quite exist, they are transitions intermediaries between two existences, unaccented beasts!'

A very real fact.

Monday, 1st July 1968

Days ago, we had had a week of gales and rain. But now, the sun is blazing down, a record of 96 degrees Fahrenheit here in Sussex. I have slept little since I started night work the previous week; I just cannot not get reoriented. Relieving the night nurse on the acutely disturbed ward of Bramber Two, the other night, I was left alone after midnight, for an hour, at one o'clock in that dark early morning; not then being used to it (my excuse), I became starkly aware that it was the *FIRST TIME ON MY OWN IN THAT WARD AT NIGHT ;* for a while I felt, fear, felt bloody, shit scared.... but it passed.

Any moment, at any moment entering a Gothic nightmare out of the darkness, a patient like a feeling-threatened Tall-John; or a wiry insane Terry attacking his evil god *Can;* any one resident might go *up-the-stick;* at me? Needless to say, those fears proved groundless and, in half-an-hour, I was immersed within that, sarcophagus, quiet. All my patients were either asleep, or appeared to be, with an occasional cough, or a patient's retort to an uncomfortable dream. I continued reading Koestler's *Spanish Testament*[39].... ears and senses primed, just in case.

The previous night, during my dinner break, stationed on Amberley One, I'd been contentedly (in between early morning patrols) engrossed, reading The Chapter on Superman, in Ouspensky's *New Model of the Universe* [40]. Nietzsche's poem *Thus Spake Zarathusa*, [41] used the icon of Zarathusa (in the Market Place) as a flawed model for a potential Superman? I pondered, was *he*, the Persian Zarathusa, a 'symbol', a myth, a cipher; or a frustrated Saint. Was he a real Persian leader, who inspired the Parsee faith with its Holy Gathas scripture and *The Zend Avesta,* [42] a two thousand years old '*Good Health and Hygiene Guide*' (Good thoughts, Good Words, Good Deeds); or, as I suspected, both. Nietzsche, poet, philosopher, was certainly such an honest human being; an *All Too Human* with his own achilles tendon.

Zend writings are full of commentary, on morals and how to potentially deter much human suffering. Sustaining good mental Health, and about Good versus Evil. I found, in the Avesta, none of the sad animosity written by other recordings and, subsequently, preached as Holy Words. Passed on as Human Law. As others with *their* interpretations of the words of God passed on to them; by others; who in turn had *read* of those before them. Bombast cast at other human groups (ethnic cleansing) and manifest in certain warlike factions, which to me dishonoured their own image of God; as Go'od, as in love and harmony in writings of the medieval Sufi poet Rumi.

And, in The Market Place, am I; like my maternal Great grandfather James Leigh Manton, and his brother George Leigh Manton who died in Victorian 1880s India (he was a real, true, Kiplingesque *Tommy Atkins* (as written into the pages of this Victorian army AB 64 pay books); aware of being fallible as 'an 'ooman-being' ; not Supermen, but in other ranks, as most of our charges. Poor Toms and Bets o'Bedlam; long-term patients in Asylum hospitals and Sanctuary care; and on this acute ward.

A new time system is to be introduced, next week at the hospital. It means four nights on duty, at eight pm till seven am; then three nights off duty, two officially for me, as one day was a Study Day. Overtime had been very difficult to fit in, during these night-shifts, since rest was always so lacking. However, I will get used to it. This week, Sunday, Monday and Tuesday, I was on duty *nights*; Thursday I was at day-school. Saturday night and, if possible, next Wednesday morning shift, I agreed to do overtime (no gap after nights!); and, then again, another Friday day-shift, on overtime. We'll see...

Now to dress and depart for this night's shift. Oh, erm, I placed my frugal monthly salary cheque in the Chichester bank, to eradicate some red ink. I browsed, for half-an-hour or so, in town before embarking for home. Whilst shopping, I picked up a Penguin Classic of Albert Camus's *The Outsider* [43] from Meynell's in Chi. Didn't Colin Wilson use this same title?

Wednesday, 3rd July 1968
On Patrol

Another night over. Little out of routine. Couple of *wet-and-dirties*. One chap, had gone *up-the-stick*. Routine, ninety-five per-cent as repetition, with five per-cent interest. This past week, I have been on Amberley and Bramber patrol duties. I arrived at the hospital around eight-thirty pm and was immediately placed, as a relief, on the long-stay ward of Amberley Two, which comprised of patients who, for the main part, could look after their bodily selves and got up, dressed, washed, shaved and ate breakfast without assistance. A number of patients worked, either within the hospital, or outside in the grounds. That brief relief was completed by eight fifty five pm. I then went downstairs to Amberley One; ward base for the night.

Commencing piquet patrol, from the MA1 base, I pulled on my white-coat about me, picked up a torch and unlocked the ward door, which was always locked at eight pm till six am, just like home. I re-checked upstairs on A2, and then went back downstairs and moved onwards to another, singularly under-staffed, mostly geriatric ward of Bramber One.

That chronic, long-stay, ward resided many, once upon a time, manic cum active type patients who had, long ago, burnt themselves out. There were schizophrenics, maladjusted elderly eps (epileptics), one or two sub-normals and psychotics — all for the main part now helpless, inadequate personalities; those unfortunates we too often and, unhappily, too truly, labelled cabbages; large but empty!? Having checked 'all' bedded and no apparently impending trouble, or beds and bodies to change, I then retraced my steps to the corridor, locked the door and proceeded upstairs to B2, the refractory ward.

At night time, at that time, only a single nurse was usually on duty up here, on Bramber Two, and why only one puzzled many of us no end, knowing the work? It was an acute ward. Up there were, basically, two types of patient; those who were known potentially violent and others who, though not aggressive, were deemed dangerous a social risk outside confinement of the hospital ward, at that time.

Having checked with the night nurse of this ward, I returned to my base for roughly one hour. Then, once-an-hour, except when relieving night-nurses for their dinner-breaks and my own dinner-break, just after midnight. In addition to the patrols, I always had to be available, for any emergencies. At five thirty that morning, I woke an A2 patient for his work and opened the kitchen for another patient, who would lay the tables for breakfast. Then, onto B1 long stay ward, where I entered to assist another nurse in upping, dressing, and directing the patients; and then, changing the, inevitable, foul linen from the numerous incontinents. At this time, we always checked for any new symptoms, sores, ulcers or new physical sickness. The air, on most chronic psycho-geriatric wards, was unfortunately permanently foetid, from the constant streams of urine and faecal matter permeating bed-linen and clothing.

The warm foetid air was, at first, almost unbearable, when one entered those wards for the very first time, but though one was always aware of it, you did get used to it. And, 'soaking', the urine was often found, in pools in and around the bed area and well creased into the well wrinkled flesh of those (doubly incontinent) patients. One disposed all into the red-linen bags, remade the beds with clean linen and washed and cleaned up the helpless patient ...

Phew! The hospital laundry bills must have been absolutely fantastic, reminded that, since its inception back in 1897, the hospital had continuously housed its own large laundry. Hospital staff were, only too well, aware of the *only* available clothes chronic long-stay patients uniformly wore around the hospital grounds. A number of 'long stays' seldom ever went out of the grounds; though in no way forbidden...

And those particular patients? Any naive visitor, might say, 'Tut! Tut! Shocking the condition of *those* patients', unaware of the inadequacies due to, then, almost permanent lacking funds, not enough made available to dress our indigent more humanely. As one patient soiled his garments etc., into the laundry basket; another patient died, clothes into the laundry bag; bath time, dirty clothes into the laundry bag and, year, after year, after year, until but relatively clean rags, undressable, remained. Those old worn clothes, were recycled and returned time and time again.

After half hour, to three quarters, the majority of our all too silent patients were up, their beds remade, and I, once more, moved on and continued my patrol. Up again, to B2 refractory ward, to see if all was well. Time was then six fifteen am. It'd been earlier, around midnight, that one patient had lost control, went *up-the-stick* (violent) and was eventually subdued and temporarily placed, for his own safety and especially that of the surrounding patients, into a side room.

On a subsequent piquet, I found him still sleeping it off. Most patients who had had night sedation, Mogadon or Sodium Amytal for most, were awake at six-fifteen am and were then, if not up and gasping for their fags and cuppa teas, in the act of getting up. Six thirty. I returned to the Admission Ward, assisted in raising its patients and helped to make the beds, whilst chatting to the residents. My five per cent interest? Mancurian university student Dave had wandered off, from his own ward, and eagerly sought me out at the beginning of the previous evening; or so it seemed. After our usual chit-chat about Kant, Kafka and other abstract *bon mots* of Philosophy, Religion, Arts, Sociology or Psychology... whatever myriad questions he presented to me.

On inspiration, I left Dave with an interesting Psychotherapeutic exercise. A question of attitudes. A picture cartoon, extracted from a *Punch* magazine,[44] portrayed an immense giant redwood tree in an American forest, with a minute ant-like group of young cubs; a scoutmaster at their head, halting his group, and shouting *Halt! Stand easy! Stand in awe!* (read its caption). It tickled me, and then, by association of ideas, I quickly brought up, from my memory vaults, a number of Tree analogies. After initially recognizing its biology and physical atomic fabric we then, together, started on more random associations. Jung, in his 'Individuality' of trees.[45] Obvious phallic innuendos. Sartre and Heideggar's utility derogatory opinions, of useless grotesque trees. Tolkein's wise old Ents. Science's dissection 'cell by cell', 'molecule by molecule', etc. Bio-sciences, Botany and tree species. My own Chair parallels (chair as tree wood). Van Gogh's *Yellow Chair;* and others...

At the back of my memory, I was only too aware of Ouspensky's dictum; '*You can go mad on examining an ash tray...*' [46] Punch's cartoon associated, at my instigation, with its minute human figures; men and trees (with a fondness approaching Louis Armstrong's musical affinities), with those natural vegetative earthly Ent cousins of ours; on Trees and Man... and. And... 'Dave', I said, a little gingerly and responding softly, silently, to his Beckett *Waiting for Godot* like eagerness. 'I want you to first just gaze at this picture, the trees and human figures and slowly, but slowly, *think of anything and everything*; every positive association and affinity, no-matter how small, with this picture of young minute humans — and this aged giant redwood tree. Think, concentrate on this picture— 'tween the tree and human figures. Look for sympathies, similes and so on. Think of all and everything, you know about them. Think positively, slowly but definitely, and *reflect* on your findings. Here you are.' I handed over the pic, taken from the *Punch* magazine.

He grinned. Was this a Lewis Carroll riddle, his puzzled creased features asserted. He replied with a laconic, 'All right! Erm! Right.... *Right On!*... Cheers. See you later.'. Dave departed, back to his Amberley One reception ward. Seven thirty am, and I had handed the ward over to Bob, the day duty Charge Nurse. I returned to collect my things; and departed on my bicycle for home, six miles away up in the downs. Sara had left a note, and already departed to adjacent fields with infants Kit and Paul, to assist a local farmer in potato-picking.

Saturday, 6th July 1968

Mid-day. Too tired, too occupied, to relate the past two days. *Thursday* was a Hospital School Day, in preparation for my Inter State exam; due on the 3rd October 1968. For the past few months, we have been without our Principal Tutor and anticipated a replacement. Mr Ilford, his assistant, was filling the gap as best he could. On that Thursday, Fourth July, we met our new Tutor, Roy Ammon, who replaced Mr Watkinson. He too was double-trained; RMN and SRN — plus teaching diploma. I informed the Nursing Office that I was 'down' for overtime am shift tomorrow (Friday). 'Do you mind working on the female side?', I was again asked by the duty female S.N.O. 'Good Lord no.', I answered. 'Send me anywhere I can be useful'. Evening, I returned, washed out! *Friday,* fifth July, I was up at quarter past four in the morning and, after one or two chores, cycled to hospital and arrived at six-twenty am.

After a rushed early breakfast, I was sent over to Richmond Two; a female long stay Geriatric Ward. In charge was an absolutely charming middle-aged ward Irish Sister; left on her own? This ward had fifty-eight patients and 'everything' had to be done or directed by Sister Brigit or, with no choice, it would remain undone.

Richmond Villa

Meal-times, here on Richmond Villa as all long-stay wards, meant a lot of work. Such labour *had* to include crisis intervention, alongside essential caring duties. Breakfast to be distributed to fifty-eight patients, under normal circumstances, an probably cumbersome necessity on such large wards; at the best of times, *but on her own*? Staff shortage the ever-ready answer of Administration, at The Office. I gathered that not only was there no other nursing staff on duty, there was no female Ward Orderly available, which meant either all laundry, washing, floor-polishing, and so on, be either carried out by her (impossible) assisted by several reasonably capable (never solely) patients, or cleaning *not* be carried out. And Sister Brigit had the Drug Rounds and considerable office paperwork to attend to....

We got on well enough together though, as an experienced nurse, Sister Brigit volunteered, *she* had her doubts and reservations at *any* male nurse working on a Female Psychiatric Ward (but no objection to females attending the male only wards or any male qualified doctor attending her ward — of course *she* would also be in attendance). And, with some eighteen to twenty-years and more nursing experience behind her, dating back to pre-war years, during the absolute segregation years of the sexes, both patients and staff, her views were she admitted somewhat biased and firmly entrenched.

I chatted up a few patients, assisted in serving breakfast, giving out the medication, and clearing up, and shortly afterwards I gave an injection, on Sister's instructions, to an non-objecting, long stay patient on her left Gluteus Minimus; upper left quadrant. Unexpectedly, a driver and hospital car turned up, to relay a patient to a Brighton Hospital Specialist. I was asked if I would kindly escort the seventy-four year-old patient. I did, and quite a rush it was, but we were still back on the ward by one-thirty pm.

In the afternoon (off duty) I spent a couple of hours in a hideaway, isolated, room on the male-side block, where I swotted up on my studies by doing a recent past, 1967 Inter Exam paper. Pleased at the effort and general events of the day, I arrived home after cycling, exhausted. Stepping into the kitchen through the back door, it was obvious that Sara had been very busy. Sara had completed a full day potato picking, collecting forty eight half hundredweight sacks, paid at ten pence a sack; and was exhausted. The boys as usual, it seems, were good; but still rather demanding. Result, on going up to see the boys, recently put to bed, Kit had pooped, pooped — and pooped. No nappy on (he'd cast it aside), it was painted over the cot-rails, over sheets, pillow case, lumps on floor (where he had been travelling over), on bricks, toys, carpet...

What a mess to be greeted with, on coming home. Worse, was the little varmint himself. His pyjama shirt (all he had on) was plastered with faecal matter, his legs, feet, hands, face, and of course, most of all his trunk. Oh well! I insisted Sara had had enough already and I set to clearing everything up. Within half-an-hour, scrubbed and wrapped anew, Kit was snug asleep. Young

Paul quietly watched, knowing the 'naughty' event. 'Use your potty next time, you naughty boy!', he helpfully advised his younger brother.

So much for *Thursday and Friday;* normal working days. In the evening, Sara's sister and her family arrived for a country weekend. *Saturday* morning, I awoke about six-thirty am, after a marvellous long sleep of six and a half hours. The four young ones were already running about the house, so we upped and started the day. I spent most of the morning with my axe, in the woods, gathering deadwood for our boiler fire.

Memories, The Time Paradox

Some months ago, I joined a Science fiction book club and, last night, finished reading *Twilight Journey* by L.P. Davies.[47] In this interesting work the hero, a Dr. Clay Solan, by means of an invention, was able to penetrate into his own brain's unexplored territory; just like Ouspensky had done, (though O had used a measured, legitimate dose of mescaline or hashish (ugh!) as a catalyst). Solan went down into his own dark night shadowed, subconscious. The novel similar, in a sense, to Colin Wilson's recent science-fiction work *The Parasites* — about dreams. Dreams paradoxically... a reality ... but, erm, not *the* reality, a true conundrum. After all... what, rather *when,* even conceptually, does one mean by *The Reality*? Surely this term must relate to *only* a passing full moment of a *living* individual?

In a much quoted allegory, by Chuang Tsu [48] Chinese Taoist philosopher, who once dreamed he was a butterfly and, when he awoke, commentated he did *not* know whether he was Chuang Tsu, who had dreamed he was a butterfly, or a butterfly now dreaming that it was Chuang Tsu? God knows we all, the Royal We but, especially referring to our legion of psychiatric patients, are further confused in trying to recall *What Actually Happened* in any singular event, back in a past life. Exploring. Examining a singular Case History.

Guesses are fraught with alterations, as there remains the mortal content, unknown and forgotten, brain hidden elements... the time paradox. Examples in Science-fiction, fantasy Ray Bradbury's 1952 *Sound of Thunder,*[49] and Robert Heinlein's 1941 *By His Bootstraps.*[50] Nineteenth century's Jules Verne and early H.G. Wells. And later, (much later!), reading time travel works of Stephen Baxter.[51] Henry James 1917 *The Sense Of The Past*[52] and Richard Burton Matheson. (There are, erm, other Richard Mathesons.) Matheson's novel *Bid Time Return,* later 1978 *Dreams May Come;* made into a feature film.[53]

And there are many, *many* other easily found examples on this conundrum, of memory being a paradox. False, or possible, gapfilling memories. Exploring a sequel of, not surface conscious, versions of past events. In substance, is one world, *our own,* just as *real* as any other, (person or planet) and, often, just as inter-dependent on one as the other. The time paradox. One is in time and dimension, philosophically *and* real, but passing, a fleeting metaphorical shadow. The other (not our) worlds, are they more permanent. Or too, *always,* also, erm... their own dimensional state of flux. And, of genealogy. All our residents have personal tales (fragmented memories) on time travel; case histories, pathways, down memory lane. Nostalgic Notes for a Case History; a variety of fact and fictional sources.

Dreams

Ouspensky [54] was of the opinion that the only way to study dreams is by a self-disciplined awareness trained in (thus in control of) 'half dream states'. I found this statement rather interesting:

> '....sleep and the waking state are not two states that succeed one another, or follow one upon the other. The names themselves are incorrect. The two states are not sleep and waking state. They may be called sleep, and sleep plus waking state. This means that when we awake there is added the waking state, which muffles the voices of dreams and makes dream images invisible.'

Ouspensky — on dreams:

> 'But all this refers to unconscious self-suggestion. The limits of voluntary self-suggestion in our ordinary state are so insignificant that it is impossible to speak of any practical application of this force.'

How did poor Bramber Two John, who had day *and* night time nightmares of descending chariots et cetera, recognise these experiences as but harmless dreams. And his were involuntary, not wishfulfillment, he loathed and feared them; night after night...

And I reflected and looked in at myself. And felt... empty.

Dimly aware, I cannot, possibly, compare present experience with *any* past total *existential* experience. I can only compare it with, *a memory,* traces and threads of that past experience. But that stored (wherever, however) memory is part of my *NOW* present total experience. All *recorded* memory is, by definition (viz. memory), a greatly distilled remembrance of all things past. Nostalgia. Yet all memories, however fragmented, are part of my total present existence, conscious and unconscious, in any *now* experience... But:

> I CAN ONLY EXIST BY A CONSCIOUS RETENTION OF MY MEMORIES AND BY CONTINUAL ASSOCIATION OF MYSELF WITH THEM.... ON ME BEING AWARE.

Am I at best always half asleep?

Phew! How odd to work at times, almost, twenty-hours a day, seven-days a week, and still *KNOW* myself to be relatively lazy? A dead match stick floating, sometimes on the crest of a wave, sometimes still in the doldrums, but always carried by the mobile current of auto-suggestibility. Sara has said that, presently, my mind has got too narrow; like a laser beam. I finished Koestler's *Spanish Testament*. (and thought a good deal more of Sartre's *Nausea* — and his accent on Freedom of choice). The following, from Koestler, [55] made me think:

> 'There is a curious mechanism at work within us which romanticizes the past; the film of past experiences is coloured by the memory. ... the colours run into one another: maybe that is why they are so fairy like. ... Most of us, are perhaps not afraid of death, but more only of the act of dying: and there were even moments in which we overcame even this fear. At such moments we are free ...'

3.15 pm Tonight I'm on Night-duty again - C Patrol.

Tuesday, 9th July 1968

Magic

I started the chapter *Magic and Mysticism;* by Ouspensky.[56] Ouspensky's self-examination of Dream and Half Dream states; and how perceptive images, visual and aural, are formed in the conscious use of memories. Half hour or so ago, I awoke, after attempting to sleep during the day. Yesterday, after being on night-duty Saturday and Sunday night, I slept only two or three hours. Today, at last, I was fortunate, having had nearly six hours sleep. I recall that dozy, semi-conscious, state — moving around *after* a session of deep-sleep.

One appears, I appear to move by sheer reflex action still; really asleep!

Even as I write this early evening, these states, half-asleep, dozy, wanting to stay asleep. Emotions are on a razor edge, not wishing to stir, and get off to work anew. Only if I could but relax, and drop into sleep again, no restraints necessary. This, my present, newly roused, body seemed to demand. But, I *MUST* stay awake, to go to work, though I am sufficiently conscious (!), any internal images are successfully suppressed in being so called awake; I am more asleep, than awake. Over tired, Sara specifies. I'm sure the muggy heat (it is quite warm, the sun is shining), must contribute to wanting to go back to sleep.

When is Real?

I wanted to Ayer-like[57] rationally, describe and categorise; be logical and pigeon hole the indescribable (not unknowable). But, I refused and would not be in denial, just because I did not have all the answers. Better to acknowledge the yet unrecognisable. Even bracketing it as Magic — whatever. Peter Ouspensky[58] segregated Magick *and* Mysticism, and divided Magic into a Concept of Concrete Knowing, through other than ordinary means. And, then, sub divided Magic into two types: Objective, with real results; and Subjective, with imaginary results. Mysticism was in all cases of intensified feeling and abstract knowing.' Ouspensky, integrity intact, said:

> 'With great amazement I became convinced that only a very small number of ideas corresponds to real facts, that actually exists. We live in an entirely unreal, fictitious world ...'

So what is real and what is un-real. But. Then I ask not what but *when is* real?
From Peter Hays *New Horizons in Psychiatry* [59]:

> 'Perceptive disorders in the schizophrenic cover more fields than size-constancy and three dimensionality; the 'existentialist' psychiatrist, interesting themselves in understanding and analysing the phenomena experienced by the schizophrenic patient, describe anomalies of perception not only of space but of time, while experimental work confirms that the schizophrenic gauges time intervals differently from the normal subject. In the field of psychological testing of the schizophrenic displays other anomalies such as 'over-inclusion', i.e. an inclination to see the trees, the sky, and the fields around rather than simply the wood, but although this may be illustrated by giving perceptual examples, it is probably a general characteristic of the kind of thinking that goes with the schizophrenic process. There are still some pathologists who aver that schizophrenia is an organic disease....'

There was a belief expressed, in the 1960s, that a schizophrenic state could be a *normal* withdrawal from and or means of coping with extreme alienation and, possibly, a direct result of bad parenting. Dr. D. Cooper [60] and Dr. R.D. Laing, [61] a radical psychiatrist and pragmatic philosopher, amongst others, subscribed, at that time, to this cause. But, I wondered, was it a response to 'combined' labilities; inherited somatic *and* emotional dysfunctions. Or was this already obvious; a which came first, the chicken or the egg? I could not, personally, subscribe to the rank belief that schizophrenia was caused by bad parenting per se. Oddness in schizophrenic behaviour, I observed, was often contrary to apparent moods (Incongruity of affect). An existence, in an *acute* phrase, of being in a world of their own. A constant flow of hallucinations, illusions, delusions; often psychopathic, persecutory, certainly not self-inflicted. Schizophrenic reasoning, to 'so called' normals was illogical; and impossible for us to follow 'their' hows, whys, whats and wherefores?

So important, one needed to often remember, that *to the psychotic, it is 'us' who are illogical for not being logical in following 'their' so obvious reasoning...* (as per G.K. Chesterton's essay - and Can Terry, on Bramber Two).

Can Terry

I quoted Schizophrenic Terry's responses to me, as well as those of his tyrannical God Can, whilst working on the Bramber Two refractory ward. Terry was convinced he was possessed by the great, but evil, god 'Can'; he being the vehicle for its voice. This, his evil God in Man, came from a planet way, way, out of this solar system. It was his Universal Space, connections with the Suns, and his known 'theory' of Evolution, of the planets from the suns, from suns, from suns. (Gurdjieff would have loved that analogy, so too Ray Bradbury?)

Terry was convinced everything was repeating itself. Without fail, every time he attempted to gain someone's understanding, agreement with him, emotional blunting (blocking?) soon led to a progressive state of aggression, as frustration, taken as rejection — accelerated into violence. Yet, to this schizophrenic, it was all *too* real to his existence. Terry felt alienated by his knowledge. He was *not* in control, but possessed by this 'other'; and could not cope with this state.....

Similarly, rare *savant* autistic schizophrenics experience religious or mathematical *obsessions*. They might 'see', 'feel', 'taste', 'smell', 'hear', 'sense', 'think of' *impressions*; and, I believed, so do Mystics. *But,* of course, the resident belief is the schiz sick former, don't know it, and are *not* in control;

but the latter true willed Mystics... do? Impressions, that most of we 'so called' normals are at any time (except in dreams) sadly, unable to generally perceive and harness. Unless, unless as fortunate mortals, *In-control...* we might be Mystics or Magicians, or perhaps unestimated; a Cocteau like poet? And, make no mistake, just because they see, perceive, them, and we don't, does not make them any the less real an existence. Shakespeare rightly said, in *The Tempest*[62]:

> 'We are such stuff ... As dreams are made on, and our little life ... Is rounded with a sleep.'

And, of Ouspensky and 'subjective' states of being as internal consideration.

Experiment

In one of Ouspensky's experiments, *sans* theoretical physics, he described in his book *A New Model Of The Universe* [63] how he succeeded in penetrating his own unconscious and observed:

> 'Each thing appeared, first of all, not as a separate whole, but as a part of another whole, in most cases incomprehensible and unknown to us....'

In a far more 'aware' state, than I could ever employ, he was able to see, sense where I could only imagine (beneath the veneer), connections of everything as mobile atoms; each balanced perfectly against another, each collection another 'thing', but still in substance perceived as atoms, molecular formations, but plus other...[64] He was aware. Expanded his consciousness. Ouspensky imaged, the dictum; '*Thinking in New Concepts*'[65] as *one* possible way of transformation (Indeed, a Transmutation). Thinking as seeing. Using this concept, *in-extremis*, the Science Fiction writer Robert Sheckley in a short story, said that:

> 'Suddenly everything moved, changed - Infinity swallowed everything - I felt - I myself disappear into infinity - this abyss.'[66]

An ultimate, terrifying experience, when not wanted. ... A cloak of Invisibility.

Friday, 12th July 1968

Morning, I intended to go into work and study awhile (on my own), I was far too tired to arise and depart. Sara and boys went potato picking; (seems some nearby Roman ruins are about to be excavated on a new site, one site was already being dug). Afternoon, I went into work for an overtime shift. Proved an interesting and worthwhile working day. In the afternoon, from 2 p m. to 6 p m., I worked on Amberley One ward with just Charge Bob and me on duty. Out of the blue, at six o'clock, another man came on the ward to assist us. I was asked if I would go up, to female Anderson Two ward, to 'chat' awhile to some disturbed patients. First, to a young, pretty, seventeen year old drug addict. And, to other patients, eventually chatting with a group of patients and playing cards at the game of 'Sevens'. At the finish, I had about seven to eight females around me, and our conversations proved most invigorating. A successful visit, I remained on the ward till 9 pm.

Saturday, 13th July 1968

Up and away at 06.10 am, a little late this morning, to do overtime work. Again asked if I would help out on the female side, Fawcett One, a long-stay geriatric ward. One ward Sister on duty (but not like Richmond 2), an untrained Spanish female ward orderly and myself, with fifty odd, mostly helpless, psycho-geriatrics; a number bedridden. We worked as a trio. Brief talks at breakfast in topical reference to the, then new, professional trend on staff and patients integration of sexes. Sister was for it, there was no doubt, but it would take time. 'Everything takes time. Change is inevitable.', as Sister Brigit had acknowledged.'

I was still *heavily* into Ouspensky and Sartre.

Nature, I learnt in Grammar School, abhors a vacuum. And 'nothing is nothing' said Shakespeare of Lear in old age, echoing his youngest daughter Cordelia, in answer to her dementing father King Lear. [67] But, as the tragic play demonstrated, it was not really true. And she could not, would *not* wear her heart upon her sleeve, and reveal her real, deep felt emotions. Physics, too, echoes that philosophy; that there is really no such reality, as nothing. It's all relative.

And no thing ever remains still.

Nothingness

'Movements never quite exist, they are transitions, intermediaries between two existences, unaccented beasts.' I thought this insight of Sartre [68] was brilliant. His historian, Roquentin, intruded upon my thoughts, on change; out of sight, electrons, positrons, neutrons, mesons, all split and joined-up sub-atomic traces

(our physics wizards inform us). Obvious, perhaps rather evading the issue. Heraclitus' state of flux, the ever-flowing river of Time. *What happens* to the closed (atomic) fist when the hand is opened. Erosion, a mould of Time... Blah! Blah! Blah! Blah!... About Nothingness And Being, and into *other* existences.

But, ah! — are these questions *only* three-dimensional, cast in stone, questions? I've neither the language of physics, or the level of experience, to pretend scientific; but I have imagination. And imagine transitional states as described by Sartre:[69]

> 'Why so many existences, since they all resemble one another? What was the use of so many trees which were all identical? ... those trees, those big clumsy bodies.?'

Why so many existences. Why so many memories. Why, *how,* one Eternal Second, and another, and another, and another; so many dimensions, perceptions— I questioned. Odd, I'd no problem with such knowledge; and accepted each verbal human, *per se,* experience with ease. But it was, and remained so, my abysmal mental block, in being unable to interpret algebraic equations and geometrical hieroglyphics. This remained as my own definite *mental handicap....yet* I find *life* (was) is of itself, *never* boring, but *exciting*, adventurous, mysterious in all its moments. Curiosity, always worth instigating an enquiry. It's man's so-many existences, to which he should continue to direct his queries. But always, always *a-priori*, enjoy the moment, *now; before* its memory, as alteration can be polluted and depressed. Before being but distorted false memories, cast out in knee-jerk limited robotic answers; no matter how fast.

Not just because there may be no topical replies, fashionable AI (artificial intelligence) robot forthcoming answers, left as residue in a recorded brain-cup centrifuge. But, perhaps, to avoid a sterile commentary... think. Ouspensky's '*Think in New Concepts*?' Not just Roquentin who found in Sartre:

> '... the World in all its nakedness which was suddenly revealing itself, and I choked with fury at that huge absurd being. ... it was not possible for it not to exist.' [70]

There was no awe, but *anger*, in Sartre's nakedness at Being. And, from this emotion, how can one assume otherwise than it was but intellectual awareness;

perceiving things as-they-are; 'things' that Roquentin became aware of, but with no emotional connection.

For many years, I have been frustrated when, in any situation or debate, I have said, 'I'm so sorry but I cannot explain it in words...' (How does one describe the content of a metaphor?), only to have the insensible unthinking reply by the listener, *'Like what?'* or, similarly, *'So what?'* Heaven and hell, how many of our unwell patients endure that frustration. Personally, I enjoyed any opportunity to debate this conundrum, in debate with Sartre and others. So many of our suffering patients instigated such questions in me.

No aesthetic emotion. No references to a 'Whiteness' occult and physic; blasting through the surface, expanding consciousness in cutting off from this naked existence, from Roquentin's 'hands on' mortality. No reference to the body released, the mind-centres slipping into the void of no-material nothingness, within the huge eternal fat *'Being'*. A void, true, yet hardly always depressing. Only incredible, to us other common men and women, who may not admit to such experiences. And, back in our world compass, if awareness in individual patients through body-chemicals dysfunction or other stimuli, give unbidden experiences of our symbiotic Huge Being, the body grammar in how they describe such happenings may be labelled a madness; and it maybe so?

> 'I had learned everything I could know about existence.'[71]

Was Roquentin satiated, or exhausted. Or labelled ill. Or unaware? But, more likely, he had learnt everything he needed to know; or wanted to know? And probably reached his full, of the moment, apex of knowledge in his mortal lifetime. Reached his human capacity to understand... All else was perhaps, too-much responsibility, too many perils implicit in accepting this natural infinity (infirmity) of ignorance; and the mysterious. To accept the mysterious, one must first accept the miraculous; the thrilling and fearful unknown... with due humility? Professor C.S. Lewis [72] said:

> 'Whatever experiences we may have, we shall not regard them as miraculous if we already hold a philosophy which excludes the supernatural.'

Sunday, 14th July 1968

Around two am young Kit woke me up and for the next hour had me cursing (for lack of sleep and rest), but very concerned. For some weeks, he had possessed a nasty hacking cough, racking his little chest, mostly prevalent during the night. I nursed him on my lap for about half an hour, then the coughing ceased completely.

Sara thought it might have been catarrh. Does catarrh originate from nervous stimuli? Eventually, I got off to sleep around 3.30 am and awoke late at 8 am, Hallelujah! But I was not, not, even tempered. I felt tension, then something I haven't suffered for many months; I felt bored. Acute boredom. What. Why. Boredom accelerated angst, discontent, more tension, self isolation and, a bout of depression. Why. Answer; perhaps because I could think of no immediate thing or action to look forward to, no spur to my being. Never mind whether a 'little' thing, like a first aid cup of tea (symbolizing both pleasure and rest); or a complex-sequence of events in the future with 'attainment' virtues.

And I certainly did *not* appreciate that; now. That moment, in hand, as it were. The fact remained, that I was bored and depressed. Why? I thought, possibly, it might be because I was unawake and the 'vital' sections of my brain had yet to stir and suggest things to be done. Typically, I was too insensitive- and I had it out on poor Sara, and worse, went 'cold' on her for about twenty-minutes, whilst that acute phase lasted. I've a distinct recollection, of a split mental condition. It was mental restraints at loggerheads, aggrieved. Whereas my body 'seemed' fully awake and yearning, autonomic.

Later, that morning, I entered the woods behind the cottage armed with my small axe. The greenery was well sodden, growth had accelerated since my last visit. Pan's sylvan wand conjured numerous storms, these past two weeks, and much rain has fallen. Hereabouts, fertility abounded. My wife's young sister (sixteen-and-a-half years) arrived yesterday, and will be glad company for Sara, whilst I'm on my next sequence of nights. Starting tonight, I am on C1 patrol. Always ready for other arrangements; whilst this nursing staff shortage worsens! Boredom gone. Normal impatience wanting to do things...

And, back to Existential John,[73] and exploration of my own human brain. Well and unwell:

> '... In each privileged situation, there are certain acts which have to be performed, certain attitudes which have to be assumed, certain words which have to be said - and other attitudes, other words are strictly prohibited. Is that it?'

Roquentin was trying to understand Anny's attachments to privileged situations. Unhappily, it turned out Anny might have been sicker than Roquentin - if indeed he was sick...

Yes, Anny remembered her moments. Having assessed a past-moment as an 'ideal' image, an icon, none could ever be so experienced again, for they, 'it', was in her past; then resident In Anny's memories. And as an ideal 'model', how could it be so again; as that past-image was, then, first experienced ? Anny lived wholly in the past, yet distanced from it, they, those precious moments; these moments, given names, could be re-arranged in any sequence she chose. Her privileged situations, had became fossilized as rite. Rite; the introverted rites of religious men and mystics and scientists and, perhaps, romantics. Every preparation had to be just so, or else nothing was achieved. Does empirical science *insist* on precise ritual games, institutionalised rules and penalties to re-create a past experience?

Ouspensky's 'experiments' were deliberately, ritually formed. Preparations. And so on. Ouspensky stipulated, '*EVERYTHING MUST BE RIGHT*.' [74] If not, on Ouspensky's level, danger lurked to the point of mental imbalance, *insanity*. A Faustian circle. To repeat only a past-event was, surely, to but evoke the dead; ghosts; would *no*t be a new, now event ?
Ah! But young Ouspensky was designing *NEW* experiences, *NOT* empirical replicas; I thought... A matter of being in control. I held a suspicion, that Roquentin's *Rite 'of Art*' was but an aesthetic point of awareness; an acknowledgment of the unexplained. Anny's duty *'to be moral*'; moral which deemed right and just. Without it, all was for nothing, and... wrong.

Monday, 15th July 1968
Insidious Death

It was early afternoon. A cloudy day. Wet, windy and generally miserable weather. Visitors still here. The women and boys downstairs in kitchen. Transistor playing. No potato picking this morning. Just gone-up-to-bed for my sleep, or at least rest? I couldn't sleep or relax at best of times, and with such a close, tense, unavoidably noisy an environment. Even when poor Sara did her damnedest to keep the noise down.

We'd had a *very* busy night, last night on the sick ward. Not unpleasant, not particularly strenuous, merely continuous and 'bitty'. Accompanying me on the ward was a female SEN, of ten years' experience (no nursing school, she insisted), a mature mother of five children 'twixt eleven years and twenty-three years old. One patient, on the sick ward, a man in his early eighties, I'd nursed on and off for some time, during his slowly depreciating state. (I didn't know his admitting diagnosis.) God, what utter human degradation and excruciating pain so 'naturally' endured. In early parlance, this state was called natural 'decay', or 'corruption'. After months in this condition; now, no speech, no movement — except occasional twitching muscle spasms; no body control; doubly incontinent and, oh God, those pressure-sores. We turn him over hourly; night and day.

No matter how much care and attention we attempt, we knew we could do nothing more to allay further pain than we do. The sores were large and ulcerated, so deep and wide that his body just could *not* ' build-up' new tissues. Brown-pus, black-pus, blood and gore. Faeces at random, to-clot and mix 'fore we remove. We prevent gangrene by constant turns, and Ickosan pink-powder 'drying' treatment. But we could not stop all his pain. He feels. His eyes just opened, just...? We wipe his eyes, clean his mouth and moisten parched lips; aware of the helpless, seeming lost soul 'wandering' in fractured thought and inward images. This fact discernible from a man who once passed sperm and played a paternal role, and a working role in life. Now, was is this living? Existence - survival - yes ...

Over his coccyx, sacral area, iliac-crests, the worst 'holes' appeared; gaping concave contours. His shoulders, feet (swaddled under the cradle) and shins all his pressure areas bound in an emaciated frame; decay impossible to deter. But, of course, we did alleviate some pain and discomfort and, as nurses, tended him as best as we could. He ate and drank, by liquid only, but little. He could do nothing for himself. How long would he last, till he drew his last breath? Exit from mortality, pain and agony!

If a human being, like a cat, dog, horse or any domestic animal, were allowed to slowly die with such nose provoking putrefaction, insulting what had been before a man; the carer could be duly prosecuted for neglect and cruelty, and forensic case, media sensationalised, with little doubt. And so we prevent that *last* flicker of human life from inevitable extinguishment. Alleviate to a maximum all pain and discomfort. But, how so, always crucial.

We'll all grow old, some day. Water under the bridge. And fate seldom discloses where ageing will conclude. Possibly, at home amongst loved ones, if lucky. But, with the gathering trend, old dismissed as mentally ill. A Geriatric or Psycho-geriatric. It might be as a helpless resident, dependent in a so-called Rest Home or terminal in Hospital? Or, found living alone and helpless, approaching death. What if, in a future Orwellian style government, there be a *policy* of rationalization, for rundown fiscal resources, deliberate gross neglect of the elderly, which becomes policy. Less, presented as more. It'd been executed in a recent past. Well within my lifetime.

Pre-war 1938, Totalitarian Germany mandated death, euthanasia (gentle, painless death? Actually evil and maximum in cruelty) for thousands of mentally ill and physically handicapped; and deemed non-aryan racially impure men women and children, including Germans.[75] I knew, a little, of other world 'cultures' where elderly, and other handicapped persons may be abandoned to the naked elements, to wither and die, alone; uncared for by anybody, and no-one, no individual deemed responsible; no elected government by, erm, wilful neglect or state policy — but in stealth, saving money over decades. Hospitals and other institutions, starved of funds. Only bank accrued interest accountable.... by Law.[76]

Our Tutor, Mr Ilford, with his own RAMC experience of sick and wounded wartime veterans' needs, indicated our prime responsibilities, now and future, of any wanton gross neglect in a duty of care to patients young or old placed in our charge, with often suddenly finding too few trained nurses to cope with our patients; and too few other necessary staff. 'I don't expect you to all be Saints', he smiled, as he added, 'But be as mindful of your sins as you go. ...'. He also added, 'Be mindful if you feel inadequate, as you or your too few colleagues, might be harassed and exhausted, unable to feed the many.' We imagined the possible scenario; too many deprived (not depraved) human beings to be fed, at breakfast, dinner, tea and/or supper. Do the beds, pot them, wash them, dress them. Attend their wounds, watch over them, apply chemotherapy. A grim picture... of wartime memories!

And *who* will have time to talk to them (psychotherapy) with thousands to consider, and not allow boredom; or despair. But, to be well enough and capable enough, to be bored? I examined the prospect needs of the elderly; in and out of hospital. Work could continue to be available for the old... as long as they wanted it so, or skills allowed. And, of course, as ordinary old age fatigue runs down. Oh I was such a naive student. Another working lived day gone!

Fragile Beings, Robb & others

Seven pm. Today, I attended a study day. The Principal Tutor was off on a course and Tutor Mr Ilford took the helm. More on the needs of the elderly in hospital. Notably, we signed our first State Exam entry forms; Harry and myself are the only two of our original intake class left (the three girls had left months ago). Mr Ilford introduced the controversial 1967 British book of Barbara Robb's *Sans Everything. A Case to Answer,*[77] which we discussed at the nursing school. Mr Ilford was answering the Minister Of Health , *Findings and Recommendations following Enquiries into Allegations concerning the Care of Elderly Patients in Certain Hospitals, 1968.* Robb's work was published, only weeks before I had entered the ranks as a student. The book in question, had painted (by critical reports) an ugly picture of *government neglect* of geriatric patients and psychogeriatric patients and their caring-staff based in long-stay hospital care; observations which certainly must have gelled with all practising physicians, psychiatrists and anti-psychiatrists alike!

Amazing! For one example. The Whittingham Long-stay Psychiatric Hospital at Preston in Lancashire had over 2,000 resident patients with considerable additional out-patients and community commitments. A later report [78] recorded that whilst on paper the large hospital had, had five psychiatric Consultants, because of its outside commitments there were usually only three to care for all its patients - and presumably to supervise all junior medical and nursing staff. And, notably, *only* one full-time consultant's services for the care of 86 per cent of the patients; who were long-stay dependent residents. If, and when, the hospital were to close down; how many qualified professional staff would be needed to replace an already dearth of essential resources. [79]

Not once have I seen brutality, or wilful neglect, in Graylingwell hospital. But, I have seen much tenderness. I've pointed out already, how one or two, possibly if lucky, three staff (one to work in office, for notes, etc.) cater physically and mentally for often over fifty patients; sixty to seventy on some villa wards, where ambulant and bedridden live, and work of a sort, with one Charge... Yet, the records show and older colleagues confirm, only twenty or so years ago (in the late 1940s) five to six staff *on each shift*, was considered *ideal*, and meagre enough - according to some of our retired staff? True, the phenothiazine group of drugs, and those chemotherapeutic other treatments; along with ECT, all helped disturbed patients who, for too many empty years, owned no hope. But many now ex-long-stay patients, in the 1960s, are able to live outside the hospital and reside in accommodation *within the community.*

Commentaries

Unhappily, the no hope theme reminded me, very much, of an initial letter in Dr. Maurice Nicoll's 1952 *Commentaries*[80] where it was pointed out back in 1941, early days of the war, that unawake man as a 'so called' cultured being had progressed *nothing* for over two thousand years. Humankind still prefers War, as opposed to Peace, as the norm. And will readily regress to savagery, when the thin swaddling robes of civilization's facade are stripped aside.

Ouspensky, in the wake of the first world war, [81] in his *1931 New Model of the Universe*, wrote all scientific progress stems from investigation into the Abnormal, the Criminal, and the Politic. Never the Good which exists of itself. Gurdjieff, in his strange, allegorical, science fiction work from 1950, *All and Everything*, makes Man look at himself; and his fear of the good.[82] So, too, did Robert Heinlein, in his 1961 *Stranger in a Strange Land.* Godness abused. What, in passing, humans dream of, and physically crave, they sadly soon corrupt, and cry for some form of power and recognition. Power and lust in lechery, power in greed, avarice and anarchy. And most, by their abuse, in crass ignorance.

Faust

Doctor Faustus attempted to repent his ills, realising that if indeed, as evidence of Evil as Mephistopheles was proven to him, then — *if there are Evil Powers, then the Good, God (*as Go'dness*) too must be also.* In guilt, the penitent Doctor believed he was damned, so he was, unlike a repentant, but faithful, Job whom God blessed, and eventually removed his Kierkegaardian boils. Temptations...

Man needs rest, sleep, a roof over his head, food and drink for his belly, a measure of security for his maintenance. And, when these basic wants are *balanced*' and satisfied, a vital sexual mate; all else is surplus, excess, above basic needs; then the higher needs and aspirations of true humans may be achieved. As so, well, illustrated by American New Existential Psychologist, Abraham Maslow's, pyramid of needs.[83] On a Swiftian, Yahoo man, level, Robb's *Sans Everything* [84], demonstrated, mechanical animal man is ever ready to take over when either 'deprivation' or 'excess' desires, are experienced; as demonstrated in the Temptations of *Doctor Faustus* et als, yielding to temptations *sans* humanity.

> 'I wanted to stop thinking about Anny.' Said Roquentin in Sartre's *Nausea.*[85] 'I started looking through the books on display in the second-hand boxes, and especially the obscene ones, because, in spite of everything, that occupies your mind.'

Poet and novelist John Cowper Powys [86] recalled suffering from this basic, physical Maslow hierarchical need deficit, which occupied his mind-and-body:

> ' On desperate lust-starved walks', *nympholeptism'* - he called his search for satisfaction ; -' solely of the idea of finding some miserable picture in a miserable window *(in a squalid little newspaper-shop*) of a girl's long legs.'

Physically and psychically out-of-sorts; Powys was recovering from an illness, 'roamed the streets' ... like a *"stygian soul* " groaning and gibbering *"for waftage.*" ... a source of some relief ('a buoyant conveyance.').

Sartre's base earthy fictional quote from *Nausea*; and Powys' honest self-observation, could comment on any, many an honest Seeker of Divine Love, who was reminded of their fleshly apparel. Satisfaction, of physical love, might be only a temptation; yet, in good health perhaps be a Tantric, inner Malkuth, gateway into their own inner non-visceral world... to potential spiritual love. And be able to surrender to God, en-route to en-soph... And bliss!

But *sans* any mystique, now but a shell of a former self, many of our sad hospital residents had, at one time, perhaps tried this and that way... but without the *capacity,* and in natural corruption, fell by the wayside. Too many patients subdued and life sustained by prescribed drugs and in dementia — are inevitably it seems, *not able to knowingly*, receive love; or the personal, natural lust of a healthy-mind-and-body. And, by a gross *involuntary* deficit of sensual fulfilment, in the husk's knee-jerk pursuit of survival — terminal, these alluded to such unfortunates. Existence *only* as an abstract, head in the clouds, with their long lost *capacity* to seek further *conscious* fulfilment in love and lust in living, in this life; and have need to be cared for until their departure. We owe them, while they wait, a just Duty Of Care.

Friday, 19th July 1968
Refractory

Overtime shift. 9 pm. This morning, I did overtime on the refractory ward of Bramber Two, presently with twenty *acute* psychiatric patients. Several new guests, since my last visit to the ward, including a seventeen-year old youth whom I knew from the Admission Ward, a DA - It was Spider, and he'd just been re-admitted into Bramber Two ward. Spider was *discharged*' months ago, and recently asked to come in again, as an informal patient, though he had previously been resident on a compulsory, Section 26, for almost a whole year. A Heroin and Cocaine cocktail addict, he was also taking Phenecytin and Methadrine – *all,* at one time. He'd started at fourteen years of age and now, for the first time, had what *'he'* felt was, incentive. Spider updated me on recent events. 'But *not* like this... Barry. She brought me here, yesterday. She's lovely looking,' he said to me in sad conversation... God, I hope *this* time he'll make it.

This refractory ward, is the one difficult ward, where grossly and sometimes incurably disturbed patients were resident. Even this ward had to be split, those men who were sometimes psychotic, and many, mostly socially undesirables to the public at large. Those who would not, and had not been able, to tolerate idiosyncrasies. And the ever-ready-to explode, more sometime violent, patients. Of what? Twelve hundred odd patients?

Surely no more than a handful of hundreds, a hypothetical ten or so patients, could be labelled *sometimes dangerous,* and equate with the lay public's ideas of the psychotic. The rest are sick with depression, or disordered and *unable* to cope with life, in some *capacity* or other, but no way harmful to others. Rather, the opposite reason was so, and Asylum was sought; so they entered hospital for 'help', 'understanding' and 'hope'; qualities which their illnesses could not (and seldom do) gain sympathy amongst the so-called *normal* society. Today, the four side-rooms were all occupied, with severely disturbed patients. No quantity of drugs alone would presently cure them, or even, (being young), hold back at times their explosions.

On Bramber Two, Tall John had attacked patients and staff so many times that, at one time, for a period, a record was kept of his unprovoked attacks on people and property damaged — but the list got far too long and attacks as unpredictable as the weather, but as regular. Last week, whilst most of the patients had retired to bed, this patient suddenly upped himself and strode over to a sleeping patient and then, unprovoked, he set about him, before help arrived. He moved very fast. The attacked patient's face was a mess. There was a chance that he might have been taken in to some Security Hospital, for ours cannot cater safely for such exceptionally severe patients. Perhaps Broadmoor or Rampton? (He never did go.) Three of the four severe patients in these side rooms could not always be separated from the rest of the patients on the ward; who were at times terrified of them.

Afternoon shift completed, I gathered wood for our kitchen fire. And, in the evening, repaired my bicycle. Sara was typing. Both the boys were asleep. The following morning, *Saturday*, I was on an overtime morning shift. Again, much needed overtime. Refractory ward, again... Sara's potato picking was also helping to resolve our, perpetual, financial crisis. Couple of days ago, our Chichester Bank Manager sent a demanding letter, and reminded us that we were ten pounds overdrawn on our account. Another day...

Sunday, 21st July 1968

Ten am. A hot restless night. One of those nights, when one doesn't appear to settle down; until *forced* to get up. Sleep, but so little, as dawn crawled in. But first, a passing note, on yesterday's night-duty. *Saturday* morning. I had got up, easily enough, at five fifteen am but on starting out on the 'much trouble recently repaired' bicycle, and twenty-five yards down the road, the damned rear wheel had seized up; apparently it was buckled. Ugh! Needless to say, off to a sour start. Half hour late at hospital, on this day's overtime, again taking it on my wife's small bike. Darned hard work on that machine; as the past week's cycling has demonstrated. From seven to quarter past eight in the morning, I was designated to be working on the Refractory ward. Bramber Two staff nurse was off duty, so I had to serve the medicines; assist in giving out the breakfasts and had just finished helping with the washing-up, when we received a 'phone call from the duty SNO at the General Nursing Office.

Urgent request, would I mind going over right away to the Summersdale Day Hospital, Female side, 'As we know You *don't mind.';* and that I had no objection to working anywhere in the hospital. At this time, formal staff integration of male-and-female nursing staff had not yet become policy. A harassed Sister Trees had thirty-two, very active, mostly young patients resident throughout the block; Summersdale's facilities being different from that over at the more Acute and Chronic long-stay *Main Building,* hospital side.

Summersdale villa housed, temporarily, acute neurotics, phobics and milder psychiatric illnesses. Essentially, they were (male and female sides) short-stayers, and day-patients, attending ECT treatment, similar to Amberley One Admission Ward; over at the Main Building. It was a *very* busy morning, and perhaps the most notable thing I had enjoyed on working there was *talking-out* a new admitted patient, a Mrs. A., who was recovering from acute hysteria and severe clinical depression. This young woman had been mute, eating nothing for the past two-to-three days, almost catatonic, her eyes half-glazed, barely open; with it, but only just.

Breaking ground only, initially, I talked but little, busying myself around her to indicate *friendly* actions. First opportunity came by attempting to give her breakfast. Small fare. I offered a cup of tea and two marmalade sandwiches, cut in four even squares. Sitting her up, I began to coax her, talking gently but audibly. After succeeding in getting her to drink some tea — moving herself, I departed, stating that I would return shortly, and would she '*try hard to eat a little something*; never mind if she couldn't; just try; it's the effort which will count.'

On my return, a little after moving some patients around, changing beds and creating vacancies, to my pleasure Mrs. A. had nibbled away full half of a sandwich, two squares. I smiled and praised her for her successful effort, her eyes raised a little, the corners of her mouth attempting a turn of a smile. By the time I went off duty at two o'clock., she had also digested a few mouths full of milk pudding at dinner-time. Most important, I had her talking very quietly, wistfully, and answering in-a-fashion to most of my softly, softly, drawn out questions. She was married with two children. Her husband had been in to see her just the night before. They were in the midst of moving house. As to what was worrying her, she had been trying to cope with too much, at one-time. I initially gained little success, but heard the repetitive sentence. She was no longer mute.

'*I AM CONFUSED. HELP ME ...*' uttered pitifully, and often. Her pleading mantra.

Her husband was all right; her children were all right; the house move progressing well. Softly, I said, 'You relax, Mrs. A., and take advantage of your temporary stay in hospital and rest whilst here you have no further cause to worry.' My mantra. Her need.

I learned... Mrs. A. did *not* take sugar in her tea... from her!

Without doubt, just talking had, in *this* instance, worked well. She was smiling by the time I left, and waved a glad 'good-bye' and said '*Thank you*!', when I went off-duty. But, this was just overtime, and the chances of seeing the patient again were slight, as by the time I go over there again she will have been discharged (I hope)!

I was thankful for the great help given to me, by one young female patient, an ex-nurse herself, who knew all the patients' names, having been in hospital a couple of months. She helped me make up beds, fill in charts, transfer patients, with the hysteric, Mrs. A. And, culminating the day's work with serving of dinner and sweet I'd served out, she distributed the necessary fare.

On return home I busied about nothing; collecting fire wood out of the wood. The blasted axe-shaft had broken. One more little thing gone wrong *this* week. Isn't it damnable, that a quick aggregate of little things going wrong, one on top of the other, soon combined with 'fatigue', reduces oneself to a bout of depression. Still, it'll pass...

I recalled frail Mrs. A., unable to cope, had very quietly sussurated, and oh so meaningfully, chaos pleaded - *'I'm too confused; all the voices they're mixed up; I can't tell who is who, what is what; too many changes.'* I thought I knew how she might have felt, when one is confused with an admixture of such overwhelming mixed emotions. Guilt for this, or that, desire for this and that, but settling for that; hating this, but loving it really. Such angst. Anguish, frustration, showing off, in a restrained fit of temper, a tightened band around the head, headaches.

This night, I'm on Admission and Bramber wards' patrols.

Tuesday, 23rd July 1968

Returned from a a much needed therapeutic visit into the wood, for firewood. A visit into another womb, peace, think, and anew, to ponder! Last night, I was on A. & B. patrols; again tonight. I learnt Manchester Dave of the Admission ward had been (hooray), transferred to a Rehabilitation Centre. The old patient on Lister ward, of whom I had spoken a few days ago, had, at last, passed away from this earth, because of the degree of his suffering. So too, in the same sick-ward, another severe patient who attempted suicide a long while back but didn't succeed, and took the top of his head off; his brain-pus has been constantly oozing out ever since, (I have wiped the brown pus up enough times) - he too has passed away from his suffering. The weather outside is stormy, gale winds blowing hard, and darkening, but the rain just holding off.

Deja Vu

Last night, on dinner-break, I rested my aching feet, in the wee small hours of the morning, and digested more of P.D. Ouspensky's feast in *A New Model of the Universe*, and read a Chapter on *Eternal Recurrence.* [87] About memories. Several days ago, I had read most of Chapter One of a Pelican paper-back called *Memory: Facts and Fallacies* by Dr. Ian M.C. Hunter.[88] In Hunter's memorable chapter on *'What is Memory*', I was intrigued by a discussion on 'paramnesia' and *'deja vu*'; literally, *'already seen*', Hunter's definition of deja vu. At first, the comparative (to Hunter) chapter's passage in Ouspensky's *Eternal Recurrence* could only, of course, be meta-physical; and written in a psychological perspective, rather than in the nebulous language of philosophy; but, then on page 480,[89] Ouspensky, with some clarity on past memories, said:

> 'It could not be otherwise, for theories of heredity, of Memories, experiences, etc. even of a dim faraway heredity, theories of hidden instincts, of unconscious memory, can explain certain sides of man, but other sides they cannot explain. And we find it possible to recognize that we have lived before, very much will remain in us that we shall never be able to understand.'

Wednesday, 24th July 1968

About 11.15 pm, I was on night-duty, in the small staff room, adjacent to the Observation Ward, on Amberley One, when a senior colleague entered the room. Laid on a corner of the table, was my (just completed) copy of Ouspensky's *New Model of the Universe,* which came into his vision. I thought well of that Staff Nurse, respecting his experience in the nursing field, but was quite unprepared for what followed. I knew, from past meetings with him, that life's path in the marital field had left him a very bitter, cynical streak. Picking up the book, he scanned its contents. Drawn to the chapter on Superman, and references to Nietzsche's *Thus Spake Zarathusa,*[90] he commented on the same and, in disgust, said gruffly *sub-rosa* 'I've read this 'Spake Zarathusa'. And, leaving the room, slammed the book back on the corner of the table and muttered, emphatically, but audibly, 'Load of bloody tripe!', turned his back, and marched out and left the ward.

A knife in my back. I felt what any sincere, Christian, Moslem, Hindu, Buddhist, Tao, Zen, Jew, albeit *any* Seeker, Sufi Mystic — whatever; *any believer*, in whatever pathway, whatever philosophic system of beliefs, might feel when, dogmatically, any other person, patient or other, but especially a trusted other, in a gut-reaction, trivialises or worse, actually, attacks one's core beliefs. And says to their face: 'Nothing but bloody out of date superstitious nonsense'. *Intolerance* — well yes, at root any person *does* have the right to their own opinion. It's if, and how, *they* in turn express it, eh? Shoot them. Decapitate them. Burn them at the stake. Treat the offender as heretic as subhuman, *not* one of us (not as me.) Such expressed insults to *their* own supposed *true* faith? Preaching. No way! Realities. Cliche — 'cause it bloody is. But, too often, it causes much fear, pain, suffering, conflict, and too much stupid, bloody, war... bloodshed.... a rank cause of mental illness. I carried on.

New experience

In the morning, I was unable to cycle home straight away, after seven am, as I had to wait around till ten o'clock when the bank opened in Chichester. But, as I cycled back, exhausted, finding each mile a million, each tread a supreme effort, I pondered on my night-time mood. Without, whilst cycling between Chichester and Chilgrove, any detrimental continuing stimuli, my *mind* relaxed, and retained some order, for a few precious moments, but my tired body couldn't... sustain it. The countryside was still Summer green, still and peaceful, a fair light wind breathed into my face, stroked and soothed me, and I remembered, knew, that only my own fears and prejudices sown by circumstance and repetitive centrifuged, memories, were responsible for the quick gathering mood of despondency. But, still, I could *not* always prevent the fatigue tightening band around my forehead, emotional centres and willed restraints — yes, I know... I felt momentarily, powerless.

S' funny, dressing a mute sub-normal patient on Bramber One at five-forty am that quiet morning; I remembered feeling a strong pang of brotherly sympathy towards him, as I drew garments onto his cabbage-like, but so dependent, frame. 'You know, George, 'ole son' I said, to myself *and* to him in my mind, for he was mute and would not (I thought) have understood: 'In a definite way, both you and I are just as much automatons; I, too, have to follow *strict* routines in everything I do... without it, I too would have my chaos, and be out of control...'

Stress

Exhausted, in a daze, another busy night-shift completed, the time around eleven-thirty am when I wheeled my bicycle into the shed at the rear of the Chilgrove cottage. As I entered the shed the boys, bless 'em, welcomed me, as per usual, in great enthusiasm. Sara too, greeted me in high spirits — then it happened. Timing was such, I guess, that at that moment, I rejected even her apparent happiness. God forgive me (*If* you're there) I resented her, envied her, her good evident feelings — for a depression was almost upon me. Sara said something or other; I, caught off balance, appeared (to her) to give a negative reply to a request, she then resented me. I felt worse and, escalation, it happened. Loss of self-control. Mine.

Chaos reigned, confusion, and seething with misery and depression I *stalked off* upstairs to bed. My poor wife was heartbroken, and had no idea *'why'* (and neither did I know *why*). I then took it, not unnaturally, personally, and *depression,* being then contagious between us, Sara too momentarily contracted it. Eventually I went to sleep; and awoke about six pm, still very miserable. In a hazy daze of sleepiness and dulled emotions, I staggered down the stairs. We rowed on contact — and inevitably her tears came down like torrents (God I hated myself at times like these, and would do for too many years ahead, for here, there, was my major flaw).

But, those same tears brought, instantaneously, a mutual concern and, with love then existent between us, spontaneously ignited a resolution. And, slowly, the depression's depth, lifted, slowly, but definitely so... I was still tired and vulnerable, as was she, but we were over the row, forged by my build-up of depression. God, I remember a few tears, and feeling, saying to myself, 'What's the use! Work, sleep, work, sleep! And then nothing but trouble soon comes up, even when things seem to be going smoothly.'

Me - gripe, gripe, gripe...

That deep feeling of hopelessness.

Sara, in tearful mood, understandably hits out and threatens to leave me. Too tired at this instance, surprised for *words* — the right words were beyond me. Aches and pains then soon come about, in the guts and head, some sharp jabs were felt, and... We soon found out that I had had a nasty bout of influenza on the way. Yet, I was *aware,* even at that deepest moment of depression, of analysing, attempting to self-remember; internally, I was sometimes, *then,* able to *self-observe* my own condition. Giving this commentary on it, suggesting — what's what, an almost schizoid presence? Yet, it was *this* sane streak that allowed the chaos to abate. Then, we both wanted, *willed,* dearly to make up, and passion declared how sorry we were, *'what's the real matte*r' and so on.

I concluded '*Sex and Evolution*' in *New Model of the Universe* [91] last night; and will record notes in due course. Ouspensky drew great emphasis on *connections* between the physical and emotional impacts of love and sex and the Mystical, aesthetic feelings that may *Tantric* Kundalini (whatever yoga it is) snake-like rise up in a surge of silent *Power*. Sex... beyond mud and dirt some people in the market place throw on *definition* of sex and love (in collating... I was amazed reading literary agent proposal advisors in Text Books insisting words (sorry *Freud* Jung Laing you're taboo) Sex and Bible Plato &

Shakespeare never, *never*, ever be used... in books: if the cap fits...) and, of *abuse* and negation, of this incredibly powerful yet, oh so vulnerable force, how much harm is done to mental health. Periodicals in the 1960s, like *The International Times* and *Playboy,*[92] and other ephemera; were educating facts about achieving full satisfaction in a physical *Orgasm.* The mags enlightening the male population, loved female partners equally entitled to full sexual satisfaction. And, us Yahoo males *not* just satisfy, selfish macho needs — alone. And, further liberation, this media when explicit, indicated the existence of the female *Clitoris* (male penis) and other hotspots be tenderly approached.

Time, ten thirty pm, and Sara contented, typing; her young sister nearby reading. Occasionally sipping a cup of coffee. I immersed my frame in a hot bath, washed and shaved; always good therapy. Relaxed my consciousness; sleepy. The following day's a school day, at the hospital, and I'd completed pre-exam homework on — Consciousness.

Thursday, 25th July 1968
Atavist

Last night, I slept well, and departed for a Study Day feeling a deal better. We revised some past examination questions. On finishing at five pm, we were informed that, starting the *following* Thursday, we would have a series of eight lectures *On Psychiatry* by resident Psychiatrists.

The next morning's shift, I would be doing overtime; and afterwards, in the afternoon, intended to study awhile, by doing a whole past Examination Paper (January 1968), in a two-and-a-half-hour's run; a good day!

Late evening, I entered the wood, to gather in a few fallen broken branches. It was getting dark and, at the top of the wood, where the trees were much thicker, an incline rose, and the ground was difficult to traverse through its thick tangled bramble of bedded green and saplings. On the narrow twisted path, I noticed deep imprints of what was a fair-sized deer's foot-prints. Nothing unnatural, quite common in those woods. The night was darkening fast, and bubbling up into mind I recalled discussions I had with a Sergeant of the Metropolitan Police back at Teddington, with regard to a puma at large in the South of England. The officer knew what he was talking about. And, to my knowledge, I believed it was still at large. I recognised (scout like) pad prints as deer paws on the woodland ground behind our cottage. But, the slight doubt added to an already grey gloom. And, as I trudged, I found myself *alert* and, so childishly, looking behind and about me, as I bent-kneed, tip-toed, and crouched crept as I moved on — *just in case.*

As the minutes ticked by, with my quiet seconds slow footfalls, the somewhere, everywhere, waiting hidden puma, in my imagination, childishly, superstitiously, changed into a darker, threatening, night misted, cold shrouded shade. At first, friend Shakespeare faun but then, as fiend opposite, in an invisible satanic form. I recall being quite conscious, and all too aware of darkening surroundings during those frightened moments, in my temporary furtive state of mind. When I'd gathered sufficient dead-wood, I straightened up and quickly hopped it back home to our small, hidden, sanctuary in Chilgrove' *Stonerock* cottage - below.

S' funny how innate atavistic fears can be resurrected. I'd been in the wood many times before, when it has been black, and had never felt, or suspected, anything superstitious. Too much stimuli. Mentally, momentary, unconditioned. Who knows. Know thyself... Anyway, the thing was to carry on regardless, as in such puerile moments of fear.

Friday, 26th July 1968

Much too tired to write! More Relief Work...

Saturday, 27th July 1968

Yesterday morning was a split morning's overtime. I was preparing for breakfast, on Male Bramber Two ward, when a call from the general office requested, would I mind going up to female Anderson Two admission ward? Most of that morning, I spent specialising (prevent from running away and doing harm to self, or others) a young patient down at Occupational Therapy. OT was an essential, albeit mandatory, form of practical rehabilitation treatment for certain patients, who had psychiatric trouble working, continuously, outside in the community. After dinner was served, I enjoyed proving useful, in applying, Psychotherapy, talking-out, to two depressed patients. One young woman had, up to recently, been a practising State Registered Nurse; another new patient was a young mother who had severe clinical depression, which pressure had driven her to nearly killing her infant child.

In the afternoon, with that shift completed, I had worked for two and a half hours on the January 1968 Intermediate RMN State Exam. The last question; what would I say to a patient who was violently upset on reading a newspaper reference to *lunatics*. I was interested to see how the principal tutor commented on my completed exam paper. Since that paper was homework, I felt (though I was mentally exhausted), it'd been another good day. The following morning, I spent half a shift, on Female Fawcett Two, a long stay chronic geriatric ward. It was just like looking after forty four very elderly grandmothers, old ladies, every one of them was helpless; every one of 'em. After the ward's own 'missing' nurse turned up, I was returned to the general nursing office, and laboured awhile for them; for the rest of that shift I covered five wards on the male side in a form of patient *paper* census.

Wednesday, 31st July 1968

Seven-thirty pm. On the *Sunday* and *Monday* — nights, I worked on Amberley One admission Ward, and its patrols. And, on *Tuesday* night, I was number two man on Bramber Two refractory Ward. At one o'clock, in the early morning, we had had an emergency admission. A gentleman who was well *Up the stick.* This day, *Wednesday,* I was far too fatigued, to write any further lines of note.

Thursday, 1st August 1968

At school all day. Nothing exceptional.

Friday, 2nd August 1968

Seven-fifty pm. Shattered. *Friday 2nd Aug,* morning, I was again employed on the locked Refractory Ward of Bramber Two. We'd another new patient, an unusual admission.[93] He was a *very* large psychotic youth, who'd been quite difficult to contain. Tall, athletic, and *very strong, a* young fourteen-year old boy. That morning, the national newspapers, *Daily Mirror, Daily Sketch,* and *Daily Telegraph,* (I don't think the *Daily Mail*) had all carried a number of paragraphs on our new admission. His father had complained, not unjustly, that the boy (which later seemed a misnomer) had *had* to be admitted to our adult ward, solely because there was *nowhere* else available, which could cope with his psychopathy. There was then no available *special* place for violent sick youngsters like his son. Instead, by default, he had had to mix with much older patients. (Later, I learnt this was not, in itself, an unusual event.)

At around nine am, yet another emergency occurred, with one of our residents, an acute disturbed schizophrenic, a twenty-eight year old *immature* boy (for so he was); a lean, ill tempered strong gauche and demanding fellow, who went right *up the stick.* His name was John, Tall John. Did the noisy appearance, of our fourteen year old giant new admission, act as a threatening trigger for Tall John? Probably. Yes.

All of a sudden, John attacked another chronic and frightened patient, drawing blood from the other patient's brow by the weight of Tall John's fist. Tall John was one of the lads who, unhappily, far, far too often attacked staff and patients, at times quite viciously and, frequently damaged property. This furore had happened *in front* of our fourteen year old new admission. Eventually, I was able to steer him away from Tall John, by confiding in him that that patient was feeling rather unwell. Which was of course quite true.

Sadly they both were.

Once Tall John was *up the stick*, unless checked immediately, his condition worsened at an alarming rate as other patients soon become involved, and likewise would too, in rank fear, go *up the stick.* Fortunately, we *reassured* them both, and quietened things down. Sooner or later, Tall John (one of a relative minority), unless an improved technique is discovered, could severely maim someone or even, as could happen, accidentally kill in one of his frequent furores. To demonstrate Tall John's toxic absorption, he was then on medication of one-hundred mg of sodium Amytal; four times (QDS) a day. And prescribed five-hundred to 1000mg chlorpromazine (largactil) for emergencies, PRN.

On that day, the duty doctor instructed that we inject a substantial dose of 500 mg of chlorpromazine and, though he was a *little* subdued by that dosage, Tall John remained quite active. We were always rather reluctant to give him the whole prescribed PRN; one thousand mgs during a bad episode (fear of toxcidity). Odd, it was on record he was more rapidly subdued when on other medication, paraldehyde, but this was now redundant.

Now, a fraction of the sodium amytal, alone, would put an average patient to sleep for a number of hours. With Tall John's absorption, it often took *three* of us to hold him and prevent him hurting anyone else (let alone hurting himself), whilst attempting to administer the PRN injection of his prescribed medication. From 500 to 1000 mgs of liquid chlorpromazine was more than ample to relax the average patient. *The two together*! From this fact alone, the psychotic state and strength of our very disturbed patient can in retrospect be easily gauged.

After our emergency, another nurse and I took half a dozen patients off the ward, for a long, one-and-a-half-hour walk, and since three of them had no money, I bought three cups of tea, at the end of our crocodile stroll, at our Naunton Pavilion cafe (the prefabricated portakabin where patients could buy coffee, tea and sundries, overlooking the wide lawns of the Havenstoke Parkland and adjacent gardens).

Sunday, 5th August 1968

Five-thirty pm. Well, only a matter of hours, then I'm on night-duty again. *Saturday,* 3rd August. I was on a morning shift, overtime on Lister, the sick ward — a busy but uneventful morning. In the evening, Pete, a ward orderly colleague on Chilgrove One ward, kindly drove Sara, our two excited little boys and I into Chichester, for a visit to the East Street cinema. We enjoyed Kipling's *Mowgli* stories, in Disney's cartoon film *Jungle Book.*

Wednesday, 6th August, 8 pm
Ghost

Catching up. Last *Sunday* night I was on A & B patrols. *Monday* night... A & B patrols. *Tuesday* night; on *Lister* and *Chilgrove* block. Last night (Tues 5th Aug.)... on Lister sick-ward. It was just after midnight, and I had just returned from an un-eventful piquet to the Chilgrove wards. Mike, the duty Senior double-trained staff nurse, had been based on nights on Lister for a very long time. He was full of interesting anecdotes and had proved excellent company. I was reporting back. 'I got the dark shivers, Mike, as I came down the cold concrete back-stairs of Chilgrove Two. Especially *mid-way* under that cornered tall-window. Do you know the place?', I prattled on. 'The window was firmly closed, so I don't believe it was a draft that caused it?' He lent forward, from his white, sheet padded, seated, long-back and slowly, as if in confidence, he said, whispered, quietly, 'You don't know then... don't know; about the resident apparition ...?'

'Know what...?' I was intrigued.

'As you do know, Barry, ward attendants, before the war, slept on their own wards when they came off duty.' I did know that, as fact, for Bob on Amberley One had told me he had, at one time, been resident in that very room. 'But he... *The ghost...* if it is one... is harmless.', Mike continued in earnest. 'At the bottom of Chilgrove, two back stairs, separated between the long-stay ward and the main south corridor, boxed-in, as-it-were, are two small side-rooms, one was used as a store room. The other single room, was used as staff quarters. At some time, *before* the last war, a member of staff, one night (and afterwards, others), had confirmed they had seen *a ghost*, a transparent man, on *that* very spot you described, on *that* small bare concrete landing, located between the upstairs and downstairs Chilgrove' wards.'

I thought of Crabbe's Parish Poor Houses, with their early 1800s Napoleonic, crude wood, wattle and earth floors.[94] And contrast with Surrey's, middle class, mid Victorian *Holloway Sanatorium.*[95] And Edinburgh's WW1 Military Hospital *Craiglockhart.*[96] Ex-RAMC psychiatrist, Dr. Joyce, told me about the Scot's building, with its prolific marble floors and colonnaded staircases. All those old buildings too had, p'haps still had, have *benign* site ghosts. Mike admitted, he himself had not *seen* that entity, but had experienced that weird, cold feeling, that I had just experienced, on my ward piquet round. I'd always sustained mixed feelings, about perceiving an authentic ghost, and wanted to see one; yet did not want to see one... or its implications

The learned Dr. Johnson, Mike related, had all through his life-time wanted to see such an authentic ghost, and had been seen tapping on coffin lids in the church vaults off Cock Lane, in the churchyard near St. Paul's in London... 'I do not know whether he ever did get his wish ...?' Thomas Carlyle, in commentary, had said:

> 'Foolish Doctor! ... The good doctor was a ghost as actual and authentic as heart could wish; well-nigh a million of Ghosts were travelling the streets by his side ... Are we not Spirits, that are shaped into a body, into an Appearance; and that fade away into air and invisibility...?' [97]

NUPE Mike

Mike was ramrod tall, in late middle-age, with a thick thatch of, recently shampooed, white hair; carpeted wide window bushy eye brows — over two, very sharp green, intelligent eyes — *and*, a dry sharp wit. His lean face topped an always well-turned-out smartly dressed lean fit frame, noticeably, in his immaculate sheathed uniform, and stark white overall, covering his charcoal grey hospital suit — complimented, by an always clean (I had met Mike on an number of occasions), white shirt. He regularly wore either an NUPE union tie or, as during this night, an army RAMC neat knotted narrow tie and, in completion, *always,* well polished, black Oxford shoes. He was then close to retirement, but was still active, in all Union and political involvements, regarding staff and patients; '*Always put the Patient First,*' was his much mooted motto... and Mike's gentle, firm care and store of well applied knowledge, tallied well with his other hospital' ex-war service, pre-war trained, psychiatric and general trained, long-service, nursing colleagues. Very dependable and, I thought, a privilege to work with (and learn from), to assist in serving our patients' needs.

Robb's topical book, *Sans Everything* [98] was, if I remember correctly, the subject of one of our early morning discourses passed in debate which Mike and I had explored. 'Sans eyes, sans taste, sans reason, sans everything?...' Mike, too, had read the substance of that long essay, and the government white paper issued in reply.

As part of our *rounds,* around the bedded patients in the ward, we changed the incontinents' beds and treated their (where valid) bed sores, where the skin has become so soft that, no matter how much regular *turning*, some frail patients inevitably developed a pattern of wrinkled skin, flesh breaking down, and produced infamous bed-sores, sadly producing much pain and discomfort. We did our maximum best, to arrest and heal those damaged tissues, but found that some erosion continued.

As we moved away, out of one patient's earshot (just in case), Mike sadly commented, 'Poor devil — look at him', he whispered respectfully. 'That is something you seldom ever read about, seldom, even, in the Nursing Mirror. The perpetual tide, of faeces and urine, to be cleaned up off of body and bed. The terrific quantity. How many times was it, that you and I have cleaned up the shit and urine torrents this-night, and last night — on the Geriatric wards, and this Lister sick-ward and, tomorrow night and... well, Barry, you know what I mean...'

Our conversation drifted, into multiplying psycho geriatrics and geriatrics as a whole. Since the advent of National Health Service, in 1948, and a vast improvement, in subsequent preventive medicine and domestic welfare, in the community, it was believed there was a post-war increase, of surviving old people who, in past generations, would probably have long since died. We both agreed, that much tabloid, media *paper* publicity, is given, about the needs of our old people — but, generally, only in a sensational vein. That man pursues, in theory and practice, the cult of the young and beautiful and discards as ugly, old age. Yet, how soon, will *all'* of us, well most, reach this inevitable stage; if we are fortunate.

We discussed the agenda, of a *Mental Health Film Forum,* that I attended last June (1968), up in London. Even that programme was almost, solely, about adolescent's problems. Little, of a growing aged population's needs, depression an exception. A few podium references, to the needs of long-term schizophrenics, and dementia, given in oratory, but a *glib* mention. Already, our needy elderly take up half of all hospital beds throughout the country, and the media bombard its readers, with such sober information. To no avail. The aged, as undead.

Visited the Chichester Market, earlier that day and, at one stall, purchased three second hand books. One item was in hardback, *Mathematics for the Million*, by Lancelot Hogben and, two oddments, a small paperback volume *What is Buddhism?* issued during the 1920s by a Buddhist Lodge. And, a lone Volume 3 (complete in itself), in the 'Everyman' Edition, of Robert Burton's classic *The Anatomy of Melancholy*. [99] Tomorrow morning, another lecture On Psychiatry at Nursing School. *Sunday*. Why can't I get off to sleep ?

Monday, 12th August 1968
Sleepless Days

DAMN, DAMN, DAMN! I have not written for days, for the one simple reason, *I am too darn tired*, mentally and physically; lacking rest, and much needed sleep. I have the one side of me (shades of reason), ever analysing all the others. My thoughts, those seeming closeted, un-ending, mind chattering commentaries *on all and everything,* just will *not* abstain and grant me any proper meditation; and much needed sleep. We have guests staying. They, along with Sara and our boys, have all gone for a drive. I don't know whether this was *tact* or no, for they were all too aware, that I was on night-duty last night, and had not yet slept a wink. Further, I was on duty again, that night, and again the following night...

Circumstances allotted me only two to three hours sleep yesterday, having been on duty the night before (*Saturday*). Needless to say, what with *not* having a *whole* day off, since I started my block of mandatory night-duty — and this continuous battle, in attempting some rest and sleep — these facets tend to more than just aggravate my aspirations, on literary and orthodox studies; both of which I wish to continue. And, so self-evident, its inevitable effect on our domestic daily life routines.

But first, another quick look back.

Last Thursday, after the day at nursing-school, I remained in the hospital and, of necessity, studied for two more hours in the early evening. *Friday*, I served fourteen hours overtime, two whole shifts, as follows; morning, six-thirty to two pm, I was on Eastergate One long-stay ward. And, on the afternoon shift, that was split, first half of that afternoon I was on Bramber Two ward when two residents, went right *up the stick* — one of whom, reached the state of a raging tiger. God, what can be done, without the benefit of chemotherapy, toning down that turbulent violence? The second half, of that afternoon into evening's shift, I was on duty, on Chilgrove One ward, where mostly elderly long stay bedridden patients were in residence.

Saturday, I was on my night shift. I was on the Amberley One admission patrol (normal patrol piqueting A1, A2, B1, B2). We were, that night, *two* part-time nursing staff absent, so, additionally, at specific times, I was detailed as relief for assistance on Chilgrove One and Lister wards, and that in addition to the Admission ward patrol work. I was on duty at the Summersdale Day Hospital on *Sunday* 11th Aug. '68 (last night) and, on Admission ward patrols. One man was absent from night duty, off the nursing staff of Cavell One, and I had to fill in *his* duties, attending some rehabilitation patients. Also, included in the night's travels, I was allocated two wards sole responsibility, for (to the general nursing office) Amberley Two and Cavell One Rehab wards... Jeez we were busy... bloody shattered.

Why can't I sleep?

Noise, *any* unwelcome noise, infiltrated my fast, pulsing, head. Who said that I should have no trouble sleeping, on days in the countryside, should hear the large harvester, at work in the large field behind me... ugh! However, when I am well rested and fed; well slept, well fed, well sexually satisfied and conscience appeased towards *orthodox* studies, then, to all mankind (my family especially), I feel a keen emanation of loving, wanting and willingness. Eagerness to participate and mix with others, to share my satisfaction.

The loving is quick to disappear, in the Pavlovian plea for 'Quiet', 'Rest', 'Love', 'Sleep', 'Satisfaction' — *all* in an a-priori state of Being, to any work of improvement on the self. Damning myself afterwards, I'll bawl at the children, act curtly towards my wife, be apathetic towards other things and people for whom I truly cared for. When the goads that prevented rest and sleep were continually at work, the idiocy of this was that, invariably, it always was also exacerbated by any movement and noise of anything, affected, even, by the run of necessary ordinary household family affairs; children playing, wife cooking, traffic passing, etc. A pin, dropped, would be as a loud peal of thunder.

I recall, sometime, hearing comedian Spike Milligan talking on a BBC radio programme, about one of his hospital admissions — when he craved some peace and quiet, and in that desperate need for rest and quiet laid in bed, at the hospital. But, it was *not* to be. Spike recalled the agony caused by the outside dustbin men, clanging about in their duties in emptying the hospital garbage; and of the terrible torture, caused by city road engineers in their seemed constant cacophony with their necessary electric road drills, excavating concrete on the road; all outside the hospital walls.

Beelzebub's Babylonian buzzing great blow-fly; for me, summer symbolized those goaded Pavlovian pricks, which continually *prevented* my sorely needed rest.,. and so necessary quota of mortal sleep.

Why? Unable to sleep, at long, long last all seemed blissfully quiet, when a bloody, great big, noisy, blue bottle insisted on settling on a naked shoulder, hand, face, and buzzed incredibly *loud*; and, then, the fly insisted on sadistically goading me, on and on and on. So close to slumber, laid at last comfortable abed, and *came the huge bluebottle*, eventually this provoked a fit of *anger*, more at my petty unquiet self not coping — than at The Fly — and out of bed I jumped, *determined to kill the fly*, so that final peace and tranquillity might be finally allowed, and that oh so wanted sleep and rest and which, oh bliss slumber finally arrived...

Flies

I experienced some peace, in the green woods at the rear of the cottage. Garbed in gumboots, jeans and sweater. It happened, when I felt pleasantly warm, settled, drinking in that lovely air; enthused by the kind swaying boughs, thickly set around me, just when I felt that emanation, a feeling of some unexplained unity pact with Dionysus, quiet greenery and wild life — when, there they were *again*, those so megaphone loud-loud filthy buzzing bloody buzzing flies — buzz, buzzing all around me and, settling on my face and body, determined to suck the salty sweat from my naked brow... This was not in a desert heat...

I know, that even the fly must have a part to play, in nature's incredibly infinite complex pattern of delicate balance — but try telling my physical cravings that, when I am utterly then ruled by fatigue. When the mind is frail, weak, the body most vulnerable; oh yes, afterwards, I might regret killing the flies, but if I succeeded in dismissing that dire swarm I was, at that moment, content. This anecdote epitomized, for me, flawed mankind in the marketplace — and I was truly flawed. Any man may boldly stress and strut how super-animal, mankind — he is, being so above the ranks of Yahoos and primitive historical forebears; but he, too, may too often feel an' need to kill, and swat the fly.

Five pm. Still, the farm harvester machines were at work, a loud, cranking, crackling, cacophony of noise — another form of large fly, but one that I could *not* still and *must* learn to live with. A distant hammering somewhere, an aircraft flying overhead, but, *at last*, no more bluebottles about my head. Oops, family returned; *still no sleep*, but this writing has been good therapy, a form of rest. Work in a couple of hours' time. No sleep at all... this day.

Wednesday, 14th August 1968

Eight pm, *Monday* night, was spent on C. Patrol; but I had worked mostly on Lister sick ward. All that night, Mike and I awaited the death of an 80 year old patient. Throughout the slowly passing hours we listened; other patients heard his erratic, loud, anguished tones. Far from comatose, he was obviously aware of his dire condition, and attempted voicing his anguish; unfortunately he couldn't, only a choked rasping emanated from his vocal chords. His face was rather of a sixty to seventy year old, rather than eighty years, but was then closely concaved where once full cheeks had contentedly masticated.

His eyes were pitiful, alien matter oozing around his eyelids and corners, the eyes half-closed. The pupils were down to needle-points in size, and a hand waved across his face gave no response. Asking him questions (for orientation and consciousness) only provoked more suspicions of persecution, already of a paranoid nature. Worst of all, his whole body was racked with obvious internal pain. We did out utmost to alleviate his suffering, but mostly we were powerless.

We injected him with some *Pethadine* to reduce his pain and discomfort, which we hoped might help a little; and, as to his bedsores, continuous turning did not help — why? Simply because now, unable to take any solids and very little liquids, new cells could not, would *not* form; and all we could do was keep him clean of urine and faeces, and treat skin surface with pink *Ickosan* powder, which certainly helped — but could *not* rebuild and regenerate dead cells in this process. In between rounds, I continued reading on *Existentialism.* And inevitably — I asked again and again; *why* this need for terrestrial suffering? Is *all* life in movement — and friction? And, in mobility, must this and that — essential all good life, by movement — have an ultimate alchemic cost in angst and suffering?

Fechner

Questions of pre-birth, life, death and *what then;* coincided with glimpses towards our dying patient? In a small published work *On Life After Death*[100], the physicist Gustav Fechner (1801-1887) described, summarily, a belief that:

> 'Man lives on earth not once, but three times. The first stage of his life was (is) in 'continual sleep' and is pre-birth. The second stage, sleeping and waking by turns and mortal. The third stage waking forever after death.'

Which made perfect sense, but explained nothing to me. However, I found Gustav Fechner's optimistic work fascinating; though it *might,* for me, have been another gripping H.G. Wells' Science Fiction fantasy.

Our sick and dying, disabled 80 year old patient had lingered in bed physically and mentally sick... *for over two years*. Surely, an end to a present miserable existence, with no hope of ever again being on his feet but, always buts, one measures by degrees?

Further. In his case notes history, he could have been anyone's grandfather. He had been married twice, had five children, and had an unsuccessful relationship with most of them. Surely, a lonely man indeed. He had, at his dying, *nothing*, as he no longer had anyone mortal, but us, to anchor onto in this, his departing life. Everyone, surely, needs something, or someone, to adhere to — like lichen, growing on stone in a vacuum. Who would have doubted the poor fellow's intent, to battle for his life's spark, as it, despite his conscious efforts, slowly extinguished. And, how he fought, his hand indicating bewilderment, as he frequently passed it up to his brow, as cells nuclei slowly gained less and less oxygen. We consoled him, as best we could, but he did not recognize us, or our standing by. And alone, he fought, and in mind alone he died, but fifteen minutes *after* I had finished my shift in the morning. One extreme — in his dire departure, sad so typical an exit of many persons; like comparison of a death in a Victorian parish workhouse: David Lean's powerful bleak opening scene of a poor woman dying, in his Dickensian' black-and-white film 1946 *Oliver Twist.*

My Grandmother *Beatrice* (aka Beat) *Manton* recently died, aged 80 (Grandfather died in 1966) in North London. Devoted, her youngest son Arthur had refused a doctor's recommendation that she should enter hospital, to die. Much loved Nan had died, *not* alone, but passed away in her own home. I have no memories of my paternal divorced Australian Vaudeville father, or of *his* own emigrant Austrian artist father and relatives. As with our dying patient's absent relatives, I have no casework memories of my own *namesake* and forebears.

Tuesday, 13th August 1968

Night shift. Again on Lister sick ward, same patrol. A quiet night, after the night before, but I finished my shift at seven am. Sara knew I had decided to pop into Chi., before cycling home, as I had the day off from usual routines; so I visited Chichester market-place. At nearby Meynell's bookshop, in East Street, I had acquired Jean-Paul Sartre's *Plays* in a Penguin paper-back edition, which included *Altona...* and *Flies.*

Thursday, 15th August 1968

Continued lectures on *Psychiatry* (No.3), *Classification and Initial Diagnosis.* A rather interesting film, on the *Mind of a Schizophrenic*, French-made and in colour, it brought to debate interesting issues. A well crafted film, but... ugh! 'Horrible', was my first response. I referred to substance of the film — of a young man persecuted by delusions, illusions and florid hallucinations, and most by his 'incongruity of effect'. 'Surely', I enquired, of our tutor, Mr Ilford, *all* schizophrenics don't suffer like that, all the time? Is their schizophrenic sense of time, distorted, as drugs may distort time, as in our sleep. Why, I've seen many schizophrenics enjoying things...? 'Ah', he replied, 'But *how many* untreated schizophrenics, naked and unashamed, as it were, have you known seen in this hospital?'

'Well, eh?', I stammered, not cottoning on. He continued, 'You see them when, already, their General Practitioners (GPs) or other hospitals have commenced treating them with tranquillisers — and so on. Have you ever honestly seen them completely untreated?' I realized I hadn't and, humbly, got his point.

Monday, 19th August 1968
Existential Dave

Late pm. Brief resume of time, since last notes of *Friday* 16th August. On the morning of Friday, the Sixteenth of August, I had made a routine trip into the woods, at the rear of our rented cottage, to stock-up a supply of fire wood for the kitchen Aga boiler. In the afternoon, I departed for an overtime shift, on

Amberley One. During my shift, Mancurian David, engaged me in conversation. Dave was a philosophy student, in as a possible *borderline* schizophrenic, (but, from what I gathered, it was an uncertain diagnosis), suffering with hallucinations, and some delusions — primary diagnosis Simple Schizophrenia.

Now well into Dave's book, *Existentialism as Philosophy* by Fernando Molina. [101] I'd recently been introduced to Kierkegaard, Nietzsche, Husserl and Heideggar (Colin Wilson's *Outsider* [102] cycle had earlier been most helpful), and I was presently immersed in a good commentary on Heideggar[103] and Sartre's works. I listened to our recovering university student, Mancurian Dave. We chatted about the conundrum of *Man and his Being*[104], it being uppermost, in his mind — and in mine. In getting better, he is able to presently express himself more and more clearly. And, from the philosopher's Preface, I interpreted Heideggar's 'being', a referral to actual life existence. And 'of *time'* as the possible horizon, for any understanding whatever of Being. Philosopher Dave said, he believed *only* rational analysis (empirical — to be seen), could explain art poetry and the emotions. I disagreed.

In analysis, surely anyone from Heideggar[105] from Being There (aka Dasein) — erm! Then Being — here, *from* There (what, rather than where) *must* be limited according to mortal *capacity* (quality) at *any* given moment in one's lifetime. The foregoing made me think, of Fechner's three stages of (known) living on earth. Heideggar's Dasein presented as a meaningful metaphor (*not* knowable quantity of onion levels); *and,* as part of that onion, a singular perceptual *matrix* of the senses; the range of just how far one can... explore, think, see, hear, smell, touch, create. But I, presently, can only dip in those learned tomes.

With the Heideggar added definition as: 'something which we can neither widen, nor go beyond, but which provides the limits for certain intellectual activities performed "within it."' I presume *it* as the body of the Being, and its absolute *capacity,* and functional minimum, in one lifeline. How many humans have attained *their* full potential (how to evaluate), introduces the conundrum, once more, of everyone's *limitations* in each unique mortal existence at its functional peak and lows — in sickness and good health. Intellectual Questionnaire (IQ) forms can only be a starting point in such a fulsome analysis. But, in honesty, Alice and the white rabbit... Charles Dodgson (1832-98) — where are you?

'When I was very bad', Dave said, 'everything was so-unreal. I could *not* believe in the reality of anything about me, even and especially about myself.'

Falling in line with his description, of his pre-morbid etiology, his recent and untreated illness origins. 'Can you tell me', I enquired, 'Did *you* feel as if everyone was against you, or that objects had symbolic meanings...?'

He replied, 'Well *no,* not really. I couldn't concentrate on anything. My mind would continuously be distracted. I *wanted* to join in with people, *but just couldn't.* I was continuously alone in my upstairs room, where I would gaze out of the window to the horizon, for hours on end, and just wish that I could cycle there. Eventually, I remember I did — and I was *very* disappointed and unhappy afterwards.'

'Oh, why?', I asked.

'Well... the horizon... it just wasn't there! It was all so *unreal,* as if it didn't exist at all. The trees I was aiming for, I touched, and even *they* didn't seem real. It's, it's *this feeling* I had, have; it prevents me enjoying anything, *keeps* everything away. Only when I eventually came to this hospital, and had treatment, tablets, did I feel myself really, once more, as a person existing. I know I'm *still* sick and can't *yet* read anything; except Kafka, that is, who I feel a strong affinity with... I've a long way to go...' A few weeks back, the day after his admission, I'd noticed articulate David, when he was attempting to read Kafka's *Castle.*[106] Dave had considerably improved, since our first meeting that time on the admission ward.

Now, it's true, Rosetta Stone textbooks tell us much. But how much easier it is to attempt some understanding (as tutor Mr Ilford had suggested to me), *when* I can experience rapport with a patient, *WHEN THE INFORMATION COMES FIRST HAND.* I seldom read Case Notes, until *after* I have met the patient. (In retrospect, I found this aspect sometimes questionable.) Where possible, I first talked to the patient myself. Odd, though, this was about the third or fourth young (i.e. in twenties) schizophrenic I had met, who had more than a passing existential interest in Kafka. Erm?

Saturday, 17th August 1968

Continued wet, miserable weather. During the day, I laboured in the woods, gathering somewhat soggy, dead, wood as logs for a few days' supply. It's hard work, but therapeutic.

Last night, Sara finished her typed manuscript, of 301 pages of adult fantasy. I promised to read it, all next week.

The boys were very active, and appeared, thank God, happy and healthy. That *Saturday* night, I had been on Chilgrove and Eastergate long-stay wards' piquet patrols, and was again based on Lister sick ward, with reliable Mike. We had a man *out*, so his wards too had to be covered; it then meant I had to include four reliefs.

Sunday, 18th August 1968

What a day! Cold, wet, miserable and very stormy. And this is Summer. How unhappily typical, an English Summer day of late. It's a funny thing, but in writing notes, one is doing just that, tiny specks of flotsam, black dust, shadows cast out from the mind; the bulk of the experienced moment dissipated, its details *already* in the past, even the writing never possible, to touch pen or paper, in *that* consciousness again. At writing, I am attempting existential, that is (was) paradoxically recording, often, impressions of those exact *now* moments. Yet, conscious, that each fraction of time in doing so, had already become but commentary, memories. And yet, I am indeed often aware of, in not otherwise thinking, of *watching* myself, that mortal self, in those acts. *Sunday* night, again, on Amberley admission ward patrols. And, another man out. I'd also been requested to assist, on Chilgrove One long-stay geriatric ward, early in the morning. This ongoing 'self analysis' habit of mine, does it, *en-toto*, have more virtues than vices... or vice-versa?

Monday, 19th August 1968

Weather still temperamental. Night patrol again on Amberley One admission ward.

Friday, 30th August 1968

Late pm. A great deal had happened. To summarise... on *Tuesday,* the twentieth of August, I'd been detailed night-duty on Amberley One, and its patrols. No problems at work, but.... arriving back home on *Wednesday* morning, of the Twenty-first August, I was greeted by a host of activities. Our home 'guests' drove us into Portsmouth, where we saw my mother and my Dublin' born step-father, at their confectionery shop in Southsea. Sara and I had collected an old television set, from my former bachelor days, which I had paid for eight years ago.

On the way back to Chilgrove, at Sara's request, we collected a deserted guard dog, from a Portsmouth branch of the RSPCA. Within hours of collection, the poor fella was already snapping... at everyone. *Thursday*, twenty-second of August, I attended the hospital school and, on return, learnt the disturbed dog had become *too* aggressive yet, oddly, very good, but *only* amongst us. Our bruised guests returned to London.

We had had another excellent lecture on Psychiatry at the hospital, but tension was mounting, at home. *Friday*, the twenty-third August, instead of doing some overtime, I'd decided it was more prudent to stay home. And proved a very rough day. *Saturday*, the twenty-fourth August. Poor Sara, we'd had no choice, and had to return Rex back to Portsmouth. He'd proved he was — was — too *good* a guard dog. Tears, masses of tears, and a resultant reactive family depression. I had to work that night, on Amberley One and its patrols. *Sunday*, the twenty-fifth August. Slightly better day. Amberley One and its patrols again... That day, my In-laws arrived, along with news that my brother-in-law had been admitted to hospital, for an emergency operation. *Monday*, the twenty-sixth August. Sara, and the children, left for Lancing, to comfort her sister, and help to look after their children; I shall fend for myself awhile. I was on A Patrol night-patrol, that night. T*uesday,* the twenty seventh August. News. Brother in law's operation, had proved successful. But a need to stay awhile, in hospital. Sara staying over at Lancing, to support her sister and young family. Again on Amberley One night-piquet patrols. *Thursday*, the Twenty-ninth August, was a hospital day; school. Good lectures.

And, what a week it was, internationally. On 21st August 1968, a fascist invasion of Czechoslovakia, by the bear of USSR Russia. And, of brutality in America led by purported exploiting elements. So, both ends of the coin, the pendulum left-and-right. Ugly Fascism. I saw the memories on film, of Munich 1938. I'd presently lost all interest in any obligatory form of *study,* but not for long.... Last *Wednesday, 21st Aug,* visiting Meynell's bookshop in East Street Chichester, I casually remarked (looking through the art books shelves) to the book-seller, there was a lack of Surrealist illustrations on view. I mentioned the French surrealist pics in Louis Pauvels' book on *Gurdjieff'*[107]. The Shop Manager commented that he thought, sadly, some Surrealist artists and thinkers had died, through a *mental excess* in attempting — too much willed isolation. I thought, whimsically, of surrealist eccentric collector Edward James, our absentee landlord, who was out in Mexico (our Estate Rent Office Manager believed) — and James' interest in Surrealist painters. I thought of two of our patients back on Bramber Two, who'd been Professional surrealist artists — before their breakdown.

On the way back home, cycling through the prolific wind-spewn rain, I thought awhile, of that bookshop verbal exchange. And reflected, parallels reaching into my sea of mind, looking for a matrix, an island of *solid* experience, that similarity — and still I knew, helpless, that *I know nothing*. Practically every bicycle-trip to and from the cottage, I'd been vividly aware of my mortal passage, mechanically moving on, through along a wormlike tunnel; a speck of matter through a mostly grey-green morass, guided by habit and memorised geographical landmark symbols. *But* how bloody *marvellous,* when *size* and *measured* distance [108] is really truly considered! How wonderful. A teleological mote, in an infinite and eternal unknown cosmology. Me. Whatever my tentative fabric.

Tuesday, 3rd September 1968
A Drug is a Drug

Saturday, 31st August, was spent on a long cycle ride to Shoreham, to visit Sara and our boys. I stayed the night with Sara, Paul and Kit, at her sister's, and returned on *Sunday,* the First of September. Last *Sunday* night, the 1st September 1968, I'd been on Amberley One, duty and its patrols. *Monday* 2nd September — night-duty again on Amberley One patrol. That night, I concluded reading an interesting novel, by Colin Wilson, called *Necessary Doubt*.[109] In Wilson's detective book he used, as its theme, a Professor Zweig, an ardent Existentialist Philosopher. An excellent mouthpiece, for Wilson's eye opening commentaries, on the existential enigmas of life.

For me, most noticeable a note on his new work, perhaps, it repeated a theme used in his *Mind Parasites*[110], adding to his superb *Outsider*[111] cycle of books. He'd introduced into his text, a soma like Huxley drug, that cleansed the perceptions. Perhaps I'm merely prejudiced, by my recent awareness of its *abusers*, young drug addicts — which included LSD and Hash addicts. I had my doubts. I was convinced, that most *contrived* chemical stimuli, used *for kicks*, was a toxic entry to the body's metabolism. No matter what catalyst buzz arguments were set forward. In particular, I had thus far concluded, that any such dialogue had to be about proper homeopathic like use — or acknowledged abuse, by any defined ingested food substance.

Most LSD, or other substance addiction, indicated a *potential* toxic abuse, or so I then believed. I realised perceptions need to be cleansed. But drug (and what is a drug) abuse in excess, if self-inflicted, can never be of lasting aesthetic value, but a craving physical dependence of which I was already aware of, in many young addicts among our patients. Surely, any so called Seeker, in depending on synthetic drugs as a mystical short cut, was pretentious; if all they really wanted was a short-term substance buzz. However if it, the cleansing, even moving on temporarily, is ultimately achieved by application of the credit will, *then* it might be, may be, positive. But, a qualified mentor is surely necessary. It's easy in principle, to abuse others in manipulation of others, *against their will* and, albeit, without any self-knowledge and deliberate ill intent.

From sparse experience and observation, I believed it, the emotional font, was that which predominately controlled brain aspects of the will. But, in drug (substance) abuse, with any described 'Incongruity of affect', being out of sync, emotional turbulence, perhaps leave a person as but a chaotic shell in a zombie like description... living, yet dead. And, though it may seem cliched, it was a far deeper aspect, I thought I'd commentated on as a student. A search for an alternative pathway, a system, one chosen method of self discipline that *had* to be taught, learnt and practised.... an aspect of a true, higher man.

Wednesday, 4th September 1968

Morning. I concluded another Amberley One patrol, and wearily cycled back home.

After some bed rest, I decided to do necessary wood sawing, then some study; and a little serious reading. After completing several Exam questions, I decided I'd had enough, and commenced, attempted, a perusal of an *Introduction* of Kierkegaard's *Five Edifying Discourses*. (Job. The ram in the thicket et cetera...) I began the *new* reading; and, suddenly, felt *very* irritated by the nearby antics of Shasa, our recently acquired lovable little ginger brown kitten. But why? On checking my petty annoyance. Clearly, I was quite *cross* with myself, and my irresponsible responses to little Shasa. Why so ...? And concluded;

I WAS TRYING TO CONCENTRATE ON TOO MANY THINGS AT ONCE!

Having just finished the *specific* substance, of Psychiatric and Nursing questions. And received uninvited data, which I had running through my brain, from a BBC television Western then being shown (its soundtrack permeating my concentration). *Idiot;* I should have turned the TV set *off,* long ago. And then, there was my subsequent attempts to concentrate and comprehend — *both* complexities, *at the same time*. In addition, I was *also* attempting multifarious questions-and-answers, provoked by Kierkegaard's Introduction; *and* its appraisal of his commentaries on Christian Ethics; and maintain awareness of the environment — in and about me....

The ever *waiting, for something to happen,* made the inoffensive noise of the little ginger kitten all too audible and unbearable. Most important, too much Superego, made me feel guilty for attempting not to concentrate *only* at the psychiatric work but, instead, I gained pleasure from other mental diversions. And perhaps then, most important, the loneliness put my emotions and perceptions on tenterhooks — hoping Sara *might* telephone... I stopped the Kierkegaard discourses, as these needed far more singular concentration. Man is gregarious by nature, but much too fickle by temperament. Well I am... Isn't life moving on, *one* damn great game of Patience.

Friday, 6th September 1968

Had a la-zee day, doing little work at home. No overtime. Day off. On my own. Workbook recorded I'd officially finished my block of *Night-Duty.*

Exam

Yesterday was the *last,* of our intake's First Year study-days and, although we had had an interesting lecture on Psychiatry, the peak events of the day centred around our Internal Hospital Examination, which preceded the real thing.

The Exam was in three parts, Written, Practical and Oral.

Unusual too, we (my colleague and I) were told we were but guinea-pigs — as this Exam procedure had *not* been done before (to his knowledge), at this Hospital.

My internal practical included, supervising and participating, in giving a blanket-bath on Chilgrove One ward to an old, believed *difficult,* bed-patient (i.e. potentially aggressive) with a delicate congestive heart condition, on three week Mersaryl dosage. I chuckled privately, for the tutor had chosen, in advance, dear old Boxer, who I already knew quite well and had a real soft spot for and, predictably, it all went well.

Psychology

I downed Kierkegaard, and decided to study orthodox (not existential) Psychology for a while; I had already started William James' *Principles of Psychology* [112], and intended to move on to William McDougall's *An Outline of Psychology* [113] on completion of James' book.

Experience made me query, why more accent (in Psychiatry) is not placed on 'habitual Depression', very much apart from 'Endogenous' or 'Reactive Depression'; habitual depression, it seemed, it meant, *to me*, that one is *not* really miserable or depressed, but from a cumulative past does *not* allow the central nervous system, happiness. That elusive butterfly... *It doesn't know it enough*—to replicate.

1st October 1968
Intermediate State Exam

On the first of October, I sat the important intermediate State RMN Exam. No student could continue the course, towards the state finals, without having *first* passed that necessary, elementary examination (reproduced below).

THE GENERAL NURSING COUNCIL FOR ENGLAND & WALES
INTERMEDIATE EXAMINATION FOR MENTAL NURSES
TUESDAY 1st OCTOBER 1968

Time allowed: 2 hours

IMPORTANT:Read the questions carefully, and answer only what is asked as no marks will be given for irrelevant matter.
The percentages shown on the right of this paper denote the weighting allocated to each section of the question.
NOTE Candidates MUST attempt ALL questions.

1. A newly admitted elderly patient has a very dirty mouth and a full set of neglected false teeth.
(a) How would you clean this patient's mouth and teeth? 25%
(b) What advice and retraining might you need to give the patient on care of the mouth? 30%
(c) What different types of human teeth are there and what are their function? 15%
(d) In what ways may a dirty mouth and bad teeth affect health? 30%

2. A rehabilitation programme is being designed for a middle-aged patient who is finishing a course of electroplexy (ECY)
(a) What occupational facilities should the hospital be able to offer? 20%
(b) What factors would influence your selection for this particular patient? 40%

(c) If this patient is reluctant to participate what part could you play? 40%

3. A patient is found unconscious in a secluded part of the hospital garden. An empty tablet container is nearby.
(a) What immediate action would you take? 30%
(b) What possible causes would you consider for loss of consciousness in this patient? 25%
(c) In what psychiatric disorders is attempted suicide a common risk? 15%
(d) What effect may an attempted suicide by a patient have on the other patients in the ward? 30%

4. What are the factors that you would expect to find in a "good secure family" with two children, aged eight and ten years? 40%
What special problems would be experienced by the family in each of the following situations:-
(a) an aged relative comes to live with them: 30%
(b) a widowed aunt dies and her ten year old child is fostered with them? 30%

5. Describe the psychological and physical needs of elderly people in the community.
Discuss ways in which these needs can be met. 100%

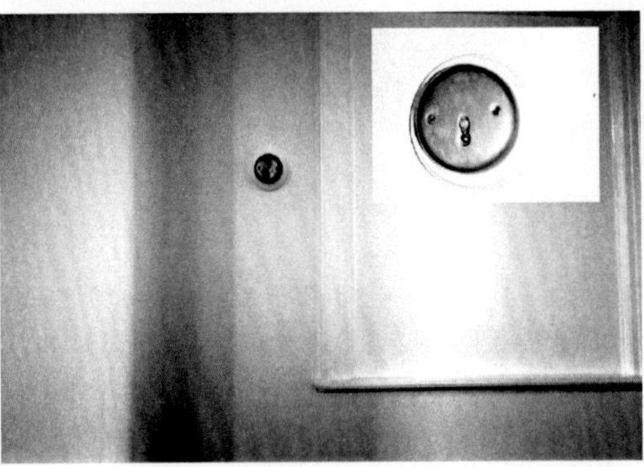

Night-time disused, staff piquet clock-in security boss (for detail, see closeup on right). Few chronic wards were staffed at nights and so a duty nurse would cover a number of those wards - every night. Every long-stay pre-sixties ward owned one. The hospital piquet night nurse, on his rounds had to clock in with a key, at specific times. The electric boss was connected to end on a paper roll in the Superintendent's office. Woe betide the night-nurse who missed recording an essential nocturnal visit.

GRAYLINGWELL HOSPITAL

CONFIDENTIAL .... WARD .... Hospital/Clinic

REPORT of Accidents or other Untoward Occurrences to Patients, Staff, or other Persons on the Premises.

Patient/Staff/Visitor *(delete as appropriate)*

Name in full .... Case No. .... *(Where appropriate)*

Home address .... Date of birth ....

.... Sex ....

....

PARTICULARS OF OCCURRENCE

Date .... Time of accident ....

Time of reporting ....

Description of nature of accident or occurrence:

Where accident or occurrence took place:

How caused:

In case of staff was person on or off duty at the time? On/Off *(Delete as appropriate)*

In case of patients and visitors, were they authorised to be in this place and engaged in the activity? Yes/No *(Delete as appropriate)*

Names and addresses and status of witnesses:

....

....

....

Description of apparatus or equipment involved: ....

Has it been retained for inspection? ....

Signature of person reporting incident ....

TO BE COMPLETED BY DUTY DOCTOR

Nature of injuries Slight Moderate Severe *(Delete as appropriate)*

Description of injuries:

Treatment prescribed:

Disposal of injured person recommended: *e.g.*, Referred to G.P. to stay on duty. put to bed.

Signed ....
Medical Officer

This Copy to Hospital Secretary

Mandatory Accident form (aka. *Incident Form*). In use 1967 to 1971. Used for Tall John (many times); The Major; William; and countless other patients during our Hospital's existence. Other caring institutions have their equivalent; but, in Psychiatric services, such 'Duty of Care' forms were in frequent use.

Chapter Eight
Summersdale Villa

'... The best of a bad job is all any of us make of it - Except of course, the saints - such as those who go ... To the sanatorium ...' [1]
T.S. Eliot. The Cocktail Party.

14th September 1968 to 7th December 1968

Summersdale Villa—Ole Bill—History—Poor Law, 1930—Not-be-'druv—Tour—Baths—Laurie & Julie—Chico—Playtime—The Rev & ECT—Eyes of Horus—And Collect—Air Castles—Dr. Ferring Technician—Dr. Harrod Psychologist—Mr Ricks—Rorschach—Phobic Jack—Art or Science—Thirty-nine Steps—Dr. William Sargant—Not Cricket—RAF Brian—Ipcress—Black Art—Propaganda—Crow—William James—Incident

14 September 1968
Summersdale Villa

I'd no idea what he meant, to start with. Third year Alternative Bob didn't sound critical, neither was he mickey-taking, judging by the affable matter-of-fact tone of his voice, as we chatted strolling, along the North Drive, towards Summersdale Villa, (which was an admission block for short-terms, out-patients, and upstairs base for the Clinical Psychology Department, and academic Medical Research Council unit, aka MRC). I was about to start my first morning, on a *new* three-month placement, and he was on his way to the Nursing School. Bob was in his early twenties, and recently married to Jean, who was another psychiatric nurse.

'Bit of a loner aren't you Barry... *odd*... you know...', Bob grinned, sagely, and nodded his head with a shake of his thick mane of neat, tied-back, long black-hair, and tight goatee, which tightly wagged, minutely, up-an'-down, as he anticipated no objection, rightly so, from me — then curious.

'What ...', I started to reply, but Bob persisted, his sharp blue-eyes piercing with intensity, atop his lean frame. 'You know... well... so, so serious; an' sort of, well, yeah, eccentric... different...'. He chuckled in apparent approval.

I looked across at him for explanation, as we continued strolling from the Main Building front-entrance, en-route to our destinations.

'Oh?', I queried, perhaps pompously, defensive. But I knew what was coming, leastway I thought I did. And it wasn't anything unpleasant, mere commentary in affable conversation. Bob was into Alternative Medicine and Sociology, in a big way.

'You do a heck of a lot of reading, don't you?', he said. I recalled he had visited me, in my room, on some alchemic Gurdjieff enquiry, a few months back.

'Art and literature Folklore, Science Fiction, Novels, Philosophy and stuff; don't you?', Bob added, in some conclusion. I didn't see anything odd, in my extra-curriculum reading, but clearly he did, and perhaps other student colleagues did too, but so what....

And then Alternative Bob's point:

'Well... I'm fascinated by Arthurian lore, and Social History, myself', he offered, by way of dove and palm. Something offered in common.

Ole Bill

At that moment, abruptly interrupted, we were stopped by Ole Bill, a long-stay nomad patient, who had been a child resident here since before the first-world war; rumoured, since 1906. I recalled, when I was being escorted around the grounds, during my interview, on that first day, Ole Bill had been introduced to me then...

He was crookedly tall, with well-weathered lean-cheeks, a hawk-nose, concave small twinkling eyes on a lean-body, and very, *very* large hands. We'd been warned that Ole Bill in horse-play might, for instance, twist our arms behind our backs with considerable force, but respond, content to talk, and be ill-advised to be persuaded by him to *box* a little...

'You heard?', Ole Bill solemnly sussurated, as we agreed to stop the moment and be sociable.

'What's that, Bill?' we asked. He was a well known eavesdropper who played dumb, when around strangers and known officials, but retained bits of, often telling, information.

'Gonna be a lotta changes with Salmon, you know.', he winked knowingly. 'Doctor Crampton told me. In confidence it were.' Ole Bill shoulder edged into us, a bit closer.

'Some nurses might be sacked.' He lowered his otherwise, loud voice, even more so, bidden under his own private, hush Holy, sub-rosa canopy. And, raised his long, crooked, right forefinger, touching his lower lip.

And looked Janus about us.

'S' right', Ole Bill concluded. And, as if to dramatise this secret messenger delivery, he about turned and slowly stalked off; perhaps on another mission.

Bob and I grinned at each other, but said nothing about Ole Bill's confidential titbits. After all, we were only RMN students, and any hierarchical changes were unlikely to affect us; though it was already common knowledge that senior staff had had to re-apply for their own jobs, on the hospital establishment. The Salmon he referred to, was the latest Ministry Of Health *Report of The Committee on Senior Nursing Staff Structure*[2], which was to be shortly phased in at the hospital, and removed the iconic *status quo,* of *the* hospital Matron.

A dry, gentle, balmy breeze delivered sweet autumn smells from uncrushed pollen, and fallen leaves, which stuck to our feet, as we slow walked and chatted. 'One thing about Ole Bill', Bob mused, as we passed the Naunton Pavilion cafe. 'He's very much a part of this hospital's history, perhaps one of its principal revered characters. Someone tried to discharge him out of the hospital, a while back. Didn't happen. He was that upset. Said, 'this is *my* home! Hands off !' Anyway, they got the message and left him alone after that.'

'Yeah. He gets everywhere about the hospital grounds, is well known in Chichester and clearly feels, no... knows, he is important, and is a principal representative, living on this Hospital Estate. And, I reckon, he has just cause, erm, don't you...?', I added, with not a little bemusement, 'I mean... really, *here* since 1906. It's his home.'

'Number One', Bob continued. 'When they opened the Naunton in sixty-six, Ole Bill was formally introduced to some visiting dignitaries; Duke of Richmond himself, I think.'

Bob concluded this anecdote, and we realized our historical pursuit had brought us to our separate ways, as he turned right towards the School.

I carried on down the North Drive, still full of Ole Bill, and musing on the historical background of this Hospital Estate; Ole Bill's long-stay Home and Manor.

Summersdale History

Before the Roman settlement of Chichester, Belgic tribes from Brittany across the English Channel had settled on the low coastland, between the sea and southern slopes of the South Down hills. The then heavy forested hills, and northward terrain, was populated by earlier resident Britons; I believed they were shorter in stature. Pure Kipling.

Occasional conflict, between the lowland Belgics and those hillside Britons off Goodwood Trundle and thereabouts, instigated a substantial amount of Belgic (or earlier) front-line earthwork fortifications and trench work (like modern ha-ha's), much evidence of which survived into the twentieth century. Those trenches, rather eroded, crossed the present Graylingwell Estate northwards, and a little further north (outside the Estate), the trenches extended westwards across modern Summersdale.

In the Thirteenth century, the grounds of Graylingwell was the site of a Royal hunting warren; later, given over to the Chichester ecclesiastical establishment, it was converted to farming and became the Estate of the Graylingwell Manor, which it remained until the Nineteenth century. Anna Sewell [3] author of *Black Beauty: his grooms and companions. The autobiography of a horse* lived for several years with her Quaker parents at the rented Grayling Wells Chichester, *Farm House,* in the mid-1850s.

In the latter Nineteenth century, the Chichester Ecclesiastical owners of the Estate re-sold it, to a newly elected West Sussex County Council — which, itself, was recently formed after the passing of the Local Government Act of 1888. The West Sussex County Asylum construction begun in 1893 under the benign powers of the new County Council — this then opened, in 1897.

Poor Law, 1930

In response to post-war demands, The Poor Law, in existence since 1601, was amended in 1930[4], which instigated the *Mental Treatment Act*. Previously, only compulsory certified patients could have been admitted into the hospital. This effectively meant that until an indigent person became too mentally ill, to be kept in a Workhouse ward, they were unable to be admitted into the public asylum — for more appropriate care and treatment.

The enlightened new act followed upon the focus of the Great War aftermath, of a need to diagnose, and treat, rate-aided people still suffering from the effects of Shell-shock and Neurasthenia. Other civilians, who needed treatment *without certification,* could be admitted as Temporary Patients under Section 5 of this act. Summersdale Villa (*Summersdale* being a local parish to the North of Chichester), was built in Graylingwell on the already so-named, farm-field, in response to the new act. The villa was then opened in 1933.

After my experiences on Bramber Two, and completion of Night-Duty, Summersdale Villa beckoned as comparative light-relief. What was self-evident, was its immediate surrounding landscape. When the old Asylum buildings were constructed, the wards and enclosed airing-courts anticipated any, and all, *severe* psychiatric conditions to be catered for, with few clinical treatments available. Only custodial care was provided.

Summersdale, in 1933, introduced wards with unlocked doors, airing-courts with no enclosing railings; and personal (their own) clothing permitted. Several, singular end-rooms could, as pads, be locked when emergencies were called for; but these odd, though essential, side-rooms were, in general, exceptions. Pads were still in use, in the mid 1960s.

As I separated from Bob, he went off to the nursing school. I continued along the North Drive and entered the hedge-lined driveway, to the front entrance of Summersdale. I would later own copies of early rustic photos (donated by a retired head gardener), which showed a hospital shepherd, with sheep, about this same area where I now walked between trees and flowering shrubs. Down the central front drive, with parked cars on either side, after climbing two concrete steps I entered, and turned left into the Male side, of this admission ward.

On the right, divided, was the Female side. Males and females met at the kitchen and dining-room areas only; exactly at the centre — before the front entrance. Each side had official social half-hours, when the opposite sex were invited across the divide.

Integration of the sexes was not yet complete. Since 1949, some sort of joint-eating arrangements in Summersdale had been accommodated; aided by organized mixed social half hours. and other informal (not obligatory) initiatives, willingly exchanged by staff and patients from each side. Today, a mixed gathering in the male ward-lounge, by planned invitation and, next time, on the female ward-lounge. This occasional exchange was still operating, when I entered for my placement, in the autumn of 1968.

Summersdale Bill was my new Charge, another old soldier, an amiable, broad shouldered man, with dark hair; a bald patch just appearing, where his forehead tide receded. He was average height, five-feet-eight or so; most noticeable feature, an narrow face and sharp Roman nose and, most, his gravel (not grave) voice giving strong Sussex boom commands which, I soon learnt, belied a sensitive man; a bit like Big Jim, on Chilgrove One, though without the ramrod approach of the latter.

Red was my Summersdale staff-nurse. He was a tall, thin, athletic young man, and an ardent sportsman, with short red hair and, very lively, with his long, fast walking strides, which were soon familiar to me, down the ward corridors.

Not-be-druv

Charge nurse Bill and Staff nurse Red were Sussex men, who '*would-not-be-druv*' as Sussex dialect suggested; they could not, would not, be intimidated—least ways I thought that was the inference. And, as strong, just carers, Summersdale Villa was thus also (as Main Building) a refuge, an Asylum, for the vulnerable.

Although I had visited this unit, for various reasons, over the past few months, I had never had a full tour; and was grateful when Red was detailed for this chore after breakfast, and early medication was completed.

And Red and I began walkabout, on male Summersdale, as colleagues.

Tour

'Summersdale has four wards; two on the male side, and two on the women's side, with other facilities in the building, upstairs', Red prefaced our leisured tour.

'Our male-side has one ward downstairs, and a second ward upstairs. The Female side has the same. So our wards are Summersdale One, Two, Three and Four. One and two are Male wards...', he continued.

'The MRC , Medical Research Council, is Summersdale Four, upstairs on the female side. They share ward space with Summersdale Three's female residents.'

A narrow wooden well, spiral staircase by the side of the central ground floor, dining-space and kitchen area, led upstairs to the female side. Two other, but concrete, stairways, were at each end of the ground floor, male and female wards. Red and I left the front entrance, and proceeded along the ground floor male-corridor of Summersdale One. Adjoining the front entrance, a corner room was used as an small storage room (later to be converted to a single bedroom). Next, on the male side, was its Nursing Office. Within it, the (then customary) large board, up on a wall by the desk, with basic details of resident inpatients, listed for admin. The board properly listed :

Names, Age, Consultant, Special (Section or Special Diet etc.), Leave column. The Consultants' names would indicate the firm they were admitted from; Worthing, Horsham or Chichester districts. Taking up space, the ward drugs trolley was chained, and locked, in one corner of the nursing office; several green filing cabinets, and the usual office furniture of wooden desk and chairs; a loose carpet mat completed the scene.

A small interviewing room was next, adjacent to the nursing office, used by visiting doctors or for other more formal purposes, and locked when not in specific use.

Next, still on the left, was a large Male lounge, with a full size billiard table and its scoreboard; and lounge chairs on the periphery. A radio, and portable record player, was placed on a corner table, with records scattered or piled alongside.

There were three young men playing snooker, as we entered the lounge; and a fourth, somewhat small, older man, with a trim white van dyke beard (I thought of young Bob and his pointed black beard), the patient sat mournfully on a cane-chair in the opposite corner.

'Hi Red', echoed two of the players in greeting. One was in bright sports jacket and flannels; the other in red-shirt and brown corduroys. A third person, standing, was a spectator who was trying to tell a joke, in the midst of their play; dressed in white shirt and summer shorts.

'Hello Mick,Tony', answered Red. And, turning towards the stand up comic, clearly the youngest of the four residents, he smiled, and added, 'Our own joker, Lawrence - Laurie'. And, no way intending to ignore the fourth man, depressed in the corner.

'Morning Rev.' The dour Reverent looked up, nodded, and smiled in a tight, tortured effort, in unspoken response to Red's acknowledgement of him.

'Ten minutes gentlemen. And off to OT, okay?', Red said to the group. 'And, let me introduce Barry here. A student with us, for the next few months. Treat him well, eh?', Red concluded.

Laurie distinctly giggled and grinned as if, well, he'd met other students in passing during his stay. And then, they all grinned in unison, except the Vicar, who had his head down again, head in hands; apparently in despair or, in deep introspection; but more likely the former.

Red and I moved out, back into the corridor, and entered the first of the dormitory bedrooms on our left.

As we came through the doorway — there were no keys for this dormitory door, just four small square glass-panes set in wood-panels, and a white lace curtain — the voice of the popular Scot folk-singer, Donovan, greeted us; out of concern, the protest song alluded, for the active war in Vietnam, and on behalf of the record owner, young Michael. He was a fair-haired, twenty-one year old patient, laid, apparently relaxed, fully-clothed on his bed (no-one else in the dorm) with a portable player on top of his bedside locker. '*... Just a Universal Soldier - And The War Drags On.*' Perhaps, Donovan's tuneful, meaningful dirge, reflected Mike's sympathetic feelings; but, true, an assumption on my part in meeting him for the first time. Michael was holding an open paperback on *Zen,* by Alan Watts, from which we had obviously interrupted his reading.

'Wotcha Red. All right?', he asked good naturedly, of Red. As I was introduced, Mike nodded in reciprocation and laconic. 'Hiya!', in welcome to me.

'Oh yes, Mike. Almost forgot. You're waiting to see the duty doctor, aren't you?', Red recalled as we paused at the bottom of his bed.

'Yup', Zen Mike confirmed.

And we moved on along, the clean, recent polished, light coloured, pine wood floor (care of the ward orderly), through this well furnished, well kept, homely dormitory.

I noted the long backed blue curtains, even net curtains; but, most, the delightful view of the lawn and front gardens, framed by the cream painted window frames, and clearly all windows, facing this south aspect, reflected the same peaceful scenes.

Internally, each bed had its own green draw curtain, that hung from a tubular-frame attached to the ceiling and, with its castors and eyelets, allowed a degree of privacy, whenever a resident wished to (for whatever reason) shut off from other patients or staff, outside this barrier.

The furnishings suggested the ward was being 'upgraded' which, periodically, through frequent use and when budget or necessity insisted, all hospital premises needed to be improved.

And, as we left the dorm and entered the bathroom, across the corridor, I recalled being shown this ablution, during my intake's lightning tour the previous autumn. Notably, there was a vertical circular tube metal scaffolding (sort of iron-maiden but without spikes or torture), with minute holes throughout its plumbed thin pipes; and it was explained, 'that' was the last remnant of old hydrotherapy shower facilities. That shower was now removed. The bathroom, or rather its four baths and surrounding sink and mirror units, was still being decorated.

Bill, Charge of Male Summersdale, later recalled to me, that a few years back (viz in 1940s and 1950s), these baths had detachable top wooden fittings, that enabled disturbed or anxiety ridden residents to experience 'continuous baths'; another benign water therapy (hydrotherapy), the warm water in a staff controlled therapeutic agitation.

This method of immersing distressed patients, in a controlled, agitated warm water bath, was well depicted by American journalist Mary Jane Ward's[5] 1946 book, *The Snake Pit*. The work, graphic, albeit sad, dramatic, dark (deliberately drawn so), and so depicted in the movie set of *The Snake Pit,* (unhelped by past fiscal depression, slavery and racism cultural origins); the film was released in 1948, a post war semi documentary, and raw, celluloid faction on (then) contemporary American treatment of Mental Illness. Psychotherapy was, when available, a key to unlocking traumatic memories, — and, in a patient's recovery.

Just what *do* we do, with trauma in our locked memories? Philosopher poet and dramatist T.S. Eliot [6] wrote on this same theme, in his classic *Four Quartets*, *Burnt Norton*:

> 'Go, go, go, said the bird : human kind / Cannot bear very much reality.'

Eliot, like Charlotte Bronte before him, had it *well* sussed!

Baths

In later, post-war decades, agitated *continuous baths treatment,* warming up cocktails of memory, would be viewed as an expensive luxury piece of domestic bathroom furniture (without the wooden boards) — a *Jacuzzi*.

I recall reading patients' pre war case notes, and other written notes, on the therapeutic practice of wrapping a person up in tight warmed sheets, a wet sheet pack, to calm down an agitated state. A pre war, American journalist, had broken down, through too much, experienced, harsh reality; and drink. Travel-writer William Seabrook[7], for a while suffering from a bout of alcoholism, was admitted, in an acute episode, and hospitalised. Seabrook successfully experienced this tight wet sheet pack 'swaddling' treatment, which experience he later wrote up in his book — *Asylum*. There is also, on record, the story of a new born child; 'Wrapped in swaddling clothes and laid on a bed of clean straw, in a manger.'... but that's another story.

The ground-floor male bathroom, complete with the now mandatory curtains, was once again converted, to just baths; though I noted the taps still had the solid hexagonal — male female — key controlled units, that I had first experienced on Amberley and Bramber wards, keys kept in the nursing office.

Several corridor doors, adjacent to the bathroom, were cupboards and storage spaces, though one single only bathroom suggested a past private facility; this door was generally locked. Red told me the key was also held in the nursing office (of course - where else), but the other main bathroom as all other ablutions, was open at all times; the whole regularly cleaned by our daily, brown coated, ward orderly.

Back to the other side of the ground floor corridor, Red showed me another, and smaller dormitory, of (then unoccupied) four beds, overlooking the garden.

And finally, at the end of this corridor on the left, were two adjacent unlocked side rooms (no longer pads, as they were originally constructed), complete with one bed and cabinet in each. The old fashioned, thick panelled door, had a vertical slot in the top panel, to enable its temporary resident to be viewed, from the corridor. This thick, self-evident, well-marked and inside kicked and battered door, was painted cream. The concrete steps, to the upstairs dormitories, was opposite the end room. A sad historical reminder, of some of its, past, more disturbed and violent encounters.

A ward upgrading was clearly not yet completed, though, like the proverbial Forth Bridge painting (viz so large it needed perpetual renovation, in one area or other), even before completion new planning would likely be under a future consideration.

'That's the lot on this level. There's more upstairs, Barry.' Red led me up the flight of concrete steps onto the first (and top) floor ward corridor, of SH2.

Up here were other doors and short shaded corridors, with pictures on the walls at regular intervals, so as to be seen symmetrically spaced, throughout all main well-lit corridors; gentle paintings of mostly rural scenes, with one or two well known Canaletto and Gainsborough coloured prints — all a uniform size.

Red mentioned, in passing, that several male nursing staff lived in bedsitters off those short corridors, and behind those private closed doors.

On this upstairs floor were two dormitories, duplicating downstairs (but no end-side-rooms) with similar furnishings. He explained that once per week, usually Thursday mornings, in-patients and visiting outpatients would attend for ECT (and I would often be assisting); most of these patients would also attend a second weekly ECT session, held across in the Main Building, on Amberley One ward on Tuesday mornings; I had already been introduced to those sessions, on my first placement.

This long top-corridor ended abruptly, in a glass and wood partition and a locked-door, exactly half-way down its length. This obstacle, was the locked wall-divide, for there was a locked door in this partition; this was between the block's Male and Female sides. Downstairs too, at the front entrance, was the divider. Female giggles emanated from the 'other ' side of the partition. The upstairs main-dormitory decor duplicated its peer downstairs and proved it, too, had recently been upgraded and renovated.

The prospect, through upstairs windows, overlooked the landscape of the Havenstoke Field and, more across the North Drive, the immense, well cut, green lawn of all the parkland presented a huge, oval, island with trees around its entire perimeter.

Through a curtain gap, clearly viewed, was part of the wide, green, ditch of the Belgic remains, extending southwards, towards the South Drive and beyond, towards the city of Chichester; cutting a sunken pathway. A 1912 map showed it as Roman Entrenchment.

It took little imagination to realise the hundreds of residents and staff who, since 1933, had so recently looked down onto that rural green, seen and heard uncounted stockmen, shepherds, horses, cows, sheep and other livestock, tended during its recent farm years. And cared for by staff and patients alike — until closure of hospital farm in 1957.

As we descended the stairs, and headed back towards the office base, there was a noticeable babble of voices, male and female, from continuous day patients arriving at the front entrance, and vehicles driving off after their safe deliveries; and so, later, they would be collected in the mid to late afternoon.

Few activities took place within this Day Hospital building, except where clinical treatments, doctors interviews and organized tests were arranged for the patients. Most arrivals, after registering their presence, would then be re-directed to whatever OT, IT, or other daily activities areas. The out-patients would then later return to the Day Hospital, to join other in-patients for meal times and prescribed medications.

It was dinnertime, after midday, when I realized what a social meeting point the dining rooms and kitchen areas provided, for staff and residents.

Physically, half a dozen long tables and chairs were set, males separate from females; a half wooden partition still separating them from each others' contact. The women patients too ate separate, at their half a dozen oblong tables, with chairs, laid apart for meal times. And male staff thus served male patients, and female staff served women patients needs.

And the medication trolleys wheeled up, adjacent to the separate enclosed — rather, half-enclosed — spaces, of the Summersdale dining-room area

The kitchen area itself, behind the dining spaces, was not distributed as strictly male and female, though each side had their own locked cupboards. And fraternization, in the kitchen area, was an acceptable norm, during the cleaning of the red-stone tiled floor and, after each meal, washing up and clearing away was organized — just (sort of) like home.

A separate rear-entrance, with a concrete ramp for kitchen deliveries, was behind, exiting to the circular back drive and across; seen through a clump of trees, the two nissan-huts of the in hospital nursing school, and OT art facility.

Laurie & Julie

Red handed me the tablets.

'Pete. Two largactil. One disipal', I took the pills, and put them into the plastic measure-cup in my hand, as Red then ticked off the appropriate entry adhered to the underside of the Drugs Trolley.

'Right'; I said, and I sought Peter out. Pete was a middle-aged ex-fireman, presently a resident with depression, from Midhurst. He was at the end of the third table, halfway through his bacon, egg, and Italian tinned tomatoes, soaked into a limp piece of fried bread, which was then about to enter his reluctant mouth.

'Here you are, Pete. Two pills. Do you want a drink of orange with it, or is your tea enough?'

'S' all right Barry. Tea's okay', and I dutifully watched him swallow the pills, one at a time. I then returned to the trolley and Red, for the next delivery.

There was a fair hub of gossip going on, during the meal time and, from behind the partition, we could hear the bubble of conversations over the female side.

Laurie was feeling rather pleasantly high, and had already wolfed down his breakfast, followed by three cups of tea, heaped with shovel loads of sugar.

'Jack?' Red paused and looked to his place where his chair remained vacant, his cereal still untouched at his place.

'I think I know where he is', offered Laurie, 'I'll fetch him for you, Red.' Without waiting for a no no, he sped off in the direction of the bathroom.

Whilst awaiting their return, I delivered the next medication, and minutes later Laurie returned, alone.

'Sorry Red.' Laurie looked a bit crestfallen, puzzled why his eager good-will had proved insufficient to bring Jack back to the table.

'Think he's rather uptight, e's at the sink, scrubbing his hands like they're on fire, or something, and muttering to 'imself', he concluded.

'Thanks for trying, Laurie. I'd better go and get him. Mind the trolley, would you Barry?'

And Red strode off, his white coat trailing behind him. Jack was an obsessional phobic, who just could not cleanse himself of microbes which, he believed, were digging their dirt into his skin. He was an apprentice carpenter, only twenty-one years old, the single son, of a single-parent mother, living alone in a small neglected farm cottage.

Suddenly, a pretty young woman appeared, from the kitchen side and called out to Laurie across the food trolley. It was Julie.

'Thought I heard you Lorr', she said affectionately.

'Good-night, last-night wasn't it?'

Laurie and Julie had visited the 'Wellington Arms' the night before, and then returned to the hospital, to orchestrate a sing-song of folk-and-pop music in the male-lounge; much to the pleasure of all present. I had been on the late shift the day before, and helped organise this informal event, with Bill's encouragement.

'Be good experience for you, Barry!', Bill said, repeated like a mantra, For many times in the weeks ahead, I was to hear this stock encouraging reassurance.

'And, eh, thanks. Barry, in't it?', added Julie, as she noticed my presence.

I nodded. Smiled. 'Any time', I said, as I delivered another round of prescribed medication. But aware of my reserved, if slightly pompous, reply.

And Julie disappeared, behind the dividing screen, out of view again, with 'Catch you later Lorr.'

And she was gone.

And we resumed our round, with Red. A sullen Jack, now present, examined his breakfast for pollution.

An hour or so later, Bill called me into the office; the Daybook diary opened up on the desk, as Day attenders began to arrive at the hospital.

'Barry. I'd like you to accompany a couple of patients to IT this morning; just for the experience. Though I think we'd better special the Reverend awhile longer, as he's very low at the moment and might mutilate himself.'

'It's possible we might have to transfer him across to the Main Building — if his condition worsens,' he added gravely.

'Yes of course, Bill. Anything else?' I replied, a little over eager to please.

'Oh yes, one other thing. Could you deliver two bundles to Chico? You know — at the Poultry Farm? '

Bill realized, although now a second-year student, I still may not have heard of Chico, let alone met him down at the Poultry pens. But I had heard of him — though true enough — I'd never yet been into the unit and spoken with him.

'Laurie!'. He was just passing the office in the corridor, in the midst of one of his stable of jokes to someone or other.

He entered, lively and grinning into the office. 'Yup, Bill Barry', in acknowledgment.

'You're going down The Yard this morning, aren't you. Could you take Barry to Chico, at the Poultry Farm, on the way in?'

'No bother, Bill. Consider he's arrived.'

'Oh, and he'll be taking the Reverend with him, so if that's all right then. Ten minutes okay?'

On the button, Laurie arrived at the office to collect me, and an unhappy (but willing) Reverend. I was carrying a large brown paper parcel, and a bundle of what appeared to be case notes — from Charge Bill, to his colleague Chico.

Laurie had changed, and was wearing a short-sleeved T-shirt, with a logo, 'JAW NOT WAR', in a bold red and printed on the white cotton cloth background, over white shorts, brown bare knees, and sandals below.

The Reverend, trying to be inconspicuous, was propped up against the wall outside the office entrance, awaiting guidance.

'Right. Let's go', I said decisively as we three led off, Laurie, The Rev, and myself, towards the Poultry Farm and then the IT Yard.

Laurie was still full of bounce and good-cheer, at face, one could not imagine that both Laurie and The Rev had a common, psychiatric diagnosis — Manic Depression.

At extremes, the malady would lead into psychosis, an apparent, wholly, unawareness, of their behaviour, and body activity.

At the bottom, in a suicidal depression, and at the other extreme, of utter mania, masqueraded as a happy-go-lucky, anything goes, everything's all right attitude, towards one's self and all the world outside them — whatever mayhem, at that time, was revealed.

At this time, The Rev was clinically worse-off than Laurie who, whilst quite lively, was not really manic, merely youthful enthusiasm at being better, than he had lately been, on admission.

As we entered the North Drive, opposite the Naunton, we passed four middle-aged men dressed in gardening clothes, and uniform grey Wellington boots, armed with large sharp spades, broad-forks, and long-pronged rakes which, when not in use, were neatly placed in the two rubber-wheeled trolley, with its detachable wooden plank sides, and two substantial metal handles, one at each end. We saw the gang, so silently at work, on the gardens at the corners of Summersdale and the Pinewood, female nurses' home.

We passed the gardeners by and moved on and around, into the main Carriage Drive and the Farm Road, and approached the front of the OT huts opposite the other-side Main Buildings.

There was then considerable to'ing and fro'ing; traffic, humans, cars and bicycles, moving in all directions, but most in our direction.

Just ahead of us were half-dozen male patients from Bramber Two, accompanied by two staff, seen en-route for IT. I noticed Harry and Manny and Jim, and Fred was there, his tall girth and white coat in their centre and, at the rear, was Bob who was working on the ward, to cover someone off sick — he looked back at me, as did Jim, as they waved and quickly strode on, down the road and out of sight.

Our small group was dawdling, there was no hurry, and all other human traffic appeared to be moving quite leisurely. Indeed, we noticed behind, and to the front, of the OT huts, amongst the numerous trees and abundant vegetation, were sat numbers of patients, some waiting to enter the OT and IT huts, others just passing-the time.

The long avenue of lime trees, alongside the South Farm Drive, continued till the Main Entrance and then, almost opposite, the handsome Sussex Flint hospital church. The Church was marked by an adjacent substantial thick cedar, Cedrus Deodora, with a green garden seat at its base (which was occupied by several male patients), — south and front of the church wall.

This tranquil panoramic scene, pictured close by a number of small oaks, a weeping elm, dark yew trees and several coniferous firs.

A well manicured green lawn, then surrounded by jig-saws of cultivated shrubs and flower beds, more scattered occupied garden seats, and other sheltering trees gently towering over them. And yet, none of those healthy looking trees appeared to be even as high as the nearby brick water-tower, of one-hundred-feet or so height. A recent planned landscape.

A large broad Acer Maple, coupled space close by with a substantial Copper Beech, and a smaller but brilliant red-leafed tree, overlooked the front of the OT huts and adjacent farm roads. Behind the huts, and left of the kitchen-gardens' gateway, loomed three slim light green leafed Lombardy Poplars, with other mostly coniferous trees in their line; all bordering the OT and church perimeter.

Within this picture-postcard scene, a loud female voice hailed us, or rather Laurie, as young Julie suddenly stood up, from the company of two other female patients; they were sat immediately to the side of the OT huts front entrance, and up off a garden seat under a young long leafed sweet-chestnut.

The whole garden area was ablaze of colour with green, purple and golden shades, reflecting sun, wind and early autumn. A playful soothing breeze made music of sorts about the scattered tree tops and played to our hospital audience below.

We stopped and were, for a minute, hypnotized in the vision of fair Julie; like something out of an Ancient Greek fable, a nymph hip-hopping over the grass towards us. Noticeably, with two older women behind her; one quite large lady held up a guitar, as they followed in her wake.

Fair Julie was Twiggy slim, her outline thickened slightly by her long dark-hair, which was secured by a red-silk ribbon headband, laying the lengths down behind her soft narrow shoulders. Her milk-white complexion was enhanced by the even whiter-tone of her thin cotton-mesh tank-top. As was then quite fashionable, she was bra-less. A thick ribbon of bare flesh was visible, like a uniform cumberbund around a narrow waist; her visible button was seen sunk and symmetrical, as natural pearl in a clear sea-bed.

Julie's paper-tissue thin cotton-white mini-skirt was, in size, almost non-existent, but with such slim legs and figure to carry it off, it enhanced the almost childlike image of her nineteen summers. Below, she was barefooted, with narrow tinkling thin brass anklet decorations, tiny bells and stars minute around their frames.

Her opened over-blouse (almost a stole) was the crowning item, a beautiful, short-sleeved, mosaic silk of psychedelic colours, patterned in red, blue, emerald green and thin purple spirals. It had no buttons, but a single toggle and loop, undone, more decoration than a fastening.

Her ultra lean frame enabled Julie to be easily bra-less, conical breasts clearly visible through the semi-transparent mesh-top, but not conspicuously so. She appeared to have no make-up on, none visible that is. And, no watch or rings, but wore a simple necklace string of blue love-beads, which completed the surface picture of Julie. Well almost.

And why was Fair Julie here?

What brought her into hospital? As she caught up to us, evidence of why became clear. The noticeable white-bandages around her slim wrists, reminded of what Bill had relayed to me the day before.

Only a month ago or so, Julie was a happy family member; one of three children of two Chichester school teachers; one older brother who had recently graduated at University, and a younger sister of fifteen years preparing for her '0' levels. Julie had completed her first year at a University when, at an end-of-term undergraduate party, in addition to then routine smoking, a well meaning student gave her some LSD — it was too much, and nearly killed her, admitting her first into the General Hospital, but subsequently needing her admission into our hospital, following sense distortion, colours and shapes 'out of this world' (to normal responses), and subsequent emotional trauma. Julie had insisted she heard God talking to her, and God-talk, as she sometimes now referred to these occasional voices, was a part of her experienced changes.

But it was the terrible flashbacks, and sudden suicidal mood changes, which produced her terrible, black bouts of incomprehensible depression; this disorder had brought Julie into the psychiatric hospital.

In two weeks, Julie had attempted suicide twice. Once, by attempting to jump out of an upstairs bedroom window in her nightdress; and saved by her sister and mother pulling back in the room. And next, after a terrifying attack of depression. which led to her cutting her wrists in the bathroom.

And, since admission, only last week, she appeared happy and buoyant one minute, and only minutes later, another patient found her, with the recent wrist wounds cut open, crouched, cowering, on her haunches in the ladies toilet — absolutely terrified of the visions and ugly thoughts in her head.

Chico

'Where you going Lorr', said fair Julie, as she placed her arms round a delighted but surprised Laurie's, not resisting neck.

'Off to the Barn. Stopping off at the Poultry Farm with Barry and The Rev.', he replied.

'Can I come?' she asked quietly, almost lisped — looking sideways at me, standing behind Laurie. As he looked to me for a reply, I grinned and nodded back at him.

'Course you can. That your guitar, Sadie's carrying behind you?'

'Oops. Yeah. Almost forgot.' Julie took it from her, with thanks. Sadie retreated back towards the huts and her other friend. Julie then promptly off-loaded the guitar to a willing Laurie, and off we trooped.

Past the Greenhouses, and Sandown behind them, down a slope towards the Drove, on a right fork past the Female side of the Main Buildings, as groups and individuals continued down into the IT yard.

The Poultry Farm was several hundred yards on, behind the Kingsmead Villa. It was one of two, other, 1933 built buildings, used as a long-stay residence for female patients. A hundred or so yards further on down, behind the site of the Poultry Farm, below, meandered a brook of the River Lavant. The brook was also an eastern perimeter of the hospital estate. Another farm existed on the other side of the Lavant tributary — once, it too had belonged to the Asylum' Estate.

Ole Bill, it happened, had placed himself on point-duty, outside the entrance to the Farmhouse drive-in, which also happened to be an unmarked roundabout spot since, from this spot, one could proceed onwards to the Farmhouse itself, left, down into the cobble-stoned Yard; or stay on the narrow road left, leading behind the Farm Yard buildings onwards; or last, down to the right through the

Drove — our destination — past Richmond Villa (once the Infirmary) and around behind Kingsmead, by the narrow road with trees and hedgerows bordering the route.

Ole Bill would stop, and waylay walkers if he could — even stopped a black Austin and gave its driver directions — but mostly, as we passed him by, we too, as others, just called out the expected greeting.

'Hi Bill. Keep the good work up.' We waved to him and moved on.

Little John was a staff nurse. He was called Smiler, by many of us, as he always appeared to be smiling, whatever the circumstances — and it was genuine too. Little John used to work on the farm, with selected patients, and had told Laurie about Chico and the Chicken Farm...

Not long ago, a-couple-of-years-or-so, this whole area reverberated with the noise of turkeys, geese and not just chickens but then, very suddenly, as Christmas time approached, relative silence then occurred; the reason being all too obvious, as the size of the Turkey Farm population, in particular, was almost brought to zero.

Little John had arrived as a probationer, back in 1952, when the farm was still complete, but already fated for run-down and closure in 1957.

Laurie and Julie were up front, and The Rev, who was still quiet, only occasionally nodding or shaking his beard in any replies, and I were located at the rear. The two anonymous parcels, that I had under each arm, were already rather cumbersome. The larger package kept slipping. The Rev had twice, already, stepped up and rescued the packages; once, as I had tripped over a large grass clump on the side of the road.

As we approached the Poultry Farm, the seeming acres of wire netting, broken woodwork doors, window frames and small sheds, revealed hundreds of large chickens — in sum, giving one loud cacophony, distributed about the whole area.

There was a wire bound door, with a bell which worked. I rang it, and a rather small, wiry man came to the entrance of the pen, to let us in. It was RMPA Nurse Chico, extraordinarily dressed.

Chico wore a large, old, grubby and battered dark-serge peaked uniform cap which, I was later informed, was part of his uniform of years ago, when he used to work on the wards — before he went and returned from war service, in 1946.

No white-coat, as I had to wear, but Chico had a long, brown, ex-army leather jerkin, over his old, onc-time, dark-serge uniform trousers and waistcoat, with an old hospital' issued whistle and key-bunch. Instead of the charcoal grey tie, he displayed a broad Biggles white silk scarf. Whilst, below, were the now familiar Wellington boots. His uniform was very necessary, in view of the acres and tonnage of excreta, dust, small grit, grime and innumerable feathers stuck about the area.

'Eh. Nurse Chico?' He grinned. Bit obvious who, formality, politeness seemed appropriate since I had never met him before.

'Yes?', he replied, looking at me expectedly.

'Bill, Charge Nurse Summersdale, asked me to give you something.'

He nodded and asked me to step over the plank threshold. The Rev, still quiet, was obliged to follow me but, just as we were about to move over the low threshold, Julie let out a howl. 'Me foot, me foot' she yelped, propping up against the wire fence outside the entrance.

'Barry. Eh! Hold this for me', said quick-thinking Laurie, going to her rescue. White knight Laurie. Androcles and the lioness' paw by Daniel's... eh... chicken den no less.

It was a small stone, trodden into her naked right foot. Laurie handed over Julie's guitar, or rather he dropped it over my right shoulder (my arms already being occupied with the two parcels). I was already committed to step over the wooden plank threshold of the chicken pen, albeit most gingerly. To prevent any chickens escaping onto the road, Chico was obliged to immediately close the gate, behind The Rev and I, leaving Laurie and Julie outside.

But, for me, Chico's automatic, so casual act, caught me unawares, and I froze. Indeed, it was so abrupt that I tripped, or rather I stumbled and, determined not to drop the precious parcels, let the guitar swing on its harness. I hit the edge of the wired inner-fence, and the strings of the frail instrument loudly thronged, as it caught on a strand of wire mesh.

The Rev, and Chico, stood stock still, as they witnessed this awkward comic entrance.

This was made even worse (for me) as, pulling myself up straight, several chickens panicked about me (probably, the noise of the guitar was just too much); one large fowl decided to fly up, on top of my head of all places. Another agile bird duly stamped on my foot, before flapping up and over me, leaving a wake of minute white feathers, some of which joined his comrades', already giving me unwelcome camouflage, about my face and person (hopefully not the packages). I was well feathered but not tarred.

Chico, with the Rev stood next to him, was rooted, and just gazed in unspoken amazement.

Outside the cage, Julie and Laurie stopped their own private engagement and, too, were mesmerised by my quite unexpected antics.

But, I was determined to keep my dignity and professional bearing.

'Splutter. Splutter... Bill... Phttt...' (as I spat foul feathers from my mouth), '...said to give you these... Phttt ... two parcels and, I think... Phttt... his notes.' And, relieved, I handed him the (surprisingly intact) parcels. Chico chuckled, but the Rev was Buster Keaton, unmoved with total restraint. Chico replied, after a momentary pause, aided by another meaningful grin, 'And I have something for Bill. Couple of dozen eggs. Do you think you could take them back?' He exchanged them for the case notes whatever. 'Bill phoned, while you were on the way... eh... Barry isn't it...?' Chico waited.

He sounded somewhat doubtful; who could blame him after that entrance. And, a little bemused, I thought,... phoned him...? Where was his telephone... In one of his poultry sheds...?

'No problem, Chico', I concluded. I felt my dignity was again intact, exit chaos, and the Rev and I stepped back, over the threshold and out of the pens. Julie's guitar was still miraculously balanced behind my back, as I held Bill's box of eggs out before me... Julie and Laurie, most concerned, were ready to receive the guitar back, with profuse apologies.

'You all right Barry?', they asked with genuine concern, though, clearly, I was not hurt. My white coat was now torn, at the elbow of my right arm, where I had collided with the fence. In retrospect, it must have been quite a humorous episode to them outside.

We resumed our journey, back down the Drove towards the Yard. Chico went back to his charges. (His nickname so obviously derived from Chicken;- it could have been Foul or Poultice.)

All the fittings and signs of livestock about the area would soon, quickly, be returned to grass wasteland. The end of the farm era, so subtle not even a whimper. One would recall that this Estate had been home to agriculture and livestock since possibly Belgic or Saxon times. And now with Chico and his flock, soon to be gone from its location on the slope, to the rear of Kingsmead Villa.

Playtime

Ole Bill was still at his post, as we four entered the brick gateway, into the old cobbled farmyard, which had not yet been upgraded to its new identity, as an Industrial Therapy Centre. Its courtyard was a square, each side designated in numbers, thus One, Two, Three, Four, and No. Five Sheds — with a smaller Number Six shed outside the perimeter.

Bramber Two patients, and I, had lately visited No. 2 Shed with Fred and Bob. That very morning, we sat with our charges at the wooden work tables, on the cheap red plastic umbrella seats, assembling or disassembling bits of old wireless apparatus and other odd-like tasks.

Laurie, Julie, Rev and I, with guitar and, now, eggs to the fore, then entered No. 5 Shed, so lately better known as The Barn — which it was...

Beryl, the Art Therapist, had for several months been allowed to utilize this large farm building, with its original hard beaten earth floor. Paintings and other works of patients' art were visible, about the four walls in advertisement.

Today was a special event, it appeared, and Beryl had a guest OT art drama instructor, to entertain and instruct any interested staff and patients.

She was a chorus girl, a young lady, Rita. I reckoned she was about twenty-eight years or so.

'Hello', said Beryl. 'Come to join us, have you?'

Surprised, when the event was explained, we agreed to join the forthcoming fun.

There were about ten other patients altogether, and I spotted two female staff at the back. I found a safe spot for the eggs, and removed my torn white coat. And returned to The Rev, Laurie and Julie at one side of the large Barn.

The gathering in The Barn had already experienced a discussion, and was about to act out some agreed scenario, which suggested a Zen version of *The Magic Roundabout* [8]; a television show for children, but which, at that time, had an extraordinary cult appeal to adults. Someone had been delegated to monitor a record machine, with art therapist Beryl at hand, in case of need ...

And the music began. It was *Catch The Wind,* followed by *Colours,* sung by Bob Dylan[9] — much to Julie's delight. And it did seem somewhat, well different, from that TV show; to say the least.

Hostess Rita explained to our assembly; 'I would like you all to relax. Select a farm animal, or other creature, and pretend to be it for a moment; clown, get down on all fours if it fills the part.' The object was *not* to belittle any of us but rather to be happy, silly and yet be constructively so. Indeed, to loosen up and enjoy, to be meaningfully funny, if possible. Hence, a reference to characters out of *The Magic Roundabout*, by which we understood this impending play. I thought the whole idea was surreal. And it seemed to totally challenge the stiff posture of my *new* Professionalism, at that point — especially as a student.

I had, only a few years before, ceased to be a Professional dancing instructor, pounding the pines (1960-1962) for *Arthur Murray's Dance Inc.*[10] at 167 Oxford Street, situated on the corner of Poland Street and Oxford Street, in London, over the *Marquee* Jazz Club and adjacent to an *Academy* cinema; and indulged my love of music and dance. I'd, deliberately, shut off in 1968 all *that* recent, past life existence, as I entered the role of a full time Professional carer. It didn't subscribe to this new image (I thought at the time) about to be put out on this old barn floor, at Graylingwell...

Laughter and frivolity was becoming a riotous mayhem, as Rita confronted each person present to offer to pretend and demonstrate something — other than of themselves; and the music played on in its 'flower power' litany.

There were dogs and cats (very popular), horses, cows and one or two farmers, and Rita arrived at our waiting group.

Laurie and Julie were already enraptured. We were, in fact, last in and last to perform, and I still felt very conspicuous. Heaven knows what the poor Rev felt, standing by my side.

'I know', said an inspired Julie, 'Barry and I will be sheep, and Laurie and The Rev can be Shepherds — or whatever else they want.'

Innocent of any other intent certainly, but to us men we could hardly be blamed for initially seeing what we saw. An attractive young woman, scantily clad in loose mesh tank-top and so brief mini-skirt, on hands and knees and baa-baa-ing. More, as she dropped down only feet away in front of me, Rev and Laurie standing, myself uncomfortably on my hands and knees. And an (apparently) oblivious Rita, choreographing the event.

On her hands and knees, Julie's brief bright-red underpants, whilst still sufficient to retain decency (but only just), revealed two fluffy cheeks. I was embarrassed at first, but the gentle inoffensive absurdity of it all worked; we baa-baa'd and laughed, together.

After that surprised moment, when this nubile reminded us of her womanhood, the childlike fun image rebounded as, indeed, the experiment appeared to have intended. Not to take ourselves, myself, too serious.

But what did bring about a natural, momentary, collapse, of my own assumed guise, was The Rev suddenly standing there and laughing, laughing and laughing, his eyes wet with tears as they cascaded down his cheeks, and his beard shook, not with hysteria; but with delight. A delightful moment... The events at the Poultry Farm, and now our Magic Roundabout, were too much for The Rev to hold back. We all laughed with him.

'Good experience for you.' said Bill, on our return.

The Rev, and ECT

Three weeks later, on a Thursday morning shortly before 9 am, I was busy upstairs in the main dormitory assisting final preparations to receive outpatients for ECT. We were also presently expecting two patients, over from Amberley One.

Red, our staff, was very busily preparing the two-tier metal trolley; on the top surface he filled syringes with anaesthetics, atropine, and scoline on one-side; and placed the black ECT box on the other side; also placed, were the necessary sterilized gauze-squares, cotton-wool balls and white plastic galley pots, packaged by the CSSD and vacuum sterilized as needed. These items were now packed, pre-sterilisation, down at the IT yard premises in one of the sheds.

Also in place were tweezers, scissors in a chrome kidney-dish, a portion of disinfection and a saline solution.

Underneath, Red had placed a range of ECT drugs and Emergency (in case) ephemera, to support the Treatment.

I sat down, on one of the beds, to look up my pocket notebook, where I had recorded, as Red had described, most of those essential items:

'ECT Drugs: Amp. Bemegride (Meglamide) an antidote to Barbiturates i.e. Sodium Brietol. Adrenaline - heart lung (Respiratory), a stimulant. Aminophylline and Nikethamide, also stimulants for heart and lungs. Atropine Sulphate - drys secretion. Hyalase - assists absorption of any infection i.e. as catalyst. Phenobarb Sol - a sedative (i.e. for anxiety states).' All of these preparations were in labelled tubes ampoules or variously coloured bottles.

'Procaine Hydro - local anaesthetic. Hydro-cortisone Univ. Relief and stimulant - incl. brain and respiratory. Suxamethomium chloride (Scoline) the muscle relaxant. Methadrine the amphetamine. Spirit for infection. Duncaine a local anaesthetic.'

Red had been very helpful, the week before, at another ECT session preparation and, added to my ECT notes, under a sub-heading of 'Resuscitating Drugs', (several of these items had cross-referenced with the general listing of ECT prescribed drugs):

'Aminophyiline IM (bronchial dilator) - Given IM 5m, or Iv 25m. Aramine 1% (raises bp when rock bottom):

Methylamphetamine (a Resuscitative): Adrenaline 1/1,000 (anti-encephelagic) IM, slowly and stylistic - apply by swab - constricts blood - local. Hydrocortisone Sodium (given in prostrate illness when bp so low that adrenal glands are incorrect): Nikethamide 2 cc IM (Coramine), a heart stimulant: Lanoxin, inj of Digoxin IM: Phenobarb Na. (anti-convulsive): Amyl Nitrite, inhalation, a capsule broken and held under nose, angina pectoris - muscle spasms of coronary arteries: Atropine Sulph. increases heart-rate as side-effects; drys secretion of mouth: Mersalyl (diuretic): Duncaine Lignocaine (local anaesthetics) - and Procaine and xylocaine.'

'Barry', Red interrupted my brief swot of the notes, as I tried to make sense of them. 'We've got a few minutes. I know you've completed the beds, but you'd better put the portable screens up. They're over in the far corner.'

'Right, Red', I acknowledged, and proceeded to place a green-cloth screen, tied to hollow metal frames on castors and in hinged sections, around each bed to be used for ECT patients. Privacy for patients being essential, whenever practical. I had almost finished this task, when the loud noise of a fire engine, no, must have been two of them in-train, appeared to be travelling over to the Main Building. (Later, I learnt it was a false alarm — a patient had broken a glass and set an alarm off.)

Red just carried on his chores at the trolley, as I went to a window in time to see the second fire engine, going up the South Drive. As it disappeared out of sight, I could not miss an isolated book on the window ledge, adjacent, I believed, to be the Rev's bed space. The subject added to this belief.

The book, a Victorian hardback, was titled *Cheque Book of Bank of Faith* by C.H. Spurgeon [11]. One of Spurgeon's fervent supporters had (unknown to my single-parent mother and, of course, to myself, during six years as a young inmate — and the orphanage itself) been an evangelist and East End (of London)

Missionary and District Visitor (now known more appropriately as a Social Worker). He, the Rev. John Manton-Smith, was first cousin to my maternal great-grand-father James Leigh Manton (1849-1914). A small world.

The past. Roots. Recent past and present genealogy became a vital part of day to day investigations, for case notes and in psychotherapy, in assisting patients towards initial diagnosis and a hopeful recovery. I learnt about different case histories, inherited assets and latent deficits donated in a patient's genes. Also fragments of data, from relatives and friends. Memory traces from whatever,- pre-morbid, social and biological sources, that preceded a person's entry into the hospital — patients, visitors and staff. *Manton* was my mother's maiden name, and my cousin Barbara, ten years my junior, was the last of our line to bear this family branch surname.

Wholly incongruent. But, *only* the week before I'd, by pure coincidence, picked up another book, a paper-back, off this same window sill, while attending the ECT session. The item was not, necessarily, the Rev's. On its dramatic front-cover, tinged in red, disclosed under its title and author's name, was a lurid picture of a crouching woman in a slip, her right-hand with long bony-fingers up to her mouth, and frightened eyes looking upwards. The book's title was *City Psychiatric* by Frank Leonard. [12] It was an American novel pb. owned by a patient probably on this ward. And, captioned beneath the obvious deliberate horror pic, said: *Mercilessly reveals the sinister secrets of public mental wards.*

'Sinister secrets?'. Absolutely no way, could 'my' experience of our English 1960s public mental wards, subscribe to such awful inferences. The opposite, in fact. Patient's acute, inner fears, sadly, yes; such as why they were hospitalised. But not the hospital itself!

But that Insight was an eye-opener for me as, intrigued, I scanned the contents and arrested my gaze at the three paragraphed Preface — signed, at its foot, F.L. New York, February 1966. It was by an American author, a Social Worker, who had experienced a time as an attendant, at several American public mental hospitals, including a large metropolitan receiving hospital, in the USA. As if to anticipate questions, and initial disbelief, at the novel's graphic real-life based introductions, Frank Leonard's *Preface* disclosed :

> 'I want to present a small bouquet of praise to the British. Great Britain is ten to twenty years ahead of the United States in its treatment of the mentally

ill. A 1961 study by the American Psychiatric Association found in Europe, in comparison to the United States: A greater respect for the patient as an individual... in nearly all psychiatric institutions. British psychiatric hospitals were singled out for special comment by the author. Treatment in small hospital units within the patient's home community is far advanced in Britain. It is only beginning to be implemented in the United States. Britain has acknowledged the severe limitations imposed upon treatment when a patient is locked up against his will. Only about ten per cent of British mental patients are involuntarily hospitalized. In the United States, the figure is closer to ninety per cent.'

A few years later in 1975, and an academy award winning American film of Ken Kesey's *One Flew Over The Cuckoos Nest* [13] appeared to confirm this strong anti-psychiatry trend was underway, in the states. I was amazed about stories from colleagues, who had visited such USA prison-like described institutions, as well as learning of public State Mental Hospitals where *armed* guards were felt necessary, on public wards. Putting the paperback down, I completed putting the screens out, while Red checked the black (white patch at its top) oxygen cylinder, in its iron-trolley, and wheeled it beside where the first ECT patient would be treated. The visiting doctor Anaesthetist, from the general hospital, again also checked out the contents of the cylinder and ensured all the parts functioned correctly.

Our patients were congregating downstairs in the lounge, with Bill, our Charge, receiving them, assisted by a willing volunteer which happened to be The Rev; who was due his fifth (out of eight) ECT treatment and was well on the road to a relative recovery.

Upstairs, Red and I remained alone, in the now prepared ECT room, with a distant sound of voices from downstairs; the cacophony mostly coming through several of the half-open windows. Next door, from the women's side, the sound of light music and muted chatter easily permeated the thin partitions, and completed our backcloth.

First to arrive upstairs was Tom, Staff Nurse from Amberley, who delivered two patients, and their notes; these notes were placed on a corner table, awaiting our medical colleagues. Tom's white-coat clearly identified him as "staff" as Red, Bill and my own.

Moments later and The Rev, in an open necked white shirt and white cotton trousers, came up to convey a message to Red and I. He said 'Bill asks — are you ready to receive the patients?'

'Oh — and Barry.', Rev smiled broadly and peered through his large round glasses — which he wore most of thc time to read, write and now generally function socially, as his depression was in retreat. 'Thanks for the long-chat yesterday... much appreciated.'

'S' all right Rev. I must thank *you;* 'specially for the loan of your booklet. Most impressed. Yes. Honestly.' He blinked, as if the remark was but to patronize. 'I'll report back to Bill, and come back myself.' He departed back, downstairs.

I'd learnt quite a lot about our Rev. What I had learnt, I liked — vulnerable, he certainly was, but he was a genuine article, and had suffered in staying true to himself; and over forty years had given much of that self for-others, despite periodic bouts of manic-depressive illness.

Born at the early part of the century, in the Edwardian era of 1904, Rev was of genteel, middle-class origins; and a sensitivity that brought on his first breakdown in 1925, when he dipped Exams as a student at Cambridge; and, four years later, suffered a second breakdown, following a failed attempt to get into the publishing business.

It was as a recovering patient in 1925-26, that The Rev's intellect had taken to exploring 'others' of a similar diagnosed disorder — Manic Depression.

'He knew what it was to go through a period of elation, just as well as he knew what it was to endure a period of depression'; his booklet described, and with clear insight Rev then found (in a textbook) and concluded, 'the etiology of this disorder is unknown'.

And though the cause, or causes, which precipitated his inability to sustain stress was unknown, he readily admitted to owning the ailment. But, despite setbacks, he had later qualified as a clergyman and was married; and, for a substantial time, held down a successful living, at a coastal town in East Sussex.

The Rev told me how, long-ago, he had met a person diagnosed 'dementia praecox', for whom there was too little (then) known treatment (1926); and only a transfer existed, from the General Hospital and their family doctor into Hellingly, his then local public Mental Hospital. And so, he consulted his Bishop, who endorsed an offer of pastoral support, working out of the church vestry, and vicarage — for as many persons as he could (with support) help out; that pastoral care was in the form of an informal Day Centre (In later parlance) and sounded a great success, for that time.

The Rev's last major breakdown had occurred in 1960 when, in a period of immense self-doubt, he was unable to suppress his overwhelming feelings that he had become more actively interested in Manic-depressive Insanity and in Schizophrenia, than in Jesus Christ. He then resigned from the Ministry.

Rev continued to pursue what was the true relationship between Body-and-Mind, and what of the connections between Feeling and Thoughts; both aspects were, of course, fundamental, in a definition of Schizophrenia where they became wrongly connected (Incongruent); and not under control.

I found most interesting the Rev's belief (based very much on his own experiences), that Schizophrenia was, to him, a state of mind marked by an 'extreme' lack of self-confidence (viz loss of same); and, in a lack of insight (psychosis), coped with by fantasy and self-deceit; alternatives as delusions of grandeur — or of persecution. To me, I considered that that condition may have been a collective result of his illness (if so), rather than the root cause? But how to divine and divide such variables, was then beyond me.

But, most, in all his literary efforts, Rev realized, with integrity, the value of self-knowledge — however painful that might be.

The importance of up to date written case-notes was always clear, as they included contra-indications of giving ECT (viz cautionary notes, or 'not to be given' because). *The Red Handbook* specified, that if a patient had active tuberculosis, or was in cardiac failure, then it was preferable to await an improved physical state. If a patient's agitated depression, was becoming too severe, then treatment was advocated sooner, rather than later. Age itself was no bar to ECT; indeed, many elderly patients made a good recovery.

Some absolutes were clear contra-indications; after a very recent cardiac infarction, the heart was very vulnerable, and treatment must be delayed for some weeks, preferably (if viable) a wait of two months was best, and women, after child-birth (no matter what depression in a puerperal psychosis for e.g.) — if there was a real risk of embolism from the uterus. With the sensible use of muscle relaxants, ECT might have been given to patients with fractures, severe hypertension or arteriosclerosis.

Frail, close to retirement age, The Rev's case-notes revealed that he suffered from arteriosclerosis; but, as ECT had well proven (for him) its ability to lift his depression and better prepare him to resume real contact with himself and with the world around him, he welcomed it. The impact of Shock, emotional and/ or physical trauma on a body had, in one form or another, been recognised since early classical times; shock could be morbid and deadly — or benign catalyst.

Modern convulsive treatments had their origins linked with the research of a Hungarian, Dr. von Meduna, who observed, in 1933, that epilepsy appeared to occur less frequently with schizophrenia than mere chance could account for. He concluded that epileptic fits might inhibit the development of schizophrenia; and shock back into reality. Initially, convulsion treatments were introduced for diagnosed schizophrenic sufferers, but it was soon realized that it was more effective in those patients with deep depression; shaking them (viz biochemical reactions) out of their anomie.

And The Rev (this confirmed in his booklet) praised the merits of ECT, whilst allowing for the debit side, of possible loss of (at least) short-term memories.

Rev's chronological history, or rather brief summary, was thus supplied to me by his own written hand — published (at his own expense) booklet — and by his file notes; but, most directly, from his own word of mouth, and observed patterns of behaviour.

Tom had led his patients over, onto the first two prepared beds - and was almost, at a whisper, speaking reassurance and general light banter with them. But first, the patients were asked to take-off their shoes; these were neatly placed beneath the bed. As they came across, in dressing gowns over pyjamas, there was little likelihood of any metal clasps on belts or other such hard objects, though wrist watches were removed; and, as one of his patients was somewhat elderly, a set of false teeth was also taken-out and placed in a tumbler with water, and placed alongside his watch on the adjacent bedside cupboard.

In the final moments, before the rest of our patients (mostly outpatients, though Rev and two other men were Summersdale residents) arrived on the ECT ward, I surveyed the whole room, and looked across to Red for any last minute instructions.

'All right Barry. Wheel 'em in', he said good naturedly, and he proceeded to put on the radio a light programme of music, at a low volume — no more music emanated from the women's wards next door.

I saw, felt, a well prepared clean ward, warm in temperature, in decor, and with colourful personal furnishings attached to bed areas.

There was no austerity or sanitary bleakness apparent (as 1940s and 50s photos depict); nor cold clinical apparatus, despite the placed screens. There were safe, earthed and waterproof, rubber sheets, underneath the white over-sheets, with singular folded blankets on the made-up ECT beds; and, especially, the so visible metal trolley, with its ECT treatment apparatus and oxygen cylinders (one, a spare).

And, of course, the nursing staff, in clean pressed working white coats and polished black shoes; wearing sincere smiles, and temperate subdued (but purposeful) church-quiet conducting manners. It was all *genuine* a setting; a stage it would have been, but the ascribed roles, in this meaningful drama, were too much respected to be abused by any of its players — staff and patients.

And it worked well, like clockwork.

Oncoming footfalls. A low hum of voices, and The Rev and remaining ECT patients entered the room. The large dormitory had two doors, one at each end onto the singular corridor.

And the out-patients arrived.

Adjacent to the corner table stood a locum doctor, he was in the company of Bill, our Charge Nurse. After nodding to me to take-over direction of our patients, Bill and the locum, after gathering up the collected case-files, went over to Staff Red, to have words about something or other.

The Rev appeared to know everybody present (or so it seemed). Again, it was a truism, that everybody grouped in their assortative set (like with like); patients off the same ward, or age set, or others with something in common, would offer each other emotional (even physical if needed) support. But, our Rev had a definite, additional, matter-of-fact, soothing presence amongst us all; and quietly, certainly reverently (no pun intended), respectfully reassured, alongside my own ready reassurance where needed. He led, and set a good example, as I attempted to shepherd them all; and distributed a patient to each allocated bed space. The Rev requested place number three, in the lineup.

In one of my ascribed nursing roles I checked up, on each person, whether they had just visited the toilet, or had forgotten and had a breakfast, or drink, in the hours before arrival; whether a cold, or other malady, had evolved this morning or any other possible contra-indications to be responded to by me; also, shoes on floor, belts and buckles loosened or removed as appropriate, clothing loosened, ties and jackets off, shirt-sleeves rolled up, and any false teeth removed along with spectacles, wrist watches or other jewellery or ephemera; any article which could inadvertently cause injury during the seizures, or internally choke or obstruct the airways and gut. And, finally, all was quiet and settled, as the Consultant Psychiatrist Dr. Mendez, and the Anaesthetist Dr. Zohar, arrived on the scene to commence the ECT treatment programme...

Only the low hum of subdued light background music, from a portable radio, punctured by occasional whispers of the participants, altered the silent primed tension as each awaited their turn; waited to get better.

Tom returned to the Main Building, to await a phone-call when his two patients were ready to be escorted back to Amberley. Bill departed downstairs, to resume his other normal charge duties of the day. Red liaised between the two doctors and the patient due service; whilst I moved from bed to bed, to firmly hold down legs which were beneath a blanket during the convulsions, and to turn them over onto their side, when the treatment was done.

Before the ECT began, Red, in company with the locum, gave an injection of atropine (about 1/100 gr) to all the dozen supine patients. By the time they had finished their round, the Consultant had checked the notes and, briefly, chatted up each person to ensure they all needed ECT (and double-checked their signed consent forms, where placed among the case notes).

Shortly before we began the treatment, it began to rain and a light wind rose, accompanied by a darkened sky, floated occasional multi-coloured leaves and minute flotsam; these seen to dance about outside and on the window panes, the latter frames unhurriedly closed by The Rev, and I. Red put the lights on. The light pitter-patter of the rain had a rhythm of its own, as if dancing, on the glass panes and window sills; mixed with a just audible patter from the tannoy radio — left playing inside the ward.

As the first patient was prepared by Dr. Mendez, given an anaesthetic from one syringe, and scoline from a second syringe, Red passed these items direct from the trolley. All the patients had their firm-pillowed heads facing the windows, thus all heads were placed back and pointed towards the room's centre; as they lost consciousness, the pleasant light music, and rain-tattoo, probably helped to soothe any remaining natural anxiety.

The anaesthetist took a cotton-wool swab, dipped in saline solution, and dabbed a circular spot one each side of the head (bilateral) to receive the headband, which carried a mild but even-distributed electro-shock; it simulated a gran-mal seizure, when the red button on the black box was pressed by the Consultant.

A mouth-gag was inserted, to protect teeth and jaw during the simulated convulsion, for the duration of the seizure. On its completion, the anaesthetist then placed an oxygen mask over the patient's mouth, for a set-time. With normal breathing restored, an airway was then placed in the still unconscious patient's mouth before he was then turned over onto his side; the head back, placed to doubly ensure no accidental obstruction would impede breathing; the atropine had earlier removed all accumulated mouth secretion so there was no prospect, no risk, of any drowning by inhalation during the ritual.

No risks whatever were taken, and each professional methodically played their part in the procedure. With surprise, I would recall that there were no loud grunts, or noisy unconscious responses, during the treatment; this was comforting for those other patients still waiting supine for their turn; out of sight; and, as the treatment was silent, the only sounds were in the soporific tones of the radio and free rainfall.

So slowly, almost gracefully where the staff movements were concerned, all twelve patients treatment were completed without any untoward incident; and, as I turned the last man onto his side and wrapped a top blanket snugly about him; he too slept on peacefully; another session of treatment completed.

Red and I then drew the ends of all the curtains back, so the bed heads and the patients' heads on their pillows could be observed; but the sides of the curtains remained drawn, as they slept on in private. And, as the first few, including The Rev, stirred and awoke, we gently assisted them up, and out of the room (all airways removed, when it was okayed by Red to do so), to the small dormitory next door, where tea-and-biscuits awaited; and another lay-down, or sat down, as the patients filed in during the next half hour or so — to complete their recovery.

Surprise surprise, as soon as The Rev was fully recovered,he insisted on helping to dish out the tea-and-biscuits, and help watch over the other recovering patients. In the treatment room, Red watched the remaining few drowsy recovering patients, as he began to clear up any debris from the treatment.

A decade or so earlier, in the 1950s, I adored an BBC television show called - '*Hancock's 'alf-'our*' [14] starring Tony Hancock, and Sid James. One episode I recalled, *The Blood Donor*, was so funny that it was repeated on numerous subsequent occasions. I recall that one scene, where the after care tea and biscuits were offered to Tony, for his pinprick blood donation. When I attended those numerous ECT sessions, and their after-care offers of tea-and-biscuits. I would, privately, chuckle to myself at 'ancock's scenario, as I recalled that delightful TV comedy — and of our different levels of reality.

Beryl, The Rev's devoted wife, arrived whilst he was still assisting in the tea-and-biscuits distribution; and other friends and relatives appeared to collect, or meet up, with the out-patients who had received ECT, and they would depart, but not before checking in at the nurses' office downstairs, with Bill and the locum, to book any remaining treatments. Tom (phoned by Bill) duly arrived with a pupil nurse (in case of need), to escort his two patients, now the rain had stopped, back to the Main Building.

Rev (a truly good man) was discharged the following weekend to finish his course of ECT as an out-patient. Laurie and Julie and numerous other patients would miss his affable presence — as too, did myself and the staff.

Eyes of Horus

Summersdale Two Mavis had an enthused gathering around her — sat in the Female Lounge, at the conclusion of another successful evening's social-hour. Fair Julie had brought Joker Laurie and Zen Michael across. And Bill had sent me over to help socialize — and gain further experience in the value of social therapy...

Tea, cake and biscuits had been served, with optional evening supper, and Mavis — in her early fifties or so, with greying hair, a black dress, pressed clean low-cut white-frilly blouse over a generous bust, with a large coloured bead necklace. Leaning forward, her bosom was a leaning tower of Pisa, as she sat on a settee, an eager audience about her.

Mavis sure looked the part, as slowly and dramatically she read the tea-leaves in a cup, for another eager enquirer. 'I see it... yes... there it is', and her right fore-finger pointed within, to the black-leaf pictographs, spread about the inner surface of the vessel. 'Something good about to happen.... Mmm! Yes definitely...'

Mavis paused for effect and looked up, towards Mrs. Celia Mount, like a still from a Noel Coward production. Celia, in a florid pink dressing-gown: a recovering reactive depressed widow, who was glad of this impending cheerful augury. 'Perhaps some money - a windfall due?' Mused a most helpful Mavis,

'Tax Rebate!' interrupted fair Julie, 'At least, I reckon, Celia'.

Not long afterward, I returned to our office and prepared to go off duty. As I chatted to Bill about Mavis' popular tea-leaf readings, I added in good humour:

'Well it certainly beats having to read a sheep's entrails, or other ancient methods of divinity, eh Bill?' He grinned and nodded to Bob, who was on overtime with us for this shift, as he too prepared to go off duty as the night nurse arrived for handover.

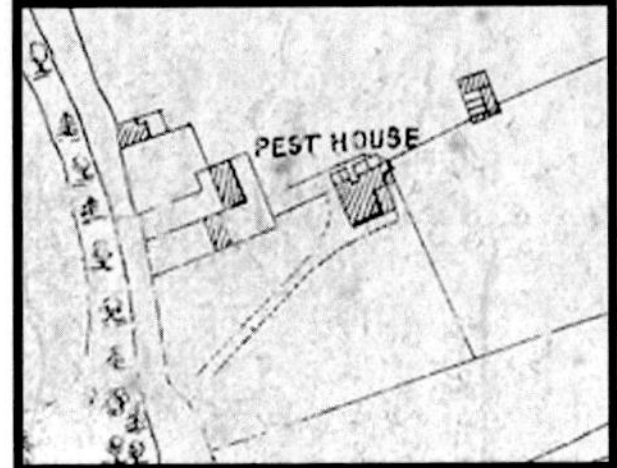

1787. (Above.)The Pest House, Love Lane, North Chichester. Note Cottage .

1908. (Right.) A gateway in a field opposite (to pest house site), led to a Chichester workhouse's back gardens and a Labour yard. Love Lane (later Bishop Otter, College Lane) led upwards to Summersdale, and The Drive to Graylingwell Farm House - and the recently erected Hospital asylum.

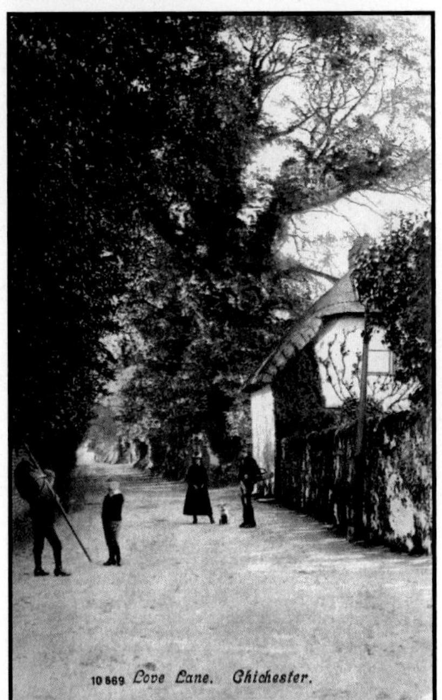

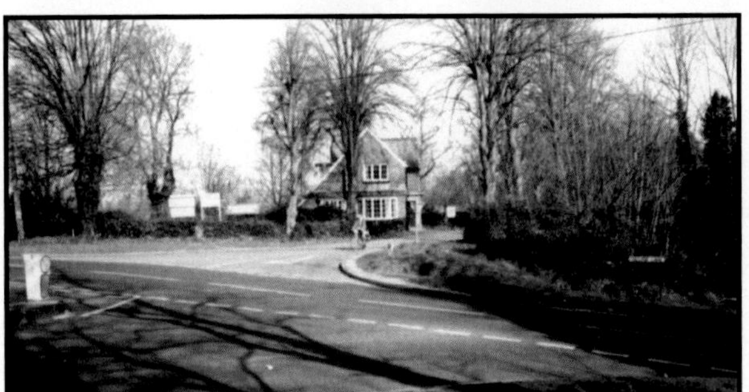

1980. Graylingwell Hospital, South Lodge Entrance, off College Lane - on the right. Love Lane renamed College Lane, after former local school, Bishop Otter College.

"The main entrance to the asylum grounds where a lodge is being erected is at the top of Love Lane, or if the visitor arrives by train he drives or walks straight through the city until he reaches the Wellington Inn, where a short turn to the right brings him to the spot. At present the grounds are in the hands of the landscape gardener, and in the planting season an avenue of limes will be planted from the lodge gate bordering the road to the asylum. The gardens and grounds arranged according to the plans of Mr. Lloyd, of the Surrey County Asylum, at Brookwood, are being rapidly and skilfully laid out by the head gardener, Mr Peacock, who has 22 men working under him. Creepers of various kinds will soon soften the sharp new lines of the pile of buildings." (W.S.G. Aug.1897 p7 column 6)

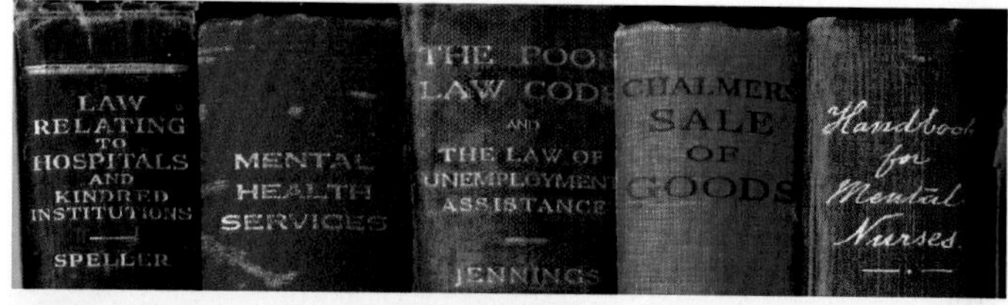

THE

LAW OF AND PRACTICE IN LUNACY

WITH THE

LUNACY ACTS 1890-91 (CONSOLIDATED AND ANNOTATED): THE RULES OF THE LUNACY COMMISSIONERS 1895: THE IDIOTS ACT 1886: THE VACATING OF SEATS ACT 1886: THE RULES IN LUNACY 1892-93 (CONSOLIDATED): THE LANCASHIRE COUNTY (ASYLUMS AND OTHER POWERS) ACT 1891: THE INEBRIATES ACTS 1879 AND 1888 (CONSOLIDATED AND ANNOTATED): THE CRIMINAL LUNATICS ACTS 1800-1884: THE RULES IN MACNAUGHTON'S CASE: AND A COLLECTION OF FORMS, PRECEDENTS, ETC.

BY

A. WOOD RENTON, M.A., LL.B.

OF GRAY'S INN, AND OF THE OXFORD CIRCUIT, BARRISTER-AT-LAW

EDINBURGH
WM. GREEN & SONS,
18 AND 20 ST. GILES STREET

LONDON
STEVENS & HAYNES,
13 BELL YARD, TEMPLE BAR

1896

1896. *Law of and Practice in Lunacy.* Not just a Law Book - it was **THE** poor law reference work, used to decide exact fate, due, *duty of care*, protection, for many thousands of staff and patients, to inhabit Graylingwell Hospital (all hospitals) during the last years of the existent 1601 Poor Law - till 1948 and introduction of the UK National Health Service.

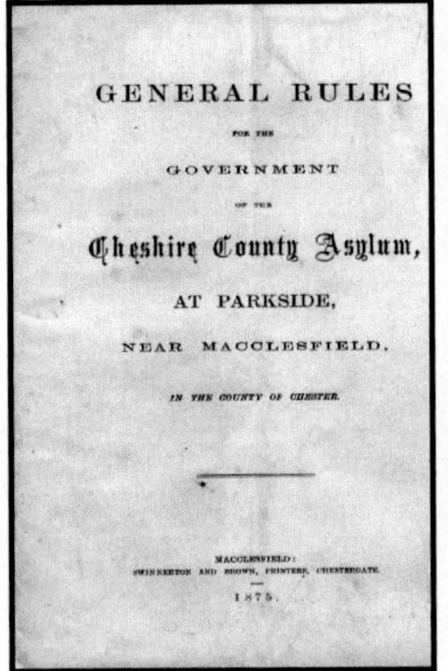

GENERAL RULES

FOR THE

GOVERNMENT

OF THE

Cheshire County Asylum,

AT PARKSIDE,

NEAR MACCLESFIELD,

IN THE COUNTY OF CHESTER.

MACCLESFIELD:
SWINNERTON AND BROWN, PRINTERS, CHESTERGATE.

1875.

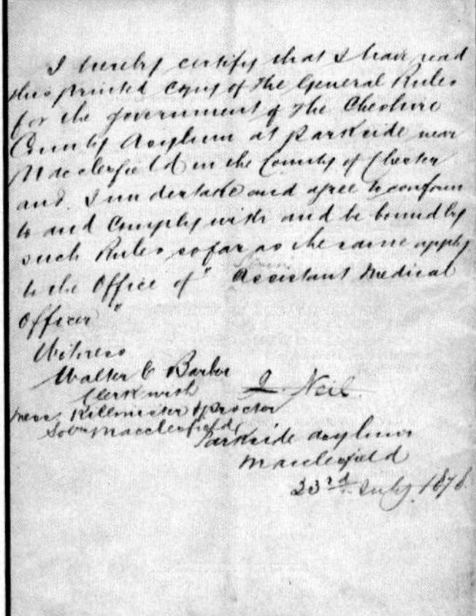

I hereby certify that I have read this printed Copy of the General Rules for the government of the Cheshire County Asylum at Parkside near Macclesfield in the County of Chester and I undertake and agree to conform to and Comply with and be bound by such Rules so far as the same apply to the Office of [illegible] Assistant Medical Officer

Witness
Walter C Barber
Clerk with
Messrs [illegible]
[illegible] Macclesfield

J. Neil
Parkside Asylum
Macclesfield
23rd July 187[illegible]

General Rules 1875. Cheshire County Asylum. Aka Parkside Macclesfield - buildings completed 1871 . Now closed.

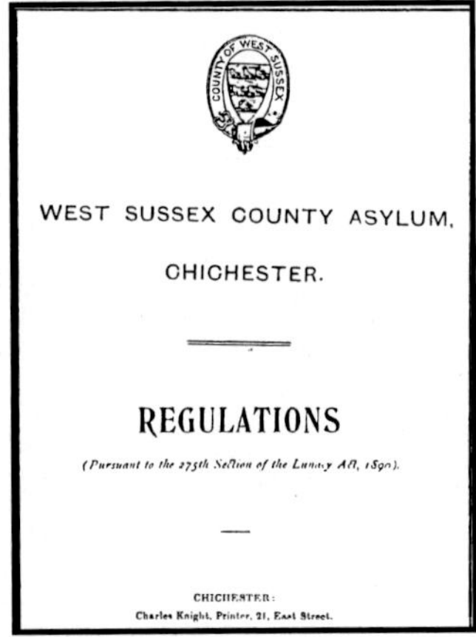

WEST SUSSEX COUNTY ASYLUM,

CHICHESTER.

REGULATIONS

(Pursuant to the 275th Section of the Lunacy Act, 1890).

CHICHESTER:
Charles Knight, Printer, 21, East Street.

Graylingwell Hospital. West Sussex County Asylum. 1897- 2001

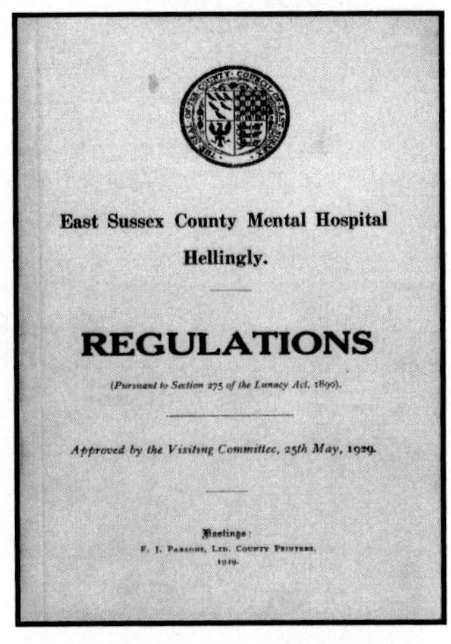

East Sussex County Mental Hospital
Hellingly.

REGULATIONS

(Pursuant to Section 275 of the Lunacy Act, 1890).

Approved by the Visiting Committee, 25th May, 1929.

Hastings:
F. J. Parsons, Ltd. County Printers.
1929.

Hellingly Hospital. East Sussex County Asylum. 1902 - 1995.

In no way was abuse tolerated in the Asylums of the United Kingdom (despite media myths to the contrary). And to ensure safety, there were established Mandatory strict Rules and Regulations at all English, Scots and Welsh County Asylums. On entry to employment in a County Asylum, *all staff* were expected to read and observe the moral rules and regulations pertaining to good conduct - subject to instant dismissal - or indicted for a felony - if found guilty of wilful abuse to patients - or to staff colleagues. All Senior hospital staff were required to sign on completion of reading the Rules. .

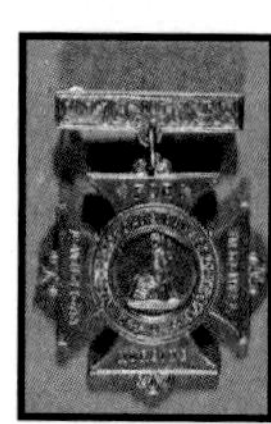

Vera Lewington's Graylingwell Hospital qualification, from 1923. (rear shown below)

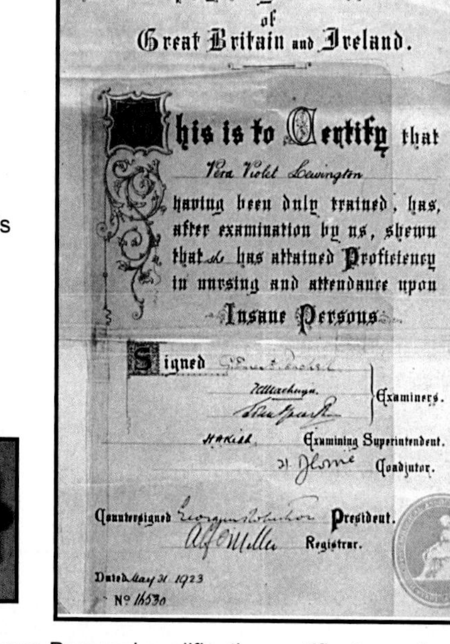

Medico-Psychological Association
of
Great Britain and Ireland.

This is to Certify that
Vera Violet Lewington
having been duly trained, has, after examination by us, shewn that she has attained Proficiency in nursing and attendance upon
Insane Persons.

Signed [illegible]
[illegible]
[illegible] Examiners.
H.A.Kidd Examining Superintendent.
[illegible] Coadjutor.

Countersigned [illegible] President.
[illegible] Registrar.

Dated May 31 1923
No 16530

V.V. LEWINGTON

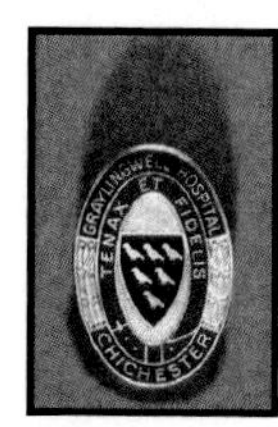

The author's own Graylingwell Hospital RMN badge, from 1970.

Vera Lewington's 'Insane Persons' qualification certificate — signed by (Supt.) H.A. Kidd. A Probationer, aged 19 years, on November 14th, 1919. Vera qualified as a staff nurse in 1923.

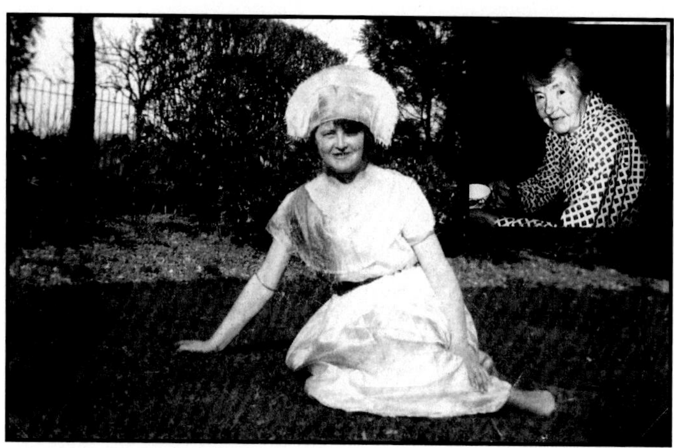

Vera (23 years old), now a staff nurse, in fancy dress, in 1923. **Inset**: widow, Mrs. Vera Searle (neé Lewington) aged 86 years, in Worthing. She was a schoolgirl at Bishop Otter, in the early 20th century. When I interviewed her, in 1986, she said that in the 1920s *only* probationers and qualified staff were allowed to nurse patients; no nursing assistants, or ward maids, in those years, nurses cleaned their own wards.

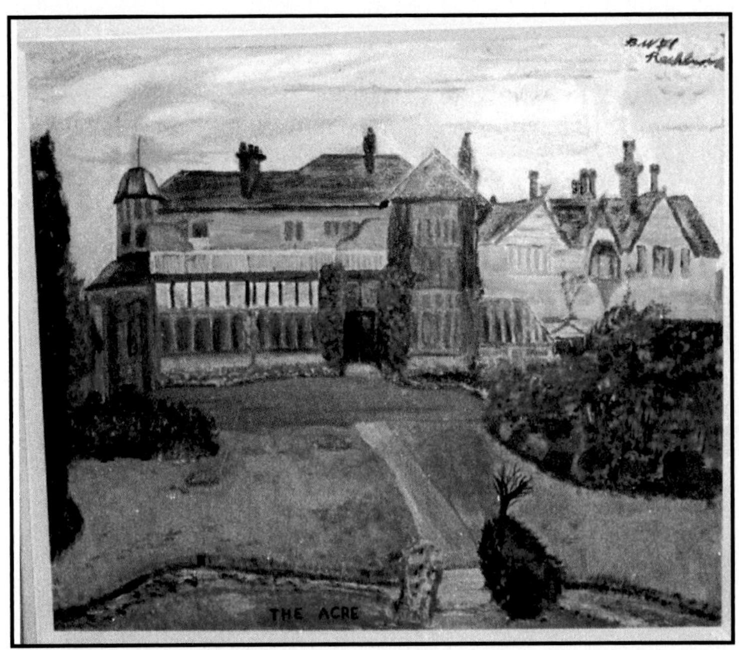

1981. The Acre. Home of *The Worthing Experiment* 1st Jan 1957 - 31st Dec 1958. Painting by day patient Barry Rashbrook - 1971. Artwork rescued from ruins in stable loft - by author.

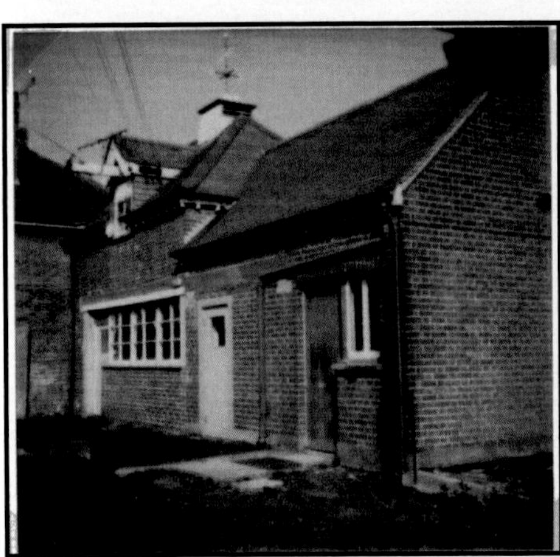

'The Acres' Worthing Day Hospital - The Old Coach House, used as Social Therapy Occupational Therapy Unit.

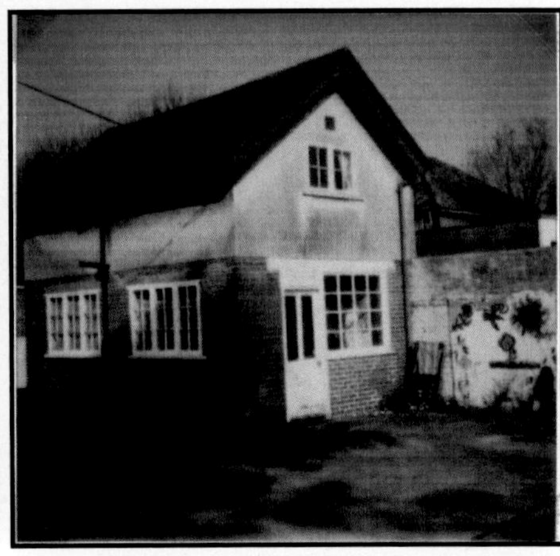

The Acres' two horse Stable - An inner-sanctum, upstairs (loft, through trap door) and downstairs adapted for Art Therapy.

'The Acres' and all its community care outbuildings were demolished after a fire in the main building during the night of 7th April 1981. The Boundary Road site has been re-developed.

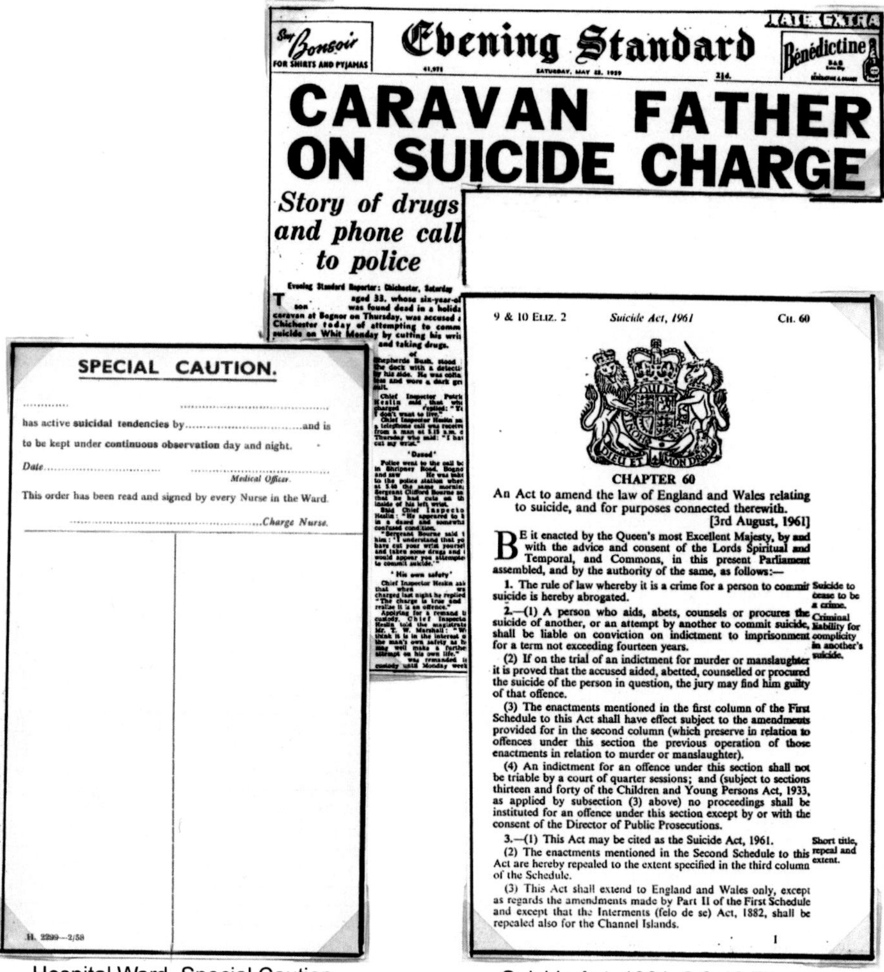

Say Bonsoir FOR SHIRTS AND PYJAMAS

Evening Standard

LATE EXTRA

Bénédictine

SATURDAY, MAY 23, 1959

CARAVAN FATHER ON SUICIDE CHARGE

Story of drugs and phone call to police

Evening Standard Reporter: Chichester, Saturday

T... aged 33, whose six-year-ol[d] son ... was found dead in a holida[y] caravan at Bognor on Thursday, was accused a[t] Chichester today of attempting to comm[it] suicide on Whit Monday by cutting his wri[st] and taking drugs.

... of Shepherds Bush, stood [in] the dock with a detecti[ve] by his side. He was colla[r]less and wore a dark gr[ey] suit.

Chief Inspector Patri[ck] Healin said that wh[en] charged ... replied: "Y[es] I don't want to live."

Chief Inspector Healin sa[id] a telephone call was receiv[ed] from a man at 5.15 a.m. o[n] Thursday who said: "I ha[ve] cut my wrist."

'Dazed'

Police went to the call bo[x] in Shripney Road, Bogno[r] and saw ... He was take[n] to the police station wher[e] at 5.40 the same mornin[g] Sergeant Clifford Bourne sa[w] that he had cuts on th[e] inside of his left wrist.

Said Chief Inspecto[r] Healin: "He appeared to b[e] in a dazed and somewha[t] confused condition.

"Sergeant Bourne said t[o] him: 'I understand that yo[u] have cut your wrist yoursel[f] and taken some drugs and i[t] would appear you attempte[d] to commit suicide.'"

'His own safety'

Chief Inspector Healin sai[d] that when ... wa[s] charged last night he replied "The charge is true and ... realise it is an offence."

Applying for a remand i[n] custody, Chief Inspecto[r] Healin told the magistrate Mr. T. W. Marshall: "W[e] think it is in the interest o[f] the man's own safety as h[e] may well make a furthe[r] attempt on his own life."

... was remanded i[n] custody until Monday week

SPECIAL CAUTION.

....

has active **suicidal tendencies** by.................................and is

to be kept under **continuous observation** day and night.

Date.................................. ....

Medical Officer.

This order has been read and signed by every Nurse in the Ward.

....*Charge Nurse.*

H. 2299—2/58

Hospital Ward, Special Caution Card. Feb. 1958

9 & 10 ELIZ. 2 *Suicide Act, 1961* CH. 60

CHAPTER 60

An Act to amend the law of England and Wales relating to suicide, and for purposes connected therewith.

[3rd August, 1961]

BE it enacted by the Queen's most Excellent Majesty, by and with the advice and consent of the Lords Spiritual and Temporal, and Commons, in this present Parliament assembled, and by the authority of the same, as follows:—

1. The rule of law whereby it is a crime for a person to commit suicide is hereby abrogated. **Suicide to cease to be a crime.**

2.—(1) A person who aids, abets, counsels or procures the suicide of another, or an attempt by another to commit suicide, shall be liable on conviction on indictment to imprisonment for a term not exceeding fourteen years. **Criminal liability for complicity in another's suicide.**

(2) If on the trial of an indictment for murder or manslaughter it is proved that the accused aided, abetted, counselled or procured the suicide of the person in question, the jury may find him guilty of that offence.

(3) The enactments mentioned in the first column of the First Schedule to this Act shall have effect subject to the amendments provided for in the second column (which preserve in relation to offences under this section the previous operation of those enactments in relation to murder or manslaughter).

(4) An indictment for an offence under this section shall not be triable by a court of quarter sessions; and (subject to sections thirteen and forty of the Children and Young Persons Act, 1933, as applied by subsection (3) above) no proceedings shall be instituted for an offence under this section except by or with the consent of the Director of Public Prosecutions.

3.—(1) This Act may be cited as the Suicide Act, 1961. **Short title, repeal and extent.**

(2) The enactments mentioned in the Second Schedule to this Act are hereby repealed to the extent specified in the third column of the Schedule.

(3) This Act shall extend to England and Wales only, except as regards the amendments made by Part II of the First Schedule and except that the Interments (felo de se) Act, 1882, shall be repealed also for the Channel Islands.

1

Suicide Act, 1961. 9 & 10 Eliz.2

Alive or dead, for centuries to attempt suicide (whatever sad reason), was made indictable, and declared a crime, a felony, against God and Man, and accountable to law - after death. **Until 1961** all personal belongings of the offender could be confiscated by the state (no inheritance). To suffer alive was not then enough; and dead, for too long, only burial on unhallowed ground and internment at a crossroads with the body a wooden stake through its lost heart. But, after 1961, to assist another person in a suicide remained a crime.

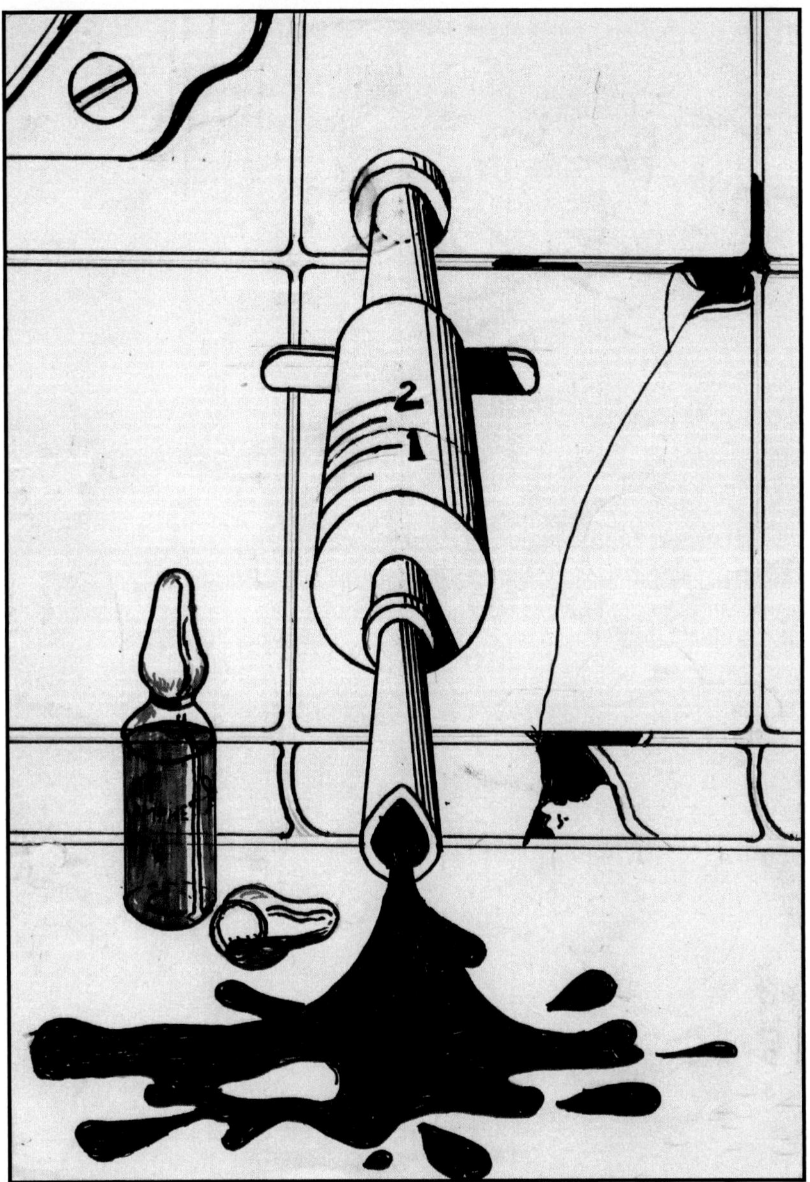

Young patients (I never encountered *old* drug offenders), were in hospital having been given a choice by the Court (Prison or Hospital), for infringing the various formal Drug Acts, and treated (detained) under *Section 26* of the *1959 Mental Health Act* - at the hospital. These mostly teenagers or in early twenties, were NOT necessarily seen as addicts (dependents), but appeared motivated to get off their *'stuff'*. This original drawing was drawn by a day patient working in IT No 5 shed, given to the author, during **Spring 1970**. ... *Better Court Than Coroners.*

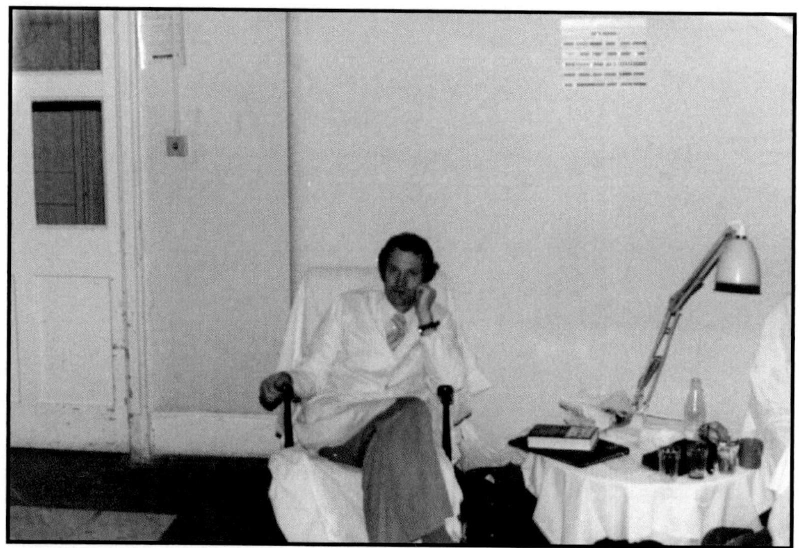

1980. Night Duty. Author, Registered Mental Nurse & qualified Mental Health, Senior Social Worker Barone Hopper, aka Barry, as part-time Staff Nurse, on a Saturday Night Duty - based on Edgeworth & Fawcett block in Graylingwell Hospital Summer.1980.

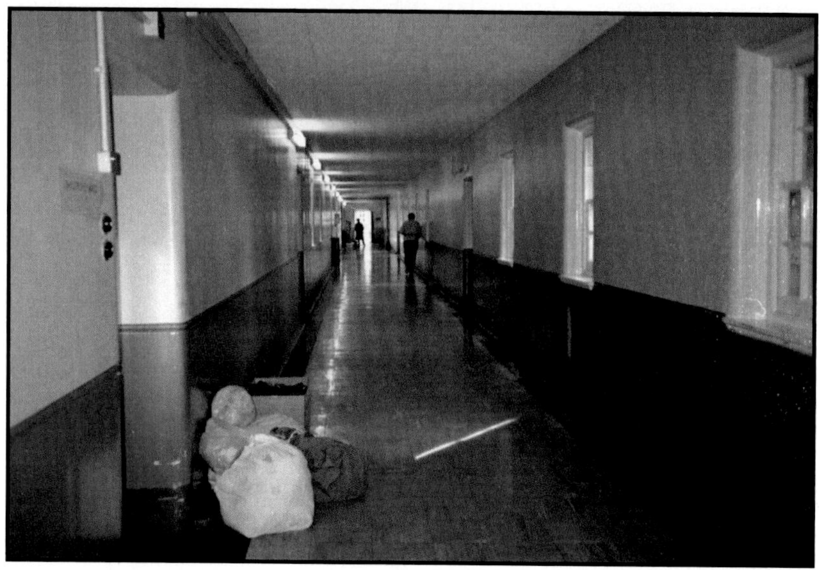

1980. Early morning. Night dirty laundry awaiting collection outside a ward block in one of the many long Graylingwell Hospital corridors 1980..

The handover began, and Alternative Bob and I, with a few more minutes to go, walked a last-round to check all's-well — and chatted en-route.

'Are you still studying up in that room over the old dispensary, Barry?'

'S' right; I reckon it used to be one of the rooms of an old assistant medical officer's quarters. Anyway it's a recreation room for a while, and I find it very useful.'

'What do you do?'

'Oh I try and do at least one past Exam paper per week up there, before going home. Burn me some joss, study and relax'.

'Jean said you were meeting with her and a couple of other students, over at the Nurses Home, for exam question times or something.'

'S' right!', I replied.

I'd agreed to meet up with a number of other students, after a morning shift, at the Pinewood Nurses Home, downstairs' lounge.

It was a standing taboo to all males, that male visitors to Pinewood were strictly, and *only*, allowed before 10 pm, and then only if they remained downstairs. Under *no* circumstances were men allowed upstairs, in the vicinity of the nurses' bedrooms — common to most nurses' quarters, at other hospitals and hostels in the U.K. I did hear of some entertaining experiences of forbidden rendezvous, that had taken place in this Nurses Home... but not for this essay.

The long, two storeyed building, was completed in 1933; as part of the same project as Summersdale Villa. I never did go upstairs; but, on several occasions, I met up with colleagues, usually to study — or to attend a birthday celebration, or other event held in the lounge.

For many years, male staff had been rigorously kept apart from contact with female staff, as the system separated their respective patient charges.

Many memories and anecdotes survived, amongst my senior and recent retired colleagues. Part-time Staff, Vic, one-time Deputy Chief Male Nurse, retired for some years, had been a hospital Dispensary boy, at this hospital, way back in 1918.

Vic described his early 1930s courtship, with his nurse colleague and wife to be, who, despite The Regulations, met on the hospital's tennis courts; and continued to meet illegally at numerous assignations, as the strict rules forbade *any* fraternisation with the opposite sex on the hospital' Estate.

Summary dismissal was possible if caught offending the standing orders; and, if a marriage resulted... well, *no* two married staff were allowed to *both* be employed — then one resignation reluctantly followed. This latter practice, of no two married staff allowed to be working together, was still common in some other professional locations.

We'd been at our Revision, at the Nurse's Home, for an hour; the girls had finished their round of questions and answers. And it was Alternative Bob's turn (his Final was due) — I asked the Question.

'What is Neurology?'

'It's a branch of a biological science, 'erm — which studies the nature; structure and functions of the nervous system...'

'Anything else Bob?'

' ... eh, yes; it's specific only to — to practical, applied aspects, in diagnosis and treatment, of identified disorders of the nervous system. Neurology lies outside the field of the psychiatrist —'

The girls giggled and clapped light-heartedly, in their approval.

It was my turn. Bob read a question out.

'All right then... What are the major features in an Anxiety Neurosis?'

'A pathological anxiety, which symptoms are... fear, a rapid pulse, sweating (body, face, neck, palms) trembling; loss of appetite and sleep...', I rattled off.

As I replied, it recalled introductory lectures on Breuer, Freud, Pavlov and Watson; and my own on Gurdjieff, Jones, Jung, Mcdougall, Nicholl, Ouspensky, Rivers, and others; in detailed discourses on the cause and effect (stick and carrot) stimulation on the body's systems; of biological truisms pertaining to pleasure, fear — ecstasy, as responses to whatever, triggered both internal and external to the body corporate.

And, also, the earthbound emphasis on biochemical constituents of the neuron synapses, as the connections in our own electro-chemical network. How they were easily rendered dysfunctional, by too much or too little salt (for example). And naturally, the anticipated contributions of prescribed drugs (or illegal drugs), in affecting the neurological pathways, and their properties in, like magic, changing perceptions and feelings... food from the gods, or in deceit by hidden demons.

Bob had to depart, for home and a quick meal, before going off to Chichester College for his *Sociology* lectures; this was a title new to me, then, but to mean a great deal in the near future (as I would take the same A level (with others) and pass at a reasonable Grade B plus), as well as to Bob and wife Jean; Sociology was *not* part of their formal student curriculum. But, soon, for a while, this would, in future years, be mandatory alongside Clinical and Social Psychology.

On Bob's departure, there were two other girls, besides Jean, left for the Tarot session. Barbara (aka Babs) and Gillian were, like Jean, third-year student RMs. All of them were in their early, or late-twenties. And as Babs went off to make our cuppas, Gill was gently chiding me. 'Come on Barry? Please...?' Face, hand and gestures playfully adding to her plea for a game. 'You promised you would bring your pack last week, when we agreed to meet? '

'I know.' I grinned and pretended to have forgotten.

'We did promise NOT to take your readings too seriously.' Gill playfully shook her long dark hair and fluttered her eyes mockingly — her hands out to me, in mock plea. 'That's right, you did too.', Babs' voice called out from the nearby Kitchen, just out of sight. It was now mid-afternoon, and I had promised to be home before six and, so, time to relax a little after the study session. I reached into my sling over shoulder-bag, which was used to carry books and wet gear on my cycle trips, to and fro to work. 'Here it is then', and I produced a green boxed Marseille pack of well worn Tarot cards — to play.

'He's got them. Barry's got 'em', responded Gill gleefully.

Jean and Gill placed themselves, around the low-long veneer covered coffee-table. Babs arrived with filled coffee mugs, and placed the tray at one end of the rigid table.

Unusual, but there was no music or other noise about the building; we did not want music for our study session, and other nurses were either away on duties or off duty — and just not visible.

We chatted about this and that, while drinking our coffee or tea — and I shuffled the cards a few times, in anticipation. A sudden loud noisy interruption, caused by the house telephone, heard ringing at the foot of the stairs and close by — only ten or so feet in front of us. Jean got up to answer it. 'Hello?... Who... oh, Eileen, you mean? Think she's on nights....?'

Before she finished, a loud slam from above indicated a room door being closed, and the patter of bare feet slapping, slamming their way down the stairs. 'Is it for me?' It was indeed Eileen, one of our other third year colleagues, who had clearly been waiting for a phone call. As she came into view, it looked as if she'd just bounded out of bed, as she appeared somewhat breathless on the scene.

'Thanks Jean... oh... eh... hello, Barry', she beamed across at us as she took the phone to reply. Eileen's nightdress, a brief fabric, was a worn torn, diaphanous blue-fleece, which openly displayed a Titian well-rounded nakedness, thinly veiled beneath.

A good job the heating was ample, about the home and hearth. And, equally clear, from our ten feet or so distance, was that her mature body was more covered by her long red gold hair, than her nightie, as she shifted about the phone.

'Oh... Ye-s. But, but, when... I could... no-no... eh, we could...?', full of too obvious uncertainty. Such was the tone of her conversation, as she would lift one leg up, placing the sole of one foot against the calf of the other leg, and then reverse it; in her restlessness, moving constantly.

At Eileen's presence, we reduced our conversation to a trickle, so as not to prevent her from hearing her caller. And we all knew our Eileen well; she was most vulnerable, in more ways than one. Vulnerable indeed... Always bubbling, a frenetic party goer, love to all not none, Eileen was having great difficulty in her academic work; she was a great carer on the wards and outside them, but too often chaotic and open to one misunderstanding, after another misunderstanding; as she had described to us earlier on her seemed numerous past relationships. And now — we suspected another breakup; and she was pregnant.

The Tarot cardboard box, with its instructions inside, lay empty on the table, said *Ancient Tarot De Marseille,* printed by B.P. Grimaud. (there are many different face packs) [15] ; on its green cover was drawn a dark triangle, equidistant in a circle, a pentagram, veiling uninitiated august events, and delightful hidden secrets yet to come.

I had owned this pack for several years or so, having purchased it from Watkins, in Cecil Court off the Charring Cross Road — where I had obtained much of my literature; Jung and Gurdjieff' related material; coupled with a sweet smelling supply of joss sticks in their long colourful Indian export packs. Although I was then fast drifting away, from that font of esoteric knowledge, to concentrate on orthodox psychology and other chosen subjects; the little know-how I had accrued, had provided a little entertainment, during the past few months and more. Eileen had been to one or two brief sittings after previous post-study encounters; indeed she took them more serious than any of the others, I concluded.

Sure enough as soon as the telephone call finished Eileen bounded over to our company, and sat next to Babs, opposite me, on a pulled up pile of cushions. 'Erm... erm...' We looked meaningfully at her vaporous undress —

uninhibited (but not denied) presence. But, but... she was fragile; and not, *not* to be rejected by our chaste company. 'Oh. It's all right. As long as Barry doesn't mind eh?' I said nothing at this plea. And, reassured, Eileen collapsed and relaxed, as she grinned child-mischief at us all, and sat down opposite me, upon naked haunches, as she crossed bare feet in a take-for-granted acceptance... I ignored her state... just!

And we contemplated The Tarot pack. Babs, Gill and Jean were still wearing their nurses' uniform, from working in the morning; and I, too, remained in my grey-suit uniform, but minus the white-coat and jacket, cast over the back of a chair. Outside was dark and dismal, though not raining; a wind was getting up and we had the lights on in the lounge. It was mid winter cold; though warm in our company.

The girls were quiet as they settled down, sat around the coffee table, and waited for me to commence the play. Gill, Jean and Babs slowly sipped their mugs of tea; whilst Eileen sat most pensive, a hand to her mouth. Eileen appeared to be sucking her right thumb, whilst her left hand dropped down onto her left thigh. Almost still, but her feet were twitching, as tapping toes set ripples up her calves. She looked so serious. And appeared so eager.

'Who's first for the draw then', I asked, breaking the heavy suspense.

'Me, please Barry. Eh, if that's all right?', Jean quickly echoed, to our surprise.

'Right, you know the Rules....' I began. ... 'Uh-huh. Shuffle them first..' Said Jean.

'S' right, three times circularly from right to left. And lay them, without looking, all of the cards; each card separately face down, on the table in front of you', I confirmed.

As always, I felt a bit of a fraud, though I always, as referee, reminded the players of my real ignorance of the Tarot; and thus, for us, to abide strictly by the written guidance supplied with every pack of the *Ancient Tarot of Marseilles* — rigid to Grimaud's book of Rules... But the seekers were indifferent to this honest declaration... after all, they said, *it's just a game*.

'Right, here we go then', said Jean, with a noticeable quiver in her voice. 'Shuffle done. I'll lay them out.' Fascinated, they leaned towards the set being presented.

An Introduction detailed two games; a purely symbolic set, in 22 cards, with twenty one cards numbered in Roman Numerals at the top; the last, but not least, the Joker or Fool being the twenty second, and unnumbered. And a second, a further fifty-six cards (making 78 in all) which were, then, sub-divided into four suits, similar to ordinary playing cards, except that instead of Spades, Hearts, Diamonds and Clubs, there were Swords, Cups, Coins and Clubs. Their symbols were believed of, at least, medieval origin, their symbolism, of ancient pedigree.

Our twenty-two Tarot cards in play, were called the Major Arcana. The Minor Arcana was a complete draw which used all 78 cards. The previous decade, I'd been fascinated by comparative religion and historical folklore; especially of ancient civilizations — *Epic of Gilgamesh.* Wallis' *Egyptian Book of the Dead.* The Zohar. Greek Dionysus rites. Buddha. Confucius. Robert Graves Celtic Hu. Especially, Graves *White Goddess.* Such data I'd stored in my fragile cranium as a few *symbols,* which came within my own brief anthology.

In youth, I had had a flirtation in reading widely on the occult, which started with Wheatley, Butler, Crowley and Blavatsky; but then moved away from the Yogas, and Cabbala — to Plato's *Dialogues*, and Bertrand Russell's works; which led me further away, to travel up an alternative Path. Of light and dark; surreal, real, unreal... and here.

I wasn't very good, at ordinary card playing, though for a brief time in HM Forces I experienced a few good 'bluff ' hands at three-card brag and five-card stud; but it was left hand stuff to me. And I vividly recalled, after one severe money loss, tearing a pack of cards up and scattering them to the four-winds back into our troopship's wake, on a return journey with others, from overseas service.

The Major Arcana card faces which appeared, were of largely medieval to 18th century woodcut illustrations, and with definite Tarot and astrological leanings. And, as with the tabloid newspapers daily readings, the stars influence was a general interpretation, based on the Sun - or so I believed. So, my readings were otherwise unpretentious and, as they laid, they were interpreted using the book as a rosetta stone, well, almost, by me. Jean finished putting the Tarot cards down on the table and was now ready for her selection. The others remained quiet and still.

'Now?' Jean looked up. I smiled, nodded.

'One.' And the first card was raised by her right hand.

'Put it face up on your left.' I said.

'Two'. 'On your right. A space between.'

'Third'. 'Place above the space.' And...

'Four' Jean anticipated 'On the bottom', I replied.
And her cards?

They were a mix. First down was No.18. The Moon. Next was No. 10, The Wheel of Fortune (two doubtfuls): Third No. 5, The Pope (a strong one): and her fourth card was No. 16, The Tower of Destruction, also known as '*The Tower Struck by Lightning*.' 'Well... well. Good? Bad? Barry? The suspense is killing', pleaded Jean, who knew I would read The Book — before personalising the reading.

And, even as I began the reading, I had a foreboding; and reflected on the little I really knew, of married Jean and, by association, of husband Bob. 'But first, we must total up the numbers, to disclose the centre card of influence: 18, 10, 5, 16; that makes 49. So four and 9 equals 13! And thirteen, Jean, is, oh...', I looked it up and read it out. 'The Death card - in the centre.'

Immediately defensive, I felt, as much as heard, the intakes of all four girls. 'Not so bad as it seems, Jean, *it's a symbol of change*.' 'Oh!' I could feel her drawn in breath, and the others meaningful silence.... I began the reading, which I did in clockwise formation. I started with the right (or from the East), then South, West, North, and to the centre.

After reading the commentary out; however I dressed her words, I was not able to change her cards. '*Secrets revealed* — and change: with a very strong card of influence. The Pope — a positive card Jean. It's quite a mixed hand.'

'Eh. Yes. Wonder what it all means, Barry. Have to wait and see...?'

The girls sat back and relaxed, a trifle, at the natural interlude. Jean looked puzzled, yet satiated, as if to accept — what? It was, after all, but a light hearted game of let's-pretend, fortune-telling; wasn't it?... Not at all scientific.

Gill had put her glasses on, when the cards were revealed, and only removed them when Jean's play was concluded. A simple act, taken absolutely for granted. So normal — 'put her glasses on', in order for her to see, and follow, a key metaphysical use, an interpretation of the picture-cards displayed below; and follow a set of albeit alchemical ascribed rules.

What was so different in such selected drawn symbols from yore, and Summersdale patient Mavis' abstract tea-leaf pictographs? Taken further, on reflection. Gill's glasses equally transformed otherwise meaningless bordered colours and shapes, into named human metaphors; and all written texts even in her own English language could not be 'read' - unless she had her reading glasses on her nose. I too, took this latter point equally for granted, in the presentation of any 'foreign' language of symbols (written and spoke); not understood but still 'pigeon holed' accepted as 'of such and such', summarily dismissed.

It would be in late middle-age before I would need glasses to read, and 'know' of what I could be missing out. Any new language, new code, new range of information would be foreign, different, but certainly *not* of itself alien; that would be a dark set in its use. How many patients had I already encountered, whose personal sets of information (whatever origins) too frequently read alien, hostile, for foreign or different. And, in fear, set in motion anti-social acts and personal tragedies.

The interlude, in our game, was brief, and no-one appeared to want to interrupt the sequence; and, to our surprise, Eileen had not uttered a word throughout Jean's act, but remained still, with her thumb sucked-tight like a proverbial taut nipple.

Barbara elected to be next. I knew even less about Babs than I did of Jean; about twenty-three years old, quite petite, blonde (I was uncertain whether it was peroxide), sparkling blue eyes and a slight build. We had met three or four times, at other gatherings; including one previous Tarot game, in one sequel to a study group in this same lounge. The Ritual was repeated exactly as Jean's of only minutes before. Babs' five cards on display.

First came No.17, The Star.

Second emerged No. 6, The Lover.

Third was No.10, The Moon.

Fourth was No.11, Force.

And adding their numbers together, was No. 8, Justice.

The influence of The Moon suggested a *feet-of-clay* shadow, but the other cards diminished its influence. No.6, The Lover, was always a popular appearance with its abstract - the thought of physical love; and its practical meaning which suggested *a Card of Union*, and possible marriage. But, its corollary was also of many unions, even infidelity, and a choice to be made.... A strong positive card to be revealed. And, for a moment or so, the company echoed the appearance of Lover as a pleasant display, after all, it was one of 'the' reasons they wanted the Tarot. It was clear, from the commentary, that Babs' reading was a good experience; with its centre Justice in confirmation.

Gillian was next; and, as she put her glasses on for a third reading, shuffled the pack and laid the selected cards down upon the table; my mind was again looking out and into, down into a three dimensional world, with the laziness of my being: Only receiving a flat, two-dimensional picture; with memory traces — threads; and, my automaton instincts, holding back, *blocking*, my perceptions of the third-dimension of depth (and all other dimensions). As Peter Ouspensky's alchemical experiments alluded to and described so well, in Gurdjieff, and Jung's (all three close friends of Nicholl) works — reflected in Dr. Maurice Nicoll's day-by-day diaries in his *Commentaries.*[16] And, of which, Nicholl's friend and colleague surgeon, author Dr. Kenneth Walker suggested how to ... '*Know, to Shape and Liberate – The Mind....*'. I re-focussed my attention, my will, at Gill's five cards: and, as with Babs, I saw quite a good set to read out.

First was No. 3, The Empress
Second was No. 11, Force.
Third led No. 7, The Chariot
Fourth said No. 11, Temperance
And together, No. 8, Justice.

We started, startled, at the re-appearance of Justice, again being a centre inference. Interesting, that the Empress preceded the Chariot, to read *Victory* (of what, her Final Exam, Life, what?). Force complemented this trend, a practical meaning; '*If you have will-power, events will be overcome. When right is on your side the situation will be mastered.*', and so on. No. 14, Temperance, suggested a delay in whatever ultimately was suggested by her set. And Justice; this reflected a successful, honest, outcome at whatever Gillian would put out in the future. Gill was well happy with this layout and slapped her knees in emphasis, 'And I do have plans', she declared, matter of factly to us all: but gave no clue as to what.

And now — it was Eileen's turn.

She was the known youngest of our group, just approaching twenty-two years old.

'My turn now, I guess — eh?', Eileen looked to me and around her for acknowledgment and approval. But her usual bubbly smile was somewhat muted, and a tension was quite visible. It was as if this make-believe show of cards would supply knowledge of all her future aspirations and even, unrealistically, perhaps change her life by the act itself?

There was no guile apparent in Eileen and, even in her almost nakedness sat there in our midst, I perceived her presence not lewdly or precocious in any way; but a living ivory flesh statuette from a cave back in prehistoric times — a sacred symbol of fertility in exaggerated roundness; her bulbous tummy in advanced pregnancy and over-large breasts, visible through her thin blue veil.

Despite this presentation, and her obvious fecundity, Eileen emanated an innocence (of worldliness) we had all come to appreciate, even wary of, at all times. And it was, generally, hands off. She began. 'I'll shuffle them extra well, I think.', and proceeded to shuffle the pack, most enthusiastically. Eileen dropped at least a dozen cards, before putting them back into the pack, and finally accepted she was ready for the lay of her cards... 'Now, to put them down', she said quite reverently. 'Slowly...' As Eileen placed the symbols below her, I momentary thought of the alchemist maxim... *'As Is Above Is Below...'*

I pondered what (or if) unknown, unseen, whatever influences could so direct a human enquirer, via these cards...? After all, to know of the world outside ourselves and, to know *something* of our own world of inner-space within, (and be aware of Others' human nature), would initially seem of a different fabric.

Superficially, we accept most brief contacts with others in life and, as with Eileen, youth and beauty were truly only skin-deep, and changed too quickly, through the lime of time. Then, in a shuddering, strange brief nauseous moment, *I perceived myself and company in a Sartrean depersonalised sculpture — as I observed all, on-view, as shapes, lines and colours,* within *an infinitely greater vessel than an inverted tea cup,* to be inadequately interpreted and read, by myself. It happened only the once. Yet *not* nauseous.

Where was I then, in that fleeting split-second moment? But that watching moment had already passed. So many of our most disturbed patients, in a horrified alienated state, would cut themselves, to see and feel the blood swell-out, beyond their single-skin surface: and so to momentarily gain their own attention; in being alive. Pain would have briefly reminded such sufferers of their real terrestrial existence...

Eileen had laid her twenty-two cards out on the table. The coffee cups were cleared away back to the kitchen. And, the table surface, like a tabula-rasa, was occupied solely by those paper shapes upon its flat surface. Perhaps inevitably, her declared cards were, at the onset, different from the other girls; at least one was presented so...

First was No. 9, The Hermit. Two, again, No. 18, The Moon. Three, surprise, No. 7, The Chariot - but Inverted. Four, no surprise, No. 6, The Lover. Eileen's centre card was thus No. 4, The Emperor, which centre influence indicated Transient wealth and Power. Despite Eileen's gregariousness, the appearance of the Tarot Hermit seemed an appropriate introduction, but what followed was even more so.

In common with other cards, The Hermit referred to her inner-life, of which (as others) suggested *a secret will be revealed.* The illusionary Moon (a normally 'bad influence' the booklet said), corresponded to a scandal, and *a secret revealed.* In my commentaries, I did not read out a 'bad card', but announced the rest of the text. Odd... I never was asked to actually show what was written, only but to read it, as if to preserve a myth of mysticism.

It was the third and fourth cards which seemed to deliver most impact. Undoubtedly, because of Eileen's shuffling the cards too much, and having dropped so many before replacement, the Chariot was Inverted. Number seven in Eileen's set, read in abstract, said it represented '*The material currents which carry man along*' — but its inverted practical value said: '*Bad News. This is a card which asserts its authority* without *being strong*.'

Again, in reading my commentary to Eileen, I did *not* add 'Bad News', but interpreted the balance. She was visibly delighted to see The Lover, and the girls again bubbled at its appearance. But with Eileen there was a rider; the book said — '*The Chariot preceding The Lover - 'Projects will be destroyed as the result of a departure*.' The booklet did not specify an alternative; 'inverted chariot preceding The Lover.' But by the Rules, clearly, it was a bad addition.

The Lover had already been declared, and I drew out the more pleasant suggestions, rather than full text, for the obvious reasons. But (to myself and to Eileen?) it was this, in-part, which seemed dishonest; like leaving an inedible part of a meal on the side of a plate, whilst pretending to eat it all. Game or not, I recollect feeling it was impossible (for me) to wilfully inflict even the possibility of psychic pain, on one so immature and vulnerable to commentary as Eileen.

It was true, that in her immature nature so essentially honest and humane, such baleful signals might not have registered anyway, but her unconscious, surely, would have stored such suggestions and that, morally, I would not chance. I concluded Eileen's reading, by repeating comment on No.4, The

Emperor: '*The Division of the Circle and practical contribution of Transient wealth and power*'; which, surely, to a so innocent optimist as Eileen, could be interpreted in numerous pleasant fantasies.

And so The Game concluded for, as agreed before, I would *not* play more than one reading at a time; for as if to change circumstances, one must keep altering the cards to suit, and keep playing to get it right.... (I would *never* use the Tarot with patients, at all... that would be obscene, I thought.)

Although one or two people had been in and out of the building, while we enjoyed (if so) our game of Tarot, we had not been interrupted during the past half-hour or so, in the lounge at the Pinewood Nurses Home. But a loud voice from the entrance completely broke the spell of our ritual, bubble, whatever of concentration; and it was someone for Jean, to collect her and drive her home. A strong cold wind blew across the lounge, as the door was opened and Eileen was starkly reminded of her almost nakedness; quickly, looking like a startled doe, she thanked me and abruptly pattered up the stairs to her room. But not before a pause and, looking back, a little lost, at a whisper, so serious, she concluded,'Not Very Good Was It My Hand. Barry?' I decided not to hear her last remark.

In my looking back, to that 1968 RMN post-studies' Tarot game at the Nurses' Home, its precise atmosphere was naturally diminished in my memory, but the outcome, though nothing whatever to do with me, was a lesson I could not forget.

Coincidence. *Jean,* a few weeks later, learnt that Bob had been having an affair, and sadly their marriage was dissolved — fortunately they had no children.

Coincidence. *Barbara,* who was single when we had participated in the game, shortly afterwards met a locum doctor whom she married some months later.

Coincidence. *Gillian* was promoted to Ward Sister, within a year of qualification after excelling at her finals, and was to experience an excellent career.

Coincidence. *Eileen* lost her boyfriend; lost her baby; and, for a time, lost her way, unable to complete her training; she was, as then customary, transferred to a neighbouring over the border hospital, after her breakdown. We all felt very sorry at her departure, but fortunately, with support, she recovered and moved on — and I heard no more of her.

Although we met a number of times in the future with other colleagues, especially in the summer time, I declined to do any more Tarot readings after our study sessions. But, I continued to respect that which I had *no* real, supernatural knowledge of, whether called Occult, Mysticism, Metaphysics — Parapsychology, or Philosophy, whatever Other deemed roots of coincidence.... To dabble in the Tarot, even for fun, was *not* an option.

It was a cautionary tale for me which, whatever my own current set of beliefs, was surely irrelevant; but, if anyone else was so influenced by such contacts, it was something I felt not inclined to dabble in, in their midst, at that time... And, as to coincidences? I considered beliefs, on the theme of what means fate and Karma. Ray Bradbury, Arthur Koestler and Carl Jung — *On Synchronicity* [17] about, freedom of choice, or none. And about hidden willpower, and hidden knowledge.

And Collect

The phone call came, late one very wet Saturday afternoon. Red was off duty, playing football for the hospital team. He was one of its best goal scorers. A number of residents were on weekend leave; and there were no day hospital visitors to cater for. A few patients were still out with relatives. I had just completed the tea-time medicines, and noticed that the ward lights had been put on, due to very dull weather, and a gathering darkness.

'Barry. Call from The Office; do you mind going out?'

'No Bill. What's it about?' I was securing the drugs trolley, in the ward office. Washing-up completed. 'But it'll leave you on your own, Bill?' I replied.

'They thought of that, they're sending Fred over.', (he was a retired charge nurse), 'to help out.'

'Oh. Right... right...', I was pleased to be asked to help out.

'Office has laid on a hospital car and driver for you. You'll meet up with the MWO., to collect a 26 absconder, gone walkabout.', Said Bill helpfully...

'Where ...?', I began....

'Bosham, Barry. Car's at the Main Front Entrance. Driver knows the way as he's been out to the house before. Better be off, eh? He's been given some details to pass on to you en-route.' On my way out, Julie and Laurie were at our Front Entrance, with young Michael; preparing to go down the Wellington Arms for an hour or so.

Alan, a late middle-aged depressive who was on Nardil, a prescribed MAO (Mono Amine Oxydase, an inhibitor and a beta-blocker), had been dissuaded from going with them; he wasn't well enough, yet. Any high protein food, in-solid or liquid form, taken with the drug in his bloodstream could have put him into a coma, or worse, and led to a fatality. Such an incident had nearly happened to him, less than a week ago.

Fred waved to me, white-coat over his arm, as he passed me by on his way over to the Villa. 'Hello Barry. Looks like rain, eh?', Fred said cheerfully, as he passed me by. And, indeed, as our hospital white Ford Estate left the hospital grounds by the South Drive, it had began to drizzle.

'Barry in't it? Jack Smith's me name.' With his left hand firm on the wheel, the driver, briefly, put his right hand across to me to shake hello, before increasing speed, away for the Portsmouth road. It was a narrow, twisted, old rutted coast road which, in places, came very close to the sea and Chichester Estuary tidal waters. Traffic was heavy and sluggish; Saturday evening loomed; and the rain increased its downfall, blurring our vision — but Jack had driven this way before.

Bosham, minute, cosy, nestled off the A27, its southern turn off only minutes past Fishbourne; the small village was almost set in Chichester Harbour itself. There was abundant stone evidence of Bosham having been a Roman port (as Fishbourne); the coastline very different from almost two thousand years ago, when the landfall was further out. Harbour waters and rills were somewhat deeper, in past centuries. Coastal erosion was always a real threat; and, each year, the sea and the seasons' clawed, claimed and buried more and more land mass.

Legends abounded about this place. King Canute was reputed to have been asked to drive a stormy sea away, at his command, and King Harold once sailed for Normandy, from this ancient site. And whatever Bosham's own history, as Jack described the area to me, he also passed on the information given him by the duty nursing officer.

Ian, a young Section 26 florid paranoid schizophrenic sufferer, had managed to abscond from Bramber Two ward, and made for home and his elderly mother. His mother lived, otherwise alone, in an old isolated house, located close off Bosham Lane. A section of coast road, during high-tides, was covered in water; a pub, and a number of houses, even had the waters lapping their outside window sills. I hoped Abbey House was not one of them.

Driver Jack cautiously made his way along the Bosham coast road, whilst the gale blew considerable spume across from the mud flats (exposed by low tide); and then across the road and our vision. The early wintry weather, despite being Saturday, appeared to be keeping people indoors; though the pub overlooking the harbour and adjacent to the road had its lights blazing out; each time a body opened and shut its front door, a searchlight probed and peppered the darkness and ragged mist. It was a blessing Jack did know the way, else we would've experienced some difficulty in finding the Abbey House — and young Ian.

I recollect, at some point, we arrived on Bosham Quay and realized through the heavy rain (or was it sea spray), there existed a long redbrick harbour wall which sides appeared steep and perilous; but our driver thought it most enjoyable. 'Not long now, mate', he chortled. About five minutes later, we stopped outside an old house, enclosed by trees, wall and tall hedgerow; and, to my surprise, four vehicles, one a police car, and another an ambulance, were stationary outside the wall, with their lights on; and passengers enclosed, and clearly waiting for us.

Jack sat tight and I got out, with my somewhat inadequate thin raincoat (taken from my bicycle saddlebag before I left the hospital), into the heavy falling rain. The two policemen and the ambulance men stayed inside their vehicles; three people emerged from two other cars. One person was a slight, well dressed, middle-aged lady with white mac, green wellies, and a red headscarf, under a black umbrella. The two men with her, introduced themselves; one was the family GP, Dr. Chalk and the other was our Mental Welfare Officer, George Pople. George introduced a student MWO colleague, Andrew, son of one of our consultants, who sat safe in the back seat of the doctor's vehicle looking most uncomfortable, and very anxious at the present goings on... George, the duty Mental Welfare Officer, was in charge of the proceedings...

The one lady present, and frightened owner of the house, was absconder Ian's mother. Mrs. Bracken was a widow who, otherwise, lived downstairs in this large, reputed early 17th century, detached house; it was built on the site of a much earlier ecclesiastical building, hence its name; and it was believed early, stone, foundations were still to be seen, in its large cellar or crypt.

The site had been continuously in use, since the second century; then, a Roman villa. Much of Bosham and district had other buildings, especially close by the church, with similar histories. Eerie the surroundings; in that biting cold wind, driving-rain and thickly swirling throat-mist, the vehicles' lights cast many moving shapes and shadows about us.

And to the house; only one light was visible, upstairs over the front entrance. Mrs. Bracken had, earlier in the afternoon, been threatened by her son soon after his fractious arrival; when he became convinced that there were Strange People, including KGB (again), occupying the house; and his mother, her son insisted, was held responsible for their intrusion. Fugitive (a misnomer) Ian had torn the telephone out, smashed the television and then broken up much of the furniture, insisting 'they' were 'taking the piss' out of him. It was only when he realized he was hungry, that he allowed his mother to depart to a local store; but promptly brandished a kitchen knife at her before locking the doors and windows, and then barricaded himself in. Terrified what he might do to himself, herself or others, in his deluded state of mind, not least as a very real fire-risk, his mother had telephoned the police and her GP for help and guidance. To do so she had had to leave the house to use an outside telephone booth.

The 1959 Mental Health Act, in law, said that any '*Sectioned*', that is, compulsory detained (life threatening) patient, who absconded from a psychiatric hospital and had survived without incident for 28 days would automatically have been eligible for discharge from their original section. Only when, and if, that patient became so acutely ill again, would a section be applied for by the relevant professionals.

Ian had 'not' survived without incident, and his Section 26 was still valid; this meant no new assessment was necessary by GP, and Consultant; but a straightforward collection and return into hospital procedure. George quickly explained the above to me, as we entered the drive. He had no need to show me his warrant card, as I already knew him. And, together, we slowly approached the front door of the house. All other persons were left out of sight, waiting in their own vehicles. And to further await instructions (if circumstances insisted) from George the Mental Welfare Officer; as he orchestrated the event.

Although I felt very wary, my trust in George's experience was absolute — but there was the otherwise unpredictable; but, again, Ian had been 'collected' by George on other occasions; though the weather was never so inclement as this winter night, he had added hastily. Ugh. I stepped into a puddle and skidded on some wet leaves; George put his hand out and helped steady me.

As I moved forward again, we could not help noticing that a second light was now on, downstairs; in a room to our left of the front entrance; and more so, the curtains were pulled aside to reveal a man watching our approach and easily seen, still clutching the large (it looked) kitchen knife, earlier described by his mother. I gulped. There was several old gnarled trees, bereft of leaves, on either side of the driveway and several shadowed clumps of shrubs, through which a few shards of jagged light came through; even such light streams were broken by the incessant rain which reflected or barred their lengths.

George and I, well sodden and still moving on. Leaving the others behind us — out of sight. Suddenly, before George even opened his mouth to call Ian's name; we heard a very loud yell from Abbey House, which stopped us dead in our tracks. But, it happened, not to be a threat or dire warning of horrors to come, but a cry of enormous joyous relief; from Ian.

We must have been easily seen on the outside, through the well lit window. We could not have been more than ten feet away, at our halt. 'Welfare... it's the man from The Welfare', shouted Ian. George and I heard his yelp of surprise; and the MWO responded quickly with well meant reassurance. 'S' right Ian. *It's me. George*, The Welfare Man.' He called out loud. 'At last. Rescue. They're going - d'yuh hear 'erm ...?', Ian shouted out to George. And Ian disappeared from the window, curtains dropped and, following a loud crashing of moving furniture, the front door flew back, and he came running out towards us, still holding his long knife aloft.

Rescued Ian only appeared to have eyes for George; and, although I was only feet away from him, he ignored (saw through) me. Only one or two seconds elapsed, as we remained still, as Ian, at a run, then approached George; knife held high as if to ward off his unseen phantoms, then he just dropped the knife, which just seemed to fall away to the earth, as he then held out both his hands towards his rescuer. Ian said no more; and, almost eagerly, allowed George to lead him out of the drive, and up to the back of the ambulance; an attendant jumped out, with a blanket ready, placing it about Ian's shoulders and, together with George, they then assisted their patient up into the back of the ambulance. And still it rained, and the mist eddied about us.

The crisis, as such, appeared to be over; and the ambulance attendant remained in the vehicle with him; whilst George, after reassuring Ian of what procedure was to follow, jumped out and spoke briefly to the driver.

George then moved over to the car with Ian's mother and Dr. Chalk, who were clearly relieved at the apparent safe outcome, of the incident. After a few brief words to them both, through a just opened car door, they then drove round the corner and down Abbey House drive; from which, only moments before, we had emerged with Ian.

Finally, George went over, to thank the two policeman for their back-up support, and confirmed that he did not think it necessary, for them to tail the ambulance back into the hospital, as Jack and I would be doing that in just a few minutes. As to George's own vehicle, he said it was only a hundred yards or so back along the road, a precaution he often took, when he anticipated there might have been special problems ahead. George, as MWO, also followed behind us, to ensure we all arrived safely back at the hospital.

Within minutes, the ambulance moved off; and we followed — not too close behind.

Getting back out, through Bosham, was even trickier than the journey in, as it soon became clear (about all that was) the tide was fast rolling in; the mud flats had disappeared and the surface of the coast road had too disappeared from view; but, fortunately, the tide was not yet high; and the ambulance driver, like Jack, our driver, knew the route and its risks. Eventually, after a few warning halts, we emerged out on the safer higher ground; and were soon back on the Portsmouth road, back towards Chichester and our hospital wards.

The rest of the journey back to Bramber Two ward was uneventful; and Ian was left contentedly drinking a mug of hot tea and awaiting a sandwich, being made for him in the kitchen, whilst he sat in the nursing office and awaited the duty Doctor. MWO George also sat in the office, with Bramber's Charge Nurse, to complete relevant paperwork.

As I trawled my way back through numerous puddles and mounds of fallen leaves from the Main Building, back to Summersdale, I was grateful the heavy rain had thinned down to a trickle. But my sodden clothing, and squelching shoes, made me shiver and shake a little with a sniffle, stifling a sneeze or two.

I was gladdened by the blazing lights of the Villa, and the loud distinct noise of music; a piano and guitar, with several voices attempting to keep time with it. The music, I noticed as I turned back onto Male Summersdale, was actually coming from the Female side. Bill said Sister Rees (his opposite peer) was pleased to accept Laurie's and Mike's offers of entertainment, for their patients.

Zen Mike was playing his guitar, and one of the ladies was gleefully accompanying him, on the piano. I noted (having quickly looked across) that Julie was sat down on a sofa, with her own guitar, and was singing most lustily

— and, well, her silent guitar appeared as, like fair Julie, a flower power dressing like her colourful outfits and partial nakedness; but well - was it ever played?... So what if it didn't!

It was getting late, and Bill was about to handover to the Night Nurse; Eric was another (like Bill) old soldier, who had worked in the hospital for well over twenty years, and seemed part of the secure furnishings, for staff and patients alike.

'Done a good job Barry. Good experience for you Eh?'

'Thanks Bill.'

Home to Stonecrock Cottages. But first, I mused, as I entered Summersdale kitchen, and absently plugged a kettle in for a cuppa tea; as I drew the water I accidentally kicked the pig-bucket (hospital pig-swill collected by a local farmer) underneath the sink.

Good hygiene was strictly maintained, as rubbish was, according to its substance, automatically separated into different lidded metal bins, or other containers. Pig swill in one (or more) dust-bins; rags and unwanted clothing in sacks; broken up cardboard cartons in another sack; milk bottles in the metal basket provided by the milkman — previously full of course; silver milk bottle cap tops kept in a pile and sold off for a charity; newspapers and paper waste in another bin. Medical waste was collected in specific, stout sealed colour coded bags, (old needles, et cetera in one, contaminated matter in another...).

Victorian, Dickensian, Boffin dust heaps and collections of 'nightsoil' were long past. Well, perhaps not completely. I had been brought up, in wartime and postwar 1940s and '50s years, when local waste collectors drove through the streets, on their horse and carts, shouting 'Old Rags And Lumber!'; and who would eagerly pay you a nominal amount, on whatever they took off you. The binmen would remove the normal 'other' unwanted rubbish and offal at least once per week; binmen renowned for their helpfulness and good cheer, during the past year; and, at Christmas, householders gladly rewarded their milkmen and binmen with cash (The Christmas Box). But, in the hospital, whilst the milkman and binmen might be generally unknown to the rank and file staff and patient — we knew, they rightly did receive their occasional perks.

And, moving the pig bucket back under the Summersdale sinks, I noticed its, almost overflowing, waste of disposable supper remains. And my action upset several pieces of discarded toast onto the floor. I felt a pang of hunger, and need for warmth, both personal and domestic; and warmly thought of Sara and our two infants back in our tithe rented cottage, out at Chilgrove. Boys probably in bed by now, I thought; and my wife, perhaps chatting with our next door neighbours (the cottage was in two halves), a young farm labourer with his wife and house dog — maybe watching television, or typing.

But first, I had to get home. As I hung my white coat up, in the office, and bid good night to Bill and Eric (Fred had gone home) and waved a goodbye to several of our patients, I collected my bicycle from one of the small back corridors, adjacent to staff bedsit quarters; and went out back into the night. I was too wet to bother with the numerous puddles and running streams; or to avoid the many piles of twigs and leaves. But I soon warmed up in the cycling, as I commenced the eight miles home, through the dark narrow country roads. It again gave me time to think. Time to contemplate...

I was cycling home on the long spindly B 2141 Petersfield Road, past the Crows Hall Farm, through Binderton and, eventual, then home stretch, turning away to the right, before the White Horse Inn of Chilgrove. And, at last, along that long unlit meandering muddied lane, and up to Stonerock. Amongst the high thickly wooded downs, close by on my left, as then, with most of my late journeys home on my travels — my reality appeared atavistic. And I responded to its emanations.

And those seeming unearthly unreal (viz not identified) feelings, gave way to more historical connections — much as, only hours ago, we experienced at Bosham; and young Ian had succumbed. Imagination easily conjured up lines of phantoms. Roman, leathered, soldiers, journeying up towards Goosehill camp; which remains I knew of, somewhere, up there on my left; up amongst those shadows in the South Down hills. There was no fear upon me, but a wonderment.

Also about me, in that damp darkness, was out of sight Kingley Vale's well hidden valley, of Ancient Yews, it too lay, on my left, the ancient forest well out of sight, but very close in distance. Were there early Neolithic settlements with benign wraiths, alongside Belgic settlers, Saxons, Vikings, Normans and Medieval yeoman; all together, in truce, mingled with Roman forebears, well in shadows about me. And I moved on as a silent witness, my own attached shadow too, amongst them all.

But it wasn't fear I felt then; but rather again a Kiplingesque wonderment; what if, if...

Little did I know, then, that also up on those close by hills, the long winding, climbing pathways from Chichester below, also led up to a hidden, isolated, 18th century Smallpox Hospital on Bow Hill; now long converted to a still-standing, private property; its memories, too, prevailed of untold hundreds of years, also walking up, and along those paths, there and back again. And, eventually, I was home. But, very soon, I would be up again at five in the morning, to cycle back again to Summersdale Villa hospital, and duty on the early shift.

Air-castles

'An American businessman walked into a restaurant in Glasgow and asked the Scots waitress, what was her speciality...'

Joker Laurie stopped his flow, briefly, to be sure no sensitive Scot was about who could (or would) take offence. Lorr was holding court in the Male Lounge, next to the billiard-table. There were three other male patients in attendance and, also present, were two females from the other side. One of them was fair Julie, who stood alongside the others, and was supported by her guitar, which she leant upon and used like a walking cane — or perhaps a Thymus magic wand ...?

And Laurie delivered the punch-line ... 'And. "She replied; 'Rr-roast and Rr-ice ....' 'He said; "I love the way you roll your r's." And she replied, "But only when I'm in high heels."...' The company guffawed (and I too at the doorway), rather than burst out laughing; and they stood their ground, looking to Laurie who concluded that, clearly, they wanted more. And moved on... 'Want another...?' Laurie suggested and without further delay, led on.

'An American schoolteacher', (it happened to be of our cousins across the deep water — it was often one of our Irish brethren across the stream) '...moved from Ohio to New York, to teach primary education. The first lesson was in sex, and one of the boys named Tommy said "I've got a crush on you, Miss". And she said "That's all right Tommy; but I don't want any children." And, *very* seriously, he softly replied: "I'll be very careful Miss... "'

Again, the group giggled. It was a pleasant, brief interlude while they waited to move on — wherever. Laurie's jokes were never intended to offer offence, or any malice and, though often about being sick (and coping), his gag-lines were never sick-jokes; rather they were standard adolescent risque suggestions.

It was another Monday morning shift; breakfasts and early medicines were over, and day patients arrived and distributed about the estate. A number of patients were held back on the ward for various reasons; one middle-aged man allowed to lay in bed, as he commenced recovery from a substantial reactive depression.

Dr. Ferring, Technician

Consulting the Day Book diary, after breakfast, Bill and Red were to be busy on a number of essential chores, whilst delegating me to also remain on the ward (not to OT or IT), and so be available as Escort, on several booked patients' diagnostic investigations. I was detailed to accompany on two visits: Zen Michael, who was due an appointment upstairs, on the brain-wave-tracing EEG machine; and, afterwards, with Mr Ricks, a visiting Chichester outpatient, who was due a First-visit to Dr. Harrod; our Clinical Psychologist, also upstairs.

These were time consuming escort duties but, as Charge Nurse Bill reminded me, they were also opportunities for further, good experience.

I looked at my watch. Ten o'clock — well, five-minutes past. I stepped into the lounge, gently eased the company out of the room, and directed them off to their work stations about the hospital. Mike was due to visit the lab technician, Dr. Ferring, at 10.15 am, so I went off to see if he was ready.

Michael was on his bed, but otherwise quite prepared, the record player was off, and his guitar placed under the bed. Mike, in T-shirt and blue jeans, was reading a paperback, about Zen. 'Time, Barry?' Mike questioned, on my arrival at his bed-end. 'No. Few minutes, Mike. And it's only upstairs.', I replied casually, time enough in my answer. No cause for anxiety.

The EEG - its full long-title 'The Electroencephalogram', was then presently found in the 'Department of Clinical Research and Neurology', upstairs at the rear of the Female side of Summersdale Villa — and adjacent to the two small rooms of the Clinical Psychologist (and his apparatus). I believed the latter was a historical offspring of the Clinical Research hospital department, and of the Medical Research Council (MRC).

'Do you know anything about your EEG investigation. What it is, Mike?' I enquired, partly to fill time, but more to link it directly to what, and why it was being recommended. And we both knew the answer to that important fact; but it was useful to be reminded of his last incident.

'Bit.... Enough, I think.', Mike said, with clearly no bother, no apparent anxiety about this physical investigation; some patients were terrified of it, indeed, fearful of all physical apparatus or investigations — however painless and benign their intention. 'Last weekend wasn't it, Mike?', I asked. He replied matter of factly, 'Yeah. Again – just blacked out. No fits, no warning. Just out cold.' I asked him, 'How often has it happened, well, approximately anyway, Mike?' He paused, then replied, 'Too often. At least dozen times. It's getting a bit too frequent now. And its been ages since I've had any stuff, Barry.' Stuff was an overdose of illegal drugs.

Several months ago, Mike had been first admitted as one of the drug addicts, on a Section 26 of the 1959 Mental Health Act, and was offered treatment in hospital, or a custodial sentence at Lewes prison. Mike decided to reside at our hospital. The blackouts had begun shortly before he was admitted onto Amberley One; and, subsequently, he was transferred over here to Summersdale Villa. Though officially a resident, he was not in prison, and was relatively free to wander as he pleased about the grounds — indeed, as were all the Summersdale patients. It was accepted that he would let The Office know, if he was going on a walkabout. Mike also enjoyed regular approved leave periods. He was here specifically for Treatment, and *not* for criminal acts, though he had, originally, broken current Drug Laws.

Zen Mike was only twenty one and, apart from those 'blackouts', appeared otherwise quite healthy; unlike poor Julie (who he was friends with) who experienced terrible freakouts, and young Spider, whose body systems were well invaded by toxins and with considerable tissue damaged organs, due to his too many cocktails of unprescribed drugs. Collectively, the only buzzes they now received were from Beelzebub's domain — most unwelcome.

We continued chatting, as we went upstairs to Dr. Ferring. The good doctor, or rather his assistant, a lady in a white laboratory-coat, sat Mike down, after introductions were completed, before a long complicated looking panel-box of machinery.

Although briefly summarizing what the apparatus was expected to do, namely to record Mike's brainwave patterns, which would be recorded by electric pulses (I thought of radar) onto a long-roll of moving paper; various wavy lines equated with different areas of his brain. Any unexpected, not normal, up or downward motions (spikes) recorded on that paper, might indicate an area needing further enquiry. It all sounded very simple and mechanical;

but yet it was mapping out responses from a human brain, Mike's, and, for me, that was quite extraordinary (he appeared to be just accepting an inevitable necessity).

On a large white-card overhead of the electroencephalogram machine, and attached to the wall behind it, was a boldly printed explanation of the clinical psychology's EEG; a legend of what-it was-not:

> (1) It does NOT pass electricity into the head.
> (2) It does NOT read your thoughts.
> (3) It is NOT a detector.
> (4) It does NOT enable you to select a husband or wife.
> 'Everybody's brain is constantly producing electrical activity,
> which this machine records. The tracings from different people are similar
> but not exactly alike.'

I wondered what our involuntary, florid, schizophrenic sufferers would interpret from that factual information. I was constantly reminded of the truism, that the difference between a person's being ill, or not ill, could depend on a detected pH toxic imbalance in the body's metabolism, too little water intake or too much; too much salt or too little salt affecting the electrolytes. Thus affected, the mortal brain could instigate dehydration, and produce fever, hallucinations and eventual death. Or, by the voluntary intrusion of other foreign and toxic substances, *stuff* taken to artificially induce changes, in a level of surface consciousness; food or drink, like alcohol which by and increasing intake interferes with the brain's sugar glucose and essential oxygen supply, this will have direct affect on thinking, emotional feelings, aural tactile and visual perceptions and mobility; as I say — these truism facts easily gauged by human analysts.

I learnt that, in the examination of extra sensory perception (ESP), practitioners have been tested; recording studies of braincell functions, during ESP cognition taken from the EEG machine's readings; wavelength patterns interpreted under Scientific laboratory conditions. For example, trance and hallucinatory states, triggered by so-called Magic Mushrooms; ambrosia of the Ancient Greeks with sips of dionysian alcohol and other hallucinatory forms of deliberate intoxication, taken voluntarily, and following a strict diet of mind and body cleansing; what of a water diviner? Questions? Ouspensky's *controlled* use of hashish; Huxley's experimental homeopathic doses of mescaline; results of laboratory EEGs investigations on chosen individuals. And to any honest observer, with an open mind, *trace* results may seem quite extraordinary — not just biological — but other implications? And, pertinent, what did *not* show up on a paper roll-out?

Of course they are *not,* here, directly relevant to the reason for Mike's attending the clinic. But, to Mike and I most certainly pertinent, was later to be found at the rear of Colin Wilson's monumental work *Mysteries*[18]; read evidence of the *Electromagnetic Induction of Psi States: The Way Forward in Parapsychology.* Contributed By Peter Maddock.[19]

And though I had read, a little, on a number of these extra-mural examinations, I accepted. This was *not* what Zen Mike and I anticipated we were here for; this EEG apparatus was deemed to investigate for *neurological* dysfunctions, thus confirming he did *not* fit a Psychiatric, per se diagnosis. And, after all, the Court had duly authorised hospitalisation, for Investigations and Treatment, which, properly, he was in receipt of... instead of being a prison inmate, detained in Lewes Prison.

Alongside the apparatus was a two-tier trolley on castors, identical to others used on our wards. There was also a pedal-bin disposal tin, on the floor alongside the trolley. On the trolley were several galley pots, a bottle of spirit; and the usual Central Sterilised Supplies Department (CSSD) packages, of cotton-wool balls and swabs. And, what appeared like a tall upright mobile spring held-arm with cables (like a dentist's), with a sort of large hairnet with attachments to be fitted over the head, at its end.

It reminded me, in part, of the ECT metal headband procedure, when the cotton-wool balls, dipped in saline solution, were put about the head where the contacts were to be laid upon; and, at its conclusion, the cleaning spirit would remove the evidence of those sites. Mike was experiencing this exploratory investigation for neurological purposes, rather than to pursue any aspects of mental illness, found in his current patterns of behaviour.

And, sure enough, another large whitecard, a little further along the wall from its twin; its legend read:

> 'This is an Electroencephalograph. What it does ... 'The machine traces on paper the electrical impulses produced by the brain. This tracing is called an EEG and is used to aid in the diagnosis of some illnesses of the nervous system and to help to control treatment. It is also used for Research in Neurology and Mental Illness.'

The hairnet, of sorts, was placed over the top of Mike's head, whilst Doctor Ferring continued to chat light-heartedly to him. Mike and I just listened, interested in proceedings. The whole incident took some time — more than we thought. After the examination, several recorded waves were explained to us.

'Those small spikes are your eye-lids flickering. And, you recollect, you coughed a couple of times — there'.

But, mostly, it remained an esoteric experience (to us) rather than scientific. After all, it did not demonstrate human feelings, as such, or even conscious (or unconsciousness) — though its 'impulses' acknowledged life-currents, in this or that believed site of the brain. And, despite the reassuring factual legends on the wall, it was attempting to read specific biological brain impulses, as a benign instrument of exploration.

The EEG machine, was also described as an oscillograph instrument, which duly recorded 'wave-forms' of electrical oscillations — from the brain. Mike and I would later chat about this experience; and we discussed how many other types of 'wave-forms' there are — all unseen, about, in and through the air; noted on some designed recorder: whether from, or into, outer-space; from one instrument (communicating) with and to another container, radio television; and other machines: various other scientific medical apparatus; from earthquakes, to micro and macro distributed planetary echoes and, of (most extreme) undetected wavelengths, of other (to earthbound) dimensions. But, this was from in his brain.

Sometime later, *an area of unusual disturbance*, or rather non-disturbance and non-activity, was identified, and *brain damage* was believed to be a possibility. This possible diagnosis was 'read', from Mike's very lengthy EEG paper tracings. Mike was later to be transferred to a Neurological Unit for further investigations. I wondered what treatment could then be offered to counter such brain-damage; but it remained another unanswered question. We were informed that EEG's, in reading impulses from the cortex (in particular) would identify *abnormal* pulse rhythms, as possibly of epilepsy, or cerebral tumours; in which case it could be treated. I wondered what Mike thought of the whole experience, as he returned to his Zen paperback and a cup of tea, prior to my departure. 'Another of life's mysteries' he grinned in reply; when I asked him what he thought about it all. *'But, if it works...?'*, Mike concluded, in his Zen philosophy.

We wondered and talked, briefly, about other than accepted normal and abnormal patterns; if people with particular above normal talents (and healthy) had been mapped out? We agreed that 'Yes' was the probable answer to that question. What, for example, of formal explorations of persons in Parapsychological Research? Always, here, about the unknown, at least to us, and in the Market Place — amidst the general populace. And so, for a little while longer, we chatted about the perhaps more esoteric and metaphysic; than physic. I excused myself to Mike, and left him reading, sat up on his bed, as I had discovered him, not so long ago. And I returned to the Nursing Office, for my next appointed duty.

Mr and Mrs. James Ricks were waiting in the Nursing Office, as I returned from Mike's visit to Doctor Ferring. We were only a few minutes late, and a phone call upstairs to Doctor Harrod reassured Mr Ricks he was still expected, in five minutes. Mrs. Ricks had an appointment, and needed to drive-off, reassured that 'Someone' will stay with her husband 'Jim' — a visiting Out-patient — throughout his Psychology visit. And Bill introduced me, as that person.

I had never seen or heard of Mr Ricks, but he had (Bill said) a range of 'psychological fears and phobias', which Dr. Harrod Graylingwell's Clinical Psychologist (and Forensic specialist) was prepared to investigate; before recommending any specific remedies.

And I again journeyed up the wooden flight of stairs, adjacent to the kitchen.

Dr. Harrod was an intense, tall broad shouldered man, dressed in a white suit, in his late fifties; he spoke with a soft, slow voice, as if to ensure each uttered syllable was giving a lesson in itself. He, too, was scientific, as were his colleagues in the adjacent Research Department, with Dr. Ferring his technician colleague. He also presented as a caring man, who was not to be rushed — nor would he rush you as a potential client, under his consideration and care.

After our introductions, I was sat behind Mr Ricks against the wall, by the door; and separated from the desk table, Dr. Harrod and Mr Ricks. File notes and ephemera were on the table before the Psychologist; the ground rules were laid for the forthcoming dialogue and, to be agreed, contract work with Mr Ricks. Much as not so long ago, he had presented himself to our student intake on his first series of psychology lectures and subsequent Exams.

I had sat an internal Psychology Exam (set by Dr. Harrod) only a couple of weeks ago; and so, he knew me in a group, but not as an individual. Mr Ricks had never met Dr. Harrod, though his GP had introduced him by letter and phone, and induced certain expectations of the clinical psychologist. 'Unlike the Psychiatrist, I am *not* a medical qualified doctor; but own a doctorate in the scientific studies of normal and abnormal mental processes, and knowledge of human development and behaviour.' He introduced. 'There are psychologists in other fields; with animals, or in industry. I am a specialist in working with people who suffer mental illness... and your doctor has referred you to me, in the hope we can together (you and I) find a few solutions, to at least some of your problems.'

I grinned good naturally to myself, having heard similar words before from Doctor Harrod. But, equally, I well approved its purpose. From the outset, Mr Ricks was given ground rules, which were already committed to helping him. The good Doctor continued, 'But before we begin to explore your problems, I need to learn a few things about you, and the way you think and feel about yourself and, perhaps, aspects of your life in general. If that's all right by you, Mr Ricks?'

'Yes, yes of course, Dr. Harrod', he nodded eagerly, perched on his chair and leaned forward, towards this bearer of future good tidings. I could not help but ponder on the mass of information, so enthusiastically and expertly given to our student intake by Dr. Harrod, over the past fifteen months or so; and with another two years instruction, yet to come; on the fields of human behaviour and in a wide spectrum of human affairs.

The RMN syllabus included a very detailed delivery on development of predicted ages and stages, and aetiology, of human beings; individual and within a family; and in social groupings: a broad description of psychological concepts: human biology; psycho-physical disturbances and physical illnesses: and patterns of behaviour in relation specifically to mental illness. I was full of the language of William James' and our introduction to psychology, and the physiology of emotions — Jame-Lange (Rage is external); Cannon-Bard (physiological, internal). About innate genetic mechanisms and various learned patterns; and, of instincts, habits, memory, maturation, conditioning (and neurological patterns), About IQs (intelligence quotients) potential, static and the type casting of personality, by social performance tests — tests and, more tests — by many written papers. But one psychological truism our senior psychologist taught us, was just how powerful words are in our belief systems as Dr. Harrod had said; back in 1968. It is extraordinary, and ironic, that,

'*The Word Is More Powerful Than The Real Thing.*'

Memories are made of such unfortunate truisms. If the biological body with its brain tissue records, robot-like, what it reads and hears in word formations. How does it (The Brain) differentiate as to what was is a truth, on experience — or automaton acceptance? I would ponder much on this conundrum later on. But not at this moment in time? Dr. Harrod had supplied numerous examples of this learned concept, and related specifically to Dr. Hans Eysenck's belief that Neurosis was only 'learned' maladjustment and could be re-learned, deconditioned; as too had said — Professor Skinner and Dr. Pavlov.

As I sat with Mr Ricks and the clinical psychologist, I was then unaware how vociferous the two main opposing schools of psychology were; the *behaviourist* which members Skinner[20] et als, purported to suggest mankind was 'only' disposable limited 'bags of bones' and chemicals — sans will. And the *psycho-analytical* school, which appeared to believe that Freudian and Jungian unconscious (UCs.) was itself a valid subject — additional to, rather than only, a net result of a brain's biological property, soul, spirit — as an intangible metaphor. Why Either Or?... Surely both studies should be integrated — as they are in existential life. The metaphors — that demonstrated other humans, other links with all and everything; without and within my own body corporate, are.... All and Everything.

Rorschach

The Inner Self is worthy of study. I pondered — again, why either, or?

'We'll start with a little test. I think you might find amusing, Mr Ricks. It's called a *Rorschach Test*', continued Dr. Harrod. And he produced several coloured print-cards, of the well known 'ink-blot' impressions — including, the expected butterfly shape (or vampire...). 'What do *you* think this picture could represent, Mr Ricks?', Dr. Harrod said, good naturedly, as he produced the first illustrated card out of *his* pack of cards — intended to project visual images and feelings out of Mr Ricks' thoughts and direct them towards the psychologist, as interpreter (I thought a little of my recent Tarot card readings). The first session was then underway, and lasted about three quarters of an hour. As we left the room, we passed a machine in the narrow corridor (smaller than the EEG instrument) with a young man sat in front of it, lights flashing on and off and projected pictures, apparently at his control, on a screen before him.

An assistant of Dr. Harrod's (another psychologist) was hovering about the young man; and, as we passed by, his assistant — a junior psychologist — looked up and smiled acknowledgment at us, as we passed by. And the earnest young man remained glued, in concentration, at a selection of buttons which produced selected projected pictures. I knew not that young man; but that machine had previously been introduced, to our student intake, on one of our walkabouts. To my (our) initial disbelief, that machine appeared to be a potential source of self-inflicted pain and pleasure.

Homosexuality, in a dictionary, is defined as love exchanged between members of the same sex. Until the mid-1960s, such love was judged as 'abnormal' and a punishable statute offence. If a person was found guilty of breaking this law, especially in public, then the legal machine would have implemented a choice of prison-custody; or, if placed on probation, be offered (or else) specific psychological help — voluntarily, through a psychiatric hospital service — as corrective treatment.

It appeared an obvious moral dilemma, even to us naive Registered Mental Nurse students. It was one thing to inflict 'uninvited' homo-sexual, or hetero-sexual attentions on anyone, man, woman or child, in a pornography of *rape* and *violence* — and warrant censure (however the law agreed that measure). And quite another aspect, to expect a person to 'legally' be instructed to change their adult physiological emotions and, (to them) ordered to change honest, real, biological instincts? In short, how can you instigate, legislate, an Orwellian love on demand? Not prostitution — which answers to biological need. It's certainly *not* love. Rather by brainwashing, through fear, and politic manipulation. Again, that is not love, but a form of state social control.

The Times [21] recently queried. '*Men cannot be* made *good by legislation.'* That legal instrument's intention was, according to the person's inclination, to be *voluntarily* wired to a machine which could self inflict pain in producing graphic pictures, including of naked, at least provocative, attractive Apollos and Venuses? I found this practice rather bizarre. It was one applied application of 1960s clinical, behavioural psychology; in the use of accepted technology. However, a new law had been passed only last year[22], which made 'sexual behaviour between consenting adults no longer an offence, so long as it was conducted in private and both consenting participants over twenty one years of age.' Another conundrum had thus been passed, which really bothered a number of patients, and not a few members of staff. A few years ago, it was deemed okay, for over sixteen year old boys and girls (men and women), to get married and conceive. And over 18 years of age, one could smoke cigarettes, drink alcohol, and fight and die for your country. But, only if you were over 21 years old, really recognised as an legal adult.... Erm! Erm!

On this principle of *antibuse,* by self-inflicted (self-abuse) electric-shock to the body systems — as supplied to drug addicts and alcoholics, who wanted, or needed, to arrest their legislated, deemed, anti-social habits; to bring them under their own control. Or was it correct social control? The 'right', the 'correct' accepted, correlated projection, could prove an oxymoron supposedly and perhaps, produce masochistic pleasure. Reward was by default — by 'not' producing a self-inflicted mild electric shock. On the other hand, any socially unwanted pictures when selected and projected onto the screen before him (or her) was coupled with a *self*-imposed, controlled electric-shock-wave. A flagellation. Self inflicted punishment ?

Dr. Harrod's Clinical Psychology Department was well up to date with modern forms of treatment, in the mid-sixties. A psychologist, named Stanley Milgram, had published a paper on '*Obedience To Authority*'[23], which used a similar machine to the one on display in Summersdale Villa, on our visit to the department... *But,* here, there was one immense difference, so far as we could make out, to the Milgram programme.

Milgram's previous 1960s experiments, were of one (unseen) person deliberately inflicting graduated shock to a wired other; assured that the other person (victim-patient) was not actually having any pain, as the controls were manipulated by — the other. A third person in Milgram's experiment, The Doctor (teacher or other), was giving the instructions to one person, inflicting pain, on the not really suffering patient which, in the media, was being compared to the thousands of wartime (e.g.) Nazi torturers who insisted, as at the Nuremberg Trials and current ex-SS Adolph Eichmann trial in Israel, that they were only carrying out their horrific actions in obedience to orders. Not as a matter of kill or be killed, but as instigators of wanton torture itself.

Now in Dr. Harrod's department, he (Dr. Harrod) was *not* at all at the controls, as we passed the young man sitting alone at the machine. The patient had, in isolation, the option to play with the instrument as if it was a Church or studio electric-organ, and was playing for sound. Or so it looked to us, in passing The Treatment. I gather it was not around for long, but soon made redundant. We had already been well introduced to the work of Watson, Pavlov, Eysenck, Sargant, Skinner, and other, clinical psychologists.

In sad silent contrast to the above, about this time, I first saw an under-rated English 1965 black-and-white fiction movie called *The Hill,* starring Sean Connery, in a World-war Two North African army prison.[24] One prisoner, Connery, played an ex-Regimental Sergeant-Major who had *refused* to order his men into certain death, a clearly defined suicide battle... but was overruled by his so-called superior and, indeed, *all the soldiers* subsequently died; except Connery who was, ironically, demoted and sent to military prison *for disobeying an order*. And, worse, was accused, in retro, of being *a malingerer* coward, responsible for his ghost company's demise. Very reminiscent of the first world war, and many such suicidal battles. This film made a great impression on me.

Mr Ricks, out-patient attending Summersdale Clinical Psychology department, was to have no such Milgram aversion instrument put at his disposal — his fears, and phobias, were related to different, other unwanted-by-him, personal and social habits. Here all was confidential (one-to-one psychotherapeutic), between his personal psychologist, Doctor Harrod — and himself. (I would not be in attendance on subsequent visits.)

He could refuse any offered treatment, at any time, by just not attending the hospital and, without censure, unless his wife or others would apply such alternative pressures. And at least he did have a choice — to be or not to be treated.

And, at least in principle, so did the young man in front of the simulator; that machine which, at his choice, here in the hospital, was his treatment. He could just not turn up. But, if it was Court directed. What then? I suspect Dr. Harrod would always side with his patient. Our Hospital owned a variety of available psychological treatments, which included a number of *aversion* models — for kleptomaniacs, compulsive shoplifters; compulsive gamblers; sexual deviationists — even, according to one source, potentially, for husbands who were unfaithful to their wives; compulsively. [25]

It was lunchtime when we descended the stairs, and I assisted in mid-day medications as Mr Ricks sat down for his dinner; apparently well satisfied with the first of his visits, to our clinical psychologist. Like the young man at the simulator, and other such voluntary visitors, they were set apart from our day-attenders, as they had specifically attended the hospital Psychology Department for treatment — then left the hospital grounds and went home.

Jack

The Handover was concluded and my morning shift over, as I left the vicinity of the front entrance. It was a brisk clear winter sunny day, and fair Julie and young Laurie were looking up, at a large black late-winter bird, flying high up and away — overhead. Laurie was on a high, feeling good; he had learnt that morning he could proceed on a weeks leave from Friday; and Julie was to go on a long-weekend to her family, also from Friday afternoon. 'Bill said my doctor believes I'm doing great, Julie.', he passed on to his friend; as together, they stood stationary to one side of the front Summersdale steps.

At this moment, they were joined by a sullen, Phobic Jack who echoed, he had just seen his doctor; but still felt down — and needed a lift. Concerned, Joker Laurie responded, 'Cheer up Jack, things really could be *much* worse.... Tell you what, back in December, Nineteen-thirty-three, it was a bad winter in China. They sent a cablegram to Moscow, asking for wheat. Russia's reply was, "Short of Wheat. Pull in belts.". China's reply was, "Send belts..."' Julie gave a loud chuckle; Jack didn't. 'Come on Jack', she sympathised, 'Listen to our Doctor Lorr, eh.'. Laurie took his cue, 'Yup! Jack, after all, you're on Summersdale; not so ill as a need to be over in the Main Building — where the *very* ill are?'

'Em', relenting a little, Jack smiled minutely at this clinical fact.

Laurie tapped his library of wisdom for reinforcement. 'You know Jack, what they say don't you, our doctors and friends ...?' 'What?' Jack looked up to Laurie (who was six-inches taller than him); and wanly gave one of his 'there's no hope for me' looks. Undaunted, Joker replied, *'A Psychotic builds castles in the air; a Neurotic lives in castles in the air; and a Psychiatrist collects the rent ....'*. In unison, all laughed at this punch line...

Jack recalled that his own malady had been labelled as Psycho-neurosis. He was a sane Neurotic, he concluded. And Jack gained momentary comfort, from pretend Doctor Laurie's stand-up pearls of wisdom. As they moved off towards the Naunton Pavilion, I went off for my lunch-break, stepped out for the Grill Room and, afterwards, back to work, for a study session up in that small room, over the old dispensary in the Main Building. Much later — home.

Art or Science.

Over at last. Doctor Alison, our First-year Neurology lecturer, had drawn out of Mike's spine, into a syringe, an exact quantity of spinal fluid to go on to the path-lab. Poor ole Mike; how many times had he regretted his over-indulgence in the past, treating drugs, particularly the LSD tabs, like sweets; and, now, with this suspected brain-damage; for some reason foreign to me, it was necessary to obtain a specimen; and, presently, I was attendant on Charge Bill and the ward doctor, throughout this clinical procedure.

I'd recently completed the first five chapters of Altschul's *Neurology for Nurses* [26] at the request of Doctor Alison; and had dutifully memorised the XII cranial nerves and the recommended routine tests, including the standard battery of allergy tests — a box which had samples of various substances which a subject was tested on — and, of course, there was always Babinski's reflex (or not) in bending the soles of the feet.

Although elementary, our knowledge of the anatomy and physiology of the nervous system neatly juxtapositioned with the more esoteric Psychology, led by our good Doctor (later Professor at the University of Surrey) Harrod — aided by Bickerstaff's *Psychology for Nurses* [27], which was then *mandatory* study, as an elementary introduction on the subject.

Something was clearly wrong with Mike's biological makeup. This was proven to Mike himself, and the physician; he had then willingly submitted to the bed being put-up — its two front feet lifted up onto wooden blocks, with indentations to sit the base secure against any unwanted motion during this elementary, but tricky, exploratory operation.

It was mid-morning and no-one else was in his dormitory, but still the curtains were drawn-round; a full CSSD and necessary equipment on an adjacent trolley. I noted that the site on Mike's lower spine, to draw the fluid, was marked with iodine for Doctor Alison (this was a very delicate operation); then it was done. What was normal, and what was abnormal, was established in these regular biological pursuits; and, if evidence of something wrong was to be seen, hopefully this would be alleviated — such was the province of Neurology as a biological science. (Sometime after this routine incident, I had cause to write to a hospital in Surrey on a research project on the history of psychiatric hospitals. To my surprise, I received a brief (but polite) reminder that it was a Neurology Hospital, and not at all connected with Psychiatry.)

I left the curtain surround drawn, as Dr. Alison and Charge Bill strode off back to the office. Mike was left to rest awhile before lunch, to recover from the local spinal anaesthetic; and his trauma.

Zen Mike was still asleep at lunchtime, so we kept his meal for later, whilst other patients and staff moved quietly about him. Despite most media hype and much public ignorance, I was already all too familiar that our hospital patients' and staff (with a few inevitable different apples in the barrel) were, in-general, considerate of the ongoing needs of others' around them. The social reality, of large numbers of people to be cared for by normally, too few staff to service their treatment needs, was equally another known factor; and an austerity and general paucity of resources too, was one norm needing no declaration.

Housed in a large public hospital institution, it was expected that its staff were not deemed to be Supermen and Superwomen, with bottomless assets to indulge their patient charges. The patients, therefore, had to be trusted as normal social human beings — but with their own limitations. Before the 1960s and early 1970s, a high proportion of our hospital residents and visitors had *considerable* experience of the bleak austerity of pre-war, wartime, and post-war unemployment; and likely austere stark home circumstances — often a chronic want. Few people then owned such comfortable assets which included accommodation with carpets; indoor bathroom suites; more than one suit (even so) of clothes and, even, a measure of security.

Our ward culture, subculture, was most of the popular media experience — and *not,* directly, of academic, clinical, press, or scholastic appraisals. There were, of course, statistical exceptions, day to day norms — art, books, education, films, pop-music icons... and villains. And a few luxuries. Changes, wilful change of one's circumstances, could convert those norms; but, if beliefs of our patients' norms — were *not* so; and rank deceit led one to doubt mistrust of root norms then abuse, The Abnormal, appeared. Julie, Laurie and Mike, had knowingly abused their norms, but hoped, expected, to improve and get better; their norms and mine (at least), were so constant. But, always, there was the unexpected.

Thirty-nine Steps

After our patients' lunch and medication was completed, I was joined by Alternative Bob, my third-year student colleague, on overtime. As we climbed the Summersdale stairway, Bob was just behind me. I heard him amusing himself in counting, out loud, the number of the grey concrete steps.

'Do you know Buchan [28] and *The Thirty-Nine-Steps*? Film was on in Chi, at *The Corn Exchange* in East Street, just a couple of weeks ago?', Bob introduced meaningfully. 'Em - Yeah. Great film with Robert Donat. Nineteen thirty five, I think', I replied. We'd stopped at the top of the concrete stairway, at the end of male Summersdale One, and continued a conversation. I added,

'Book published about Nineteen-fifteen, I think?', my knee jerk reply. Alternative Bob had something to say. Why... what?'

It was a few years, since I had enjoyed reading that espionage classic; and I could not remember much detail. He continued, with some intensity, 'The Black Stone was Scudder's term for a foreign spy network - foreign devils I think ?'. Bob, loud, well into his theme. Interesting, but... so what. What was his point?

We laughed at the *Boy's Own Paper* (BOP) references. In times of armed conflict, The Enemy is always committing atrocities, demonised, and vilified en masse. The more *they,* the enemy, are depicted ugly and horrific — the blacker such norms (viz of enemy). And, too, the darker, our reflected inner-imagery — the better to motivate fighting as just cause; to kill, and instill fear into anyone. The panic of war. Kill innocents.... kill strangers on sight. If they're *not* actively with us, then they must be against us — thus supporting The Enemy and, of course, become of the enemy. (Ouch!) Deliberate lies and propaganda. The process triggered killers, at a signal threat to National Peace; and to Family and self when threatened by others — or so we believed. Didn't Clinical Psychologist Eysenck talk about 'Normal responses to the Abnormal.', or was it McDougall? (And what of abnormal responses to the abnormal — is that pathology.) We were off again about our hero, Richard Hannay, and his story.

Battle Exhaustion WW2

Recent readings and school chats with Mr Ilford, on Freud and Jung, and extra-mural readings of some of the classics, including works of Robert Graves. One friend of Graves was Dr. Will Sargant, another Clinical Psychologist working in Psychological Medicine, who had mounted *these* same Buchan-like steps that Bob and I were standing on. Dr. Sargant had worked here, during the recent Second World War, in the 1940s. Last year Dr. Sargant published a volume of Memoirs, entitled, *The Unquiet Mind.*[29] In that book, he described his involvement with treating casualties, direct from the battleground of war-torn Europe, at this Hospital — treated them *here* in Chichester. ' Our Graylingwell centre,', Sargant referred to it. That centre was in *this* building, where his military team treated hundreds of WW2 casualties with - '... acute states of neurotic disturbances.' In WW1, it had included the generic term *Shell Shock* and its symptoms. In WW2, it was *Battle Fatigue* (fugue) aka Exhaustion.

It was the Summer of 1944, near to the June 6th Normandy D-Day Landings; and, anticipating heavy casualties, Dr. Sargant and his team had been switched, from *Belmont Hospital* in Surrey to the EMS block of Summersdale Hospital; incoming patients first shipped across to Chichester Harbour, or Southampton, and thence moved on into nearby Graylingwell. A substantial provenance for affable Dr. Harrod, and his 1960s colleagues, in the Psychology Department — on this floor, adjacent to nursing facilities on SH4 ward for the Medical Research Council (MRC).

Dr. Sargant was relevant to our 1967 debate on the physiology of the use — about use and abuse in Pavlovian and Skinner behavioural conversion. And of brain-washing, and war trauma, especially use of Talking Therapies as previously adopted in the 1940s, under the clinical blanket of '*The Department of Psychological Medicine*' — the unit temporarily occupied in Graylingwell Hospital. but administered by the military authorities.

Not Cricket

We were rambling, in our random free associations, and returned to Buchan's *39 steps*. Bob had clearly identified this theme, and reflected on the *Black Stone* as a literary, fictitious, 1915 icon representing deliberate deceit. Jim, a temporary day-patient, passed us by, while chatting with Harold a resident and, observing our lunchtime exchange, they grinned across to each other, as they continued down the stairs.

'Hannay knew, like Conan Doyle's Holmes, eh Bob... by *fine* differences in behaviour. The Secret was a coded map reference, to a Norfolk cliff's number of steps, connected to the spies' planned escape by sea, after theft of the secret war plans....', I said. Bob broke in, 'Hitchcock's film changed the substance of the plot, but retained the wartime code as a trigger — *What Are The Thirty Nine Steps*? A Palladium theatre *savant* performer, had committed (without understanding) by rote to memory, specific facts about a secret organisation. The phrase '*What Are The Thirty Nine Steps*', triggered the entertainer, *against his will,* to respond to the question.' And I replied, excited by the obvious... '*Hypnotised...* You know, sort of waking trance... man's unconscious used, then abused... by The Enemy.'

Bob had something to say....

'Oh, I see', I concluded. 'By deceit, and Hannay's detective work, they used Conscious Norms — on both sides. Sort of agreed rules, in the game of espionage?'

'Right. *Right*', Bob assented. I'd got *his* drift.... It was about The Black Arts.

'Hitchcock's film, and Buchan's novel, used — the Enemy *abused* — the Memory Man's unconscious, against his will...? Broke the rules. Couldn't stop himself...'

Bob softly — sub-rosa — '*Not Cricket eh?*... Just not cricket! Such is war.'

A call from downstairs by Red, from the foot of the concrete steps, brought us both down to earth, and the ground floor of the hospital ward, and ended our discourse on the unconscious, espionage, and The 39 Steps, as we resumed our duties of care.

Into November 1968, and my Summersdale Villa placement was almost at an end. I was well ridden with a stuffy cold and dodgy stomach pains, but not enough to go off sick out of necessity. Winter... Not all our patients went out to OT or IT, as indicated earlier; a number were too depressed, or too disturbed, for the minimum of concentration and commitment required to attend day activities. Several patients were allowed to just occupy themselves between meals, medications and tests, as required.

Laurie was still away on extended leave; it was unlikely that he would meet up with fair Julie as, effectively, they lived in different social worlds, as well as distanced miles apart from each other, without transport. Anyway, it was *not* really a romance, as such, but, as good friends in hospital, they often joined with Mike and others, their peers of similar age. A recovering middle aged, depressed resident, Brian, was waiting for a visitor and transport, as he waited, Jack the young phobic (one of Laurie and Julie's friends) sat down next to him in the ward lounge — whilst the older man was trying to teach him how to play a game of patience, with a well worn pack of playing cards.

The pack was one of a number of packs left in the lounge, amongst a variety of indoor games; draughts, chess, scrabble, dominoes, snakes-and-ladders and ludo. Most of these quiet games were well used at lunch breaks, evenings and weekends. Also available were battered paperbacks, which were constantly restacked in a small glass-fronted bookcase. Two newspapers were delivered each day to every ward, usually one tabloid and one broadsheet. Summersdale presently had a *Daily Sketch,* and a *Daily Telegraph* (other wards — other choices). And, for the so inclined, the Billiard Table was constantly in use as relaxation. Brian and Jack were together, in the ward lounge,

RAF Brian and The Ipcress

As I went into the Television Lounge to deliver a message for Brian (and check on Jack), I noticed an upside down, opened paperback, with a half filled mug of tea placed alongside it, on a low table. The book was Len Deighton's popular 1962, *The Ipcress File*.[30] Yes, Brian was clearly feeling much brighter; his depression had almost disappeared. Brian produced a rolled-up cigarette, and an RAF embossed lighter; its blue letters raised on a flat silver polished metal base. He absently set the moulded tube between his thin lips, thin chevron trimmed moustache above bristling a trifle, as he bent over the flame, cupped, and turned to smile at Jack.

'Patience is what its called, Jack — and patience is what we need to play the game', Brian stated, as he slowly sucked, then blew a small smoke spiral upwards — holding his rollup in his right hand, with his left hand turning a picture card face up. 'I don't think I can finish... can't concentrate... ', said doleful Jack, who was interested, but in need of reassurance.

'Nonsense lad! Practice often enough, even every now and then, it'll get easier.'

'Do you think so?', Jack mused. It was nice to witness the credence, given to this war-time veteran. And, it was well deserved... 'Yes, I do.' Brian was gently giving what, he felt, was a proxy... sort of fatherly advice. 'I wish I could believe you, Brian...'

Stood only a few feet away, watching the pair play their game and hearing their dialogue, I thought Jack's negative response was typical — but at least he hadn't got up and rushed out of the room, as he often did. Brian, then almost fifty years old, had been an RAF rear gunner, at one time placed at nearby Tangmere Airfield — from where the two towers of Graylingwell and Chichester Cathedral were both clearly viewed, as local landmarks.

A number of our staff still remembered, affectionately, when bus loads of servicemen, of many different nationalities, were brought over into the Graylingwell Recreation Hall, for wartime dances. I wondered if RAF Brian was one of The Few, back in the early 1940s... one of Lord Dowding's Battle Of Britain's — own Chicks.

Wartime memories abounded and, since earliest childhood, I'd never known a time when some such ugly conflict was not ongoing somewhere. The Second world war was quickly followed by the Korean campaign, which, as a squaddie, I had missed by only a couple of years as, too, I'd just missed (thankfully) the Mau Mau and Malayan campaigns (there were others). And, presently, the sad media fever, over Vietnam and Cambodia, was very much in evidence. I followed the 1960s writings of Cassandra (O'Connor); and, especially, James Cameron, a journalist writing in the *Evening Standard* and broad sheets; *The Picture Post,* with Bert Hardy and Robert Capa photos and, later, the incredible records of US oral historian Studs Terkel and 'witness' accounts of thousands of persons — pertinent to this text.

We were all daily media fed on whatever ongoing death and destruction was enjoyed by much of the media, as guaranteed copy; so too, were all our patients and staff daily confronted; which minute facts were often fused with unpleasant fantasies and, to some, confirmed their own paranoid fears and repugnant memories. From childhood reading, I recalled heroes like the gallant *Rockfist Rogan* — an RAF Spitfire pilot in the English 1940s and 1950s *Champion* comic-paper. Such icons were reinforced by the exploits of Captain W.E. Johns' RAF Officer, *Biggles,* his friend Ginger and comrades. And, *here,* was *RAF Brian*. Brian was an alcoholic, who had dried-out on Amberley One, and been transferred across to Summersdale Villa, whilst he awaited a vacancy at the nearby Therapeutic Unit of *Sandown House*. Feet of clay. There were other ex-servicemen in the hospital, both staff and patients. Even one German ex-paratrooper, who had served in the German armed-forces, and numerous, silent, elderly Great War and WW2 veterans.

Black Art, Bad Faith

Facts and fiction, anecdotes and stories, always mingled and shaped our personal beliefs and symbols. Shaped our role-models... and, our fears. And, inevitably, what one person believed and experienced was often vastly different from another's. Such differences often led to confusion, but were *not* at all necessarily evidence of *The Black Art* of deceit. Integrity was all. *Deliberate* deceit was about wilful harm and being BRAINWASHED.[31] This was about psychology, and the propaganda of the Black Art... what Sartre referred to as abuse — in Bad Faith.

'*If you want to learn to concentrate, you have to listen, Jack.*' Our kind veteran spoke, in Good Faith with integrity. 'Now *listen to me*, Jack, *listen to me*. I know how difficult concentrating is.'

Brian was talking, and reminded himself again, again and again; he'd too often lost *that* vital capacity, a need *to concentrate,* in the past. And drink had too long clouded his thoughts, muted his dreams and, physically, slowed him to a halt. But now Brian was becoming mobile, once more. Jack was in awe of ex-RAF Brian and, so, he listened with considerable respect, integrity and trust... with Brian, rightly so.

Bob, Brian, Mike and myself had recently seen the recent English IPCRESS film, in the hospital recreation hall. We'd all read the book, of the anti cold war fiction, *Ipcress File*.[32] That work was reinforced by an even more powerful post-war, Korean based 1959 novel (and subsequent film-version, in 1962) titled *The Manchurian Candidate,* by Richard Condon[33]. Both contemporary works presented gross abuse of any, and many, mechanical methods in changing human behaviour — using, exploiting, the onion layers of consciousness, against one's will — or unknowing. Of Jungian coincidence[35], about incredible *Synchronicity.* Both, Condon and Deighton's novels and films, presented in a similar way, showed how to block out and abuse man's conditioned reflexes.

Condon's work updated a long-standing Orwellian fear (sadly, reciprocated by distant foreigners — the Tweedledum and Tweedledee syndrome)[35], fearing the same, about the polluted West. About alien Reds (or black, green, red, or yellow and other, white men), lurking Under The Bed. Decades earlier, of fears of an *invasion,* by multiplying Asiatic 'yellow-men' invading Australia[36], Asia, Europe, and... erm... Sussex. I recall one *Case note* in the archives, of a woman; a fearful pauper lunatic, transferred from the East Preston (Worthing) Union Workhouse, into Graylingwell. The unhappy lady believed that *she* had really seen a 'Yellow man' under her bed. It was in the early 1900s (perhaps in the wake of the Boxer Rebellion). The case note was kept, in one of the early pigskin volumes, with two photos of her; one on admission and the second on her discharge. The data was attached to the front sheet, where I recall seeing the admitting note on her file.

Closer, to our modern times. We heard much of American fears, in postwar 1950s McCarthyism, which the USA media believed in home grown fifth columnist, communist (Russian) terrorists, rampant in their midst. And discovered *reds,* in their subsequent politically motivated witch hunts. Memories... Of the real OGPU, and abundant forensic evidence of 1930s and 1940s Nazi *Fifth Column At Work.*[37] Updates of *The Thirty Nine Steps* Great War 1915 novel, and hidden enemies; and into today, and the 1960s (and early Seventies). Also, the post-Korea and present Vietnam conflict, and of fiction or factually based *The Manchurian Candidate,* and the dark workings of the CIA.[38] Paranoia or hidden truisms; to us in Graylingwell and Summersdale it all seemed so surreal and so far away.

We didn't doubt that military regimes daily openly (and covertly) exploit and experiment with the Black Arts. Perhaps dubiously, they illegally practised in the name of Empirical Science.... Medicine or in aggressive self-defence. Result; gross paranoia and mental illness. Very much around, in the hospital life of the 1960s, care of the media. Both *The Ipcress File,* and *The Manchurian Candidate,* focused on abusive Brainwashing (Conversion, Normalisation, Re-education — Thought Reform). Such graphic works certainly influenced public attitude, and policy makers, on *any* psychiatric treatment; both in and out of our hospital institutions. This, inevitably, affected a few of our patients in Graylingwell — and Summersdale Villa.

Zen Mike (as I had come to think of him) had read, and chatted, on the book of *Ipcress*, with Brian and myself; and observed, although the theme was similar, much of the content was different, in substance, between The Book and The Film. Mike, looking most serious, his right hand stroking a wispy fuzz of a beard, had said, 'Ah, Barry, but they're *not* the same, are they'. It was *not* about the proper use of Insulin, ECT, Psychotherapy, Clinical Psychology and Neurology, and Rehabilitation — as of the Graylingwell ITU unit down at The Yard (used with integrity and proper care — applied in Good Faith). Mike, Brian and I had agreed on this, as fact. The title of the Book, and Film of the same, was an acronym; *'Induction of Psycho neuroses by Conditioned Reflex with Stress'* - IPCRESS.[39] The subject of that fictitious graphic work, was The Enemy's use-and-abuse of Pavlovian' conditioning processes, about brainwashing techniques. But, *how* did Palmer escape from his captors, and their wilful, involuntary conditioning.

A telling phrase; *'I hurt, therefore I am.'* Psychiatric patients, who blood let by self-mutilation, in cutting into their own flesh are called, designated Cutters. They might give a reason, that their self-harm was *not* to gain attention of others, rather, it was to remind, render themselves, momentarily self-aware. To *know* they exist: *If I prick, do I not bleed.* And, paraphrased, the maxim of the Cartesian '*Cogito, ergo-sum';* ' I think, therefore I am.'. This suggested how Palmer had survived his torture, with foreknowledge; a rusty nail and application, and his subsequent, self inflicted, hand wound...

'I had enough information about their methods, to make an informal guess' (what was happening to him) ... and, certainly, sickness, frailty and considerable anxieties were part of our patients' low vulnerable conditions in hospital; as were the contrived conditions of our fictional victims. So, I recollect *Ipcress* as a topical trigger, on the merits and debits of use and abuse, of Pavlovian'

conditioning, and of other methods of psychiatric (psychological) behavioural treatment; as understood by laymen and media in the 1960s. I doubted young phobic Jack (he couldn't concentrate) had read the book *The Ipcress File;* though he had probably seen the cinematic version at the *Corn Exchange* Cinema in Chichester.

On the way out of the patients' lounge that day, I espied a thin worn Mayflower paperback on the top of Summersdale bookcase (amongst popular crime and cowboy novels) about the renowned detective and adventurer, Sexton Blake. The book's title was *Brainwashed* [40]. It was about an ex-Vietnam prisoner, who threatens the entire Western World. Hmm! I still have that book somewhere, as a memento.

The Black Art was renowned for its spells, which put unwilling subjects into trances; bewitched. This was always carried out by some knowledgeable person. But, since the advent of scientific knowledge (technology), it's generally believed by most of the populace (so the media report) that no-one could really be put to sleep, and hypnotised into a trance, against their will. I had my doubts. What of the subliminal mind, in operant conditioning ...

Propaganda

Bertrand Russell, in his 1952 *Dictionary of Mind, Matter and Morals* [41] said:

> 'Advertising is the art of producing belief by reiterated and striking assertions, wholly divorced from all appeal to reason. Experience shows that the average man, if he is told a hundred times a day that A's soap is the best, and fifty times a day that B's is the best, will buy A's, although he knows that A is making the assertion for the sake of his own pocket, not from a disinterested love of truth.'

Russell stipulated, then qualified his definition -

> 'Propaganda is only successful when it is in harmony with something in the patient: his desire for an immortal soul, for health, for the greatness of his nation, or what not.'

Therapeutic conditioning, re-learning, was a proper option for a patient who wanted to change for the better. Whereas, in the unconscious conditioning processes alluded to by Condon' and Deighton's excellent literary works, and the behaviourists, such processes could be experienced as a heretical form of abuse by others (as reported by John Marks). Certainly, as a mature student, I was of that opinion. There is use... and there's abuse.

It was in watching Brian and Jack, playing that innocent game of patience, that I could not help but recall Deighton's cinematic, unconscious, conditioned, trigger phase, contained in a specific spectral tone of voice and sound, *'Now Listen To Me. Listen to Me....'* [42] And, similarly, in Condon's powerful conditioned reflex — triggered in Raymond Shaw:

'Raymond, why don't you pass the time by playing a little solitaire?', which, by card play, was intended to produce a further, unconscious conditioned response, when the red Queen of Diamonds face-card appeared. It seemed, to me, to be all about the use of icons, meaningful symbols. And, sometimes, about *abused* Kabbalistic inner-mind gateways.

Given that dementia (irreversible memory loss) is a consistent fear, and reality, for all too many of our psychiatric patients; sadly, our media led culture appeared to thrive on bad-faith attitudes. And, many aspects of the good were given over, for myth and fairy tales alone (or so it seemed to me, in a lay analysis). Many of our patients had developed numerous fears, phobias and mental illnesses, as a result of their own experiences of life; and, now, needed a duty of care, self-control and, where possible, obtain relief. Inevitably, as neurotic Jack's game of patience, solitaire, progressed, he turned up various face cards. And yes, a black King of Spades was exposed, and allowed his red *Queen of Diamonds,* pointed out by Brian, to be laid on top of his King.

Shortly afterwards was Jack's time for a regular visit upstairs, as part of the ongoing treatment for his phobias, to the good Dr. Harrod's Clinical Psychology Department. Also, Brian departed with his visitor for the rest of the afternoon. I never attended Jack's behavioural treatment upstairs; and I wondered how long Jack's '*Deconditioning Programme*' would take, and even if it would ultimately be a success, and remove his pathological fear of microbes and dirt, contaminating his body, every moment of the day, every day.

Psychiatric Nurses were, in the Sixties, only just beginning to get involved with Behaviourist programmes; working in tandem with physicians, psychiatrists, psychologists, relatives and patient; both in hospital and, later, in the community. More sophisticated behavioural programmes would soon to be introduced, to combat many fears and phobias. But, they were *not* yet an option, during my three years RMN training programme.

Dr. Harrod had lectured us that conditioning didn't decrease with time, and, presumably, as habits, left alone, would possibly often be reinforcing an original programme — unless interrupted. Deconditioning was removal of reinforcement, and could take twice as long to cancel out, as it took the original programme to be implemented. Since Pavlovian' conditioning did not necessarily involve the cortex, it was a process of learning a formation of New Habits and in the retraining of instincts; as well as acknowledgment of new, metaphorical, knee jerk responses. Lengthy reading, lectures and observations provided an introduction, a little understanding, of behavioural programmes, as given by Dr. Harrod, in tandem with my experiences of Aversion Therapies (mechanical) in the main hospital setting.

Familiarisation. First, was the need to relax the patient as much as possible, the Doctor instructed. To establish a rapport and *trust* (not fear) between therapist and client patient; a safe, slow introduction to positive, possible change, as a viable concept. Then, acquaintance and friendly discussion, using graphics, whatever; and progress to 'safely' work on whatever outcome was required. And, so, to begin. Clearly, I had a great deal yet to learn, both conceptually and by experience. But often, as time dictates, events occur, whether one feels competent or not. And one has to do the best one can, in the circumstances.... As with our Jack, and myself.

Mid-day, I left Summersdale, on an errand to the Main Building. It was dark out. Someone, him, (or is it a Her), hadn't drawn the morning curtains. It was heavy going, with a persistent drizzle, making me keep my head down, and feet avoiding the zigzags of numerous rain pools, and slippery leaf patches. All about was dark evidence, of a late November day, towards the end of 1968.

At work — surely, for me, it had already been a good year, a successful, stimulating time. The hospital's 67th Annual, and last formal published, Report would include routine changes in 1967-8, such as the addition of extra toilets, at The Acre in Worthing, on the receipt of Architects' plans for the upgrading of Chilgrove One Ward, (adjacent to the Farm House, and close by the IT Yard and The Barn) on which I had lately been, formerly, a first-year student. The much photographed farm-pond, in front of the enclosed Graylingwell's Well, had been filled in, and the surface had been bulldozed, to enable students to landscape the area. A Nursing Cadet scheme was also proposed, for pre RMN training; youngsters of 16 years plus were to be eligible.

Advertised world events included the assassination of another of the American Kennedy family, Robert Kennedy, murdered in June 1968. Much closer, in origin, to home was the death of the English comedian Tony Hancock (of BBC's 'Hancock's Half hour' fame) in June, away in Sydney, Australia; distanced - but partings no less. And yet *another* global assassination had taken place, of the great humanitarian blacks' civil-rights leader Dr. Martin Luther King — who was murdered, in April of 1968. A terrible loss to the world.

In nearby Europe in August, Russian troops had invaded Czechoslovakia, after a too brief experience of a hard won democratic freedom. Two young refugee women, both nurses, had recently appeared in our hospital, having fled from that Czechoslovakian conflict — though I knew nothing of their circumstances. I had seen them, briefly, over the female side in Summersdale Villa, and in the Grill Room canteen. Their free-leader, Alexander Dubcek, was to be feted as initiator of that proud Prague Spring of '68. But, to us — patients and staff, and our relatives and friends — to most of us. Those mostly fractious world events, were as distanced from us as was the war in Vietnam and Civil Rights movements in USA. But, closer to home, home grown conflict was sadly escalating in nearby Northern Ireland...

Crow

'Caw, Caw,' — A singularly loud bird-call, echoed from, I presumed, a black Crow, either a Jay, Jackdaw, Raven or Rook, which sat high up on a tree, in its saucer nest, close to the road entrance to the Occupational Therapy Huts — where fair Julie had risen, from a garden seat, early in the autumn, to greet the Rev, Laurie and I, on our way to Chico at the poultry farm. English poet Ted Hughes [43] had written that 'A crow is a sign of life. Even though it sits motionless.'

That singular, black, bird drew me back, from my reflections on the past year's activities; and I looked up, defying the rain droplets; up into the stark then bare branches, high up, where a group of large saucer nests seemed otherwise abandoned — up in the highest reaches of that beech tree... But though I could well hear that loud raucous, visceral call, still I could *not* see that bird. All birds do not fly abroad in the winter-time, I thought; my knowledge of bird life species was sparse, rather than trite. Another 'Caw', loud, again raucous, which echoed, hollowing, seemed coarse, raw, jagged — certainly not lyrical — but Crow was up there, perhaps on his (or her) own, out of sight... Somewhere...?

Ole Bill was not deterred by the bleak melancholic weather, and was out on one of his daily constitutional walkabouts; no doubt to try and catch up on the hospital's bush telegraph. He spotted me, just as I approached the Front Entrance. 'Have you heard? Seen you with 'er, and Rev and Laurie...!' Directed at me, knowingly, as he stepped up close, to convey his latest bit of eaves-dropping. 'No...', distantly... for I was still *up there*... with Crow. 'What's that, Bill ?' I asked. Not that interested.

'Julie, I think she was, on Summersdale', said sympathetic ole Bill, in a low sussurated grave tone. I was immediately rooted. 'Was?', I thought. And asked, 'What about her, Bill?'. Matter of fact, Bill replied, '*Dead she is*. Sad, eh?'.

'But how, Bill. How do you know?', I asked, incredulous. I fervently prayed that he'd misheard something or other. 'Not sure. Heard she'd tried to fly out of a window, whilst she was on leave. Nothing on, she 'ad I 'eard... Fell like a stone she did ...' 'And where did you hear that, Bill?', I lisped.'Heard it from Doctor Crampton, talking to someone in the passage, just now', Ole Bill explained so authoritatively.

I was stunned. Fair Julie — dead?

Surely it can't be true, I pondered, disbelievingly. After all, she seemed so much better when she had gone on leave; when I last saw her, and Laurie, they were chatting outside Summersdale. Such a short time ago... But, I already well knew the (sometimes terrible) after effects, of overdosing on LSD tabs (or other hallucinogens) and, yes, yes it was possible, for such an event to happen, during an acute flashback attack.

'Eh. Thanks Bill', I said, *not* wanting to offer any comments; and he about turned, and continued his slow walkabout.

It was still dark, and raining, as I entered the Main Entrance into the hospital. A little later it was confirmed, yes, Fair Julie was gone. And, whilst I had no way of really knowing, it was ,just speculating, *highly improbable,* that she killed herself wilfully. Indeed, Julie had probably tried to fly like a bird — answering either to her God-voice, or in response to one of her flashback, centred delusions. Gone on her last flight, to wherever...

Many other 'versions', of why Fair Julie died, were cited; but that truth could never be learnt; only, as the local press reported, was one truth self evident — she was dead, and had recently been a psychiatric hospital patient, suffering from the effects of LSD drug abuse (viz her body). And, had indeed thrown her naked body, out of her bedroom window. Thrown, or flown, she had fallen. And it would never be known which preceded that sad event.

There were no suspicious circumstances...

A few days later,during my last week on my three-month placement at Summersdale Villa, I heard from Charge Nurse Bill that Lawrence, Laurie, had been re-admitted, and was presently on Bramber Two ward, over in the Main Building, having threatened to kill himself in his despair. He had read in the papers, of Julie's demise, and it had triggered another relapse back into hospital.

RAF Brian, and Zen Mike, were quite philosophical about the news; but most other patients, like Phobic Jack, remained somewhat distanced from the sad event, as too many other such world-horrors were reported daily, and insisted that they were already polluted, and wholly self-centred (to survive) and encapsulated, in whatever pathological conditions ensued; it confirmed their reasons, for not being.

On my penultimate shift, feeling rather low and iffy; but strictly somatic. Red, who was in charge that afternoon, asked me to take a large bouquet of flowers, In Memoriam, which had arrived from The Rev, to be given over for display, with a black embossed sympathy card for the staff and residents, over on the female side.

Sister Rees was on duty, with one of the Czech nurses, in their Summersdale Two ward office. The flowers were well received (Sister had attended the funeral). I couldn't help noticing, over in one corner, isolated and laying akimbo, was Fair Julie's guitar — a string was broken, one-end curled upwards, propped up, forlorn, in a dark corner....

Back home, in our tithe cottage at Chilgrove, I contemplated my next due student placement, on the hospital's new male Sick Ward — replacing Lister Ward, christened England Ward, and named after a popular Hospital Secretary.

That weekend, as I routinely trod the upland woodland paths behind us, in search of fuel, I noticed how empty the wood seemed; almost bare of animal life, green-sward and vegetation.

The tall elms and beeches, on top of the higher ground displayed, up-top, numerous circular bird nests (Rooks I think), but no sounds came from any occupants. The uneven black earth slopes of the dells were most pockmarked by chalk, and white flint-stones; and numerous holes in the concave sides; burrows, buries and setts, I knew not for sure, but hopefully, even probably, snug inside those warrens were various creatures of these woods; rabbits and hares, moles and badgers; and about, too, were their enemies; Reynards, ferrets, stoats, weasels; and in tight balls under hedgerows, wherever, were hedgehogs.

On the upper slopes of this neck of the woods, occasional Bambi deer were known to be 'hidden' amongst clumps of (out of place) large rhododendron bushes. The silver-birch-tree copses were too thin, too young to give cover; though the brambles and bracken beneath, and the humps of leaf-mould below, harboured considerable small life. I noticed, then, no singing bird life; all was wintertime. Silent... for the moment ...

And December was upon us.

William James

Progress in reading has been fruitful. I completed an abridged 1892 introductory edition of William James' *Text Book of Psychology*[44]. James contemporary, H.G. Wells, published his first book, a *Textbook Of Biology* (1893) shortly afterwards; but I'd not read, or was ever to see, a copy of *that* milestone. Wonderful, wonderful stuff. I found James work the most exciting adventurous book I had — at this time in 1968, ever appreciated. Everything, *so* lucidly written. I found it *impossible,* not to mentally ingest any and every morsel of enquiry. Taken from the last eight-page abridged chapter on *Psychology and Philosophy*, the following metaphysical quotes summed up James' primary investigation - for me:

> '... *referring beyond themselves.* Although they also possess an immediately given 'content', they have a 'fringe' beyond it ... and claim to 'represent' something else than it. Our non-sensational, or conceptual states of mind, on the other hand, seem to obey a different law. They present themselves immediately as referring beyond themselves ... how long may a state last and still be treated as one state? Things' have been doubted, but thoughts and feelings have never been doubted ... who the knower really is ... it is indeed strange to hear people talk triumphantly of the *'New Psychology'*, and write Histories of Psychology, when into the real elements and forces which the word covers not the first glimpse of clear insight exists. This is no science, it is only the hope of a science. The necessities of the case will make them metaphysical. ... *'If we could only forget our scruples, our doubts, our fears, what exultant energy we should for a while display...'*

If only !!!

Incident

Sara was working in the fields that afternoon, potato gathering — young Kit was with her. Paul was, at that moment, with me, as he had a nasty fall the day before — typical of climbing where they shouldn't, inquisitive little boys. Paul had fallen on a piece of wood, with a large six inch rusty nail protruding. First aid. I cleaned the wound, and put on a temporary bandage. A little later, having calmed Paul, and his (rightly anxious) mother, my in laws had arrived, in their car. And so, accompanied by my father-in-law, we took Paul down to St. Richard's Hospital in Chichester where, after an hour's fretting, two stitches were inserted over the wound in his right thigh.

Poor little Paul. I shall never forget those torturing screams, for those few moments, when the wound was actually given attention. A local anaesthetic helped immensely. I hugged him tight, and comforted as best I could; re-assured him of the briefness of the incident, sitting him on my lap as the doctor sutured, and the nurse and I held his thrashing limbs. Moments after leaving the hospital, 'knowing' it was all over, as I promised — and was promptly reminded by young Paul — I obtained a chocolate ice-cream, for him. Thank Heavens, he was as happy as anything by the time we arrived home, full of '*Mummee - I had an ice-cream*'.

Whilst the wound heals, and to prevent damaging or dirtying the stitches, I'll keep him rested and in sight of my person, securely 'wrapped up'; playing with his cars and coloured toy bricks. Kit was very happy, and extremely active all day. Together, we put up a fence at the rear of the garden, by the wood; this was to prevent seeing the eyesore of the chemical cesspit, as well as to corral it. Kit helped, carrying wood off just as we were about to nail it up, filling the holes up, as we were about to place poles in them, taking nails off just as they were about to be used, and generally happily underfoot; scoffing buns in between, whilst being watched by the three sitting females, Sara, her mother and young sister.

On duty at Summersdale. I recently experienced two attempts at suicide.... one event, a week ago, and the other, two days later. Both involved incidents by the same impulsive nineteen-year-old youth, Phobic Jack. This unhappy lad had taken two overdoses of aspirin, the first of 150 tabs, and, in his later gesture, second attempt, eighty tablets.... He took them (he told me), as he could never mix with boys and girls of his own age group, without feeling inadequate. 'I felt 'what's the use.'' Two years ago, he slit his wrist. He has been coming and going to and from the hospital, for some years. From first-aid and treatment and investigations, I had gained some useful experience...

I was doing the afternoon 'teatime' medicines at that time in Summersdale Day Hospital. It was Jack — having queued up, he reached me, and as I gathered his tablets he calmly, with a proud grin, said: 'I took one hundred and fifty aspirins just after dinner-time...'. Charge Nurse Bill and I swung into action. First, the Charge went off for some salt and water, as an emetic — whilst I escorted him off, to the toilet area.

'Right', I said. 'Now we've got to try and get those tablets up from your stomach, by vomiting. I'm going to place my fingers down the back of your throat.' And I did! He brought a little up, but not much. Charge arrived with the salt water emetic. 'Right, lad, now drink this. Force it down.' With protest, he commenced, but to little avail. As I held the patient and administered the emetic, Charge went off to phone the duty doctor, first aid thus being applied.

On the doctor's arrival, after a few questions, I 'phoned the Path Lab for a technician, to come over and extract a blood-sample for urgent analysis. The duty doctor phoned the General Hospital, located down the road, 'The Royal West Sussex' Casualty Department, and an ambulance was called in. The ambulance was to make a rapid appearance. Meanwhile, as much fluid as possible was attempted, to dilute his stomach's content. At the General, a complete stomach wash out was to be given, and he was soon to be bedded down for several days, on observations and treatment. I accompanied our patient, in the ambulance.

On Jack's later return, to Summersdale Day Hospital, he said, cheerily to me, how nice it was to have young ladies looking after him. I commended appropriately and he grinned approval.

But, by nature of his so-called 'immature personality' and complete unpredictability, two days later Jack gave a repeat performance, at the same medicine-giving time, he again glibly boasted; 'This morning, about nine, I took eighty aspirins — I'd have taken more — but I couldn't keep them down....'

'Oh yes,', I replied, unsure of the truth in this matter of fact blithe statement. 'Why...? No way would we take a chance of it not being true — and answering to a later Chichester Coroner's Court.' Jack answered why. 'Because I didn't want to see my Dad.' It was a visiting day, and his father was seen coming up the drive. And so Jack promptly ran out into the rain; and disappeared for the next two hours, until he was sure of his father's departure, from the hospital grounds. Home life was but one, of his problems. A different Charge Nurse was on this second re-run, at that time, and though the time limit demonstrated (six hours had passed) that the tablets taken would have, or should have, passed out of his stomach, and into the blood stream. He'd vomited some up (he told us), and urinated a fair deal, during the course of the day.

Next we put him to bed in pyjamas, and sent for the duty doctor. Whilst waiting developments, we started a quarter-hourly TPR. chart and bp count. I attended to this detail, whilst the Charge returned to the office to await the doctor, and any other urgent details. The aspirins had fetched his temperature down, at first taking 97.2, pulse 106, respiration 26..

Perspiration on his brow, he complained of a continuous ringing in his ears. If.... if, the aspirins' overdose eventually reached the cerebral regions, by way of the blood-stream, 'fits' would ensue and, eventually, death be inevitable. I took his blood pressure, as a matter of routine — and couldn't believe it! The systolic (upper) beat, the strium contraction was 110 — nothing so unusual (approximately 100 plus age for an adult) — but the diastolic (lower) beat, the ventricles, was zero — not registering.

I checked the diaphragm of the stethoscope. Tapped my fingers on its drum. Ouch! The echo confirmed it was ok. I looked at the manual sphygnamometer mercury movement, OK, and repeated the blood pressure count. I'm not the world's best, at this routine check — it was the same. Erm.... Concerned. I calmly put the instrument down, and walked out to the Charge Nurse's office. He followed me back and checked it for himself.

I was right. He was mystified too — anyway, no time for debate. We agreed, it was too low. Tactfully, the doctor was 'geed up'. He arrived, and ordered — stat — the blood sample (we, as nurses, even as first-aid procedures, may not ask for such). Later, the salicylic count was at a critical level of 53, one major difference, before the critical time gap. No time for stomach wash-out though, as a matter of course, we made him drink a jugful of salted water, to no avail. The doctor ordered an intravenous saline drip, in the hope of neutralizing the blood's content; meanwhile, time marched on. Temperature now just below 96 degrees. After some fast cycling, to the Main Building sick-ward, and seconding a drip and cannula from England Ward, I returned to Summersdale....

Eventually, I was relieved from my sentinel duty and, leaving the night-nurse at the helm, our patient safe and sound asleep (not-in-a-coma), I left work about nine-fifteen pm... Another long day; but who knows what consequences might have ensued, had we taken 'any' chances. I learnt a fair deal, that day.

One of the questions, in my RMN Intermediate State Exam, related to a.... '*patient found unconscious on the drive, with an empty tablet bottle by his side*'. As Charge Bill affably concluded — 'Good Experience, eh?'

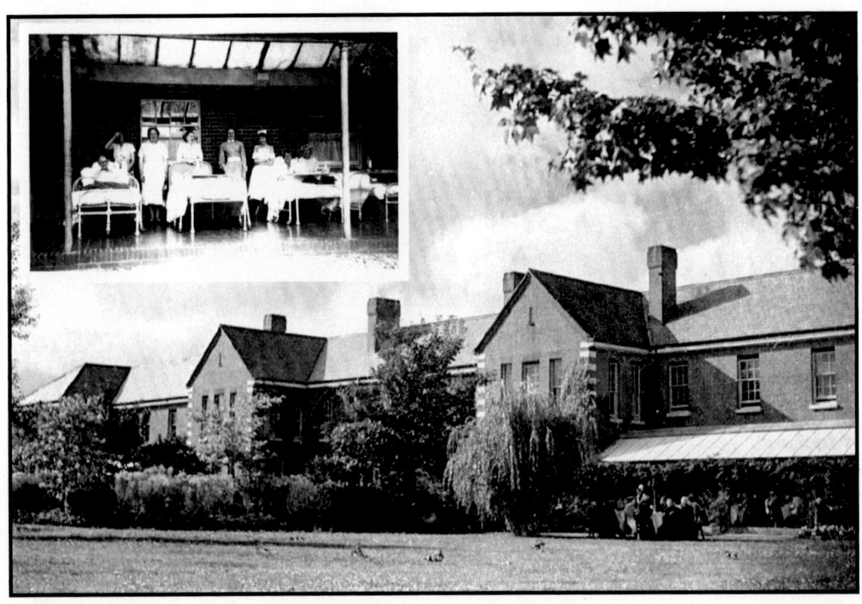

Front view, Summersdale Villa Hospital, Graylingwell, built 1933. Two pictures above, taken during the 1950s. In the 1960s and seventies — wards as follows; **left side**, two male wards; ground floor, MS1; top floor, MS2; **right side**, female wards; ground floor FS3; top floor, FS4 — including MRC (research) and Psychology dept; staff quarters at rear, upstairs. **Inset**: outside, on verandah, female ward; centre, Nurse Green, during summer of 1953.

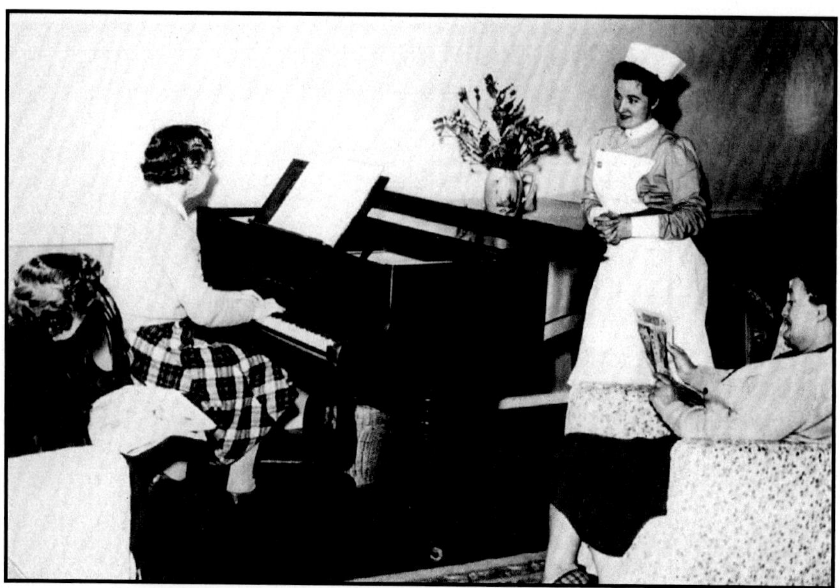

Summersale Admission & Day Hospital. Social Hour (males invited) on ground floor ward FSH2, female side, probably during early 1960s: Sister P. Weeks (wife of Charge Nurse Norman Weeks Amberley One reception ward over the main building) on duty..

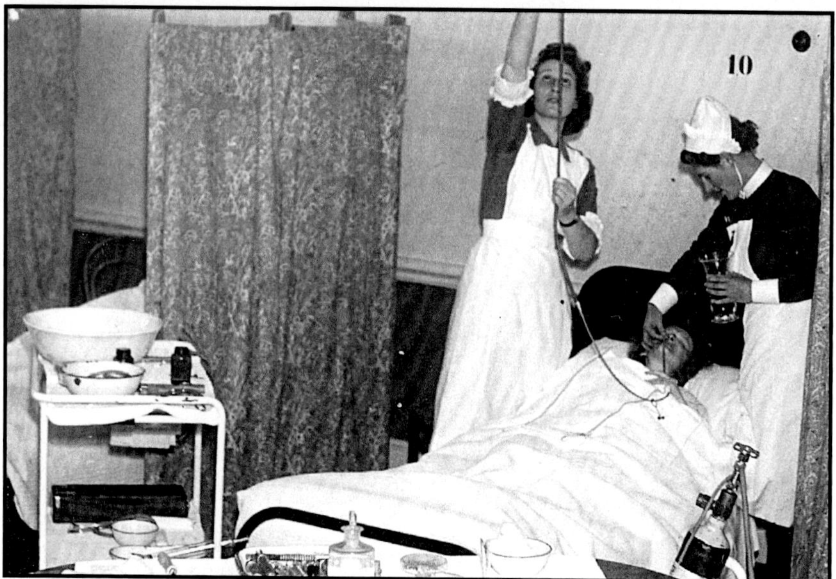

Summersdale Admission & Day Hospital. Ward Sister **(R),** and **(L),** Staff Nurse Green RMN, attending *Modified Insulin treatment* poss late 1950s early 60s.Note, enamel vessels on treatment trolley (not late 60s CSSD sterilised plastic pots et cetera).

Chapter Nine
England Ward

' Our personal memory is so often a false, distorted thing. The point is we remember very little - let us say, one hundred-millionth part of all that happened. I often doubt if we ever can remember anything as it actually was. Our memory depends on our powers of reception and is by no means objective. Do you remember, for instance, all that happened outside and inside you in the external world and in your mind even yesterday? Or last week? Or last year?' Dr. Maurice Nicoll. 1946.[1]

8th December 1968 to 12th April 1969

England Ward—Setting—Staff—The Major—Ablutions—Desert Ablution—Karl Jaspers—Departure—The Colonel—Incident—Case notes—Changes—Another Incident—Non Verbal Communication—Table talk

8th December 1968
England Ward

As a nowhere child, living in an austere wartime orphan institution, I believed the safest, most pleasant place, in its milieu, was the haven of Sister Webb and the Sick Bay. But one could only be there for genuine reasons, any pretence was (in retrospect) just not on — the value of that relief was otherwise lost. Sickbay as a refuge. Historically; Asylum, Hospital and Sanctuary were synonymous, blessed by church and state. For blessed, read as protected, those within. Those benign institutions were for oppressed, sick and vulnerable patients. Whereas, the church Sanctuary' altar was the spiritual sanction, perhaps in the civic-sense, whatever the institution, in whatever age, the model infirmary block, the sickbay, hospital ward and lazarette, was an inner sanctum. Mankind respects or even reveres, or *should* so, the good Church, Mosque, Synagogue, Temple — whatever, and *wherever,* holy icon core of any true domain.... not of War.

Our hospital's records, its architect's plans, the topical social policy, during seventy-five or so years, easily disclosed how medically *self-contained* the Asylum had been. Why, till only this past decade (1960s), it had its own general-hospital equipment. And its Forms; Graylingwell's headed paperwork reflected this level of autonomy; its administration, its operating theatres, x-ray department, pathological laboratory, dispensary (pharmacy), research and, as topical, *new* treatment facilities.

Many of the hospital's facilities that existed in the early 1960s, such as the operating theatres, had closed down, and new facilities made available *down-the-road*. First at The Royal West Sussex (General Hospital), in Broyle Road, Chichester and, a few years later (but after I left) moved again, down to St. Richard's Hospital on the site, hitherto but fields, once owned by nearby ecclesiastical, medieval *St. James Hospital.*

Post-war policies, introduced after the mandates of the National Health Service after 1946, and 1948, were mostly full of optimism; and Mental Illness, for a while, superficially disappeared in the mantle of general hospitals...

Graylingwell's last Medical Superintendent, the tall charismatic pioneer Dr. Joshua Carse, retired in 1963 (he died in May 1971) and, exit local control, a new administration was implemented by The Ministry of Health. The singular Graylingwell Hospital, its records administered by Chichester's local-authority since the Asylum's inception back in 1897, gave way to radical re-organization in 1963, under a new Chairman of the Medical Advisory Committee — and The Hospital Management Committee.

At ward level, day to day hospital forms changed from *Graylingwell Hospital*, to the plural, *Chichester & Graylingwell Group Hospitals.*[2] The long stay, psychiatric hospital was directly linked, at administrative levels, to the local General and Specialised Hospitals — with their own additional respective general facilities.

For some years advertised policies, through the mass media, had recommended that *all* psychiatric facilities ought to be based out of local (or District) general hospitals; and whereas, about much of the country, this transfer had taken place, in Sussex this was then, not yet the case, and our psychiatric hospital's essential facilities (sans Labs. and Operating Theatres) still operated on their own.

Local, economic stewardship was also being reduced and removed and, as alluded to, our own general hospital equipment was being slowly removed or closed down. Such was the atmosphere on beginning my later placement on *England Ward,* the sick-bay of Graylingwell in 1968. It'd been only five years since the formal close down of the previous administration, under the benign, insular, autocracy of the Hospital Superintendent.

On arrival, I'd been a trifle confused at the removal of hospital equipment, from such a large hospital as Graylingwell, and its need to be re-located in other nearby General Hospitals. If relocation was for economy, shared-facilities, then there was a rationale: as at Summersdale Villa where outsiders (outpatients) visited the upstairs Clinical Psychology Department - and then left the site.

Even so, to isolate diagnosed *Psychiatric* patients, without their own physical facilities, surely that was to *isolate* them, en masse; rather than accept the General (read generic) Hospital mantle? A medical-model or an sector-behavioural model; based on accepted behaviour and containment - rather than *illness.*

Surely the system was *not,* then, removing a stigma (viz. generic mental-illness as generic-fevers), but denying that fact and reinforcing the anti-social stigma.

Setting

Changes. Only a few months ago, in 1968, I had worked on the old Chilgrove One H shaped ward — of which England Ward had recently been adapted from off its right-side, with its own entrance taken off the corridor below. It was in that long-stay dormitory I had then found Barney, indulging in some isolated, pleasurable relief. And, during that Summer, I assisted ex-Chilgrove' patients in carrying their ward effects, down the snake long-corridor, across and into the great-divide of The Female Side - to the, then, being newly formed Male Rehabilitation Ward of Cavell One — overhead its peer, Cavell Two, designated the new Female Rehabilitation Ward.

And so, exit Lister Ward and, in the name of progress, that part of the old Chilgrove Ward had been emptied — and, into its bare frame, the hospital's own employed skilled union craftsmen, carpenters, engineers, painters, plumbers et cetera had, in quick time, upgraded the area, to receive the physically Ill of Graylingwell — it was renamed England Ward, after a recently deceased, popular hospital secretary.

Physically ill, in 1968, had to mean something different from pre-war years, when the hospital population included patients who, *in addition* to mental illness, *also* may have suffered from *infectious* fevers, tuberculosis (aka consumption, pthisis, TB), general paralysis of the insane (GPI) and, or other infectious diseases. But, fortunately, new prescribed drugs had greatly reduced *Annual Report* logistics, on these notifiable diseases (risk to the general population), and a formal police removal out of the community. And it meant that the Handbooks and training of its psychiatric, clinical and nursing staff, during those pre-war years, reflected the professional caring needs of this group of residents.

Graylingwell's own 1897 built *Isolation Hospital* (Sandown) had pre-war barrier nursed *all* its own worst infected GPI -TB, and Fever, diagnosed psychiatric residents. Barrier nursing had, thus, been a substantial *essential* feature of this hospital's psychiatric facilities. And so those earlier Asylum, student nurse training pre-1964 RMPA textbook manuals, like *The Red Handbook*[3], had contained *considerable* extra data, mandatory learned and practised, on those infectious diseases. The thick textbooks then, also combined with the florid symptoms, deemed, in contemporary parlance, in the 1920s and 1930s and 1940s... known as *Mental Diseases*.[4]

Our tutor, Mr Ilford, had successfully drummed into us that however much a symptom, an ailment, or diagnostic feature (physical or social more) was presented; the Mind, brain and body corporate could, and would, often combine with *other* numerous ailments and side-effects to follow, with subsequent clinical and perhaps anti-social consequences to be endured by patients, and others.

A bright new signposted wall plaque identified *England Ward,* outside the glass and wood panelled, unlocked door, off the Main south corridor; another inside second door then presented — leading into our new acute Sickbay, in late 1968. Between those two doors, on the left, was a small storeroom for storing cases, baggage, whatever; adjacent, another small room — opposite and next to a flight of stairs; this room was for cleaning stores. Opposite, and the other side of the steps, was another small, single room, once used for a nurse attendant — adapted as a small ward kitchen.

A concrete flight of steps, between the doors, was a back stairs flight up to a dormitory, of the male long-stay ward of *Chilgrove Two,* and located immediately on the right, past that open door leading off the Main Corridor. The previous Summer, on night-duty, and on *Lister;* the then sick-bay (of male D-block), I'd had to include MC2 ward on my piquet round. Mike, the old-soldier and Senior staff RMN and SRN, on night duty with me on the old sick ward had, perhaps tongue in cheek, indicated the sometimes presence of a 'Night time ghost' who occasioned this upstairs back flight of stairs' area, which was now attached to England Ward. Un-afraid, I often imagined 'cold draughts' of air, giving unseen puzzle shapes.

On entering England ward, the Nurses' Office was located on the immediate left; this room, on the original 1893 architect's drawing, was labelled S, designated for a single-room, now known, colloquially, as a single side room — long occupied by a *privileged* patient, in the *past* Chilgrove MC1 dormitory. The modern new ward Nursing Office was outfitted with standard desk, lights, two-chairs, wall-bookcase, and customary wallcharts, including that map which located all named, occupied beds (none were unoccupied).

In this small ward, built for eighteen residents and now reduced for twelve bed spaces, six to a side, were newly installed bed curtains and rails; and, behind, were new green window curtains *and* white net curtains. Behind each bed space was a two-point electric-plug socket, to receive an electric shaver, or radio, during ablutions. A bedside, padded, red long back chair was placed adjacent to each brand new adjustable bed. Record progress charts hung (as to be expected) on an shiny white-painted iron-rail, at the bottom of each bed. Curved bed tables on castors were (though optional) placed one to each bed area — standard fittings in modern U.K. hospitals.

The false ceiling, and the solid walls, had been redecorated, and lighted by new hung down, evenly spaced, bright light shades and fittings. There was also one cup-shaded light, behind each individual bed-space, held on substantial metal hinges. At floor level, gone were the old, thick and much polished naked wooden planked floor-boards, numerous grey white twelve inch Marley lino tiles were now laid above that wood foundation — to provide now *policy,* non-slip, easy to clean ward-floor surfaces.

I'd worked on *Chilgrove One* elderly ward, only months before; the sick observatory ward, and solarium day rooms, were Marley lino-tiled, and resurfaced. How well I recall that original, much highly wax polished, pitch-pine long stay ward flooring; its many decades thick, wax taper surplus slivers, at each bumping, forced down between the filled floor cracks, aged, out of sight, inflammable wax-stalactites, hidden above and below, in the warren subways, below the Main hospital buildings. All those wood-floor surfaces were now covered, in the new acute *England Ward* — with new fittings.

Adjacent to each bed head were new bedside lockers on castors, and above the beds, on a small projected shelf over the lockers (not beds proper), the usual round holed thermometer holders, with one ready to hand glass and mercury measure in place, to each resident. *Underneath* each bed, and within the hand reach of each bedridden patient, attached to the underside of the bed frame of some beds, was a customary long necked male urine bottle — new, opaque, white *plastic* receptacles, rather than old heavy, cumbersome, breakable, transparent measure marked *glass* bottles. Notably, these old bottles were still to be found on most back wards — though *some* of those bottles were still in use, on this new sick ward too, loosely laid in their substantial, flat, steel banded baskets or, like chamber pots, placed on the floor under the beds and awaiting staff collection.

Just inside the dormitory, first on the left, past the nursing office, with its small clear glass observatory window looking into the dorm, was an empty long back padded chair, propped against the wall, and, adjacent, an occupied cradled bed, with an enclosed silent patient's legs and stomach area housed underneath — an essential space preventing any pressure of bed-clothing on tender body surface The foot of the top sheet, and warm Red cross red wool blanket and counterpane (all normally tucked-in), were turned back over — to expose sight of his vulnerable feet, at its bottom. I would soon learn that he had a stomach cancer, amongst other ailments — *John Brown,* his name.

Alongside this most sick occupier, of the first bed-space, apart from his bedside locker (flowers in vase, several get well cards on its top surface, and another bedside chair), was an absent bed space, where a small oblong table and two dining room type chairs were placed. At this station, a duty nurse would sit, when not otherwise occupied. At other times, a getting better, mobile, patient might sit and attempt a puzzle, read (if able to concentrate), write a letter, have their meals — or just sit vacant, and wait to get better.

Then, there were three other occupied beds, followed by a space on the left, where the ward extension occupied the remaining right side portion, of the converted half H — now partitioned, with a locked doorway into MC1 in situ. Another single room, which was previously a male nurse attendants' room, in its early occupancy as part of the MC1 (formerly known as King's Cl ward), was on the immediate left of this small area and, adjacent, a designated restroom for recovering patients, with a small, black and white television, two large chairs and a separate toilet and bathroom area. This completed this short extension of *England Ward.*

Back in the main new sick dorm, two other corner beds completed the left side of the sick ward — that top end had no door, only wide curtained windows, which overlooked the large airing court garden of *Chilgrove One* Ward. The new sick bay had no direct garden access. On the right side of the ward were six, evenly spaced, occupied beds — and their attendant furniture and fittings.

The tall windows guaranteed plenty of light, sunshine and, of course, an essential clean air supply.

Staff

It was morning, just after 9 o'clock, when I reported in to the *England* ward office and its august Charge Nurse. He was a tall, broad shouldered well confident man, of uncertain age — early middle-years, I gauged, late thirties early-forties; a well-filled frame, but certainly *not* fat; he held himself Passe Doble erect, graceful, as if dignity was *always* expressed in one's own carriage; and so appeared of strong muscular stuff. He had dark hair, full and thick, but well cut and groomed so well it set on his high-domed forehead like a beatle styled wig (which it certainly was not; at least it looked like an artist's black beret). His face was full, round and clean. His green eyes reflected from the outset a high intelligence and a warm sense of humour.

Julian was my new Charge Nurse. His large long white coat was not only immaculately clean and spotless but, from its appearance, was starched and pressed with lined creases reminding me (a little ominously) of such exact knife edge lines in my past, best army khaki uniform blouse (and trousers); in fact, at his broad back, such creases were to be seen from the top of one sleeve to the top of the other sleeve, a distinct pressed crease; and even the sleeves had matching down singular neat creases, front and rear.

At the collar line, above his white shirt, the white coat had a sewn on red patch, extending over and down, to the top of his starched front lapels, on which two nursing qualification badges were pinned — a GNC, and Psychiatric Nursing Medal. He was, I had already been informed by a colleague, no fop, but a Gold Star, doubly qualified nurse — with high standards, and a sharp tongue for any erring delinquent. His grey tie wore an Oxford knot and was clean and immaculate; below his buttoned down white-coat, his well tailored uniformed grey bags (surprise surprise) displayed knife-edges, without a stain, or badge of wear, in sight — even his slim black shoes were shining, and mirror polished.

Aware of this ward as *the* physically sick ward, I wondered how he could maintain such a level of immaculate cleanliness and graphic precision. Julian soon enlightened me on this basic point and, with his green-eyes sparkling, he spoke in a slow crisp clear pitched animated tone, and explained that he always had a number of spare coats kept on the ward — even a change of shoes kept under his desk.

The brown coated cardboard laundry boxes, that nursing staff used each week, were always full, and personally named — though Julian admitted his wife pressed his coats at home, and the red-tabbed coats were for his special office use, only. Other white coats, like mine, were for on the ward use, the utility they were designed for.

In his top pocket, several clips were visible; one a silver Parker pen (black-lead, reliable for his reports) and, another, a thermometer in its spring clip container — also, a pair of chrome scissors which, too, were securely held by another spring clip container, in that top pocket. There was no visible stopwatch, as the fob, so common, with our Sister' colleagues on the other side. But I would not've been surprised if Julian had a gold, at least a shiny, bold silver antique Hunter watch, secured by a filagree chain in one of his waistcoat side-pockets.

On the desk before me, as I sat in *England Ward's* Nursing Office, on that first morning, was a brown, wooden boxed, sphygnamometer; a polished, wood, mushroom-like blunt headed nerve testing stick (Babinski's reflex and knee jerks), and other sundry basic apparatus. There was an inevitable wall-chart, which listed each bed space and its occupant, and other divers notices and charts, very neatly clipped and spaced in view.

We'd already met on several occasions and, lately, on the customary pre-placement ward visit, to meet our to be new Charge Nurse, and his Staff Nurse; and, introduced to the next work, ward milieu — and its occupants. 'Nice to have you on board, Barry. We expect plenty from you, these next three months; and hope you enjoy your stay in *England* — and obtain plenty of knowledge during your experience with us.' He smiled, in confirmation. His voice soft, almost mellow. Slow speech, each word measured, clear and meaningful. I replied — already encouraged, 'Thanks, Julian. I'll do my best.' Standing up, Julian said, 'Well, Harry's on the ward. I'll let him introduce our patients to you ...'

Breakfasts over, and cleared away. First bed (John Brown's) on the left, had a green curtain drawn around it, and a trolley with ablution's apparatus upon it — Staff Nurse Harry was, softly softly, busy about the patient. Staff was tall (like Julian), but there any resemblance finished; he was lean and slightly stooped; cleanly attired, no starch or pressed crease in view. Harry nodded acknowledgment, as Charge Nurse Julian introduced me, during the hand over, to his delegate, a new student and temporary dependent colleague — to learn from him.

Harry's fair hair was receding, its sides wispy; loose strands about his ears, and a thin blonde moustache, straight above his lips. I would later learn from him that his leanness and apparent fragile health (he was in mid-thirties), was due to a past long bout of tuberculosis which, now cured, had left Staff Harry with that lean stooped and famished frame. His uniform complemented our own; though his shoes, in evidence of his work, were already lightly covered with a sprinkling of pink powder called *Ickosan*, then fashionable (like adult's baby-powder) to conclude a dry cleansing, ablution site. 'Hello Barry. Put a pair of gloves on, and you can give me a hand, if you would — though I've about finished with Mr Brown here (he's more asleep than awake).' Staff Harry wore a pair of thin transparent, elasticated gloves — of which I would soon be very familiar with in the months ahead, in the exercise of uncounted ablutions, and sterile treatments attending our sick charges.

John Brown (my first sick ward patient) was granted a sad, unique distinction; he was deemed the comparative most *sick* condition on the ward and, thus, his bed location, adjacent to the nursing office and (silent) nurse's station, of table and chairs. As we moved away and out of his hearing distance; Harry informs me, solemnly, that Mr Brown was dying with cancer, and was regularly sedated, with pain-killing pethidine (signed for, religiously, in the DDA and night sedations' records); hence his tranquil half sleep — but painless state. The next two beds, two and three, were occupied by patients recovering from influenza. At the top of the ward, on my left, there was a gap, which led to the drugs cupboard, toilets, and a single room (nearby, a closed partition door into the remaining ground floor observatory, Chilgrove Ward). This was where, presently, our brown-coated ward orderly was busy, clanging his wet-mop and bucket about the red-tiled toilets' floor. In the first of the two corner beds, on the left-side of the dormitory, Harry introduced me to — *The Major*.

The Major

Major Argus was an ex-World-War II, shoulders' square, retired soldier from the *Royal Artillery*; convex round faced; twinkling brown eyes which, animated, appeared to be always reflecting inwards, and reporting outwards (like the proverbial eyes on a wall painting sentinel — following you wherever you went). For most of the time, he sat, propped up against four pillows, hardly moving; a bed table was invariably in easy reach, and a *Readers Digest* or large print book, brought by his very devoted wife Marion (who never ever missed a visiting time, in thc three months I attended that ward) were, with fruit and drink, in easy arm's reach — either on the table, or adjacent bedside locker.

Major Argus reminded me of a slightly larger version of a past work-colleague; a retired army Major I knew, when I was employed, for a while, in the labs of *Agfacolor Processing* at Wimbledon, back in 1962. *That Agfa* Major, I recall, was a small, smart, and very dapper warm, amiable, sharp witted gentleman, with (despite overalls) immaculate dress, ample tidied hair (not a trace of silver white) and a well-trimmed, slim moustache. *Agfa* Major was *not* a manager, for he was but a junior lab assistant like myself, but *he* was always able to be 'one of the lads' yet always, *in-mystique*, about the *Agfa* processing lab floor, commanded respect and popularity, in our staff presence — quiet, laconic, dignified, we viewed him as *really* one of our betters, receiving respect without ever demanding it and, rightly, getting same.

England's Major Argus too, retained that *Agfa* dignity (I don't think it was just my own interpretation); and, aided by his regular visitor, his wife Rita, and my staff colleagues, in his daily ablutions, we ensured his grooming was as immaculate as possible. The Major, during ablutions, would beam, his red-cheeks puffed out; his eyes agreeing; and, as close as his speech could allow, a stuttered splutter, which somehow never ever resulted in coherent words — yet his wants, likes, and dislikes and pertinent emotions were mostly clear enough. But he couldn't, would never utter a word of definite sense.

Harry explained, in a matter of fact tone, that the Major suffered from irregular epileptic fits and was immobile, though he was occasionally able to have his glasses put on (he couldn't manage this himself) and appeared to be able to read for short periods. Loyal Rita, his loving wife, believed he was an avid reader (a compensation) rather than the too brief episodes, the staff observed.

Next to the Major's bed, in the top left-hand corner of the ward, already sat out in a chair in formal Dressing Gown Order (DGO), his hospital rainbow striped (viz. many colours) gown tied with a white cotton cord about his waist; was *Parkinson William*, a former professional accountant, who experienced a major nervous breakdown about ten years ago. He then developed Parkinsonian symptoms, which included stuttering, and a severe marked tremor in both hands. He could still walk, a few paces at a time, but invariably would collapse onto the floor, bed, patient or chair close by.

William, unlike his neighbour The Major, was able to sometimes speak, albeit staccato stuttered and often frustrated; knowing too well what he wanted to say, but unable to achieve the cadence he desired. It was sad, and sometimes a little humorous (though a little humbling to an observer), to watch the two of them trying to talk to each other, and yes, little efforts sometimes succeeded as (for example) with considerable tremors William might pass an object to him (being mobile) and, with a nodding or shaking head, The Major expressed sentiment, that he knew what his companion was trying to say, or do. Neighbours. *Good neighbours.*

It was sufficient that whatever psychiatric diagnosis brought them into the hospital, they were physically disabled as well. But William nevertheless was, in the months ahead, one of the few of the *England Ward* patients who was able to occasionally walk about, albeit very slowly, between the beds, and even to take himself to the toilets (though wee accidents occurred from time to time).

Down the right hand side of the ward, a number of men were bedded, suffering or recovering from a bout of influenza; or with a foot, or leg, injury, which prevented them from remaining on their own ward. Two low voices drew Harry and I to the small area of the television, rest area and toilets; and the inhabited side-room, wherein the ward orderly and its resident were engaged in a friendly dispute.

Harry grinned as he led me towards the hubbub; a young man in a brown overall was leaning upon the handle of a mop, as he exchanged conversation with a big, late middle-aged man with a wide girth, dressed in obvious hospital laundered clothing; the trousers at half mast, but clean no less; and in a white shirt and grey pullover. They stopped and looked to us, as we approached them. 'Oh.... Hi Harry', said the orderly, and the resident waved a hello. 'John! Introduce you to a new student, second year, Barry. And the other gentleman'. Harry continued looking to the resident, '... is *Charles Oak*, off E2 — been here long time, eh Charlie?'

'S' right, Harry... 'ere 'bout thirty year.' Charlie was beginning to go bald at the temples but, otherwise, had dark hair with not a white strand in sight. He looked as if he had recently completed his ablutions; his hair was still wet and shining pasted down flat across the crown. 'We'd better get back on our round; chat later, eh?', Harry concluded, and led me back into the dormitory ward of the sick-bay.

For the next hour, I assisted Harry, aided with small talk, about his round. Our slight stooped, pencil lean, animate Staff, took his job very seriously — but he did allow the customary ward radio to play light music. There was very little chatter, or movement, amongst the other ward residents (Charlie was an exception) — this greatly contrasted with *Summersdale Villa,* which had been very lively by comparison. And even *Chilgrove One* had had considerable more animation, amongst its mostly more elderly residents. This was indeed a Sickbay.

Ablutions

Again. Every ward had its set day-routine; similar where mealtimes, drug rounds, laundry, and so forth were concerned. But, in the matter of ablutions, *England Ward* had very considerable additional, and most essential, features that, in sum, did not apply to our other, psychiatric, hospital wards. There was a so obvious, noticeable, high level of hygiene and asepsis (where so); and increased needs of diets and prescribed drugs. Bed rest was essential to most sick residents, with an inevitable extra work-load. Some patients' needs, more frequent than others. There were TPR (temperature pulse respiration) charts to be maintained; diet charts to be kept on weight loss; fluid charts; bowels opened records; bed bath ablutions; regular records; and numerous, *special* demands, every day — according to any sick patient's individual requirements. Such legion, very basic, nursing applications are (however mundane) fundamental on general hospital wards, but, in degree, were not at all in such demand, expected on the average psychiatric hospital ward.

Lean Staff Harry, clean and sharp, complimented his senior — my new Charge Julian; who was an Encyclopedia, on whatever related subject was enquired, of his ward charges and staff colleagues. Anatomy, biology, bio-chemistry, dentistry, economics, medicine, neurology, nursing, optics, physiology (all the P's) and, from A to Z, Julian's office library and 'one liner' benign throwaways reflected the arts (music in particular); philosophy, considerable psychology, and, most gravely, occasionally of the acidity of politics. All this and more, I very soon became aware of, as a new student on the sick ward. And, to their credit, amongst this fount of knowledge I experienced, no apparent arrogance, or chest-beating ego echoes, from Julian and his right-hand Harry.

On *Chilgrove One,* I had, with Ahmed and Big Jim, first experienced shaving — wet and dries on bed-ridden patients, and this daily shaving ablution was, inevitably, an early after breakfasts task on *England Ward.* Hair cuts were executed by a regular outsider.

Volunteer Bill, the hairdresser, once per week appeared on the ward (usually in an afternoon), to offer his services gratis for our patients — along with friendly barber patter. There was one considerable ablution chore I had not anticipated which, twice per week (more for individuals), lean Harry allowed (insisted) I took on duty — the Enema Rounds. It generally took two staff, though, with effort, one could manage alone. Rectal lavage was not essential for all our bedridden patients, but was for most — the function not only cleaned the bowels, but could if necessary, introduce drugs or fluids, and was always one of the many constants for diagnostic purposes — colour of stools, uraemia, et cetera.

So, with trolley loaded, white coat on; curtains drawn; patient informed and prepared; bowl-of-water towel etc. to-hand; kidney-dish ammunition at the ready — the wax like bullet shaped (like 303 rounds) laxatives were unwrapped from their blue-paper containers, gently heated in lukewarm water; and, with thin transparent gloves on, duty commenced about the round.

The Major was always mischievous during this ablution, and (Dignity intact, Sir) would act the servant and master role well, despite being unable to verbally speak. His brow would rise, moustache and upper-lip quiver and crease into a knowing grin; Yes, it's ok, I know it needs to be done (humour, *not* mockery), which his eyes would compliment and their pupils' aimed darts of animated communication. Nightingale' Hygiene in — 'Palpable hits, Sir!' *The Mysteries of Purity.* [5] Good discipline. Sufi cleanliness — absolute ritual.... Yes, Sir!

After the allotted timespan, for the round of rectal ablutions, covering paper towels were removed, along with their contents — then examined and disposed of, as appropriate. Those sick patients, on prescribed iron tablets (for example), would discharge small, hard black bullets; to be like rabbit's deposits — others would be more colourful, as it were, even occasional blood droplets would remind of *other* possible complaints. This ablution was but one of the many so *basic,* in nursing care duties — but relatively still new to me. And there were many, more to come...

Houghton and Whittow's *Practical Nursing* [6] was well thumbed by me, in those early days. Between Julian and lean Harry I received (and welcomed) almost daily in-depth lessons, on numerous nursing exercises, and considerable extra-curriculum demonstrations, writings, drawings, books, magazines and off-ward homework — all media material given to encourage extra in depth learning — and ongoing experience in pursuance of good practise.

The radio Light Programme turned on after breakfast, drugs trolley away, essential cleaning ablutions were begun — tpr's, washings, shaving, beds, laundry, dressings, doctor's round (along with Julian or Harry), patients' clothing changed, as re-dressed sat-outs (if agreeable), all and sundry, other specialising daily duties were soon, again, in regular routine. And completed. It was all ward routine. And so, the sick ward premise, too, experienced an immaculate daily cleansing; much instigated by John, our morning ward orderly. But, most nurses assisted in the cleaning, moving furniture and patients, about the floor space.

One memorable event, I recall, Julian was off-duty, and Staff Harry in charge as Simon (the other *Charge,* on his long day) was absent, off the ward, for a while. We were expecting a Consultant, for a daily ward round. Well... lean Harry decided to be a little zealous, and informed John and I that after patients' ablutions were completed (before 10 am if possible), he wanted the ward to be *especially* clean and symmetrical — and he explained to us what he meant in an anecdote.

'Not many years ago', he said, 'the Medical Superintendent and his entourage would sometimes descend on a ward for an Inspection Tour' — (sounded like the media proverbial tour of Matron, Chief Male Nurse, Consultant, and Others; and or the military machine of CO. and train, on their dire barracks inspection).

'*And caps on*?', I, tongue-in-cheek, queried....

'Yes. Caps on, and with all staff in full serge uniform. Pressed, short, white coats. The furniture and beds were exactly lined-up. It was so immaculate; so much so, that all VIP visitors were always enchanted, with the pure cleanliness, care and attention, so *self-evident* to any outsider.'

And so... after the floor was cleaned, washed and polished, the window-ledges, door-frames and table-surfaces swiftly cleaned down (patients' most amused); lean Harry produced a large ball of white twine. 'Right John, Barry, one of you take the end, and tie it to the bed end, at the bottom; 'bout half way up the bedstead', Lean Harry instructed.

Orderly John and I obliged, with The Major's critical eyes and other bed residents eyes upon us. (Talk about a *Carry On*...) Taking up the slack, lean Harry measured it to the other end (we were on the right-side of the ward), and asked John to cut and tie a knot, when it was taut enough. With Harry standing back, John and I were then directed to line-up, exactly, every bed end onto this string line. The same exercise was carried out, on the other side of the ward. Then, to follow, all the bedside lockers were also lined up, exactly so. And all bed trays on their castors; and the drawn back curtains — even the bedside lights were all uniformly folded back to the wall, at an identical angle.

All inanimate — even animate, as our bemused and amused patients readily joined in this un-expected event — all objects, which were about the ward were, if at all possible, *neatly* put-away, or lined up and polished; whatever! Standing back. Almost finished. Outside the office, lean Harry, hummed and arred, frowning a moment and then, another decision, the half dozen sat out first bemused, then amused patients were in their chairs, also uniformly lined up. Two sat out lines (one to each side of ward) of residents, with neat tucked in blankets, about their person.

All bed clothing was smoothed out (it *was* like a barracks inspection!); and creases were uniformly stylised, so that colour schemes (white-sheets, red-blankets, counterpanes folded-back), indeed all fabrics complimented the ward picture. At last, but by no means least, all urine bottles were seen clean, ready, and empty — and any urine-bags, too, were properly presented. All in all, an immaculate ward state presentation. There was even a light polish on the Marley tiles (non-slip!) which seemed unnecessary — but a gloss maintained. Not a Faustian dust mote to be seen.

With moments to spare, the job was done, and Charge Simon appeared with our Duty Consultant and two VIP Visitors (unknown to me — but probably members of a House Committee) who, after they had quickly walked through the ward, halted by me, at John Brown's bed; and then, swiftly, moved on up the ward, to The Major and his bemused neighbour William (sat out). The Visitors were briefly out-of-sight, but heard chatting to Charlie around the top-left corner, while John and I stayed put, by the observation table — lean Harry in train had been attached to the Inspectorate. Then, it was over. A smile and a nod (of approval?) from each person, to orderly John and I, in their dignified passing, and they then disappeared into the Nursing Office — then off the ward.

But, the degree (of twine) of such a ward ablution, so time consuming, was *not* experienced again during my stay — although the high degree of ward cleanliness and asepsis remained constant. No gross infection of the residents, from a lack in cleanliness of the sick ward or its attending staff, was ever recorded, to my knowledge.

Karl Jaspers

The male side of the long snake south corridor was crowded, as I left the *Blue Lagoon* staff dining-room after lunch, with Bob and Ahmed. Close to Christmas 1968, and colourful decorations were up on all the wards; a lit up, coniferous tree, in each day-room; and both staff restaurants similarly prepared, in each room a small, potted, decorated tree on display.

One tradition detailed the hospital staff electricians to decorate a large long-ago planted coniferous annual, situated in the open-air outside the Graylingwell Front Entrance, with a substantial array of coloured lights; at night-time, this constant sign of *Peace And Goodwill To All* was instantly reassuring to our whole community. As we passed the Amberley's' entrance, we saw their Main Corridor doorway frame was well garlanded; with *Love And Peace, Goodwill To All* — the message to all passers by, letters cut out in silver and gold coloured words tacked on to that outer corridor door; the admission wards' staff and residents visible message to all ongoing human traffic, which passed its outmost door.

Bramber One had, too, similarly decorated their corridor doorways' area — its ward dormitory was located directly opposite, across the corridor, so separated from MB1 kitchen; its nursing office and dayroom; the internal corridor and the upper concrete stairway led onto Bramber Two, a route I was already familiar with. Both MB1 downstairs doorways reflected Christmas cheer and greetings to all. We moved on, jostling, down the corridor, as Staff Ahmed left to enter Chilgrove's own decorated entrance. And a doleful Alternative Bob (something was bothering him) moved on off to Summersdale Villa, and I turned into our decorated England Ward. The sick bay was peaceful, and church sanctuary quiet — only a Christmas carol threaded off the wooden boxed radio-tannoy, and gently stroked our resting patients about the ward.

Charge Nurse Julian, at my request, had begun giving me regular homework (the School was closed over the holidays). After our handover was complete, and Simon departed, lean Harry went out onto the ward; and Julian asked me to stay a few minutes in the office. My homework, to be discussed, was on the Endocrinal System and its disorders — pertinent to psychiatric practice. Bing Crosby's mellow voice crooned, *I'm dreaming of a White Christmas*, on the ward radio, as lean Staff Harry begun a routine Tpr (Temperature Pulse and Respiration) ward round.

We'd received two new admissions, during the morning shift; Charlie Oak (who had helped decorate the ward) had returned to his own home-ward, on Eastergate Two; Charlie's vacated single-room was now occupied by a small thin fellow in for observation off of ME1 ward; a Mr John Evans. And, on the left side of the ward (bed four), the previous tenant had returned to Amberley Two, and in his place a man, in his early sixties, was Mr Peter Jackson, who had been transferred across from Summersdale Villa, shortly after his admission into the hospital. The New Admission had routinely been discussed, during the handover. The new resident — as yet unknown.

Our new admission Mr Jackson's symptoms included clinical depression, possible early dementia — and confusion (Summersdale reported hallucinations); — his condition was deteriorating; if he deteriorated too much, then an urgent transfer down the road to the *Royal West,* would be advised. His wife (who had herself been unwell) was to visit sometime, in the next two days. Julian had asked me *not* to read his transferred case notes, yet — for reasons he would explain to me later on. Julian concluded his comment on the endocrinal disorders; and I completed several pages of new notes. ...

Sat in the office overhead, were two crossed paper chains; the old-fashioned multi-coloured strips, hand-pasted links, which were diagonally placed to form an X of cheer above. Alternative Bob, not for the first time, had talked with me about two New Names, American Erving Goffman (*Total Institutions*), and Scot Dr. Ronald Laing (*The Divided Self,* as Wm James). And, Bob expressed a passion in his tone, during those introductions. Several months ago, on Amberley One, I'd met Existential Dave, a young patient on long-term sick-leave from *Manchester University*. Dave had been keen on Kafka and various angst existentialists, which (already well introduced by Colin Wilson) led me into more in-depth, self-explorations — of the mind and body of others — but especially my own self-examination; and that had been quite acceptable. Such self observation was initiated out of rank humility, not shallow ego. I was puzzled, as a new, to me, *very* negative concept of mental illness was also being introduced, something called *Anti-Psychiatry* and Laing. And, additionally, out of Bob's *Sociology* classes, presented a then mandatory college *Total Institutions* by Goffman. None of these names were included in my formal RMN studies.

Why? Are *all total* Institutions mad, sad and bad, as Alternative Bob's social studies appeared to infer? This seemed, to me, as being rather absurd. If so, I had a very great deal to learn! Given experience, knowledge available, resources, and *good* levels of caring, what was wrong? Surely, with *no* benign institutions, there could only be anarchy, chaos?

Julian admitted to knowing a little of Laing, Cooper and Esterton; but, *as yet,* neither he nor I had seen, or previously heard of, Goffman and his *Sociology* textbook called *Asylums,* and that it was this American study of which, that our Third Year student, RMN colleague Bob, presently, was so affected, disturbed by... 'Hang on a mo' Barry...' On one reflection, Julian reached up onto the bookshelves behind him, and drew down a slim volume. Names, ideas, images... 'Laing read existentialism and *phenomenology,* of which I know this chap remains little known, outside Europe... I believe *you* will find him *most* relevant.' Julian smiled at me, knowingly, as of Great Expectations, well, at least potential. I left the office, and returned to ward duties.

The man's name, was Karl Jaspers.[7] It was one of the New Names introduced as an Existential Philosopher by Colin Wilson, and Existential student Dave. But *not* yet to me of Psychiatry, as being introduced by Julian — is it the same man? Jaspers with Sartre, Husserl, Heideggar and others: But duty called me out to the ward, and I departed with this new name offering me tempting New concepts; intellectual and subjective food to be digested later on. Jaspers seminal works would act as another arsenal, counter (for me), to more hostile elements of anti-psychiatry and anti-institutions. William James would have got on well with Jaspers (as did R.D. Laing), as Philosopher *and* Psychiatrist, good doctors of The Mind and body corporate.

But, again, Jaspers et al were *not* part of our 1964 RMN curriculum, or in that Bible, *The Red Handbook.* Yet, such *new* knowledge was not at all subversive, in my experience, but additional sources of fascinating knowledge. As we began our ward round, Laing was mentioned by me to Staff Nurse RMN SRN lean Harry (he'd trained some years back). But, unlike Charge Julian, he admitted never hearing of Scot Dr. R.D. Laing, or of American Goffman, anti-psychiatry and topical sociology.

Only days later (pure coincidence) at Meynell's bookshop in East Street, Chichester, I purchased two Karl Jaspers' works, second hand. The first, a post war paperback, *The Future of Mankind*? [8]; which echoed to me H.G. Wells, *Mind at the End of its Tether.* [9] And, within weeks, I was fortunate in finding an incredible, to me, Karl Jaspers work - *on Psychiatry,* and in hardback.[10] It was my first sighting of his classic, *General Psychopathology.* There'd been no mention of this gentle but giant scholar, in any of my medical or nursing reference textbooks or, as a name in an *Index,* or content in any of our school lectures; only located in the more nebulous realms of Philosophy. I didn't know, then, that the Jaspers 922 pp work, is a psychiatric bible of *immense* worth. And although I subsequently used its *Index* as a dipper, it seemed, overall, that its sheer volume proved beyond my comprehension (*like Kant*). It remained a rare Rosetta stone glossary, in depth, about the nebulous *realities* of human emotions, feelings, and perceptions, pertaining to the human mind — to an open mind, ready for exploration. Jaspers, like the Sufi mystic poet and saint the Persian Rumi, *'exalted love as highest form of existence,'* [11].

And I put Jaspers' clinical psychiatric tome, too, amongst other *dipper* books to refer to, better digested later on. Another source of threads. It was alchemic pure gold. And, giant Jaspers became a compliment, to Jung, Gurdjieff, Ouspensky, Sartre and now questioning Psychiatrists, like our good Dr. Joyce and the (mis-named) anti-psychiatrist Doctor R.D. Laing. I Later read that Laing was, indeed, a friend and post-war pupil of Jaspers. And I became an admirer of both of them, and how they, for example, worked with patients' hidden trauma (from sudden Shell Shock, or peacetime cultural shocks *in extremis* — to psychoanalysis and Post Traumatic Stress Disorder — PTSD.[12] And, for me, increased a growing interest in *New Existentialism,* as of Colin Wilson.[13] European Nobel Peace Prize winner, Karl Jaspers, was clearly of Peace and Goodwill, as I moved on, in that spirit of Christmas in 1968, from Julian, to lean Staff Harry, to assist in the early afternoon ward round. New seeds of knowledge had been well planted in my potted head, for later.

Departure

Sad. John Brown died just before Christmas, having submerged into a coma he never emerged from, whilst I was off duty; his distressed visitors' last mortal glimpse, of their father, was *not* of him in dire cancerous pain, but departed peacefully in sleep; already on his way, wherever, after life. I never did learn of his reason for being in our psychiatric hospital, but had no doubt of a legitimate origin.

Overtime was in abundance, during the run-up to Christmas, and I worked a number of extra shifts on Chilgrove and Eastergate wards, with a few faces absent from my last on duty sessions, and new bodies in situ. Such changes occurred as routine. Bouts of influenza, stomach' complaints and other ailments, were common to staff and patients, in the hospital during wintertime; and hospital record years evidenced periods when a staff shortage, due to flu, or whatever, was all too common. I experienced another bout of flu, which came and went with inconvenience; but, to others, flu was potentially more lethal.

18th January 1969

Alf, one of our long stay patients off of one of the back wards had, I understood, been ill for sometime, and developed pneumonia; he died, during an early afternoon shift, and I recorded his departure in, for me, a special, unusual way. Whereas I'd seen a wrapped cadaver in the morgue, during my six weeks intake course, this was my first experience as a witness, and, afterwards, I sketched a crude likeness to record that event, in one of my small red notebooks. For me, it was a single form of respect, on record. Deaths on duty, though only occasional, were an inevitable reality, which joined the statistics of hospital departures.

Arriving on duty, early in the crisp white frost New Year of 1969, I was greeted by an unusual sight — a young woman was assisting lean Harry in tidying up the beds, prior to the arrival of ward visitors. It was still a males only haven, female staff were still segregated, though our new PNO Principal Nursing Officer, Mr Alexander Pushkin, had, as part of his appointment brief, been instructed to integrate male and female nursing staffs throughout the hospital. What made the surprise more complete, was *who* it was — it was young Jenny, off of Barnet Two ward. Her Case History showed that, prior to her schizophrenic breakdown, Jenny had been an SRN student, at another Sussex hospital; and she still, then, experienced occasional, relative lucid periods, and was allowed to *sometimes* help out on some wards — under supervision.

Jen didn't know me, had no recollection, from that past crisis — when I was a first year student on Chilgrove One. In future encounters in the hospital, she would recognize me... But there was that day, the appearance of a new admission on the right-side (bed three); cot sides already attached. Charge Julian discretely briefed me on our new admission — a genuine VIP, our new un-named patient was an ex-WW2 war veteran, known as *The Colonel* to us ward staff.

The Colonel

He'd been a wartime serving soldier, a Colonel (wartime rank?) — that much I was informed; and, in some *capacity,* had been involved in a real-life breakout, a tragedy known as *The Great Escape*[14]; a true story about seventy-seven prisoners who escaped, in March 1944, from the German POW camp *Stalag Luft Three*. For a year two-hundred prisoners had worked at digging out three long tunnels; two of which were deliberate decoys. Very sadly, of seventy-seven escapees — who tied up numerous enemy troops and, considerable time in searching for escapees, fifty, when re-captured, were murdered by the Gestapo on the direct order of Hitler himself. I believe only three escapees eventually reached safety. I was, at this time, unsure how, and knew only what I read or seen, in the Hollywood film drama.

On our sickbay admission, the old soldier, was, unhappily, already terminal. He was in an advanced state of alcoholism, with shaking delirium tremens. And whatever role the unnamed army Colonel (his present rank) had played in that very unhappy wartime drama we, I, would never know. We, the hospital staff, made his departure as comfortable as possible. But, he never spoke. Out of respect, I didn't enquire, pry, whatever — and didn't, whenever a visitor called to see the gentleman. Yet, Julian had been informed of sufficient confidential case-history, for this brief anecdote. I never asked him. The Colonel was an unknown warrior.

Our wartime hero died shortly afterwards; and, of the truth as to his past, I knew only that as of our sad, young ex-nurse Jenny — who presently lived, but whose schizophrenic illness would worsen in the years ahead. Pain and suffering, years and years and years of it — how much *did* that poor man endure, that unknown past prisoner... and of poor Jenny, her years to come?

Mr Peter Jackson was sat out by the side of his bed, with a blanket over his knees and another draped around his shoulders. Julian had asked me to do a mid-afternoon tpr round, on several of the recent admissions. It was subnormal, 96.5° fahrenheit. Almost teatime, last visitor departed. Harry was in the office, with Julian. I was used to quiet, depressed patients who, had with inactivity and medication, become perhaps a trifle obese. But, it helped to know something of a person, what they normally (pre-morbid) looked like, and of their temperament and personality.

His face was fat and puffy, like soft pastry, with no lines of animation; and his hands and fingers were equally thick and dry (almost flaky). Mr Jackson's hair was sparse. I didn't know whether he had recently lost any or not, though the scalp was visibly, flaky dry. He mumbled rather than spoke any coherent replies; locomotion was very slow and clumsy, noticeable when he was having his meals (he kept on losing his spoon or dropping his beaker, and had to be fed).

But it was when he put his hand up to his face with those red cheeks, like a clown, rouged, as I waited to remove the thermometer, I noticed there was no indentation, in the otherwise yellowish tinged tissue — there was no-elasticity. His pulse was quite sluggish; and respiration.... so shallow, I thought. Ah. Myxoedoema. The Handover of the previous day, and my chat with Julian about the endocrinal disorders, was still quite fresh. It was not therefore so surprising that, on my return to the office, I reported my findings, and I asked Julian if Mr Jackson had been diagnosed *Myxoedoema* — a low condition resulting from a deficiency, and a lack of secretion, of the thyroid gland. Julian replied, clearly well pleased, 'Well done, Barry. Yes, it was confirmed this morning, with the lab analysis report returns.' Aside, lean Harry nodded. 'Mr Jackson's basal metabolic rate is definitely too low — a strong symptom.'

'What treatment...?' I asked Julian, though I guessed the answer from my textbook notes. Thyroid extract, with a starting dose of 30 mg, to increase slowly, to prevent toxicity. His wife visited the ward the following day, and was relieved that a diagnosis and treatment had been realized. She also confirmed the other symptoms — per textbook. I recall how delighted I was at that detection; and understood why my Charge did *not* want me to read those case notes, before seeing the patient on the ward.

Mr Jackson made a remarkable recovery, on his prescribed medication, and recommended diet, and was soon discharged. His *psychiatric episode* was fortunately brief, though not knowing the primary cause as to why his thyroid was deficient meant that he might be on a thyroid extract the rest of his life — or not. I would never know. His was a benign quick exit departure, from the hospital.

It would be twenty years on, before I read Dr. A.J. Cronin's book, *The Citadel*[15]; and of his fictional Dr. Manson's discovery, of Emylin Hughes' Myxoedoema. In time to prevent him being sectioned, into a mental hospital. I recall a chronic depressed patient, in the Shoreham, West Sussex community, who described to me his mother having treatment, in Harley Street, for Myxoedoema depression, in the mid-1920s, and her being given raw-liver extract. She too fully recovered.

Incident

Still outside. No wind. The wintry morning almost over; two of us were in quiet routine with our settled patients; and a late hour's silence, in satisfaction, as John and I prepared for the midday lunches arrival on the ward. Julian was attending the drugs trolley, (checking its recent top ups for our residents), out of sight, around the corner. Staff nurse lean Harry was off-sick, with his turn of flu; and Dick, his opposite, had been feeling out of sorts yesterday; and so, we were unsure whether, or not, he would turn in this coming afternoon. Staff shortages... again.

The BBC news readers on the ward-radio, had occasionally interrupted a routine concert of music and rapid banter with their additions to a commentary we had been experiencing for some weeks, on the media, and on-going, about preparations for a real Moon Landing by an American scientific expedition — in the near future. Helpful orderly John, moved from bed to bed, patient to patient, to genially place a customary large ward-bib around those who needed it — several rather messy eaters also needed a half draw sheet placed over their top bed clothes, to protect their tender flesh, their bed linen, and their dignity.

I was preparing the two-tier wooden trolley on castors, to transfer the filled metal food containers, on to our lighter ward trolley. The kitchen's electric trolley, when detached, was left outside the ward entrance, full of our hot-food; and we placed the right number of dinner-plates (and pudding-plates - if required) in our ward kitchen oven to heat up, in anticipation. Most important; I anticipated when our patients were satiated, stacking the used and dirty plates, and prepared for later disposal of the used cutlery. I filled a large jug with hot soapy water to put the used cutlery in — a side container was also placed underneath, to later deposit the leavings into the pig swill bucket, kept under the kitchen sink; collected and re-cycled as per contract, for a local farmer's livestock.

The nursing staff were responsible for washing up the ward plates and cutlery, depending on the ward orderly, or capable resident who would likely assist, and the kitchen flat food containers emptied (though left dirty) and stacked back on the trolleys for later collection by a kitchen staff member. It was, in-sequence, well organised at every meal-time; and (as with all wards) the prescribed drugs ward round was generally delivered, in tandem with the meal time distributions. Good humour was in full supply, as orderly John exchanged good-cheer remarks with those patients who were capable of talk.

Bed one, vacated for such a short time, was presently occupied by a youngish epileptic Michael, off Eastergate Two ward. Although prone to regular fits, he was in for observation, but had no need of a bib. Bed two, other side of the table, and sat out, was an affable chap nick named Gannet, a chronic schizophrenic, also off of Eastergate Two (and same ward as Charlie Oak); an explosive messy eater, who enjoyed his food, *all* food (anyone's food), and had been known to devour quantities of wood and paper, under the aural instruction of one of his voices that he was eating choice delicacies.

And John placed a bib around messy James — The Gannet's neck.

'Wot we got, John?'; he enthused. 'Chicken Fricassee I think, Jim.' 'Smashin — plenty eh?' The Gannet, a lively bird, grinned in anticipation, for (though at times most unhappy) when not overwhelmed by hallucinations, James was a colourful, friendly chap.

And oh, oh yes, how Jim enjoyed his food!

The past few days had been quite rough for *The Major* (and neighbour William as helpless witness), who had been infected by a virus which triggered off a sequence of heavy, erratic behaviour, loss of appetite, and several gran-mals. But, today, he was much improved and, in the settled atmosphere of the ward, was feeling his normal mischievous self. As John applied the bib, and half draw sheet, The Major spluttered and gesticulated an enthusiastic reply, to John's cadenced — 'All right Major?'

William was, if anything, unusually quiet and inactive — sat out in DGO next to his bed and his friend The Major — one book, a pack of Players and an ashtray (no matches in sight), for Bill liked his occasional smoke — Parkinson's (pyramidal dysfunction) or not; all objects were placed neatly on one side of his adjacent table. He looked blankly at John, as a bib was gently placed around his neck, in anticipation.

The food-trolley was placed almost central, in the dormitory ward and, as I completed the transfer of the dinner trays onto the ward trolley, I noticed a concerned orderly John disappear for a moment around the corner — to call on our tuberculosis suspect, as we now knew patient John Evans to be. Evans was being barrier-nursed, in the single side-room. I knew our orderly would put on the Central Sterilized Supplies Department's pre-packed items of dress — including a face-mask. A supply of CSSD packs was conveniently placed outside his door on a small table; included were sealed sputum cups, and a supply of wooden spatulas.

The ward radio was not on, at this time, and only the sound of our leather foot-falls, the occasional clatter of dinner-plates, clinking cutlery, and the sound of our occasional voices echoed about the ward. On completion of preparations for lunch, we had begun serving, when, as Julian came out to join us, the phone in the nursing office rang shrilly, and Charge returned to answer the call. Trouble...

Moments later, and Julian emerged from the ward office, holding the long white crash box under his arm. 'Sorry lads, must dash, emergency on Eastergate...', and Julian swiftly exited out of the ward. Such Emergencies were not at all unusual, as sometimes staff or patients (like out-patients) arrived on the sick-ward for first-aid treatment, or to collect equipment not available in their own ward clinic rooms.

John and I continued to serve out our bedridden patients' food. Jim Gannet received his usual substantial portion; fricassee in its white sauce, mashed potatoes and peas. The next patient was being served when I looked at the check list (specials, diets, requests), and noticed one of the dietary specials was missing. 'John could you go down to the kitchen, and collect Fred's diet order. Shouldn't take long but, if it looks as if there is going to be some delay, better leave the request, and come back to the ward.' 'No problem, Barry - shan't be a jiff ....' And orderly John left the ward.

On my own (as staff), I continued to serve the patients down the right side of the dorm. The Major was all ready contentedly, slowly (he enjoyed chicken dishes), ploughing in his way, making his usual splutter and mess but, no matter, he was prepared. William was even slower, a little out of my sight as, sat out the other side of The Major, I could only see his top half.

And then. It happened very, very quickly. Must have been two or three minutes only, after John departed for the kitchen... As I was loading another plate, from my centre point in the middle of the room, I looked up abruptly, as I heard a loud gagging, spluttering, choking noise, which was all too obvious. (The radio tannoy was off.) It was incoming from Jim Gannet. But, and *at that same moment,* as I looked out, scanned, across the ward in enquiry, I couldn't miss seeing a distinct spiral of smoke from, it seemed, about Parkinsonian Bill's bed place — it didn't register as a cigarette spiral as it was too discoloured.

What was it?

I could see The Major gesticulating, close to panic, as he pointed downwards to his neighbour; and William, well, he was incredibly, inactive — just sat. Something was clearly on fire, though only smoke was visible from my vantage point. Decisions - decisions ...?

Putting a half-filled plate down and a large serving-spoon; I quickly strode the few yards over to Gannet Jim's choking, struggling form; his two hands were up to his throat; though he was making no-attempt to pull whatever obstruction, out of his mouth or gullet. Eyes were already bulging, his face moving from bright red to purple, and sort of blueish as I reached him; sat slumped in the long-back bedside chair.

No time to waste. ...

My hands, fortunately, were rather lean, thin, and bony long-fingered. And, so holding the nape of his neck in my left hand, I adroitly reached into his mouth with my right hand and, yes, just *visible* and protruding, was a longish, thin, chicken bone, that had found its way into the supposed bone free dish. And in Gannet's rush to stuff the popular food into his mouth (in order to ask for more) too much too fast, the unwanted item was not observed, as he attempted to swallow the mass. It had jammed at the top mouth of his gullet and, fortunately for him, was still accessible from his open mouth...

Folding my hand inwards, so the finger-ends would clamp together within the tender wet cavern of his mouth; innermost reaching, I luckily, straight away, achieved meeting of my right thumb and second index finger (adjacent to the little digit), as they felt for, and then instantly clamped upon, the intruding, thin, bone; and, swiftly, I withdrew the foreign obstruction altogether — out.

Jim Gannet had all too frequently experienced *choking* episodes in the long and recent past; and, so, he suffered no panic (more acute physical discomfort) during this incident; and, bone gone, he instantly relaxed, though I insisted he kept his head down between his legs as I, again swiftly, strode off — this time towards the vicinity of William; our distressed Bill.

It couldn't have been more than a maximum of ninety seconds, from arresting Jim's choking to moving up to Bill, and the ascending smoke signals. The Major, huffed and puffed his food remainder as it was displaced onto the half-sheet; placed in his concave lap — but his urgent, sentinel eyes had well taken in my episode with The Gannet; and he flashed clear approval, and signal relief, as I arrived at his neighbour's side.

At a glance I saw that a much shaking rattling Bill had somehow obtained a light, for one of his Players, and chosen to first smoke, rather than partake of his chicken fricassee placed in front of him. But his malady had got in the way, and his head was shaking in-time with tics, twitching tremors visible in both his hands which were now still shaking, dropped for the moment, by his sides. The lighted cigarette had dropped down, into the folds of Bill's dressing gown, a sump shaped between his slightly chattering, vibrating, knees. Collected in this fold were some morsels of food, which had likely prevented the lighted, smouldering fabric of his dressing gown, from accelerating into flame.

Two strides behind Bill's chair, and I borrowed The Major's tall plastic jug of lemon barley off' the top of his bedside locker, and immediately doused an emerging flame. Soaked desperate Bill was himself unharmed, the only visible damage was to his dressing gown, rather wet and messy; and, to his dinner tray, upside down upon the floor, with its previous contents well scattered about his feet. Relief. No real harm done.

On impulse, I again returned to Jim Gannet, who to my relief had made a full recovery. As a precaution I'd decided, temporarily, to remove Bill's box of matches which appeared on the top of his opened packet of twenty Players. And as I picked the offending matches up; so obvious why; to my surprise, grateful Bill, spluttered, and stuttered out 'Th-th-anks - B-b-b-a-ree-sss-o-rr-ee...' Sympathy full, I replied, 'Accident, Bill. I'll return your matches later — okay?'

'Sh-sh-ure.' Deciding to clear up later on, I returned to the dinner trolley and its routine, to finish the interrupted distribution. Unaware, orderly John reappeared only moments later, and I briefly told him of the two ward incidents. We'd just finished the mopping up ablutions, and changed Bill's dressing gown, when Julian arrived back from his life-and-death errand. And, of necessity, the two accidents were again related, before I was instructed to fill in, as mandatory, an Accident *Incident Form* (one copy to administration, and a copy into the file) — for each event.

It was Wednesday afternoon, and Mrs. Rita Argus, The Major's good wife, was now expected, sharp at two o'clock. We were still sharing with several patients, all of us enjoying a few chocolates from her last gift, of an large two-pound box of Cadbury's Black Magic, given to the ward staff on her last visit. At home, I had two, new, red velvet cushions, made by Mrs. Argus, and purchased by me for a Christmas charity collection.

After a short break, at the afternoon Handover, I returned to duty for my overtime afternoon shift, with Charge Nurse Simon; Dick indeed off-sick with influenza (he'd phoned in). I was on another long-day.

A seconds' long loud wheezing emitted from Joseph Ferret, in bed seven, top corner end right of the dormitory; and booming sounds stormed into my ear, through the cold flat metal drum, of the ward stethoscope. Julian had asked me to attempt a respiratory reading and since this act, with this always basic but impressive clinical instrument challenged my limitations, Joe's rhythmic, or rather irregular, staccato made the task quite awkward, as he laboured so hard to breathe. It was early evening.

Amongst poor old Joe's catalogue of problems, he was catheterized, and suffering from poisonous uraemia. His lung's tidal waves were descriptive of cheyne-stokes respiration. Between, apnoea, *cessation* of breathing, and hyper apnoea *deep-breathing* desperation; his battered abdominal muscles struggled to maintain a last hold on his life existence. After completing the reading, I returned the stethoscope to a diagnostic tray; marked his chart; read his bag's urine-content level, and dutifully changed the bag, for the night.

I reported into the ward office and, then, departed to the ward kitchen to collect the dentures tray, for the evening's round assembly of patients' false-teeth. Julian reminded me of doing a Nursing Summary Case note on Mr Ferret, and several others I had been involved with, during that working shift. (Harry was about night medication.) ... A patient had died of pneumonia — whilst I was on duty. 'And, Barry, you'll have a good half hour left, before the night staff arrive and handover, why don't you look through some old Case notes?... It'll give you some insight into past Asylum life; and tell you about some old treatments. And you will learn something more about individual long-term patients; who, like old Joe Ferret, have been in and out of this hospital for up to forty years, or more.'

'Thanks Julian.'

Case notes

I rinsed the name taped plastic containers, and filled them, adding one large white, flat round steradent tablet, which dissolved in the water, ready to receive the evening's consignment of dentures to be left, overnight, in the kitchen.

I mused on how much, insidiously, the psychiatric institution had changed in recent years and was likely to continue to change, with new ideas, new politics, and hopefully some new *scientific* discoveries, on biological orientated mental illness.

And, as Julian sagely reminded, the volumes of patients' case notes were social histories in miniature, of psychiatric hospital life. It wasn't obvious (for there was no requirement to challenge, or was there?) that all Textbooks, including our *Red Handbook*, were, in their time, finite sets of information, to any New student-intake's commencement in the hospital employment. Any recent changes and *new* ideas (where so, like Doctor Laing, Dr. Cooper, Erving Goffman and Professor Michel Foucault) were far *too* recent to enter, and to challenge, as later chapters of content, in our 1960s current mandatory textbooks.

But; so many of our patients (and staff) had had *vivid* experience of *past* treatments; and the fruits of *past* legislature changes, and subsequent provisions. Back on the *Dentures Round*; moving past epileptic Michael, and Jim Gannet. John Evans was well on the road to a full recovery, now safe out of *the barrier* and watching the very popular police series *Z Cars* on television — he had no dentures.

The Major, and his neighbour friend William, owned their own teeth (the latter, as with all sat-outs, now put back to bed). The friends were already half asleep in a half light, cast through the nearby curtains drawn tall windows; outside, winter was coming to an end; strong, howling, winds and heavy sounding rain diminished the continuity of hoar frosts — but they were all, thankfully, snug.

Joe Ferret, well asleep, owned dentures, but they had already been placed in a closed container for some days — he was only able to take in occasional liquids. Several of the remaining patients needed precautionary removal of well-worn sets. It was not uncommon for sick and confused residents to choke on dislodged dentures; directing my folded-in right hand, in a clamp used not long ago in a routine rescue of Jim Gannet, wet and a bit mucky, one of the patients, alert but confused, needed two staff for a safe action - the task was soon completed. And the dentures tray was removed to the ward kitchen, then covered over with a clean-cloth for the night's duration.

Julian was on the phone, as I re-entered the office, having first made our evening tea (patients' cocoa and ovaltine or tea on request, had already been distributed), so I advanced on Julian with his cuppa. Staff Harry was sat down chatting, medicines and ablutions completed, round the corner, with John Evans. They were watching television, as I took two hot cuppas, *Ovaltine* to John, around to them.

Minutes later, I collected Volume six of Joseph Ferret's Case notes, lights on now, and, contentedly, sat down at the ward dormitory table with my own cuppa, and begun to thumb its pages and to add on my own notations, of today's date. From the seeming far-off top-right (bed seven) corner, the loud staccato echoes of old Joe's whistle, wheezing and then awesome silences in-between — distanced the nearby subdued television — and any whispers of John Evans, and lean Harry in conversation, were sussurated, in consideration of our sleeping charges.

As I perused Joe's Case notes, I was only too aware of the absent earlier other thick volumes; years of probable content, about Joe's life.

I had all ready perused, occasional, other *Case notes* files, on a variety of male and female wards, whilst on overtime; considerable historical information was self-evident, showing Medication underwent radical merit changes only a decade or so before.

Medicine Cards, kept in file, proved that, after many years use (for example), *Paraldehyde* had ceased to be the main stabilising prescribed drug; and in 1957, *Chlorpromazine,* a Major Tranquilliser, first appeared in Graylingwell, as a new stabiliser. And *Tofranil,* an Anti-depressant, with the *MAO* prescribed drugs, which followed a little later...

Between 1957 and 1960, *at least* twenty-four New prescribed drugs appeared in common use in the hospital. An Australian medical colleague reminded me that *Lithium-carbonate* (I had seen *Priadel,* its other name, in use for Manic-Depression on the Amberley Admission Ward), had been around sometime in the 1940s, used in clinical, military research, but didn't formally emerge till post war years, in the 1950s.

*Haloperidol (*seranace) and *Orphenadrine* (disipal) were two other prescribed drugs, which soon became effective for long-suffering schizophrenics. And, although side effects contra indications were an inevitability, the gross effects of those *New Drugs* was almost miraculous in subduing dire symptoms, such as being out of touch with reality. Together, they allowed many, non forensic patients a resumed, *even if occasional*, contact with a terrestrial reality, both personal and social, and enabled them to be discharged back *Into The Community;* even if there was no fantastic cure-all, for all-and-everything maladies.

Most of the patients' *Case notes* volumes recorded past, now defunct, clinical treatments; and, as an eager press media topically confirmed, from the late 1930s until the 1960s, physical based clinical treatments were *very* much in demand. And, in *all* textbooks of that period, Medical, Nursing (RMPA and RMN), and other professions, it was *essential* that qualified-staff knew and practised those then common-place psychiatric treatments.

Presently, my own *1964 Syllabus and Practice Record*, included under Section 1, a sub-heading *Nursing care in special treatments* :

(1) Electro-convulsive therapy (ECT)
(2) Narcosis-therapy
(3) Narco-analysis
(4) Special drugs
(5) Pre-frontal leucotomy
(6) Other forms of surgical treatment -

Of this list - (2), (3) and (5), I had had no personal experience of in their application. Noticeably, *Deep Insulin Therapy*, - and the sub-coma *Modified Insulin Therapy,* for a time so prevalent, had ceased to be used altogether — though the latter, too, had stopped less than a decade ago. The introduction of the new *phenothiazine drugs*, and increased application of ECT, aided the end of Insulin Therapy.

The *Case notes* disclosed that in the 1950s, *all* of the above Treatments[16] were in multiple use, for many hospital in patient residents, and for selected out patients. A New Insulin Ward was constructed, in Graylingwell, in 1957— but the room was never used, it was in the top corridor, on the east corner, and, in 1968 was used as a patients' small library. *Deep Insulin* was in use for Schizophrenia, in 1955, when one male patient had refused to go into a coma despite a high dosage, a published Annual Report recorded. He was a schizophrenic, with a severe obsessional state with many *new* delusional ideas...

Fortunately, *Case notes* disclosed that, mercifully, no more GPIs were being admitted, at this time, thankfully due to the post-war New drugs. And *leucotomy*, in use since 1942, and now very little used (not at all in this hospital now in the late 1960s) had been given to a total of 532 past patients with numerous successes, out of thousands of long-term suffering patients sadly, formerly, deemed, *in those years*, as incurable. [17]

Changes

I read, from those old Notes and Records, the frequent use of our psychiatric hospital's own Operating Theatres. The last one *in use,* was sited opposite Amberley One Admission Ward, across the corridor in what was, one time earlier still, a communal bath-house, on the 1894 plans. After the operation theatre became redundant, since its cessation in the early 1960s, it was then, in 1968, space for the Porters' lockers and changing rooms.

From the 1950s and into early 1960s, just before my arrival in '67, psychiatric student-nurses would have had to have served four-months training, at the operating theatres of the Royal West Sussex, down the road, before returning to Graylingwell. Julian, lean Harry and Staff Tom on Amberley, for example, had all had considerable experience in the operating theatres, as had most other experienced qualified psychiatric staff — and those notes indicated resident patients who had had operations in *this* hospital and experienced, over the years, a cumulative cocktail of those *past* fashionable clinical treatments...

It was also clear from residents' files, and confirmed with colleagues who trained pre 1964, that the former RMPA workload and Syllabus was *very*, very much more comprehensive, than our present agenda. Not surprising, when one realized their required knowledge of *essential* general, medical and current nursing procedures. And, aware of how many childbirths and children; and *Mentally Handicapped*, of all ages, were resident *here* before the *Mental Deficiency Acts,* emptied some wards, their residents transferred to deemed, other, *specialist* facilities, before the onset of the second world war.

A substantial amount to be cared for by pre 1960s staff, were among those numerous *infected* residents with venereal diseases; and terminal GPI residents, placed out in the isolated Sandown House. And those *older* staff, who had also cared for numerous tuberculosis patients (consumption in old notes); and a *spectrum* of ailments that were previously absorbed and treated as *sick* within the psychiatric hospital estate; and *not* sent down the road, or elsewhere.

Much was being spoken nowadays, in the late 1960s, of new *Multi-disciplinary* teamwork possibilities, with *Therapeutic* [18] regimes and *Communities...* Pre 1963 Annual Reports described an attempt to also expand *Psychoanalytic* work, in the 1950s and early 1960s, and of the numerous skilled (and unskilled) tradesmen, agricultural workers and stockmen; who were employed working sometimes alongside recovered or recovering patients - on *The Farm* ...

Now, too, gone, the farm workers dcparted.

And, further back, reflecting the outside social structure of those years — and integrated sub-culture of the hospital, employed servants (1920s and before). And those patients and staff *Archives* recorded hospital staff as bandsmen and firemen — most nurses (qualified and unqualified) and nursing attendants in then Health & Safety necessary multi roles.[19]

And more, we'll never know of...

Most older staff, and certainly many of our present patients *still* in hospital had, indeed, worked on the farm, in the laundry, tailors, carpenters, bakers, in the cookhouse, painters, printers, upholsterers... as carters, gardeners, coal-heavers, shepherds, dairymen, domestics, and about those patients'— parents, relatives, friends and their past recorded lives — how were *they* recorded, in those volumes of case-histories...?

The whole foregoing was easily reflected, in the thousands of volumes of *Case notes,* and formally audited and recorded data, for posterity, in the formal Annual Reports, Archives, Medical Records and ephemeral records of the Administration... Although the full-range of physical treatments were all, but ECT, mostly already extinct; as referred to earlier, I was expected to have knowledge of those psychiatric methods...

The following *Summary* notes were written by an anonymous senior nursing colleague when a student in the late 1940s and early '50s - on *Carbon Dioxide Therapy* , and is quite informative. [20]

> 'This treatment has been found of great advantage in early neuroses, chiefly from the point of view that except for attending an out-patient's clinic 2/ 3 times per week the patient may continue their normal activities, and this reason alone makes them more willing to have treatment. The CO2 makes the patient more susceptible to a mild form of CO2 therapy, and it does *not* give the patient any dread of their next treatment. Preparation. Oxygen 70% — CO2 30% Cylinder: Gags: Airways: Sterilized Syringes and needles: Coramine: Labeline: B.P. apparatus: French needle .... The patient should be warned *not* to have a heavy meal prior to treatment (the reason being since they will be unconscious there is the danger of vomiting — hence aspirated pneumonia).
>
> All tight clothing should be loosened, and in such a state that injections and artificial respiration may be readily carried out. At the first treatment the patient is given 10/15 inhalations, this is subsequently increased slowly at each treatment until a state of Apnoea is reached (number varies widely with different patients). Signs and Symptoms before Apnoea is reached include: profuse sweating, dilated pupils, either increase or decrease of pulse, bp pressure also varies. 30/ 60 treatments are given during each course.'

I found *Carbon Dioxide Therapy,* in reading, initially quite a puzzle. And, of the other treatments, *out of their time and context.* It was *impossible* to properly gauge, to guess or assess, for example, ECT's efficacy, controversial though it would always be. It appeared to have *proved* to me then, as witness, to have its successes with depressed patients — but always, too, I would wish for other alternatives. For a while, I became engrossed with curiosity on the merits, and demerits, of those hard, physical treatments for psychiatric maladies, which appeared at their height in the 1940s and 1950s, in the U.K. and abroad. And such was reflected in so many of those old case notes...

Hospital staff (and, later — patients) I interviewed, who'd worked or had experienced these therapies; even one Sister who had managed a *Deep Insulin* and *Modified Insulin Ward* (over on Summersdale); were very clear in their memories of its efficacy — and apparent faults. Some of those staff spoke to me about them as too, subsequently, did a number of patients, who had undergone these treatments. *Deep Insulin* was remembered, by one colleague, as '*very labour intensive, quite frightening at times, one could* never *leave a patient*'. And, quizzed on its patient value — intensity of physical care and attention appeared essential. How this awesome treatment was presented depended *very* much on attitudes *and* an essential quantity of *Qualified* attending staff; as well as its application, *and* after-care facilities. The cessation of *Deep Insulin* was (it seemed) received with considerable relief by staff (and patients?), and released numerous qualified staff, in the U.K. hospitals, for other duties.

After release of the 1948 USA Oscar film *The Snake Pit,* in an English *Picture Post,* of June 1949 a journalist, *Joan Skipsey* [21] wrote, '*I worked In A Snake Pit*' about her personal experience, *as* a volunteer at '*Topeka State Hospital, in Kansas USA*', an American state hospital, which could *not* obtain any, let alone enough, untrained ward attendants — there were no Qualified staff available. 'After just a quick briefing', Skipsey wrote, 'I was turned loose on half a dozen women emerging from insulin shock treatment.' A sad extreme... I noted, *no* mention of *any* available *qualified* USA psychiatric nursing staff, a depressing account; in great contrast to UK superior staff facilities.

Also on the USA *debit* side, Carl Solomon, an American Beat poet, quoted in 1959 book *The Beat Generation,*[22] of his experience, in receipt of *fifty* deep insulin comas. He recalled, in his memoirs, albeit dramatically, being:

> 'forcibly administered in the dead of night by white-clad, impersonal creatures who tear the subject from his bed, carry him screaming into an elevator, strap him to another bed on another floor, and who, later, recalled him from his reverie...'

Beat Poet Carl Solomon also wrote in *Neurotica.*[23] of his retrospect Kafkan fear, and poetic paranoia. He quoted, (amongst others), Hoch and Kalinowski's work, on *Shock Therapy.*[24] And, of the European, French Surrealist poet, Antonin Artaud's published prose (post-humous) of February 1949 *Les Temps Moderries* — about dire experiences, of electric and insulin shock therapies. Artaud was confined in the French' *Rodez* asylum, for nine years — and died in March 1948. Whatever extreme *debit* views Solomon, as a patient, described on *Deep* Insulin, it was sadly remembered as a *coma void* and, clearly, was most traumatic — recalled as a most unpleasant experience .

In rank contrast, *Modified Insulin* in Graylingwell Hospital, Sussex, was recorded with *merit* accounts — as my hospital staff *and* patient informants recalled — it was sometimes given as night sedation, so, when the patient awoke in the morning, they would feel absolutely ravenous; able to *enjoy* eating and being fattened up. It was then used to *increase* one's physical health, *and* vitality, and helped *decrease* depression. *Modified Insulin* appears to have been more successful. But, with the entrance of the new phenothiazines, combined with a sequence of ECT treatments (two or three in a week); so all Insulin Therapies in the United Kingdom, made their exit.

Narcosis therapy and narco analysis; otherwise known as *Continuous Narcosis;* a *continuous sleep,* in the treatment of acute anxiety (a neurotic state) followed a period of severe stress; this was another physical treatment prevalent until the late 1950s. An enforced rest, lasting up to four weeks, it was very *risky* for patients — with poor physical health.

When I asked colleagues, about this *continuous sleep* therapy, they remarked how *labour intensive* (as Insulin treatments) it was — in *their* personal experience. 'I remember', one nurse colleague informed me, 'having to wake them up regularly, to ensure they ate and drank — and the physical checks before putting them back under — it seemed always fraught with risk. Two of us holding a patient up (who wanted to get back to sleep) and, walking up and down, up and down, up and down; and of frequently turning them over...'

Even more risk-laden and controversial was *Pre-frontal Leucotomy.* I had only met one patient who had, recently, been in receipt of a *partial-leucotomy*; and, after some weeks absence I met him, on the way over to see someone in Summersdale Villa, with his head well covered in bandages; he admitted feeling very much better — at that time.

Pre-frontal leucotomy, also known as *lobotomy*, was suggested by the neurologist Moniz in 1935; as a treatment for *intractable* mental stress, tension, psychotic violence and, or suicidal depression. Selected white-fibres from the frontal-lobes were surgically removed, which reduced or removed their stress; and which surgery otherwise was believed, to minimally interfere with the patient's other faculties — and irreversible. During the first years of its use, I learnt it did, indeed, give hope to numerous diagnosed 'hopeless' chronic mentally ill patients. Introduced into Graylingwell, in October 1942 (the same year as Deep Insulin), for a selected few females only, to start with, due to an acute staff shortage. Yet, in 1946, The Graylingwell's *Annual Report* officially recorded that 319 patients who'd experienced pre-frontal leucotomy, with *236 recovered...* improved, 83 had *not* improved. Optimism, in post-war years. A popular U.K. weekly magazine, *Illustrated*[25], reported enormous optimism *at that time,* towards any new *physical* treatments. The magazine, with graphic illustrations, enthused:

> 'Leucotomy. This is the name of a brain operation which gives a new personality and a fresh outlook on life to certain sufferers from mental illness.'

And, weeks later, in follow up, published a similar enthused article — on Electrical Shock Treatment aka EST. - in 1947. [26]

I stumbled in my reading, on a Science Fiction pb novel entitled *Limbo '90.* [27] This fiction made full use of the growing new physics, called *Cybernetics* Technology. There were to be the electric machines of Norbert Wiener [28] and other post-war scientists, inventing electric and solar-fed computers, with replicated robotic-brains, extra strong false-limbs, and numerous support drugs — new bio-medicines, anticipating many moral, inevitable *legal* and political issues. They were the Shape of Things to come, which would arrive soon enough. Dr. Martine, in the novel, suggested the use of 'lobotomy', in dealing with intractable crimes of violence; forensic brain surgery, as a solution. He was, in no way, the first — or last — to suggest specific clinical psychiatric treatment, for deemed chronic, mentally-ill. In his futuristic novel, moral issues were explored, in medicine and philosophy — kept in perspective. In Wolfe's novel, towards the future (then) time of 1990 — science-fiction time, when men would have begun: 'to mutilate their minds and bodies voluntarily, in the search for a less aggressive existence.'[29] In the years ahead, I would meet, and hear, of many people who had had a leucotomy, and a number of persons who had had *more* than one such brain operation — but were well enough able to get married, and *remain* in the community.

One young woman in the 1950s, an *extreme* case, had a catalogued, seemed *hopeless,* track of violence recorded in her file, and experienced a partial leucotomy — only to need another some years later. Another anecdote had recalled a desperate father, a London surgeon who, in the 1950s surge of optimism, wanted his so sick daughter to undergo that operation.[30] *Operations,* neurological or whatever, however sad and deemed necessary, were generally *not* forensic, but prescribed *to cure* or *relieve* whatever deemed intractable an unhappy condition. Much, perhaps, as a Heart operation, or other organic op prescribed in General Medicine. If subsequent side-effects were gauged, to become a *lesser* suffering. It was deemed a risk, worth the taking; in that perspective, Surgery was a believed worthy option, filled with hope; and offered in good-faith — in its time....

As a rider; in one of many debit *and* merit letters to *Picture Post,* following an excellent published article entitled *Life In A Mental Hospital*[31], a grateful reader wrote a very long, heart rending response, whereupon they had complained that, for over a year, he or she had campaigned to obtain ECT treatment for a loved relative, who *needed* to be certified into a Mental Hospital... eventually, the patient was moved into a Private Mental Home in the community. And, after giving considerable further background, the *Grateful Reader* concluded that the patient *did* obtain a course of ECT, *and made a complete recovery.*

Cynics, reading the above quotes, on the *merit* side of critiques, could construe its invention; but a full reading of its text appeared to the contrary in the integrity of *The Picture Post.*[32] And then, English *Woman's* magazines, all published credit, and debit, commentaries. They presented balanced perspectives, on ECT, on the available treatments in Psychiatry, *and* other helpful contemporary, topical, physical and psychiatric treatments — on offer in post-war years.

There were, in addition, other physical treatments administered, from the end of the 1930s into late 1950s: and, to be found in old hospital *Case-notes* — the files still in use. *Cardiazol Treatment,* another example, was used for a short time with *Insulin* Therapy, to treat chronic schizophrenics, but soon discontinued. *Malaria* induced shock treatment for then, selected, intractable GPI (General Paralysis of the Insane) patients, resident in the *Isolation Hospital* within the hospital grounds — later called Sandown. Sufferers, with advanced syphilis venereal disease (two such patients were treated, and recorded dated 31st December 1945) published in the hospital's retrospect *Annual Report,* of 1946.

Mass readings of patients' *Case notes,* and ongoing media's reflections (sometimes frenetic convulsions upon these subjects), gave me very considerable additional insight into some background about our patients' histories. But also, it reflected prejudices, fears, the hopes and temper of the times they were introduced into. Most important I wondered, in the compass of my enquiries, *what* patients, their relatives and friends had thought, about those myriad treatments. And, with little doubt, I knew much of those social comments too, *are* written into those file case notes.

It was anathema, absurd, to expect someone to say *I enjoyed my despair.* And so, collectively, we the staff had *a duty to care*, and so much care was to be found, on perusal of those patients' notes. During many years afterwards, where so, I would hear from their own lips, what *some* of our ex-hospital patients in the community recalled, of those old physical treatments. What was often generally remarked, past patients felt, was quite positive. *'Something'*, they said, *'was at least, attempted, to make me better!* '

Another Incident

The sound of breaking glass, and a loud inclement exclamation, propelled lean Harry and I out of the office; to a source, immediately self-evident, towards The Major and friend neighbour William's corner.

A very distressed Bill lay stretched out on the floor, alongside his friend's bed, surrounded by shattered glass off a former bottle of barley water — and (how?) a cast down plastic urine-bottle, its content emptied and diluted around his upper torso. Poor Major was absolutely distraught, spluttering, shaking, his eyes blinked like castanets; and hands and arms attempting to reach downwards, as he leant over at plus forty-five degrees, legs frozen to the mattress beneath him; he was not fitting — but quite hysterical.

With Harry and I at each arm-pit we, gently, lifted frail Bill up, and helped him on to his bed. Fortunately, though uncomfortably wet, the shards had not jagged him. I went to The Major to straighten him up, and reassure him that it was '*just an accident*', adding a rider 'honestly no real harm done', for the also benefit of Bill's recovering earshot.

Lean Harry strode off to Julian in the nursing office, to phone for the duty doctor to attend, as soon as possible, to Bill and The Major. Our orderly, John, was not on duty that day and so, soon as I was satisfied they were both warm and settled (and having changed Bill's wet-things, and tucked him back into bed), I cleared the mess up off the floor.

While we waited for the doctor, I set about another bottle and bag round; and mused how very grateful I was, for the revolutionary appearance of the Central Sterilized Supplies Department (CSSD), replacing the need for the otherwise essential and previous, tedious, time consuming practices of boiling, steaming, soaking (whatever) to *sterilise* sundry instruments. And that wrapped CSSD packages were now at hand when needed but *not,* yet, for everything. Not quite....

Taking the bottles out, I collected them in the metal-container kept for that purpose, resembling a wine-basket, or milkman's hand-carrier, and passed through the connecting door 'tween Chilgrove One and our England Ward. We did not have a separate ablution apparatus for sterilising, so I placed them within next door's large round metal-drum and, after emptying the unwanted contents, pulled the handle down to release the boiling water and contain its steam.

It was not uncommon for the sterilizing steam vessel to malfunction, and the resultant, inevitable hand-washing — the debit side of all those media descriptions of chirpy nurses with bedpans, et cetera. Dr. Champion soon arrived at the ward office and, with Julian and lean Harry, attended to our most recent casualties; which, after his examinations, fortunately proved the incident was not at all serious. Parkinson Bill had attempted to remove The Major's already half-full urine bottle out of its under-bed casket, and lift it up to his friend for further use, after recognising nonverbal communications — as NVC signals, given out by his neighbour. It had then proved *too* heavy for friend Bill. And, with sudden erupted Parkinsonian hand-shakes, he had been prevented from retaining a firm grip on the bottle's neck. Bill had, almost, triumphantly succeeded in the exercise, when he, and it, slipped, accidentally knocking down an unopened bottle of barley water, off the top of the adjacent bedside locker. And Bill, and the objects, had fallen onto the floor, much to the Major's witness horror.

I was a second-year RMN student, and talking at any length with a medical Consultant colleague was for me (then) a *rare* personal event — except for brief exchanges on the telephone, or as an attendant in the company of Julian,

Harry, or other more senior colleagues, at special clinic examinations. I didn't have the opportunity to speak with Dr. Champion. There appeared to be too few doctors, for our minimum 984 residents and out-patients, and other expected duties to be covered — for all seasons. Our doctors' time was precious....

Among my own, pre-student, RMN memories, I was reminded that previous experience of hospital clinical wards, and their rarefied Doctors, related mostly to distanced childhood traumas; except, more recently, I had, had a catarrhal operation at a mid-Sixties' North London general hospital for an inhibiting breathing nasal complaint which would, years later, cause me some grief. About that op — I recall with humour, a young female staff-nurse in *that* 1965 North London hospital, was about giving me a pre-op anaesthetic injection, in the backside, when her filled-needle *snapped* and, like a shorn plume-free arrow, looking behind me I saw *it* — a broken-lance reed, or feathered dart, sticking up like a *Carry on Nurse* daffodil behind me. But, fortunately, that human error had *not* deterred the operation's success. And neither did it deter, afterwards, the young woman nurse's anecdote attending my op — who insisted, that under the full anaesthetic's effect, I had subsequently, whilst unconscious, talked non-stop philosophy, peppered with numerous Herbert Spencer' references. I had been perusing Spencer's book, *First Principles* [33], which (amongst other reading matter) I had brought onto that hospital ward.

Retrospectively, many cartoon cardboard-images had told me more about the domestic romances of doctors-and-nurses, than of ward-culture in hospital day-to-day existence. I recall the delightful light-hearted rural-life scenarios, of *Doctor Finlay's Casebook* [34], adapted homely material from author Dr. A.J. Cronin's auto-biography, *Adventure in Two Worlds.* [35] (Dr. Finlay returning from the war.) Storylines, in his biography, were mostly in between the wars tales, in the village of Tannochbrae in Scotland. A postwar television series re-adapted the theme — from WW2 years. Enjoyable fantasy episodes, but inevitably and essentially, these were limited perspectives of an otherwise seemed taboo social reality — hospital life behind closed doors.

At the time, as a student in the sixties, I shared a more common view of most members of the public, a healthy respect for members of the medical profession — an almost God-like mystic Latin veiled image, with the physician's *special* trained knowledge and skills in mind. I was aware of a Consultant's long apprenticeship, usually thirteen years total training — a minimum in the 60s, I was informed. In the near future, I would be working with called-out qualified Psychiatrists on statutory Mental Health sections. Isolated in the community often, the two-of-us found in difficult forensic scenarios — at close quarters. And I appreciated this *vulnerable* human trait — ironically, this enhanced respect, rather than diminished the image.

In the not long-ago past (Gentry apart) Doctors and nurses, like Officers and other ranks, were poles apart in the social structure — during the Victorian age. My favourite Chichester East Street bookshop produced a late Victorian magazine article, headed *Hospital Days And Hospital Ways*[36], in which the female author, a writer named Mansford, wrote a benign record of her time as a patient at London's *Royal Free Hospital,* which confirmed this awe: '*After eight o'clock prayers were read, talking forbidden, the lamp lighted*, (and) *we were told to "lie down and go to sleep*." ' Distressed, through encountering an — *'abrupt house surgeon*', Mansford was pacified by '... the night-nurse, who said to cheer her... "*One must never mind what doctors do,"* she said, *"as to them we are like so many chairs and tables."...'*

A few minutes after Dr. Champion's England Ward departure, we had two visitors down from Bramber Two; Dougie, the Charge Nurse, accompanied a distressed, slightly bloody forehead Tall John. Bramber's clinic room had run out of specific CSSD dressing packs, and Doug deemed it prudent to render First Aid at our station, and collect new supplies for their return. Tall John had several small, bleeding, cuts on his forehead. I asked him how he obtained them, he replied, more irritated and petulant than suffering any dire pain: '*Tried to stop 'em. Knock some sense into myself – Dougie stopped me...*'. It transpired no-one had hit Tall John; he had *not* been in one of his all-too common fracas with somebody else...

Tall John had, bizarrely, crashed his fore-head against a corridor ward wall, until his head bled, and, until interrupted, by Doug, who consoled him and, after a quick visit to their own ward-clinic, had subsequently made their way to our sick-bay. I assisted cleaning Tall John up and, after adhering several light-dressings, rewarded him with a cigarette (rather Doug did); and our satisfied casualty strode off back into the corridor. In bland humour Charge would later make out yet another *Incident form* on Tall John; and would include in its contents; John said to me he wanted ... "*to knock some sense into myself*"...' It was as well he didn't have his glasses on, at the time of the accident (incident), or it would have been more serious; with broken-glass fragments to extract from his wounds.

Mid-afternoon; another bed round due, before patients' tea-time. We stopped for a cuppa — Dougie, now without his satisfied casualty Tall John, joining us. Julian had his beloved large twelve-stringed Spanish-guitar in the office, and was expanding on the merits of a concert, he and his wife had recently attended at Brighton. Lean Harry's wife was a trained nurse, and contributed a dramatic, but brief, anecdote on the nursing home of which Dora (his wife) was its Matron. Doug patiently waited to collect the box of CSSD supplies, from our new locked cupboard, which was around the corner, and adjacent to the connecting partition, with Chilgrove One ward.

I introduced, in conversation, the notion of a possible move for me and my family, from Chilgrove hamlet to Littlehampton by sea, in the near future... Sara, Paul, Kit, myself, and our recently acquired farm kitten, Shasa, a lively ginger and white streaked feline hunter...

Before drinking our warm cups to a dreg, we had further visitors. This time, Alan, a patient off Eastergate Two, who had recently returned from a spell-of-leave with a burn on his right arm. Formerly, the burn had been dressed by his local GP; he was now sent down off his ward for a change of dressing. I went off, to the white cupboard, for a tube gauze cotton dressing reel, and a CSSD burns' dressing-pack, with its brown coated honey comb like centre pad. I collected Doug's package, for Bramber Two Ward.

We had had a crisis with first bed Michael, yesterday. Redhead Mike had moved into a quite dramatic sequence of *status-epilepiticus* fits, one gran mal fit, following another and another and another — exhaustion alone would have finished Mike but, unconscious, he was given an intra-muscular valium injection, which had, fortunately, been successful and had arrested the fits. We had placed young Mike on a drip. He was presently sound asleep, but at least the troublesome fits had ceased.

Jenny had been able to assist on the ward, yesterday. But their Staff had phoned down this morning; Jen was unfortunately 'not well enough' to help out, today. It was unfortunate she'd been present, as witness, when Michael had initially commenced his long epileptic sequence; though that was to presume her intrusive *voices* were not soaking up her sensibilities. The Major always made a fuss of Jen when she was about the ward...

I was soon to finish this ward placement, and my tuition with Julian during that mid-morning (before the duty doctor arrived), was my last. As I left the office, after that last ward office teaching session, I sat down to the observation table, and checked additions signed by Julian in my *Practice Records Handbook...*

'Fractures; cardiac and pulmonary diseases; infirm; air-pillows electric-pads (special) blankets; food and fluid intakes; surgery; evacuent enemas; surgical techniques; instruments, catheters; bowls and utensils; syringes; lotions; dressing trolleys and ward dressings; examination (e.g.) — rectum; urine tests; cerebro-spinal fluid evacuation; intravenous infusions; lumber puncture; artificial feeding oral, nasal, gastric lavage; sutures; catheterisation; last offices: and more, more, more ...'

It had been a great placement. Extra-curriculum reading experiences had also been numerous — and always most personal. The importance of conscious, and more so, unconscious, in-numerable aspects of what were non verbal communications — linked conceptually with my other limited readings, and occasionally put to a test...

Non Verbal Communication

Responding to The Major's on-going NVC gesticulations, and earnest mumblings, I was immersed in a cadence of pure emotions (debit words), and attempted a spontaneous experiment. Instead of routine asking if he wanted a drink, or anything else, I recall doing specific hand jives and mouthing, pitched noises (viz. like The Major's) in exaggerated cadences; no song, no mockery, but my own earnest-murmerings, offered in good-faith; and deliberate... The Major paused, posture froze, and surprise in his eyes, and hand signs, NVC answered, in a distinct affirmation at the prospect — perhaps — of a new, but pleasant, game; it was an agreed emotional code; a new agreed one off set of rules...

As I stood at the side of his bed (as per normal), I then mouthed riff noises, deliberate, yet enthusiastic, degrees in linked dissonance. Our sounds sharp, and then flat (a little sibilant from The Major), but soft and respectful; and some fast. some slow. controlled in flow — attempting a minute piece of new NVC ground. It was an attempt at emotional music cadence communication — alone. No words allowed. And so, we concluded an unusual (for me) but brief, innocent exchange.

Neither of us were blind, or deaf, and certainly didn't own any formal sign language code; and so, it depended on use of our rapport, and a shared sense of humour, and mutual trust, for interpretation of those emotive murmurings. Despite the feeling of success, at that emotive experiment, I decided it was *not* to be repeated — apart from out of respect, and a liking for The Major; I concluded something about it could be morally wrong (there was no need), however innocent my intent. In retrospect, I laughed a little at myself; at that possible image to an observer, as a non-participant. It could've easily been viewed as meaningless noise, in grunts, groans, moans and staccato — a scene in a pantomime, but of care, no less.

And so, apart from an inevitable final track of routine incidents, and ever essential, numerous ablutions, my mandatory RMN three months placement (as such), came to an end on England sick-ward — though opportunities for overtime would continue, during my employment on our hospital estate. Another departure — more partings.

Table talk

School day — and lunch break, in the Blue Lagoon Grill Room. Just after one o'clock and shifts were changing over; as evident by the long-queue at the ordering counter. Painters, engineers, workshop employees, gardeners, physiotherapists, psychologists, MRC staff (notably, there were few medical colleagues, they appeared to prefer the waitress served Restaurant); numerous nursing staff, ambulance officers and drivers, a pharmacist, and a scattering of visitors. We all competed, patiently waited, for an early place in the single, orderly, line queue.

Rose, one of my student, group colleagues (from our assortative set) in advance of lunch orders, had sat down and reserved a table. We had two tables placed together, as all of our *original* student intake was present for the last time — Audrey, Harry, Rose, Sally and myself. Also present was Andrew (he'd asked to join us), a student MWO (supervised by George) and son of one of the hospital Consultant psychiatrists.

And last, a new acquaintance (to us) of Andy's was — Magda. I had last seen Magda on Summersdale, late last summer. Andy explained, in a polite introduction, that she was recently from Czechoslovakia and, herself, a trained nurse. *'Freedom*, that's what that's all about', declared Andy to all of us. He was reading from a recent newspaper report, in *The Evening Argus* (Brighton edition). 'Seven Flower People were arrested and taken to Court, for taking part in a "*paint-in*"; a psychedelic piece of graffiti painted upon a Brighton seafront wall.'

It was about psychedelic *Pop Art*...

Asylum Magda laughed, or rather wide-grinned like a proverbial Cheshire cat, her long dark-hair hanging over a worn-brow, and down, almost into her tomato-soup. The rest of us just ate, and listened as MWO student Andy continued the anecdote... 'The seven painters were taken to the Brighton police headquarters, over the last Bank Holiday weekend, and released without being charged, after ninety minutes.'

'Why? What did they do?' asked Magda.

Andy continued his topical reading, no comment — yet ... invited.

The Flower People, as they called themselves, had organized a team of painters, to cover the arches on the Lower Esplanade with rainbows and other murals, but the police stepped in, while the painting was still in progress.'

'Oh. I think it's lovely. Lovely. So — *so English,* I fink, eh?', added Magda, looking around our group sat round the table. '*If Only...* If Freedom, could be *so* simple, and *so* care-free?' she concluded, and sighed wistfully — her face downcast, and momentarily hidden from us, down crystal ball into her now, all ready luke-warm, soup.

Andy had then, meaningfully, completed his brief reading and, silently, put the paper down onto the floor, at his feet.

'Where are you working Magda?', I asked; very aware of the unspoken questions about her arrival, from an unsuccessful result of *The Revolution,* back in her home country, during that painful *Prague Spring* of '68.

'For two weeks, I work on Summersdale, now must work on Fawcett One. And I help look after what Sister Kelly call her *Babies.*', Magda said, in great and tender earnest.

When I had first heard *that* term — aged patients referred to as '*babies*', which was sometimes used by experienced nursing staff, on the long stay *female* back wards, of the Fawcett Block — I'd recoiled with an indignant, self-righteous horror, at its use. But, later, after considerable overtime on those wards, as a (then) lone male-student helping out, I came to acknowledge it was a *strong* word of care and affection, used when tending those very elderly, and mostly helpless, ladies who'd wholly lost their applied intellectual abilities and *most* of their physical controls. But — those aged patients *did* respond to the constant on-going TLC (tender loving care), given by their ward nurse care-takers.

The word *babies* was, I found, therefore used for those mostly helpless *specific* elderly residents. Was it not an oxymoron? Given that with such an intended grace, it was an opposite; not of a malice aforethought, that ignorant critics might deduce.

It was an instant bonding of its own, with Magda, as she warmly identified with Sister Kelly's use of the word Babies on F-Block — and, in dove and palm, from her experience, she talked volubly, to us, of her nursing such elderly sick-persons, back home in Czechoslovakia. Magda, soup finished, started on her salad, and carefully, brushed her hair back over the nape of her neck, with her left hand. We could not help noticing a recent long-scar, forming over the back of that hand, and another, ragged, scar, on her forehead; this was revealed briefly, in the act of putting the hair behind her.

As nothing was alluded to by anyone, not least our Czech refugee, at the table, her fresh scars were not enquired into. True, the scars could have had an origin not at all from those ongoing revolution activities; but good manners insisted we ignored them — unless, that is, Magda herself wished to introduce her so recent, pain filled, past history.

And her blue dress hospital uniform, of an auxiliary nurse, already formally now identified her at one with us, whatever her world origins. Magda sat opposite me. Andy, with his rosy-cheeked, round-face brown-eyes, still sparkling with enthusiasm, and his own black-hair, close-cropped cut neatly in an crew-cut, was wearing a smart single-breasted dark-suit and blue-silk-tie, sat on her right. Rose was on Magda's left. Shy Rose sat quietly, with her tomato soup and a buttered roll, which she nibbled slowly, and spoke not at all, content to listen, rather than join in our table-talk.

On my right sat Harry, his smooth skin, neat tight-curled hair and dark-eyes, with a pressed hospital charcoal grey suit — matching my own. Both our white coats hung-up on hooks, just inside the Grill Room entrance. He too, as Rose, sat quietly and ate his lunch. Occasionally, he smiled.... if a little wanly. Unlike the rest of us, Harry, more than anyone else at the table, could've identified with the painful revolutionary turmoil of Magda's European origins — with *his* own recent country's troubles, tribal class disputes, and post colonial traumas, he'd told me. Talks of Freedom and of bloodshed '*Back Home*' were, in sum, too recent, and too painful, for any light-hearted, table talk conversation, for Magda and Harry.

Sally, the youngest baby, and fairest of our group, was sat on my left. Sadly, that very morning, she had told us she would be leaving next month. Ironically, it was F-Block which had contributed to her sensibilities being over-reached —'*too much for me*', she had whispered, to our tutor and us at the nursing-school. And Sally's lean frame had winced, at Magda's mention of Sister Kelly and '*The Babies*'.

'I guess I'm too sensitive to distance myself — keep becoming emotional. It's *not* the Sisters' fault that I wince, sometimes, when I'm told off by them. I... I might... perhaps, come back into nursing, later.' She'd recently lost an elderly relative, and *that* death had deeply upset her. And Sally's bereavement — coupled with other domestic traumas, back home up-north, had tipped the balance. Sad, Sal' was to leave us shortly...

Worse — Audrey, too, was going from our company. She had almost completed SRN training, before leaving nursing the last time — and *now,* with eighteen months RMN almost up, was again to leave. Aud', said some colleagues, had *no* choice — wished she was *free* to make it, but had no-choice; single parent mum, with no supporting relative, or friend, to allow otherwise. About relative freedom?

So recent into our second year and, already, our Intake reduced to three students. The school had informed us that, due to economy, two new post-grad students would probably be joining Harry, Rose and I at our lectures, in the near future. This would bump the numbers up again? Our lunch table talk concluded, and we left the Grill Room, for our separate afternoon appointments.... And, there were more partings.

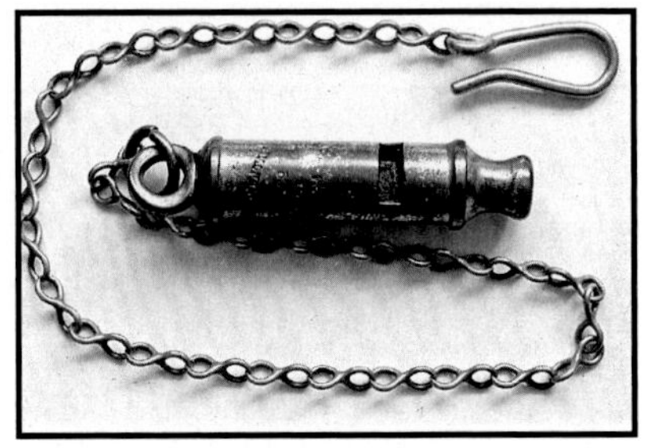

Attendants uniform whistle, from the 1920s.

[- FROM: 'ILLUSTRATED' MAG. FEB 8. 1947.]

5 CRUCIAL MOMENT IN THIS AMAZING OPERATION IS WHEN THE SURGEON, HAVING REACHED THE SKULL

LEUCOTOMY

PHOTOGRAPHED BY DESMOND LAING DESCRIBED BY STEPHEN BLACK

This is the name of a brain operation which gives a new personality and a fresh outlook on life to certain sufferers from mental illness

WHAT are mind and matter—and what, if any, is the difference between these two? For many thousands of years such problems have dominated the thoughts of philosophers and scientists alike. Have the great scientific advances of the last fifty years brought us any nearer to a solution of them?

Undoubtedly our ideas on *matter* have been greatly influenced by the atomic researches, but any advance towards a scientific understanding of the *mind* is still slow—and is often contested fiercely by those who seem to fear the illumination of tru

Nevertheless the picture is by no means as dim as it was at the beginning of the century. The cla fication is due to the work of those tradition enemies, the materialist physiologists and the psychologists.

In Russia the physiologist Pavlov rang a bell every time he offered food to his experimental dogs and noted the flow of saliva from their par glands. Then he started ringing the bell with offering food—and found that they salivated ju

1947. At the time of dire American *Snake Pit* asylum post-war reports - advanced British psychiatry had new physical treatments on trial.

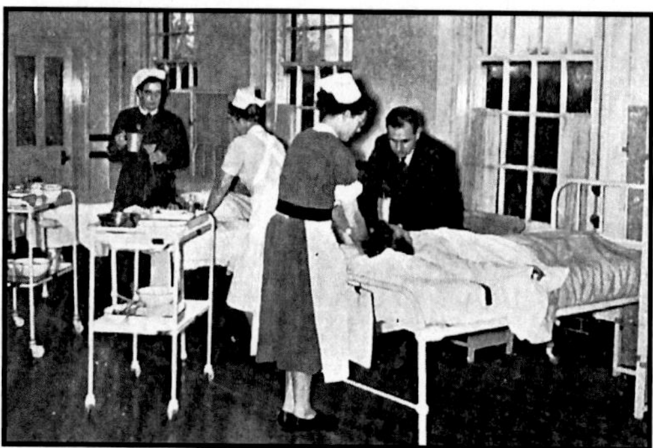

1958, Deep insulin treatment became untenable. Modified insulin combined with continued narcosis (sleep), proved invaluable, but was not practical - it tied up too many qualified hospital staff - each 24 hours. Photo source — Park Prewett Brochure.

[- FROM 'ILLUSTATED' MAG. APRIL 19TH. 1947]

Split Mind is treated by electric shock. Rest and quiet failed to bring relief to this ... six years old man, a sufferer from schizophrenia, so this new treatment was recommended. Electrodes are damped for better conductio

IT'S THE SHOCK THAT CURES THEM

A vast new field of research has been opened up by the successful application of Electrical Shock Treatment, now a recognized method of curing "split personality"

PHOTOGRAPHED BY AUGUSTO PANCALDI

DESCRIBED BY STEPHEN BLACK

1947. *Electrotherapy* (aka EST) known in WW1. After World War two, aka ECT, Electric Convulsive Therapy; given in low doses with *Scoline* (muscle relaxant) and in moderation (average six-sessions, some temp memory loss), proved, helpful in relieving clinical depression. ... But did not cure schizophrenia.

Chapter Ten
Bramber One Ward & Eastergate Block

' It is regretted that there is a tendency on the part of the Union Authorities to send children and aged persons to this institution merely because they are regarded as undesirables at the Workhouse.'
Dr. Harold Kidd. 1905.[1]

13th April 1969 to 15th January 1970

Bramber One—Leviathan—Petit mal Alan—Decay—Epileptic ward—Gentle Mike—Brieve of Ideocy—Epileptics—Elderly—Gran mal George—Experiential—Love in the fifth—Fitz—Mirrors—Dependants—Magic Corridors—Galadriel—Capacity—Two Hughs—Eastergate Block—Martin—Ex-RSM Jim—Fire—On The Carpet—Doctor Joyce—Luna-ticks and modules—Tusk—Pantomime—Brighton—Professional—Bramber Two again—Romantic Jim & Rainbow Jill—The Hall

13th April 1969
Leviathan

The hospital's long, snakelike corridors were dark tunnel ways of a deep human warren. Our asylum buildings' square box *Borges* labyrinth, I experienced as pulsing, smooth sided visceral canals. Its slow voyageurs seen doing crawl, with passing electric tugs towing metal trolleys, in and out of the Main Building, piloted towards marked ward block stops with patients' essential victuals. Wards were experienced as occupied havens, our patients refugees on Islands (like Summersdale Villa — or the Sandown islet), or living on offshore, long stay peninsulas (like the Eastergate Block) — a corporate, caterpillar body whole, large-linked, symmetrically stressed, inter dependent, a tight, throbbing, pulsing, living *Leviathan.*

The Rorschach butterfly Head was so real — until 1964, it had had a single brain, being managed by an Asylum Medical Superintendent (there has been three of them). They were accountable to their employers, the local Chichester based, West Sussex County Council, since Dr. Harold Kidd's appointment in 1893. The head, its well oiled, autonomous parts, initially located about the Front Entrance, head and neck, reception, offices, secretaries and switchboard.

Nowadays, several chimera heads were sometimes seen together, linked as the local *Hospital Management Committee* (post-1948 and the NHS), with little of the old autonomy; and now answerable, accountable, up a long, long, twisting invisible neck, upwards to a government, unseen, *Minister of Health.* The MOH had, at their official strings, numerous other hospitals, manipulated, audited, by offices and Officers, many miles distanced. Most officials were seldom (if ever) seen in any direct contact with their vulnerable charges — so far below.

With hindsight - I had to admit that the 1960s administration was almost seamless. This presented an 'infrastructure' that had taken many decades in the making, and a hierarchical thread, of *defined* responsibility, for all staff and patients in their care. And, despite the austerity of postwar, previous recent two world wars, the Asylum system was aware that to minimise costs to government, it needed to be as self-sufficient as practical. It therefore employed its own qualified Professionals and Tradesmen, and provided necessary training, food and utility services. This, for its time, meant that there would not be the otherwise uneconomic, grossly inflated costs of engaging only outside agencies, professional staff, and continuous subcontractors for Tradesmen for a large caring institution — for carpenters, carters, caterers, cleaners, cobblers, drivers, electricians, engineers, painters, pharmacists, plumbers, porters, stewards... et cetera... et cetera. Cost cutting, in obvious longterm needs, would be otherwise unwise, and would lead to needless *neglect* of the Asylum's charges.

At the top of the 1960s pyramid of accountability, was the *Department of Health*; next down was the *Regional Health Authority*, who, below them, directed (at per se Hospitals level) *The Hospital Management Committee.* Below the HMC was the hands-on, grassroots nexus of employed caring staff — among which, at the bottom of this ladder, and on the ground level, I found myself — amongst our patient charges.

Captains (or Warrant Officers) in practice, the hospital wards' Charge Nurses and Sisters were then in command of each separate Island vessel; which, with dependent on-board charges, were regularly serviced and victualled by those motor-driven trolleys; and tuned by those most-skilled visitors — the doctors, pharmacists, pathologists, psychologists and others; essential messengers, so vital to all parts of that occupied estate.

The Hospital had not been built as a palace, or prison, but a purpose-built Pavilion — belittled by some unsympathetic media critics as Barracks, or worse... The Reverend George Crabbe[2], an East-Anglian poet, in his 1810 graphic long-poem, *The Borough* [3], like Jonathan Swift before him, attacked a hostile, smug Establishment, which appeared to have openly condoned awful conditions for its own helpless, unproductive sick paupers. Crabbe wrote... of *The Poor And Their Dwellings*[4]:

'The Pauper-palace which they hate to see ...'

In the late, 19th century, this unsympathetic Dickensian attitude was *still* prevalent, amongst some of the then, in-post, parish Councillors, who were voting funds for, or not for, the new county West Sussex Asylum. And such was in evidence, during a long correspondence, in the *Sussex Daily News*[5]. One uncharitable letter said: 'He will build us an ideal palace for the feeble minded; but is a palace necessary? I trust there will be such an expression of public opinion on the matter as will enable the Asylum Committee to tell their Architect that an asylum on his present ideas is impossible. Yours, &c ...'

Fortunately, the Asylum Committee *did* approve the plans, as the hospital's flint stoned Church displayed (it was opened in 1897 and still much used in the 1960s). Outside the Main Building edifice, with its internal capillary corridors, were extensive tentacles off numerous other lanes, a connecting network of concrete-way canals, hidden subterranean passages and water courses. And, all these hospital's warm veins found Villas and ancillary islands — additional facilities, like the church, on the living hospital Estate, designated for the benefit of our patients and carers; within their time, map and compass.

Numerous visitors and ward passengers stayed awhile but, then in logistics, so many departed; for it was never a totally closed institution. Vigilance, against any wilful abuse, or neglect, was always a constant for all its members. But, as bard Bob Dylan sang; '*Times they are a'changin'*[6].

Bramber One male elderly ward was one, minute, island backstop; a remnant of a one time substantial Epileptic Block, completed in 1897. It was also my present placement. I was about to make drinks for our patients, when an angry Tall John bumped into me, in the narrow ground floor passageway, and confronted me. 'No John! I have *not* been upstairs today — fact is I'm working down here, now, and *not* on your ward.'

Tall John ignored my answer, and grimaced, his eyes tightened, narrowed — fierce, as he stared, insanely, into my perplexed face. 'You gave me that injection this morning... I'll hurt you, *if you do-it-again.*', he insisted, determined. Bemused John stood rigid, posture sideways on to me, with his left arm stretched forward, a balled-fist screwed up, shaking, just in front of my nose. John's fixed demeanour was one of hurt righteous indignation.

We were outside the Bramber One ward's kitchen, about two yards from the foot of the concrete stairwell off the MB1 ward corridor — the kitchen sited almost opposite the steps, up to Bramber Two ward. Out of habit, I kept my voice slow, wanting to understand why; not what, that was always self-evident. I looked directly at him, my face straight and equally dogged. 'What's upset you, John... you come back from IT, have you?'

Diverted. He paused, frozen a moment, fist tight, with blue veins and raised sinews at his wrist and forearm, still in threat, but not quite sure now. Clearly, he had strutted back from IT. I'd experienced that action, several times, with him before; when working up there on B2.

To confirm my suspicion, at that moment, Tom (Staff off MA1), on overtime up on Bramber Two, stepped sharpish into the ward passage, from the Main corridor, and spotted Tall John — and his posture — so self-evident. 'Ah! ... *There* you are, John — s'truth — you moved fast, from IT, I couldn't keep up with you.'

Tall John swivelled his head and glared at Tom, when, suddenly, simultaneously, from out of our adjacent MB1 day room, a second *intruder* (to John) appeared, as the already ajar door opened wide, and Charge Nurse Ron found Tall John and I, in confrontation at the foot of the steps, in an impasse sculpture, and addressed me — as Tom, but one second before, had called out to him from the other end of the ward corridor...

'Thought you'd got lost in the kitchen, Barry...', said Ron.

It was too much for Tall John, as he broke off his confrontation and, echoing loudly, stamped off upstairs, with a patient Staff Tom at his heels; and a loud crashing noise ensued. Upstairs, John's manic, caustic, shouts echoed and bounced back, down the block's concrete passage stairwell, in his now, out of sight wake. I entered Bramber One's ward kitchen, to make the patients', and then our, mid-morning drinks.

I'd been on Bramber One before, whilst on night-duty, helping to do wet rounds and assisting patients getting up and dressed, before the dayshift arrived; and, often, enroute through the passage, upwards to Bramber Two — intensive care patients overhead. Architecturally, the layout of Bramber One appeared identical with its peer upstairs; except, downstairs, the ward dormitory was separated from its ward passage offices and kitchen, by The Main Corridor: and, at its end (T), was the day room, which doubled as a dining room, with its ephemeral side-rooms and toilet; outside, adjacent, Bramber gardens.

A glimpse, at architect Blomfield's original 1894 ground-plan, disclosed how little the appearance had changed, into the late 1960s. What, pictorially, did it look like within? One of the many, real-life postcard photographs, taken of the hospital during the first-world-war, shows the Kings' MB1 dormitory, occupied with recovering soldiers; and the fabric of the ward — just as it was presented to me on this placement, in 1969.

A description of any one of the then long-stay psychiatric wards would surely have matched numerous austere asylum Psychiatric Hospitals in the U.K. I would later be puzzled why my memories of this particular ward were always of it as a *minute* unit. It definitely *felt* smaller than the upstairs rooms — at least its day room appeared so. This enclosed space was so claustrophobic, though its bricks and mortar were identical, in dimensions, to the ward Bramber Two day room — just above it?

Even the size of the two charge nurses seemed diminutive, but no less compassionate, or effective, for that fact. Ronnie — ex-soldier RAMC Ron, my new placement Charge on MB1, was close to fifty, with a full head of dark hair. Slim, small and so lithe, he'd been an ardent hospital athlete and sportsman, through most of his working life. His wife (like Bob and Norman on MA1), was a Ward Sister, employed nights on Summersdale.

Our Staff nurse was irregular, in fact, I seldom saw one on a regular basis, on this ward. Due, essentially, to an always relative staff shortage, too often he was transferred over to Summersdale or Amberley, even to upstairs, when the Staff was absent. And, often, with no staff nurse on duty, the student, Charge, and ward orderly (in the mornings) would together fill in Staff's formal duties. And, apart from the other twenty-five patients, who were essentially *all* chronic, many stabilized epileptics and mostly elderly and immobile, was lone Epileptic Alan, on Bramber One ward. With medication, he no longer suffered full blown *gran mal* epileptic fits, but did experience frequent *petit mals,* and an occasional, localised, *Jacksonian* fit — and was very much compos mentis. No savant, but with it, no less.

Epileptic Alan

Alan had been on this ward for years, but, instead of moving on or, even, moving out, had requested to stay. He had his own quarters, a single-bed side room, off the Day Room, with his own meagre personal effects clean and tidy about him — and, in 'his room', Alan's privacy, his space, was wholly respected. Unlike all other patients resident on this ward, although Alan had a life-time history of epilepsy, he was fully compos-mentis, whatever previous, earlier psychiatric case notes had recorded in his file; his occasional petit mals (just sat still for a few moments) epilepsy now appeared well stabilized. No family contacts were apparent. Alan, small, slim, dressed quite smartly in self-respect and full dignity, had had his 'jobs' about the ward fabric.

Let's be clear on this matter. As I recall, in his niched role, Alan was no unpaid servant, as such. What did he do about the ward? On receipt of his early morning call, by the night nurse, on completion of his own ablutions, his first job was in laying the tables for breakfast, preparing the battered metal tea-urns, and serrated butter tubs. Alan helped ward nursing staff, on domestic orientated tasks, until arrival of the orderly. Light duties was all the work possible for him, at this level; and Alan did get paid, albeit a relatively minute sum, under National Assistance limitations (later, DHSS. Therapeutic earnings), and it was his choice — more on long-stay resident patients' income, later.

Work completed, after breakfast, time was his own; he could attend OT, or IT, and work with any hospital tradesman; still possible, within the compass of the hospital estate But horizons were limited, and total legal income remained austere. Alan, presently, one of a number of paid auxiliaries to ward staff complements, still experienced sudden silences, usually sat down 'just staring'... not meditation, but probably one of his numerous *petit mals* — and safe within the institution. His hospital days were already numbered, with escalation of relocation facilities towards an alternative mode of care.

Care In The Community was, for the most relatively, capable residents, an endpoint to rehabilitation — but this move was to be in the near future. Such Great Expectations were questionable; so Alan, our resident, had declared. I thought he no longer belonged in this hospital, but *he* appeared to think otherwise. Perhaps, his social reality depended as much on economic, as psychological choices, in 1969.

In my rough diary I'd recorded... 'Early, on Wednesday 3rd July, 1968. Night duty. On Piquet Patrol. At five thirty in the morning — on to B1 chronic ward to assist another nurse in upping, dressing, and directing the patients. And then changing the inevitable foul linen from the numerous incontinents...' I recall, easily, such early morning chores were mostly *silent* — and very, *very* busy indeed, with many, full, red linen bags completed on each occasion.

Shortly afterwards, on Sunday September 29th 1968, I purchased a *Sunday Times*. Its supplement *Magazine* had a well illustrated article, on *One of Britain's Mental Hospitals*[7], that could equally describe a scenario on our Bramber One ward — more so, the Eastergate Block along the main corridor. Lord Snowdon's superb black and white photographs, with Jones' text, showed a caring, but austere, psychiatric hospital, as it was, neither debit or merited an account. Like ours.

Decay

Coming on duty on a morning shift, I entered Bramber One, a cramped claustrophobic cavern, to take over from whatever stage (in getting patients up) the night staff had, by then, achieved. And, it seemed to me, we had to then *again* decant all our patients, into a crammed odious stifled minute dayroom. All endured poor frail bodies, in various living stages of decay. *Sans* elasticity. *Sans* acuity and, *sans* loss of control of one's own body — in decay.

God, it's sad. Becoming aged with inevitable diminishing a capacity in necessary skills in *living,* leads to natural body 'decay' — and brain 'dementia', in later parlance. In a recent lexicon replacing the word decay, to indicate intellectual and demise of memory, Johnson[8] in 1755 defined: 'Demonate. v.a. (demento, Latin.) To make mad....'. Ouch! It's that negative use of demon — to demonise a natural state of decay, yet, probably, just a recognition of *not* being in goodness perfection, et cetera. Thus... 'Dementation. s. (dementatio, Lat.) Making mad, or frantick.' And genius Johnson, as if to clarify this point, included in his compendium: *'To Decay*. v.n. (debonair, Fr.)... To lose excellence; to decline from the state of perfection; to be gradually impaired (Pope).' Logistics and manpower inevitably defined what proper facilities existed to the caring staff and, truly, I found carers consistently responded tenderly in their duty of care. In their own future capacity, carers too might live long enough, to onetime need care by others...

Meanwhile, in the ward office, Charge Nurse Ron officiated The Handover from the duty Night Nurse. Again, that awesome ward silence; except voice-over, coughs, sneezes, wheezing grunts and occasional moans, emanating from our resident B1 patients. All the patients on the ward were infirm Elderly, except Alan, if not by exact chronology (average age) then, certainly, by their dementia and inability to move about or motivate themselves. Indeed, all *things* and temporal affections change and decay, including the mortal brain.

Most of our unfortunates had to be dressed and assisted into one of the folding canvas wheel-chairs, wheeled out of the ward, across the Main South corridor, and negotiated along through the short Bramber downstairs' passage — into the minute day room and dining room area. This was partly institutionalised, but also starved of space; the placement of (then always filled) longback chairs, backed to the wall. Fresh wrapped patients were then lifted out of their wheelchairs, and sat down, four to a table, where possible. The few almost mobile, with frail staccato carpet slippered heavy set steps, sadly shuffled — yes, definitely moved — with their shoulders hunched, head and hollow eyes fixed downward, for their next minute movement forwards; moving on into the ward day room, and to their expected, special places.

A number could *not* sit up, or sit still, and always needed to be placed directly into padded long-back chairs; a folded over osmotic draw sheet and dry porous paper incontinence pad placed under each seated resident. And, then, a chair table on its tubular support (no legs as such), partially trapping each newly sat down person in their chair place. Several residents needed assistance at meal time, to eat and in medication (most had liquid versions — there was a banana flavoured tranquillizer, to make one more acceptable). Acceptable... bless 'em. The elderly demented's internal psychic world will always be invisible — to others, incomprehensible.

A few residents were *just* able to spoon feed themselves, albeit very slowly, to survive becoming totally institutionalized (dependent). Consultants, moving on and out of the hospitals said, in the 1970s, of all the elderly (an oft topic of discussion), 'that patients became institutionalised after six weeks', and would need robot Pavlovian behaviour therapy, in re-learning, re-socialising, just to sit up to a table and negotiate a meal; afterwards, where capable, and of their own volition, re-seat themselves, about the ward dayroom. But the majority, though not logistically defined *physically ill,* (sick — down the road or into England Ward) were in *decay,* as stated, *unable,* rather than unwilling, with little *will* surviving to move on, anywhere, after meal time.

In consequence, unlike other wards where, after meals were finished, their patients, more mobile, would have some choice (no matter how mentally ill — or recovering from same) to walk out of their ward milieu, out into the Estate grounds, into town, or participate in the hospital's numerous activities — on Bramber One, its infirm Elderly remained on the ward. All things change and decay in mortal time, including our brain.

Half of the dayroom's space was taken up by the dining room furniture; the kitchen had a hatch linking into that area; the hot food, when off-loaded from the unhitched metal trolley, left in the adjacent passage. The second half of the dayroom was taken up, wholly, with longbacks and wicker chairs. I recall the children's party game, called musical chairs, where a large number (at least substantial to begin with) of seats were placed back-to-back, filling the central area of a room, in addition to all 'normal' seating around the room's periphery.

In that children's game, each time the played music stopped, one chair was removed as one person 'lost', and was obliged to remove to the perimeter. But our patients were all adults, and it was no game of playtime. Its consequence was, that after bedtime and meal times, all residents were sat around the periphery. And, all sat down, they wholly filled the centre of the dayroom and the crowded perimeter space, increasing that cavernous, thick cotton wool swaddled claustrophobia....

All hospital staff regularly attended Fire Drill lectures, and experienced the practice of checking out the numerous, seen, red-metal belled electric fire alarms. And, as the bells rung loudly in a practice during one morning's shift, I imagined, with horror, if this ward, as but example in the hospital, had a night-time fire... The press had recently reported several gruesome hospital buildings' fires — one was an old long-stay hospital, for the Mentally Subnormal — as they were still then titled.

If there was sufficient staff on duty, in Spring and Summer, during warmer weather, as many chair bound residents as possible were escorted, wheeled, out, into the adjacent garden airing court. That was, without doubt, why the architectural fabric of this Elderly downstairs' epileptic ward looked and felt considerably smaller, than its peer up above it. On B2 above, the patients were, however acute, more mobile, and usually much younger, and able to get up and about. Bramber Two had no need for such a large collection of back-to-back, longback chairs, filling up the central ward space. Patient mobility removed any need for that extra, claustrophobic, territorial body-space, so filled-up downstairs on the B1 ward. At this time, I had only been on an occasional visit to one of the many outside community Nursing Homes and General Hospital wards wherein sick Elderly long-stay patients resided.

Epileptic ward

Gently, slow, but firm, we placed George back on his low bed, having first ensured drawsheet and rubber sheet were underlaid; he'd experienced a particularly fierce gran-mal attack, and would now sleep in sequelae for sometime. Ron and I laid him on his side, knees drawn up to a partial foetal position, especially to ensure his airway was cleared for breathing. We noted (as usual for him) that loud stertorous snores emanated from rubbery lips and broad nose, which visibly vibrated with each exhalation. George was otherwise all right; at least, from this Major epileptic fit.

All right. Not life threatened, perhaps; but what quality of life did frail George and his patient peers' enjoy (surely a hollow term in this context). What life had any of these patients enjoyed, rather than endured, in respective lifetimes. And, for introduction: To be Epileptic, was a descriptive term, that was first diagnostic of a symptom, not its cause but, here in hospital, might (probably) suggest other additional semantic, social and psychological possibilities.

In a psychiatric, *Mental Hospital,* being epileptic was, in itself, defined as a somatic disorder (yes) but was the patient, therefore, in diagnosis mentally ill (no — not at all necessarily). It was more often a dominant primary symptom, which accompanied other 'problems'. And, often by default, rather than wilful design, circumstances had brought together George, Alan and their ward resident neighbours.

The Red Handbook [9], with other introductory textbooks, had well acquainted me with the various types of epileptic seizures — and of some probable etiology: petit mal; gran mal; epileptic furore; status epilepticus; Jacksonian Epilepsy; especially, psychosis with epilepsy. And of various treatments and case managements, required in a patient's care, as well as historical febrile convulsions (in infants, mostly, to evaporate with maturity). Numerous organic and cerebral trauma, could introduce one of the epilepsies at any age or stage of life. But, most *accidents* appeared to evade the psychiatric condition, and be attended in a general hospital or in the community, with relations and carers in ongoing support — in tandem with individuals' evolved personalities, and cultivated life styles.

But in the long-stay hospitals?

On Amberley admission ward, Bob, my Charge, had introduced me to some differences between a true epileptic fit and hysterical fits; bearing in mind that a patient might endure both, yet appeared to be quite different. The cause of a true epileptic seizure might have been triggered by an emotional or sensory disturbance but, in general, there need not have been an obvious cause, but a quite probable, unconscious bio-chemical origin — an idiopathic source.

In generic *hysteria* (touch of the vapours), there was probably some perceived crisis (by the sufferer) or emotional situation, from which the patient might escape by way of a pseudo-convulsion, to excite the sympathetic response of others; hence the former, an Epileptic, would fall heavily (with possible injury) *unconscious* to the floor, anywhere and any time; but rarely did an hysteric do somatic damage to themselves. The epileptic, in at least half the cases, emanated an aura — but the hysteric, never. And although the hysteric might thresh limbs about, no *loss* of consciousness was likely; and certainly bloody tongue-biting was probable in a Major Fit (gran mal), but not at all in the hysterical episode (unless visibly deliberate, or an arrested form of shell-shock). Incontinence was almost inevitable with the chronic Epileptic — but most improbable, in the bogus fit.

In coma, the epileptic seizure would render the patient deep and unrousable. The hysteric could be aroused, in a time sequence — the epileptic fit's duration was usually over in a few minutes — but a hysterical attack could linger into hours. *Babinski's' test* was positive with a true epileptic (unconscious) response, but appeared negative, in the hysteric. On Amberley One, I'd witnessed a patient appearing to collapse onto the floor, one meal time, and then throw his limbs about with noise and gusto — alarmed, I looked to experienced Charge Nurse Bob: 'Doubt that was a real fit, *he* often vies for attention — right. Take his pulse; and see if he responds to your concern.' I went over and, at that time, the patient's pulse appeared quite regular, and he visibly responded to my attention — that is, he *acknowledged* my presence.

Bob suggested, that when the patient had just experienced a seizure, it was likely a racing pulse could be felt, and if he had indeed *fallen* to the floor, even without any aura at the conclusion of the fit, he would be in a comatosed sleep — exhausted from his epileptic attack. And yet, *that* patient did occasionally experience true epileptic seizures and was on anti-convulsive (analeptic) drugs. It was helpful to know when he was in a real seizure — or when feeling in need of particular attention; and certainly that patient was *not of* a psychotic, epileptic personality.

One often spoke of an *Epileptic Personality* in those days, with particular connotations as we referred to Hysterical Personalities, the latter more neurotic, and often playing up to the gallery, as it were — both types were institutional norms. A large number of people suffered from bouts of epilepsy; but, with suitable care and treatment, most of these persons with epilepsy abided normally, *in the community*. Or *only* came into hospital, for observation, when a crisis arrived, to be re-stabilised on their prescribed drugs (as too, individuals with diabctcs).

Although certain health and safety rules were either legally or otherwise recommended, to remain *compos-mentis*, and avoid hospitalization — *no* driving, don't climb ladders, avoid alcohol and high-places, and especially avoid challenging stressful situations, was basic to the individual who had epilepsy. But they were *not* the average residents referred to as Epileptic, on our long-stay psychiatric wards.

Until recent times, and early arresting chemotherapy, a vast amount of epileptics who developed escalating fits from an early age had stood, sadly, a probable likelihood of acquiring mental disorders — and a long-stay residency, in care. In past history, early grand convulsions, which had inhibited growth and development, also evolved epileptic personalities — to adjust, survive their experienced abnormalities. A diagnosed *epileptic with insanity* (where so) revealed itself, in increasing mental-dullness, difficulty of thought, mental retardation, defective memory, irritability and abnormal behaviour — a chronic organic type of epilepsy, tended towards dementia.

And, an un-treated epileptic, in response to hallucinations *and* other phenomena which resulted from a patient's abnormal and frightening experiences. Well — it's *not* surprising, that a number of epileptics had developed paranoia, *and* a frequent concern with their bodily functions. Many early, young psychiatric epileptics, in the past, developed quarrelsome and even aggressive, superior personalities — but, often after Major convulsions, such florid behaviour, for a time, disappeared. So much — legion old *Case note Files* recorded.

Gentle Mike

Ginger haired Michael, a quiet gentle most vulnerable soul aged Nineteen summers, a teenage resident on Eastergate Two, amongst otherwise mostly older residents, was quite lively about the hospital estate, quite shy and unquarrelsome. His father had been a Japanese Prisoner Of War and experienced a very rough time in captivity. Michael suffered from an immense frequency of gran-mal fits, which he often experienced in the ward corridors, down at IT (or anywhere else), even in the grounds. With loud vocal auras Mike was often violently thrown down in his seizures and carried numerous scars about his body in evidence of this infirmity: notably, he always wore a leather helmet on his head, a thick tailored leather net which was strapped under his broad scarred neck. In previous decades it might have been possible he would have been compulsorily transferred to a more *appropriate* institution for chronic indigent epileptics. In fashionable parlance, to an *Epileptic Colony* — The Chalfont Hospital complex was one example, Epsom in Surrey, another which came to mind. Ginger Mike asked to remain in the hospital, when a move was suggested by a ward doctor. It was clear patients and staff had developed a fondness for Mike (one of the Graylingwell extended family) and he remained a resident as *no way* could he look after himself — and remained quite frail.

In contrast, on Amberley, nearly eighteen months ago, I was introduced to one new admission, Roger, a thirty five year old married man (to another e.p.) who was loud, devious and described as an aggressive Epileptic Personality. He often intimidated weaker willed patients, and *persuaded* them to part with personal belongings. However, his excessive anti social behaviour, for a time, transferred him up onto Bramber Two; before he was sufficiently re-stabilised, and later discharged once more, back into the community, to his own GP and family carers — if he had them. Someone, at one time, suggested (in his Case notes file), Roger as an amoral *Sociopath* (or Psychopath). But, I was unclear on this diagnostic judgement; there was however little doubt of his coping abilities outside — as long as he partook of prescribed analeptics. He wasn't of subnormal intelligence, no congenital idiot.

Brieve of Ideocy

By the end of the Thirteenth century, in the reign of King Henry the third, *The King's Prerogative* was established in Statute as a firm either/or difference, between 'idiocy and madness' — albeit written in Latin, as was the custom.[10] The former idiot as from birth immutable, the latter *not* necessarily a proven Lunatick (but a possible Malingerer), and a changeling as King Henry the Eighth inferred in 1541, in Lady Rochford's Trial for High Treason. Notably. And If 'issue' bore *an innocent idiot* born and entitled to a title and landed estate, he or she '*being of weak Understanding*' had their birth-right, estate and legal affairs, managed by the monarch — or more likely a relative — or other legally designated other person as guardian, for the period of the idiot's lifetime.

As a bibliophile and frequent visitor to second-hand bookshops, I found it amazing what gems can be acquired, from time to time. One item I purchased, from a South Street shop in Chichester West Sussex (close to the local Magistrates Court and backstreet Solicitors' Offices and Bus-station), was a battered, antique, tall but thin folio, entitled *Cases of The House of Lords*.[11] What attracted my curiosity, was a glimpse of its first page footnote (in mind my adopted profession):

> 'The Proceedings upon the Brieve of Ideocy , as well as this Service, are in the Custody of the Guardians or Agents of Lady Elizabeth.'[12]

The document (one of a number) belonged to the '*Sutherland Peerage Case*', from which the above asterisk footnote was extracted from the first page of this unique, well researched, collection of published 18th century papers. The case law documents involved two male peer contestants, and a third person (it was *not* a criminal proceeding). The third candidate, by proxy, was on behalf of an innocent (and *not* an idiot) infant, only one-year-old Elizabeth Sutherland: The first Brieve (brief) — '*Case of Sir Robert Gordon, Bart. (Including the Title, Honour and Dignity of) Earl of Sutherland.*' ... had an annondated footnote.

What arrested my attention was not *just* a contemporary focus, a benign lexicon historical study of the English and Scots word *idiocy* in its pre Dr. Johnson, *legal* and general use, but in the docs *'Appendices - Table of Pedigree of the Family of Sutherland'* et al, to the Case law papers... which presented a provenance dating back, at least, to the eighth and 9th Centuries. Details of the 10th and eleventh century, and the fascinating, supplementary data offered *'in evidence'*...

It was as if I had found a 'Holy Grail', an early history predating a First Folio of Shakespeare (1564-1616) — like Macbeth... At least such (at that time) recent historical material, as the Master himself might have had access to — to use and re-invent for his Shakespearean historical tragedies.

My search enquired what happened to *any* person, Noble or peasant who, through no fault of their own, was identified by others as an innocent *idiot* — or... *demented* (as became King Lear) as quixotic 'idiot and lunatic' — deprived of true reason. So, I became aware that, collectively, thousands of hospital and workhouse inmates and Private patients would be so classified over the centuries — mostly anonymous. As helpless useless idiots.

The Sutherland casebook's Eighteenth century argument, first paragraph, explained the legal situation (there were three contestants claiming the peerage). Pivot of the legal debate, dated from the early 16th century, and was about the fate of the historical named *Tenth* Earl of Sutherland, known as Earl John — who'd died *without issue* in 1514. (A conundrum surfaced in collation, when, attempting to check given facts, I compared the data to recent research off the

Google Web[13] as a Sutherland Clan source, at this time, with the objective of verifying available writing as to whether he was the 9th — or tenth Earl? ... the infant Elizabeth was listed as the 10th Countess in 1515. It remained unclear, when compared to other general historical sources of 15th and 16th century written records.

Prior to *his* (Elizabeth's father's) demise... Family history declared that, back in 1515, Elizabeth's father, too, had been declared *unfit* to manage his own affairs (it didn't say why — just inferred). His son-in-law, Adam Gordon, and his wife the deceased idiot's issue Elizabeth (who, herself, in 1493 or 1494, had, had her father, the unlucky 9th or 10th Earl John, *taken* away, along with his father, at a young age, to the Court of King James IV). The young Earl John was kept in *close confinement,* as an idiot, for 14 years - but legally succeeded his father, and was made a Ward of the Crown in 1508. The Earldom was administered[14] by Andrew Stewart, Bishop of Caithness. And, at Perth in 1514, the idiot Earl John, too, was declared 'legally incapable', *as was his father,* and he *died only one month later*, 'without issue'.... It was all most confusing. Adam Gordan's descendent, was one of the claimants in 1769. The original March 1769 published legal *Brieve*[15] on past genealogy said:

> 'The *Sutherlands*, Earls of *Sutherland*, were of great antiquity, but the precise Period when ennobled does not appear from any Record now extant. After many Descents in the Male Line, this Honour, leaving issue, came to *John* Earl of *Sutherland,* (the ninth Earl) 'who died in the Beginning of 1509' (another account says 1508) 'leaving issue, a Son and a Daughter, John and Elizabeth; which last was in her Father's life, and about the End of the 15th Century, married to *Adam Gordan*, second son of *George,* Earl of *Huntley*, Chancellor of *Scotland*, and Ancestor to the Duke of *Gordan.* Upon Earl John's death, his Title and Estate descended of course to his Son *John*, who, being of weak Understanding, was wholly managed by his brother in law *Adam Gordon;* and he, desirous to secure the Estate of his Wife, upon their brother's death without issue, and to prevent his alienating any Part thereof, took out a Writ of Ideocy against him 13 July 1514. In the Court of Proceedings wheron, Earl *John* in Presence of the jury [16] and appointed his Brother-in-law Adam Gordon and John Sutherland his curators for the Management of his Estate. *The Writ of Ideocy* was prosecuted no further; and this Earl *John* dying in *July* 1514, his Sister *Elizabeth* was, the 3rd of October following, by the Name of *Elizabeth Sutherland* served heir to the Estate.'

The outcome of the protracted proceedings in 1769, contested by the three claimants, was instigated after William, eighteenth Earl of Sutherland, had died in 1766, leaving issue a daughter and *only* child who (by proxy) won her case in the House of Lords on 21st March 1771... and rightly entitled to the *Title and Dignity* of Countess of Sutherland — and its Estates: (Elizabeth Gordon, 1765-1839. 19th Duchess-Countess of Sutherland thus held the Earldom till her death.)... A break in then custom, The Title and Estate was *not* passed on to a nearest *male* issue. The two peers contested (and lost) that the vacant title should not legally descend to the female legal heir Elizabeth, in her own right, but to one of them. But, there was no legal *brieve on ideocy* as in 1514. Indeed no need of such. No longer extant in 1769 — the feudal practice of taking and seizing an innocent's property by an illegal power ' giving in a law of Sasine' (seisin).

Epileptics

Till a late date, pauper Epileptics, *with no means or legacy,* were placed in asylums, poor houses and workhouses, and generally classified with the *Mentally Defective* — in earlier parlance, with idiots, moral imbeciles, and feeble-minded persons — housed in wards distinct from *lunatics,* per se. In 1897, at the time of our hospital's completion, Blomfield's plans included two specific Epileptic Blocks. One was the Female Block (Barnet Wards), with 32 beds on each ward; provision for sixty-four female patients. And, on the Male Block (Bramber Wards), 27 beds on each floor, provision for fifty-four male epileptics. This designation excluded all other diagnosed epileptic and mentally defective persons, resident on the other hospital wards. Bramber One was the ground floor ward that I was presently working on.

The 1913 *Mental Deficiency Act*[17] reclassified and removed (or relocated, as I've read some accounts) many of those early hospital residents. First removed, the so-called Idiot boys, and girls (Graylingwell *Annual Reports*). And, later, so-called adult idiots were also relocated; some to *Earlswood Asylum,* in Redhill, Surrey, or to other locations, perhaps an Epileptic Colony and/or other alternative institutions, such as the Epson group of asylums. They were viewed as more appropriate provisions, in later, current parlance, with *Special Needs.* Those transfers appeared to have been very slow — and perhaps costly, in human and economic terms — which, in time, transcended two world-wars, and resulted in a small residue of those vulnerable patients, now mostly elderly, being still resident in this hospital — a smaller number (in proportion) remaining on this long-stay Bramber One. But, thankfully, with passing of time Epilepsy now, in the late 1960s, was seen more as a province of Neurology, than Psychiatry.

Elderly

As early as 1905, Graylingwell, through its first Medical Superintendent Dr. Harold Kidd, protested that this Chichester Hospital:

> '... regretted that there is a tendency on the part of the Union Authorities to send children and aged persons to this Institution merely because they are regarded as undesirables at the Workhouse ...'

The Union Workhouse was, then, the only local authority residence for indigent persons, for many, many years, administered under the pre-1948 Poor Laws. By 1925, twenty years later, and one year before his retirement, Dr. Harold Kidd reported that:

> 'As an alternative to the erection of new buildings an approach was made to two Boards of Guardians in West Sussex to transfer chronic, quiet, inoffensive patients to their workhouses ...'

Forty years plus on[18], a number of Elderly patients have been transferred (discharged *out)* of the long-stay hospital, *into* old *Budgenor Lodge*, a former Public Assistance Institution (PAI), at Midhurst — historically, an original Sussex model *House of Industry,* built, pre-Dickens, in the 1790s as a Workhouse. In a change of policy, aged patients were being transferred, back into their own pre-admission, local parish. Another old workhouse was being used, to discharge elderly patients out of Graylingwell; this was The East Preston Public Assistance Institution — a local Union Workhouse and Poor Law Infirmary, since 1869, for Worthing and District residents.

In an enlightened 1960s, a Ten Year Plan was introduced by the West Sussex County Council local welfare authorities, which would enable more and more aged, and deemed *inappropriate,* mental hospital' residents, to be transferred *out*, again, into existent *Community Care* facilities. So, Safe Elderly in the 1960s (and Seventies) were being moved out, into smaller, local authority, purpose-built Homes, rather than placed in their old large poor-law institutions (workhouses) — a move Dr. Kidd had advocated back in 1905.

George

Beginning of another work-day, the radio tannoy on, not loud, its cordial banter and light pop music most welcome. I was, at this moment, nurse, staff alone (Staff was called to another ward and Ron was still in the middle of the Handover from the Night Nurse), in the Bramber One dormitory. Only the usual wheezes, grunts and coughs accompanied any distant mist radio sounds, with any ward words directed by myself, amongst this, our so sad silent minority. I'd just reached George, frail friendly mute Down's syndrome epileptic, very wet on his low, personal needs' bed (in case he fell off, in a Major convulsion, and injured himself during the night); his thoughts and emotions were invisible to me — only traces.

George smiled, in recognition of my presence, as I sat gingerly on the edge of his bed (a wee puddle and glow about its feet); and, yet again, assisted him up, and slowly dressed him, ready for breakfast and early medication. The first time was almost a year ago, when I was on Night Duty patrol. I remembered... ghost images... reflected inner visualised brain traces. Whilst dressing him, on the radio tannoy a new Hollies' pop-record was being played, the beautiful soft number lyrics and tone coincidentally so meaningful at this time.... '...He's my brother...' [19]

The lyrics could easily have been about Bramber One George, albeit all dependent Georges, and I recalled that first encounter, of which I had written in my brief *Journal,* whilst on Night Duty. A moment of irony:

> '... whilst dressing a mute subnormal patient on B1 at 0.540 am this morning, I remembered a pang of '*brotherly*' sympathy, as I drew garments onto his cabbage-like but 'felt' dependent frame. ...You know ole son' I said low and sussurated to myself and said to him in my mind, for he would not have understood (I thought);- 'In a definite way, both you-and-I are just as much automatons. I, too have to follow strict unthinking routines in everything I do, without it - I too - disorientated - would have my chaos.'

And, hereon, almost a year later, 1969, together on the ward, we heard that Hollies' record for the first time — as I assisted epileptic George up.... '*... The road is long - but I'm strong, strong enough to Care. Yeah. He ain't Heavy, He's My Brother - His welfare is my concern ...*' [20] Oh! Again, what wonderful lyrics. Underway. Another, routine day. Tomorrow — my day off, and I needed to study. George, when did *he* ever have days-off. Did he have any relative precious moments, unexpected pleasant episodes, however brief? The rest of his life — will it be unchanged in his subnormality. A fractured bird in a cage. Epilepsy, a broken wing?

Sara and our boys were in the back garden of *Stonerock,* out at Chilgrove. Sat contentedly in a chair outside the kitchen door, with prankster kitten Shasa at play between the three of them; — and, me, I was about thirty-feet away, out of sight within a hedgerow border. I was at study. For sometime, I had made use of a bracken tunnel I had carved out, ending deep within a thicket, a cleared circle shade; sufficient bush and bramble to veil playful distractions from Paul and Kit, if they had spotted me in that leafy den. As I watched over them whilst at study, I could see them, happily chasing after several bright butterflies flying towards the thick woodland.

Overhead, a tree's thick heavy branches bore overlaid green tiles, completing my seasoned shelter, as it leant comfort, and heaviness, upon my chlorophyll corridor. It was a warm, late Spring day, the sun's rays piercing the hidden darker inner space, whilst unwanted flies buzzed about my chosen naked feet and face; seeking salt in perspiration, as I completed school revision on Epilepsy, and noted, once again, that Alexander The Great was believed to have suffered from a falling sickness, or other hystero-epilepsy — and look what he achieved.

Thinking, then, of George and Bramber One's residents, I inwardly transferred back into our hospital's corridors. We experienced exquisite, changing canvases about our notable Surrealist and Namesake relative, of those two giants Henry and William James, the local Edward James' owned cottage (he was then I believe in Mexico). It was his West Dean Estate Manager, who had kindly rented this Stonerock cottage to us.

Scattered groups of isolated snowdrops, crocuses, and primroses tipped triumphantly, above our temp rented loamed carpet of mulch and were giving way to waves of colourful blue, sailing on a canvas of tall-friendly bluebells. Clumps of slim, dark-green finger-leaves with thick white squelchy stalks. Flowers submerged not only the woodland ground behind us, but much of the roadside passed, journeying to and from the hospital. Did they also exhibit for occupying Roman legions, Nineteen-hundred or so years ago.

They came by flood and trickles, into the hospital parkland — a large, colourful bouquet of swaying Spring bluebells, delivered into Bramber Block's ward-gardens. Escorting a group of our residents out into the adjacent ward-garden, a few puddles of bluebells were clearly visible about us. I hoped some patients were able to perceive something of that Spring benefit, but, sadly, few straight features reflected such a joyful reception. George was an exception. He'd meandered off, out to the Bramber garden's perimeter, now stooping over, now on his knees reaching, picking-up a bluebell bloom or two, up to feasting eyes and sensitive nose — there was no acknowledgment in words, though his face displayed a momentary pleasure. A beautiful rear-admiral butterfly was hovering, still, over the bluebell flowers' blooms, below him...

And then, a loud cry, as (damn it) George's moment ended, and he fell down heavily, into those chlorophyll arms — crushing that fragile insect and ending its then life-line, under his rendered unconscious form. But, enough, we could not take away the fact George did enjoy his experience of the bluebells, and of that lone butterfly's brief existence, then recorded in his senses. Poor George had had one of his daily quota of gran-mal fits, and so, not-so-heavy, Joe Burt, retired ex-Charge Nurse, RMN, SRN, and myself, carefully picked him up, placed him in a chair, and wheeled him back into the ward dormitory, onto his low bed, to sleep it off once more. And we returned to the garden, and our other dependent charges...

Experiential

A dark afternoon, lights on. Spring, or not, the sun was not always out shining; the air not always warm to the senses. By mid-afternoon, I had finished a round of clean-ups on the long-back patients, and one or two on the periphery. In doing so I had (again and again) in process attempted to exchange some conversation, at least response — and did evoke a smile or two, but no intelligible remarks were received in my passing.

Gran Mal George remained mute, and didn't or couldn't speak, so his non-verbal-communication (NVC) was vital. And, unable to obtain a specific ward Occupational Therapy facility, we were attempting to find somewhere that could anticipate George's personal unmet social needs, and accept his clinical care. Alan was out into town, Ron was off duty, and a drafted in Staff was busy in the office, with someone from the Nursing administration.

The ward dayroom, almost quiet, hushed, with only soft background music — its input breaking the absolute quietude of our patients, nodding off asleep in their chairs. And I had time to reflect on numerous things, and occasionally took stock of my meagre paucity of life knowledge, and of my brief experience of our dependent charges. On arrival at the hospital, a few hours before, I'd bumped into Harry, Alternative Bob and, at the side-entrance, Anita, nursing colleagues. On this ward, I had been seeing very little of my peers, except on the necessary school days behind Summersdale. And, for a while, I felt relatively alone.

Quiet. Ruminating. I often caught myself (with a shudder sometimes) cogitating upon Sartre's abstract experiences. I winced at occasional intense responses to unidentified, unpleasant, dire experiences, then distanced, through my *deliberate* alienation. Mostly through fear (and respect) of an unknown... I was conscious of trying to *disown* what, in William James' words, '... *was beyond.*' [21] I didn't, then, want to experience, possess, *whatever it was....* it was so *Unexpected.* But these are only words, in a recollection, probing The Invisible.

Love in the Fifth

At the opposite pole, sweet occasion. The classical poet Robert Graves wrote to me, in reply to a letter (anticipating an A Level in *English Literature,* but more out of absolute curiosity). I sent to Majorca asking, of him, searching questions. He was unwell, but kindly sent a laconic reply[22] to me from Majorca:

> 'Sorry; I have been ill and can't toss off answers to questions as wide-ranging as yours. All that seems to matter is to think and love in the Fifth Dimension where one uses Time as one uses Space in the Third. This gives poetic power, and all the real poets have worked that way. Yours r.s.. Robert Graves.'

I seldom experienced such rare feelings, indeed, but body hairs *had* truly stood erect, in a startled *electric* quiver. Momentary I had felt, again, in touch with — what is *beyond.* A benign experience of The Unexpected... Just raw inadequate words upon an inner reflection — shadow traces. Both experiences were, for me, *rare*, but *real,* no less. And they were physical (neither erotic or exotic, quixotic perhaps). As if, to me, new tangible feelings had accidentally penetrated into an unknown land or all God dimension; blind, somatic unseen, but remembered, felt no less — The Invisible — in touch perhaps... with me.

Such happenings were for real, and not imaginary, not in vision, or bare emotive, and mystical (cause unknown). However, for me, they would always remain unexplained... extra mural work. A little candle clear then, my mind and body senses corporate, once in a while had, through whatever accidental recent preparations, in a compound of experience — thinking, feeling, being; enabled such cursory *minute* mirrored break-throughs... albeit very briefly occur. Afterwards, on reflection, I would often, too often, in a vain attempt to understand those experiential explorations, go into denial, and sadly, ultimately, dismiss such feelings of well-being. In retrospect, I guess I was still — my loss, too afraid of *that* unknown.

I dismissed all osmotic, physical feelings, as but *only* somatic, neuro-physiological, behavioural chemical responses (revulsion or ecstasy, et cetera). Really, I could *not* explore what I felt, it was beyond my *capacity (but not my desire),* to experience in such inner-isolation. Similar, in ignorance — *bad faith* — perhaps, as sad-cynic others, who always equally dismiss as pithy descriptions, in experiencing *love*, both mortal and Divine, as *only* but attached biological elements, of our flesh. Yet, is it not *what* in, erm, in substance — it is all about. Being in an unknown land.

Within, my body corporate, just what *are* these so-called intense *feelings,* of into, or of, an unknown physiological ecology, *beneath my skin*? At my feeble *normal* consciousness level (not deemed asleep), I have *no* eye visual perception, of my own body, *beneath* its frail polyps thin skin layers, except in *good faith,* when I read or what I am told of those contours *by others* — no more than of the *outer* cosmos?

Subsequently I accepted, as valid data, knowledge as acts of faith, found in *Gray's Anatomy*[23], a sketched human universe beneath, and including, my own frail porous layers of skin on a map, broken into by Harvey.[24] A body icon, mapped out by others, to enable carers to occasionally explore and mend broken human bodies, of flesh, blood and brain. And, occasionally, ponder our, my own, mortality. Not at all in a depersonalisation, rather in a singular moment of clarity. French philosopher Maurice Merleau-Ponty[25] put this existential question, of perceiving one's own inner body as of *The Visible and the Invisible*, most eloquently, in his published *Working Notes* of — 'My body in the visible.'[26]

Fitz

Our ward-orderly's day off. Ablutions were complete at last, despite a number of interruptions. Ron was in the office, on essential paperwork. Joe had departed to the pharmacy, with the brown box and a list of requirements; pity, they'd be no possible patient TTOs (ToTakeOut) medicines for this back ward. It was quite dark outside, and I was by the window, watching the wind come up and aware of a rainfall due any time, as I stood still, seeing my own mirrored image immobile, and quiet, and listening to the low background drone of the subdued ward radio, in the dayroom. Suddenly, through the doorway, the tall lean form of Fitz (Fitzwilliams), marched in, strait-faced and, perhaps, absorbed in a sotto-voce conversation with his inner-voices, wholly unaware of other residents, and myself, in the dayroom about him... as he strode, continued down and along his own mental corridor... towards the windows.

Fitz was a patient from upstairs on Bramber Two ward. Adroit, only feet away from myself, Fitz shouted something or other and abruptly thrust his right arm through two windows, shattering the glass and, inevitably, badly cutting himself — the blood gushed out of one ragged wound. Fallen glass fragments seemed to miss patients — and myself. Fitz collapsed onto the floor. First-aid. I raised his arm up ninety degrees, to attempt and arrest the bleeding, and supply pressure in the absence of an immediate tourniquet...

'Ron, Ron...!', I shouted. But, I needn't have worried, he'd heard the noise of breaking glass, and strode out of the office — into our presence. Tenderly, Ron cleaned the jagged skin (concerned at minute fragments in situ) and placed a temporary dressing upon the wound, as I continued to hold the limb aloft. We placed a now silent, dazed Fitz into a nearby wheelchair, and I commenced wheeling him up to England sick-ward — as Charge Ron re-entered his office to phone for the duty-doctor, to meet Fitz and I down the corridor.

He then phoned through to Julian, The Sick Ward's Charge Nurse, who happened to be on duty; and let him know we were en-route. England received Fitz as I stood by, watching Staff Harry again clean the wound. Harry searched for minute particles, taut, with a sterilized pair of tweezers. Julian anticipated Doctor Joyce, and drew up a local anaesthetic dosage of lignocaine. Lean Harry spoke soothingly to Fitz (who he knew well), reassured of the procedure — and anticipating his unspoken voices — perhaps giving him a detached inner-commentary.

Doctor Joyce was most prompt and unflustered, sanctioning the nurses' actions, and on examining the wound, agreed for lean Harry to site the local — and with the ready-threaded cat-gut, applied the dozen or so sutures. Fitz, whatever motivated his dire action, was now relatively calm; still not wanting to speak, but content for his extended family to tend his wound, and offer dynamic balm. Prompt action (the doctor said) had prevented too much blood loss; and, aware of inevitable shock, Fitz was well wrapped in a warm red blanket, and accepted a cup of tea. Julian, with Doctor Joyce, went into the office, as I assisted lean Harry with the sutures and covering dressing.

I asked if Fitz would require an X-ray. Staff said the duty doctor would probably do a slip, for this check, and take a blood sample for grouping and cross-matching (just in case). Fitz's medicine card disclosed prescribed tranquillizer chlorpromazine; and, for his voices, trifluoperazine and orphenadrine; PRN medication was also detailed. By this time, a staff member off Bramber Two was with us (they were short-staffed — again), sent down by an over-busy Dougie — and so, I looked to our sad patient, and said farewell as I returned to my present ward — it, too, was under-staffed. I wasn't surprised, when Ron joined me in the dayroom, back on Bramber One. Our voices sound presently subdued, against loud heavy falling rain outside, and he said; 'Don't forget to do an *Incident Form,* Barry, before you go off-duty;' as I stacked a trolley with towels, and clean clothes, for another round of wet and dirties.

Mirrors

The evenings were lighter now, but the rain still dribbled from an overcast sky, while low puddle clouds of mist drifted about me, as I cycled home — the shift complete. Puddles of rainwater reflected what daylight survived, as I stopped to turn left off the Y fork — off the northern A286 West Dean road — onto the long-winding B211, for Chilgrove, with dark hidden ancient Kingley Vale over on my left. But, it wasn't the Roman legionaries; or Kipling Celts; nor slow walking smallpox or terminal lepers, sufferers, dragged back and forth up to that secluded hilltop Pest House; near the site of the Roman hilltop camp. Or, indeed, at that still moment, better, Sara and our boys — but my reflection was on Fitz and George, and — and...

Why did Fitz thrust his limb through those two windows, breaking glass? Did he hear commanding voices, or did he *see* (other than the ward windows, and through them, the other side of those clear panes of glass, and beyond) something, or someone (or more); a pellucid phantom, like stark Hamlet's ghost — *beyond the glass?* Or, in an illusion, did *he* see a still, real reflection, mirrored by the background darkening light, outside the dayroom, his own image reflected and changed by his mind's fragile interpreter — like *Orphee;* Cocteau's ghost, in his postwar film.[27] A tragic graphic parody, on Orpheus' descent, into the labyrinth of the underworld... Trapped between two linked, ostly hidden and clouded — sub-real worlds... truly into The Invisible.... From life into death. And back again.

I *really* wanted to have some idea of what Fitz was experiencing, during that Incident. I knew that Fitz would be unable to describe his matrix in *Rosetta Stone* codex words — what *he* had been seeing, thinking and feeling, during his recent experience. And so-called *normal* diagnostic and prescriptive terms;

as delusions, illusions, knights-move-thinking, et cetera — were, I thought, wholly inadequate as to what *he* was authentically experiencing... biological traces into and through an accidental quantum. But, and what a but — a number of other notable, highly literate, fellow sufferers, left invaluable past Rosetta Stone data, as to what Fitz might have experienced. Was Fitz' window breaking a gesture in *despair,* or an attempt to venture into the labyrinth of the dark underworld, dormant, in his mind.

In the 18th century Dr. Samuel Johnson vividly described his bouts of Melancholy[28] (as Churchill's later Black Dog).[29] One of Johnson's friends, the poet William Cowper (aka Cooper), also suffered despair — *but more so*, suffered from that deadly black-bile, his black dog of depression, which caused acute bouts of Insanity. The poet was periodically admitted into Private insane asylums. Quoting from *The Correspondence Of William Cowper.*[30] Cowper, in a 1754 poem, described his experiences of *insanity,* exacerbated by depression, from which he suffered so dreadfully throughout his life: '*As gloomy thoughts led on by spleen.*' Cowper celebrated, 'his recovery with intense thankfulness and joy.' Alluding, in this poem, to his previous dreadful state, the poet recalled, "Then what soul-distressing noises — Seemed to reach me from below, — Visionary scenes and voices, — Flames of Hell and screams of woe."[31] A Shaman lead gateway, into an alternative *other* domain.... into a nether, under-and-over-world; beckoning or threatening — benign or malign, in threat or with promise. And so, through the looking glass (broken glass) Fitz had, perhaps unknowingly, implemented pain upon himself. Perhaps, in response to such inner voices — this sudden incident, addressed in my reality, could have led to his accidental death.

In Spring 1969, sifting through some old magazines, in a box outside a Second hand Bookshop, close to the Railway Station in South Street Chichester, I discovered a lone copy of an old magazine, called *Life And Letters*,[32] which presented to me an incredible Rosetta Stone, which I related to Fitz. It included a short story called *The House Of Clouds* — brilliantly written by Antonia White about her dire experience, suffering from an acute episode of madness in the early 1920s.[33] The true short story was later graphically enlarged, detailing incredible insights — on self-observation — written later into a full length novel, *Beyond The Glass.*[34]

Antonia White[35] mirrored her awesome life experiences, recording dire occasional bouts of insanity — specifically, a ten-month acute admission in 1922-3, at The *Royal Bethlem* hospital — formerly known as *Bethlehem Hospital* — off the Lambeth Road in South London (now Imperial War Museum). Using the fictional names of 'Helen' in 1930, and 'Clara' in 1954 (*Bethlem* was called *Nazareth hospital,* in her writings.) Antonia described in *The House Of Clouds* (Bethlem), one particular long, painful memory. It followed an unwanted bath, given to her when she was very ill, by ward nursing staff. Antonia recalled:

> 'They took her out and dried her and rubbed something on her eyes and nostrils that stung like fire. She had human limbs, but she was not human; she was a horse or a stag being prepared for the hunt. On the wall was a looking-glass, dim with steam. She looked and saw a face in the glass, the face of a fairy horse or stag, sometimes with antlers, sometimes with a wild golden mane, but always with the same dark stony eyes and nostrils red as blood.' [36]

Antonia White's writing analysis, as to *what* she remembered is *was happening,* whilst she was most disturbed read, *for me,* as if of Rosetta Stone codex words — entering into the Time Travel Paradox, of Science Fiction worlds; imaginative worlds, like American Ray Bradbury's 1950s *The Martian Chronicles*; and the little known terrestrial minutiae world of Heisenberg (Quantum Physics); and backwards, to H.G. Wells 1895 *Time Machine.* I was fascinated by these written down accounts, on the influence of perspective and *distorted* experiences about *time,* involuntarily experienced by both the well and, by contrast, with many mentally unwell patients. And the various writings (apart from some Case notes content) on the subject. Of distorted time and space experiences, by science fiction writers, physicists, psychologists. How to distinguish between the real, surreal, or falsely imagined, as just so.

Desmond MacCarthy, editor of *Life and Letters*' Preface to Antonia's 1930 short story-line,[37] which introduced the subject of *The House Of Clouds* said: 'as a document... One of the marks of abnormal experience, of this kind, seems to be a loss of the sense of time.' MacCarthy said ... 'She dies perpetually and is reborn; sometimes as an animal, sometimes as another human being in some terrible predicament, a phantasmagoric shadow thrown by some painful reality. She lives through life-times. Hours or minutes are either lengthened into years, or weeks are compressed into moments. Sometimes,' Antonia said of Helen, 'it would take a whole day to lift a spoon to her mouth; at other times she would live at such a pace that she could see the leaves of the ivy on the garden wall positively opening and growing before her eyes.'

Adding evidence to the theme of all movement as quantum Time Travel (all motion *is* time travel) equation. I recall working on Graylingwell's England Ward with our patients; the affable Major, and his friendly neighbour, Parkinsonian Bill... and their erratic, slow time, somatic motions. And how, so jerky, Bill was, in his eating time — how difficult he found it, in time, to feed himself, but he did — yet, his condition would worsen, as he got slower and slower. Back, in the winter of 1918 war-torn Europe, a vicious un-identified flu-like virus killed off millions of people. But, a number survived, and, of those survivors, a number suffered severe states of Parkinsonism — this condition later named *encephalitis lethargica* (sleeping sickness). Statues, sat seemingly forever motionless, alive, existing in homes and hospitals, comatosed, like in a Brothers Grimm story, remaining speechless and frozen, from back in time, from outset of their illness — all those years ago.

Was it the summer of 1969, when a bio-miracle (not known precisely why, only how) occurred, in an American hospital. A brilliant neurologist, Dr. Oliver Sacks, published a non fiction book, called *Awakenings*.[38] This was an in depth study of twenty patients, on a new drug called laevo-dihroxyphenylalanine, *L-dopa,* and its use, on a number of hospitalised, immobile, Parkinsonian patients. With L-dopa, some of his patients, unexpectedly, made, temporarily, a remarkable recovery, and, revitalised, responded and picked up, *in time*, from *exactly* where and when they had stopped — thirty, forty, to fifty years ago.... Talk about a limited wonder drug....

Film records were made, during the treatments, and the so slow in time (for example) eating motions, such as *bringing a spoon to the mouth,* sped up graphically, showed how, very drawn out. Certain *tics* were identified as purposeful, slowed down, singular time motions — much as I read of Antonia White's self observation; though much modified. I recall watching The Major, and Parkinsonian Bill, on our England Ward. Synchronised human time, in slowed mechanical motion. (Some years later, I was working in the Community during the 1980s, employed as a hospital Senior Mental Health Social Worker, when, on one of my regular Home Visits, I met a married couple who had *both* suffered, in the 1950s, from Poliomyelitis, which had left the husband bound to a wheelchair. After the media, book, and later film of Dr. Oliver Sacks' *Awakenings*, one of the couple's enlightened GPs experimented with the prescribed drug of L-dopa and, to their amazement, the crippled husband walked for the first time — temporarily — for over twenty years; conclusion that he *may,* possibly, have been mis-diagnosed.)

Antonia White, [39] as Clara, was getting better; though not yet recovered:

> 'One day she was looking beyond the open door through the window when a bright idea struck her. Why had she never realized it before. She was in Looking-Glass Land. Of course everything was peculiar. Of course time behaved in this most extraordinary way... I've discovered where I am. In the Looking-Glass. ... I mean I've gone through. I'm like Alice Through the Looking-Glass.'

Fitz? ... His Bramber Two ward *Case-notes* reported an *Attempted Suicide* — in later jargon, a *Para-suicide,* to describe the broken glass episode. It was, then, an all too commonplace activity, amongst many of our suffering long-stay schizophrenic community. However routinely, to save a person's life was far, far from a happy activity for many a psychiatric patient, for which they might, rationally, be thankful, '*at that time*'.

Indeed, such regular routine matter-of-fact practice was exercised quite frequently about the long-stay hospital Estate by vigilant caring staff. Saving lives? I chuckled, in good faith and knowingly to myself, as on reflection I had all ready, been in the job long enough to know the score — and cycled on, pedalling my way home. Afterwards, I remained in some doubt whether, in *his* phenomenal experience, Fitz had been *really* attempting his demise. But, of course, his action of bloodletting could, indeed, have lead to an earthly departure in his possible tunnel journey, however veiled and linked within his alternative nether — even matrix — parallel world. Bluebells were disappearing into an inevitable, clockwork, darkness.

Dependants

Amiable Ron and I hush talked, as the ward breakfast concluded on a sussurated note, seated in the small Bramber One pocket-square kitchen; its thick, white door kept wide open before us. Unlike the New Names and life events exchanges I had enjoyed earlier, with musical philosopher Julian on England Ward, as well as with deep émigré Doug, on Bramber Two, this present brief conversation was unremarkable, though pleasant, cotton wool. Warm.

Adjacent, our silent mute charges nodded along friendly to soporific, metronome, dayroom radio' rhythms. A benign captive audience (those that could hear); a subdued gathering, of immaculate shrouds, sat upright, on very clean red plastic longbacks. Lively NVC George had departed, for pleasure and occupation, to a willing Social Therapy. Alan had finished a token breakfast, seated with Ron and I, then excused himself, and departed to his room oasis.

Surrounded on three sides — around us and, behind, a tall window sans curtaining — installed, cold white mellanated filled cupboards, with white clean flat surfaces; and a steel, always hot steam water-heater, adhered to the white wall on our left. Furniture materials were now constructed of synthetic, compressed, porous remnants of an unknown wood. Rubber, new easy-to-clean fabricated plastic utensils were replacing most antique wood steel and stone materials. Even this small square laid kitchen table (disguised by clean pressed tablecloth; thank you to the laundry, and Alan) was such a new innovation. The floor, kitchen floor, was an old red stone, thick, quality tiled floor, remnant of original 1894 planned fixtures. Solid. Meant to last. Being replaced by modernisation, in a world of plastic.

Back at our rented home, Sara and I had recently purchased a few square yards of a colourful pebbledash mosaic vinolay, which now covered the Chilgrove cottage kitchen flagstones. And, similar, most of this hospital's other small ward kitchens' tiles were now *protected* by overlaid rubber and plastic *non-slip,* easy-to-clean, lino floor coverings. But, not yet, on Bramber One Ward... Not Yet...

Magic Corridors

'Who?'

'Someone. A woman. Bunty, she said her name is... telephone call... in the office', said matter of fact Charge, Ron. It was on, then. Sara was, mostly for real, understanding about the visit to the Dicker. I'd visited booksellers *John. M. Watkins,* of 21 Cecil Court off the Charing Cross Road, for some years, prior to working here: and, two years ago, during one visit the son, Mr Geoffrey Watkins, [40] in that learned premises, sited in a narrow Dickensian Court, had kindly written some details, on one of his letterheads, before my departure to the hospital, and imparted a Name and Address of a *School of Alchemy*, at Upper Dicker, near Hailsham in East Sussex. He said he hoped I would continue the philosophical studies, wherever they led.

Bunty offered to take me, in her wee Morris Minor, to The Dicker. She agreed to collcct me from Chilgrove, for a short weekend at the school, and return me on Sunday evening. Dicker Bunty was a few years older than me, well dressed, a most pleasant, most serious, understanding lady. As we chatted in the car, she spoke briefly about her family life; about Petworth — and her commitment to *The Work* teachings, via the learned 1941-1953 diary *Commentaries* of physician and psychologist Dr. Maurice Nicoll — as presently interpreted by students, attending The Dicker. [41] This was real... so real.

It was early; a chilly, damp Saturday morning. We were on the road for some two hours or more, before our arrival at this, what appeared immense, sixteen acres Country Estate. Down a winding drive, through Sussex woodland, and around a man made landscaped lake, complete with ornate bridge; like a Zen blue willow plate. And thereby hangs a tale....

The Dicker premise, at the turn of the century in the early 1900s, was purchased by a colourful English Member of Parliament, an eccentric businessman, Horatio Bottomley. [42] He purchased a small country cottage at Upper Dicker, in East Sussex, after having founded pre-World War One *John Bull,* a patriotic illustrated weekly magazine; and, from his profits, purchased a small rural retreat, which he converted into a large Mansion Estate with attendant racing-stables; and substantial accommodation for his family and resident staff employees. Bottomley had had one ploughed field excavated, and an ornamental lake constructed within the grounds. To supply the water, a special well was sunk for the purpose, this was serviced by a small pumping station, which fed the delightful lake before me.

A retired Rear-Admiral was in command of the School. A learned, kind, slow speaking quiet gentleman who, in retrospect, reminded me of a benign cross, between a picture of Dr. Samuel Johnson and Charles Dickens' Samuel Pickwick. The good Admiral's office, at The Dicker, was adjacent to the School's library (to which I was introduced and allowed full access). As was customary to all new entrants (whatever agencies, schools, or institutions they had come from), I was 'interviewed' by that community's Principal.

We talked for about half-an-hour; about why I was there. About my life as a psychiatric nurse, working in a hospital. Our range of conversation covered many Names and opinions; Gurdjieff (and the Sufis), Ouspensky, Nicoll; and, related to this alchemic school, someone called Beryl Pogson, who had recently passed away (she was The Admiral's predecessor). And, together, we talked psychology and philosophy; of Jaspers, Kierkegaard, Sartre, Kafka, and Nietzsche. And of many more, Names — on Freud, Jung et als...

The Admiral showed particular interest in my early 1960s *Arthur Murray* method Dance Teaching experience, and of Music and Dance in general, especially the latter. And, again, about Yeats, Graves, Eliot, Shaw and, especially, about Tolkien... I knew minutely but enough for some questions on Gurdjieff's Sufi Exercises, Intellectual and Dance disciplines; and the Admiral offered the School's resources, potentially at my disposal...

Bunty had her own specified programme to adhere to, but promised to link up at Agape meal times. The Admiral, subsequently, as guide and weekend mentor, introduced me to a tall willow extraordinary, an elegant soft spoken lady, with just greying hair, who was to personally accompany me on a tour, of The Dicker estate and its facilities.

'Barry is particularly fond of Tolkien', he said, to the lady who was waiting for me. And, surely, he smiled knowingly, even mischievously, at her, as we departed the room? 'I'm sorry. Perhaps I ought to explain who I am? Let me introduce myself, more properly. You see, I am a cousin of Professor Tolkien. My name is Marjorie Incledon.' She was an oil-painter and stained-glass designer, and an *active* member of The Group that was, then, in part residence at the Dicker. She smiled, indeed seemed to expand, as she lightly but definitely chuckled. 'This might amuse you', she explained further, as she walked with me down a corridor en-route and escorted me around the Estate. 'One of the Halflings... one of the Hobbits, was named and modelled on me', Marjorie offered.

Galadrial

I cannot recollect which character Marjorie said she immortalized in the 1954-55 *The Lord of The Rings* (or was it in the 1937 *The Hobbit*). But that tall, sylvan Lady, certainly spiced an oxymoron — and metaphor, for me.... Surely, having met the lady, Tolkien's cousin appeared more like The Lady Galadriel, than a Halfling...? Marjorie introduced me to several Dicker resident acolytes. I noticed all the students were performing particular domestic tasks, like sweeping up leaves, house-cleaning or similar activity, or in the process of creating various handicraft and artwork. I thought, *at first,* Just Like Home, or at Work, or as necessary, in *all* institutions.

Ah!... *But...* like Sufi mystics, or cowled monks of Zen devotees, the students were *also* expected to be, quietly, silently, doing Other things, performing, practising specific Self-observation exercises and, perhaps, added difficult athletic and ancient learning signal sacred-dance movements (Good Vibrations - with appropriate music mantras) — to increase willpower, and, in Good Faith, learn to *submit* to that inner, purifying 'godness' which, by submission, honestly communed with... with all. Contact. A closer link with eternity beyond.

Oh, to be developed, into *that* savant and purer distilled capacity. ... Sigh!

It appeared, as even occasional residents, one needed to be able to commit lots and *lots* of devoted time. I sadly, quickly realised that, in continuum, I was already committed, in service and learning to The Hospital and its patients; and, of course, to my domestic life. Fortunately, *The Fourth Way*[43] allowed me to continue *some*, albeit back-up, alchemic (chuckle, Magical) learning — whilst building my new calling, and career; if only in some small part.

At the end of this initial tour of The Dicker, I was shown, anticipating my over-night stay, to the male dormitory. This was a long room, with its walls bearing beautiful large painted murals, these depicting various Great Work related iconic scenes... Tarot... Arthurian... Sufi... and other. In the morning Breakfast too, to me, experienced as unique. The large room had an occupied top table, with The Admiral and other notables (who, of course, were unknown to me) and several lower set tables where I again met up with Bunty and The Lady Galadrial (Marjorie Incledon).[44] I, a stranger, was fascinated, privileged, to share a truly, Agape breakfast.

The dining-room walls were painted with Shakespearean Heroines. Above a raised piano I saw a beautiful paper mosaic panel — all works made by members of The Group. There were side-tables, with pristine fine-white table-cloths, on which a number of large covered silver tureens and other containers and ladles, provided the 'Help Yourself' catering, for vegetarian *and* non-vegetarians. I enjoyed fried eggs, thin sausages, kidneys, tomatoes and mushrooms, with bread & butter and fresh coffee. But, before we begun eating, The Admiral stood up, and gave a short speech and prayer — and I enjoyed an awed, learned meal, chatting with people who *know.* Afterwards, each student went about their allocated morning tasks. I accompanied one regular resident out into the garden — with a large stiff broom. Before my departure from The Dicker, Marjorie took some written down details from me for her distinguished cousin, and promised to write or speak with Professor Tolkien, on my behalf, with some questions. In retrospect. Now *what,* what were those questions?

Marjorie, later, sent me a postcard, post-marked address, Ditchling, East Sussex; *dated Hassocks 29 APRIL 1970* — a brief reply sent to me at Chilgrove, which said, in an apology:

> 'JRRT was very harassed ... emphasised there was no chance of his answering any of my questions. No hope at all, as I feared' (*and added as if to echo Boehme: Every one must seek it for himself.*) "No one can do it for you, you must do it for yourselves." used to be a frequent refrain at some lectures I attended years ago. Charge 1 shilling. JRRT was very harassed when I rang — said so, wife's injections not taken. Film going badly — Could not possibly undertake anything more. Hoping to see you at the Dicker when it can be managed. To our next merry meeting ! Marjorie Incledon.'

What a lovely Lady.... Sadly, JRRT's wife, Edith, died shortly afterwards in 1971. And, within two more years, both Tolkien and his cousin Marjorie passed away into the next world. But, I was delighted to have met Marjorie, and sorry I was unable to see her as she suggested, following our merry meeting at the Dicker. I recall our last conversation at The Dicker. Tolkien's physical health was ailing; JRRT was presently, she'd said to me, 'most concerned' at a Cult interest in him, at an American University Campus'. He, also, was *not* happy for films to be made on The Hobbits — *in-his-lifetime,* she conveyed to me at The Dicker. It was years later, that I learnt how much Marjorie and her cousin influenced and supported each other, in their early lifetime out in South Africa... Magic !

Shortly after Tolkien's demise, an animated American film *The Lord of the Rings*, starring the voice of the excellent John Hurt, that was based on the first two books of the Tolkien' trilogy, was released in 1978. I thought the cartoon captured the spirit of the Hobbit's Quest, very well. But I would love to have seen a full length feature of all three books, and, of his earlier work, Bilbo's adventure in the 1937 *The Hobbit.*

Capacity

'What do *you* think, Ron?'

He wasn't convinced.... Biting his lips in concentration, he paused, as he thought out his reply. I was trying to persuade Charge that Gran Mal George, despite being mute and prone to frequent full ep attacks, was *not* so *'non-*compos mentis' as his Case notes, *Subnormal,* diagnosis disclosed. George's emotional responses, in day-to-day interactions, had persuaded me to tackle Ron on the issue. 'Okay, Barry. Contact *Social Therapy,* as you suggest. Do you know someone qualified to work with George, and our ward, in George's Education?' I'd anticipated this question and, in a kneejerk, I duly responded....

'Yup! — Cicely, over in Social Therapy. Cis is a qualified Occupational Therapist, she recently came to Graylingwell from *Oakwood.* I've spoken to her. She's as enthusiastic as I am, to break the mould for our George. And *perhaps* one or two others, later on? Cis said she'll talk to Dr. Harrod, the Clinical Psychologist, for a battery of 'Tests'...' 'I'll have a word with the ward doctor, to confirm the move.... in a way, I guess it will create a precedent', Ron said, 'to confirm *this* recommendation, *from* Bramber One ward.' He was well aware that this was rather unusual.... a bit like requesting a resurrection, from among statistical undead.

I, too, was only too aware that Bramber One was a fossil from the time of the 1890 Lunatics Act; and the subsequent Graylingwell, Blomfield 1897 *Epileptic Block* — given Poor law ward name *classifications,* dating from the time of the first world war, and postwar years. This was also true between wars, when many ex-servicemen and other paupers, by default, were first classified with *feeble-minded,* in the receiving Casual wards of local workhouses — and, later, re-classified and transferred as chronic lunatics; incurables, idiots, imbeciles, morons, sub-normals, even *severe* subnormal — all designated terms, and often *arbitrary*, demonised immutable group labels for *natural* idiots (Yet innocent — as they were believed unable to abstract, and discern, in a norm, moral sense). In time, they all became in decay, *demented,* aged. All these, our helpless patients, in whom intellect was deemed wholly inadequate, to function *alone* in the outside world.

English philosopher, John Locke [45] published a lengthy work in 1690, on an exploration of the senses, in which he described the functional IQ differences between 'Idiots and Madmen' (a matter of Capacity):

> 'Idiots ... who perceive but dully, or retain the ideas that come into their Minds but ill, who cannot readily excite or compound them, will have little Matter to think on. Those who cannot distinguish, compare and abstract, would hardly be able to understand, and make use of Language, or judge, or reason, to any tolerable Degree; but only a little, and imperfectly about Things present, and very familiar to their Senses. ... the Defect of Naturals seems to proceed from Want of Quickness, Activity, and Motion in the intellectual Faculties, whereby they are deprived of Reason: Whereas Madmen , on the

> other side, seem to suffer by the other Extreme. For they do not appear to me to have lost the Faculty of Reasoning; but having joined together some Ideas very wrongly, they mistake them for Truths; and they err as Men do that argue right from wrong Principles: For by the violence of their Imaginations, having taken their Fancies for Realities, they make Deductions from them. Thus you find a distracted Man fancying himself a King, with a right Inference, require suitable Attendance, Respect, and Obedience.' [46]

There were no self-styled fatuous Locke' designated; Insane Gods, Prophets, Kings and Queens or tyrants, who I found, expected obedience of staff on Bramber block — or other patients, about them and resident in the hospital. The Majority of long-term residents, whatever degree of insight into 'their' condition, accepted their limitations, and incapacity to achieve *any* betterment, without the assistance of those who, clearly, experience taught them that others were Superior or worse off and inferior, in being compared to themselves. Without exception, *no* two human beings, however drone like or twin like, doppelganger shadow of another they might *appear* to be... each person (despite the cliche) really is unique. And always undergoing change, by decay and anew. Obviously, I accepted myself, as of others, in that same analysis. About capacity, and true humility.

Occasional planned visits to other caring institutions were a must, as an RMN student — and two such visits, to specialist Mentally Handicapped (subnormal) hospitals, left indelible traces, in my fragile memory. On one visit to an ESN (Educational Sub-Normal) residential unit, and training school, at *Highdown* in Worthing, I recall someone, standing statuesque, like a tall tree, gently holding up a large doll in raised arms, and clasped hands on its bough — firm amongst tended flower gardens. Only, it wasn't a doll... the (obviously caring, from her demeanour) nurse, was cradling a teenager — so the nurse said. The child had an incredibly tiny pin-head, sat on top of a small, lean, dressed as a female child body. The young girl was twittering (only word to describe it) — like a sparrow on a twig. She was unique to me. Little Jane was a human *micro-encephalic*, born with a substantial portion of her brain absent; consequently, she could do absolutely nothing whatever, *willed by herself* — needing Total Care during her entire lifetime.

Another visit whilst on Community Block, in early 1970, was to a large Mentally Handicapped (aka Subnormal) long-stay Hospital, in Hampshire. The buildings, though mostly old brickwork, were supplemented by a range of single-storied long Nissan-like huts, like our own nexus of outlying

Graylingwell buildings; immaculate, clean and homely — despite the usual paucity of state resources. Our group had almost completed the tour of the wards; meeting one or two residents — most were attending their afternoon OT, and various *'educational' classes.* We were stopped at a bed. There sat on it, reading a book, was a lone teenager (mid afternoon, the ward was otherwise empty of residents) a smartly dressed young man named John, who was about 18 years old. He was introduced to us, as someone *special.*

The ward RNMH Charge Nurse proudly told us (the boy's face lit up in joy) this was because he was soon, today, to be singing, as a Soprano, at a hospital concert later in the afternoon. Just like a Pop-star. And *hydroencephalic* John spoke with us in an unusually high pitched voice. 'That's right!', he said.

John had an enormous head, like Humpty Dumpty. Almost translucent skin enhancing blue veins, on a taut stretched unblemished skin. Not unkind. He did *not* represent a clinical functional pyknic stereotype of being sub-normal, seen with a high forehead and flattened nose, as some deemed *Downs Syndrome* persons. I knew and compared our Gran-mal George on Bramber One ward, listed as a Downs syndrome, and diagnosed as subnormal (though there remained some doubt about George's original Downs diagnosis). Young Singer John, momentarily, made me think of a 1950s front-page cartoon science fiction hero, a Dan Dare image, out of the English Hulton comic *The Eagle* — a picture of *The Mekon.* The latter had a huge, blue, egg-shaped head, with small sharp blue eyes, sat atop an otherwise normal proportioned body. And compensated with an ultra high IQ — pure phenomenal *savant* brain power. Downside, more vulnerable, an *Alice in Wonderland* Tenniel pic of a large eggshell head, and body of an ultra-frail *Humpty Dumpty* sat on a wall (bed or mushroom), his eggshell thin head awaiting a fall.

Singer John had Hydrocephalus. It wasn't a Downs syndrome. He presented with but a *mild* dementia. The head with enlarged ventricles, existing in the presence of normal cerebro-spinal fluid pressure. His head and brain bearing a quantity of unwanted surplus fluid. Thankfully, he had a Spitz-holder valve in-situ, attached to his neck, which was being used to reduce the fluid and unwanted pressure. The process, I think, was called ventricle shunting. His Charge nurse said that there was a *good* prognosis, as swelling was already reducing. And no complications as infection, et cetera. Before we left, John insisted on singing several verses for us — sung, truly sounding like a Nightingale, with a slow short crisp melody, and words that held us spellbound.

Affected, we adult students walked away, impressed by the savant like experience of Coldeast's Singer John.

But our visiting group of students were ill-prepared, for what followed.

Our last port of call, before leaving the hospital, was the Charge Nurse's office at the end of Singer John's long ward, where we were invited for a cuppa and Summary of our educational visit. A female nurse was sitting down by the office desk and, otherside of her, was a large children's filled cot. Charge smiled and nodded to the nurse, as we entered and ourselves sat down; the Staff nurse knew who we were, and was ready for the inevitable questions to follow our entrance, at least we concluded this was so... 'She is three years of age', The Charge informed us, in a hushed, reverent tone, as he knew the occasion demanded. For the infant was a miniature of Singer John but, with no reducing swelling, her little (God, there's a misnomer!) head was *huge*. Jesus! And so taut, the poor thing looked like a still smooth pink balloon, about to burst. 'No valve insertion possible', Charge commented, the child unable to make *any* noises. And Charge answered an unstated question, as we looked horrified, mortified, at the vague markings of her (God!) but poor, minute, facial features, anticipating us. 'No! Angela can't close her eyes as the lids are stretched back — and stuck, I'm afraid.' And, it seemed such a futile yet then loaded, obvious remark for me to make... anything, *something,* to say, 'Is she in pain, do you think...?' And... and... hot acrid tears crept out, escaped and dropped down, from the corner of my eyes.

As in a Holy Place, in *any* world place true Sanctuary (already in one), at any altar, the ward RNMH (*Registered Nurse* in *Mentally Handicap*) Charge added in a low church voice. 'Don't know how long she's got. We can't extract the fluid, I'm afraid.... We do what we can, don't we, Maria', he said, looking across at his equally affected Staff nurse colleague. And, as she nodded, written in her face was a resignation to the inevitable.

I recall those warm, wet silent tears slowly seeping, creeping down my cheeks. As here, all these years on, I would and will *never* forget seeing that dying three year old little girl during that visit, in all my next thirty-five plus years of Professional caring that lay ahead.

Gran mal George, on Bramber One, continued to experience his fits *but* the quality of his meagre daily social life had surely improved. Each weekday he was escorted over to the *Social Therapy* nissan like hut, located North side of the Church. At first, he was wheeled over, but soon, with his escort, he walked unsupported over to the unit, and learned how to join in social activity such as the inevitable, but enjoyable, musical games. I had no Knowledge of George's responses to Dr. Harrods's Binet IQ test scores (George was Mute?) and other Clinical, but spatial, testing et cetera... There was also a range of Social Therapy tests, gauging whatever emotive or other discernable exploratory sensual *responses*. There was rightly and understandably no expectation that his increased capacity would suddenly allow him to attend the formal Occupational and Industrial Therapy units down in The Yard - he was no Mensa Charles.

Dr. Joyce told me that, for many years, there had been a block (reason unclear) on the employment of Qualified Occupational Therapists in the hospital. This fact of *no* OTs since, sometime in the 1950s when, it was discovered, the only known Qualified tall spectacled lady, then working in the OT nissan huts (located opposite the Main Hospital Front Entrance, and adjacent to the Church (no Industrial Therapy in those days)) was over 70 years old. And, no replacement in sight.... Indeed, all the time I worked with patients on IT, in the late 1960s and early 1970s, there was certainly no Qualified OT worker employed down The Yard at Industrial Therapy. I never did work in the Social Therapy unit... All IT rehab staff, were either nurses or qualified craftsmen of some sort. They were mostly employed utility tradesmen, or former dairy and cattlemen et cetera — but all, now, on The Payroll as Nursing Assistants, as they worked specifically with patients and psychiatric Nursing Staff. There were also occasional volunteers.

I wondered if qualified OT Cicely was the first, or certainly one of the first, of the new breed of invaluable employed Graylingwell occupational therapists. To my astonishment, and delight, just before I left Bramber One ward, George mouthed — 'th - th - Thanks Nurse', when I shook hands with him on that last day. Or was it wishful thinking on my part. ...

Two Hughs

June 1969. After I finished my mandatory block on Bramber One, I left hospital on two weeks leave, before moving on to the next mandatory placement, to be on the two chronic long-stay wards of the Eastergate Block... three months on Eastergate One, and three months on Eastergate Two.

Sara and I were shortly due to move to Littlehampton, from the isolated hamlet of Chilgrove but, before then, I was to travel up to London for a few days, and earn a few extra pounds. Well... In 1969, staying with ex-Agfacolor friends Pete and Veronica, in Cadogan Gardens SW3, I worked for a week with Dr. Hugh, learned bio-chemist and friend. He was based out at Fulham, Parsons Green, in a mostly derelict property — its low back-yard where the Doc's constructed apparatus was set up, for his experimentations on plant milk. Last year, April 3rd 1968, Hugh's current project — on a dubbed 'Mechanical Cow' — was the subject of a BBC TV television broadcast, with the speaker Raymond Baxter. Hugh kindly sent on to me a copy of the original typescript, aware of my continuing interest in his scientific project.[47] Hugh and his wife, Winifred, gave me enormous support and encouragement when I became a full-time student at Graylingwell Hospital — especially, on my meagre intellectual, and sceptical, spiritual plane. Hugh's Doctorate had been on *Yeast,* his thesis on wine bio-chemistry. He was presently exploring research for a recently formed company, called Plantmilk Ltd., on the development of a vegetable plant-milk, *specifically* for people who were allergic to toxicity in animal's milk — or who chose *not* to ingest dairy products (considered as toxic by them), e.g. vegans. And, of course, as an excellent natural full-cream milk addition in its own right. I found it tasted delicious (though I remained an omnivore).

In the London Fulham yard, the Plamil process, as I recall, started with a container for the raw vegetative matter. This was electrically fed into a large round metal centrifuge. A tub (it looked like a large institutional cooking drum, hospital, army, other) within this drum, which spun around at XX revolutions, had a finely meshed inner-skin, which acted as a filter to remove unwanted fibre, and the residue was forwarded to further filtration, and to have added in Hugh's formulae — the eventual product, Plantmilk. I remember Hugh's chuckle, as he indicated that, potentially, the process, which removed any and all toxic matter, could produce, at least, three products — plantmilk, de-hydrated fibre (compacted perhaps as cardboard or other), and pure alcohol (really?). Hugh gave me detailed written data, to help me have a glimmer of understanding, on the process of which the media dubbed it a Mechanical Cow.

As a general factotum, one of my numerous messenger errands (recorded in one of my erratic diary red notebooks) took me to Kew Gardens, to meet with a Sir G.T., Director of the Botanical Gardens, of No. Ten house (?) at Kew, and ask him to part with a particular comfrey, and other flora. One of a number of other-place and faces, in assisting Dr. Hugh in his research — as a labourer, I enjoyed feeding the bubbling yeast in the last box in the chain.

I'd known Hugh and Winifred since the early 1960s, when in 1960, for fun, they enrolled as my dance-students, when I'd worked at Arthur Murray's

Dance studio at 167 Oxford Street W1. Dr. Hugh F., a bio-chemist, and Winifred a retired school-teacher (an amateur painter in oils), had no children and, for a decade or so, became friends and mentors. They were both Vegans (Hugh for health reasons, I recall) but, in the many times I shared meals with them, either at their Kensington Gardens flat or dining out, they *Never* pressured me to abstain from fish, meat, or fowl, and dairy products ... but I *did* try, whilst employed at Agfacolor labs in Wimbledon.

Back in 1962. On holiday, I visited two friends of Hugh and Winifred's, living on a large seaside caravan site in Nice, South France — aided by a written introduction from H & W to a qualified GP and Homeopath Dr. G.F. (and Pat his wife); one-time a gynaecologist who had attended (the doctor told me) the beautiful former film actress Grace Kelly, then a Princess of nearby Monaco. All lovely people! Doc, afterwards and at my departure from Nice, kindly offered me a post as a *student* homeopathic pharmaceutical assistant (I was sorely tempted... he also had a Harley Street practice) in Walthamstow, London — but, I declined and decided, eventually, and five eventful years later, be an adult RMN student - at Graylingwell Hospital.

Among Hugh and Winifred's friends, was another Hugh. He was the legendary Lord Air Vice-Marshal, Hugh Dowding[48] forever, and rightly so, associated with the Battle Of Britain. I only knew of Dowding (from H & W), as a mutual vegan and anti-cruelty to animals fund raiser, an associate of Hugh and Winifred's. But... I was often not a little puzzled, by some of the earnest content of Winifred's chats, which sometimes referred, with a reverence, to their affectionate friend, Hugh Dowding; years later, as a student at Graylingwell, I began to make sense of *that* content, and most treasured long conversations.

Sunday, 15th June 1969
Eastergate Block

On the move. Sara's brother in law Mick's open-topped lorry negotiated the low, sunk, un-metalled lane, up from the Main Road, its turnoff situated close to the village green blacksmith forge, on that triangle island and adjacent sump of its one-time village pond, close-by Chilgrove's *White Horse Inn.*

Mick found the journey into the West Dean Farm Estate quite a task, fenced sides of the lane brushing tight against the battered vehicle's sides, whilst in the fields, on either side, the noisy moving metal rattled, smoked, and duly excited the curiosity of the horses, bulls and cows, sheep and other enclosed livestock. There were fractious moments, when the thin wire-fence, almost in collision, would have been inadequate in separating our tin-dragon from the farm's rightful indignant, yet awed, residents. Our short memorable stay in Stonerock tithe cottage was at an end. We were en-route for Littlehampton-on-sea, beneath, close by and south of the sentinel castle town of Arundel, atop the low South Down hills — that minute sea-town, long-time maritime port, sheltered in a crescent shaped haven, at least for one millennium. The whole rural landscape about the ancient downs a magical delight.

The mortgage deeds (our first) detailed that our new end-of-terrace home was once owned by the Duke of Norfolk Arundel estate. It was one of the his numerous properties. Indeed, the Duke's Norfolk Estate appeared to have *owned* the whole Town, *and district*, up until 1930 or so.[49] Noticeably, included in the text of our new mortgage deeds, amongst other written down banned and then deemed anti-social uses, was written a clause — *not* to use the premises as a *private lunatic asylum.* I wondered if other persons buying property, off the being sold off properties, belonging to the former Norfolk Estate also had, had this clause on their deeds.... and how, or if , this clause was to be followed up. But, after making specific legal enquiries, we heard that the clause was redundant.

16th July 1969

A letter arrived at the Front Entrance Enquiries Desk for me, sent care of Amberley One Ward. It was from Manchester Dave, who had been discharged from hospital a few months ago. It was a pleasant missive, giving me an update of his situation. No idea of whether he was intent on a return to his pre-admission University studies. I found his philosophical entries interesting.... I'd sent David a quote gleaned from Kierkegaard, and he was just *'Wondering on your intensions ie. Are you trying to safeguard me from the nihilistic thought of existentialism?'*, he wrote.

Which of course, at that time, *I was...* David stated he was to read Bertrand Russell's *History Of Western Philosophy,*[50] which I'd read about ten years ago. Dave said that he'd sought for Ouspensky's *In Search Of The Miraculous* [51] from his local library, but he'd been informed it had gone missing. He said, *he felt* Gurdjieff's philosophy[52] 'will break down on analysis from the standpoint of logical positivism of Ayer and Ryles', (he added), ' for instance, claims that the dualism between mind and body a linguistic error and called this fallacy 'The Ghost In The Machine.' What I'm saying is this that Gurdjieff's philosophy may be a lot of mystification. Would you agree ? ...'

My first response, as I recall, to his remark on Gurdjieff, is yes, *of course* it's about mystification. But, even more so, G's knowledge is about a *de-mystification* of life's tenets. And, in reference to *The Ghost In The Machine*.[53] I don't believe it's a fallacy; whatever designated words are attempted *to describe* our invisible inhabitant; dressed in terrestrial clothes. Arthur Koestler's works, on exactly this theme, on the GITM I read and found, very useful an introduction to this theme. But I thought it imprudent, even irresponsible on my part, to continue the correspondence in view of the substance, and an inability to monitor David's rehab progress.

Eastergate Block appeared massive in its dimensions, after the recent experience of the minute Bramber One ward, and its crowded elderly infirm residents. And moved on... I was about to begin a three-month mandatory third-year placement on ME1 — the large Male Eastergate One long-stay ward. Entering the narrow ward passage, through the outside doorway, I first observed, on the left side of the doorway, the usual ward plaque insignia sign posting — with a jet black raised, round nippled door bell, located on the door-post.

KE2... Eastergate Two. Upstairs. (The KE, a survival of the WW1, Kings initial, K, indicating a Male side ward); *KE1. Eastergate One. Downstairs.*

Passing into the narrow ward passage was, initially, like entering an igloo — then emerging into a high ceilinged, many windowed, Ackerman Gallery. This was a huge day-room and dining-room area and, of course, after meals, served as the patients' lounge, with their television and attendant viewing armchairs located at the far end of the gallery. Full length, green, curtains framed outside views of the airing court gardens.

Adjacent to the dayroom, was the equally large, long Main dormitory, housing over fifty longterm residents (above and below) — with additional, occupied, single side-rooms, placed at the top end of the substantial high ceilinged dormitory. One of those side rooms was an occasionally used padded room — to where, some-time back, I had helped to wheel an acutely disturbed aggressive patient, from another ward. Peripheral offices and utility side rooms, including the ward nursing office, were found from the ward entrance to the day-room — the small ward-kitchen located conveniently adjacent, to the day-room and dining area. The large toilets and baths area led off to the immediate right, as you entered the day-room — the dormitory, too, had its main doorway leading off from this threeway junction.

A Hogarth illustrated Old Bethlem Hospital, with minute straw lain cells (back in the 18th. century) gave way to Ackerman illustrated high-ceilinged galleries of St. Lukes' Hospital — also, then in London, to which numbers of Sussex patients had been sent, before the local County Asylums had been erected in the Nineteenth century. The bleak minute, dismal un-healthy cells, giving way to large contemporary hygienic galleries.

As I approached the office, that first early morning on Eastergate, I noticed the ward was already a hive of activity. Outside the kitchen corner open doorway sat out in the passage on the floor, and propped up against the low wall wainscoting, I saw two animated, middle-aged patients, engaged in eager conversation. In front of them, two other dressed patients were busied about the kitchen in tea-making, a third, about them, was busy, anticipating the ward's breakfast, delivered by the electric storage trolley's arrival in half-an'hour or so...

It was still Summertime, and daylight had risen several hours ago, but all the ward's warm, friendly lights were still switched on. And, as I entered the nursing office, I observed, through the passage and at the end of the lengthy gallery of the day room, a number of patients, some dressed, one or two still in their pyjamas, contentedly sat, watching pre-breakfast television.

'Morning Sid... Morning Vic... Johnny...'

I already knew E1 staff from numerous relief duties, over the past two years. Sid was my new ward Charge Nurse. Victor was a brown coated ward orderly. And, guitar Johnny, our RMN Staff, who qualified less than a year ago, and was already a ward fixture.

Team work was basic to the ward's stability. Its evidence well reflected in the patients' attitudes towards the staff, and generally towards each other in this long-term ward — their transient Sanctuary.

'Morning Barry. Sit *down*... Join us... have a cuppa, before you get going. *And* we *are* very pleased to have *you*... eh lads ?', Charge Sid added, as he looked to colleagues Vic and Johnny, sat down in front of him, around the office desk. Together, warmly, they responded, smiling, 'Welcome,', up at me.

Well, I'd arrived at another posting and relaxed, ready for work...

As we talked, the office door properly ajar, patients drifted in and out of the office, with numerous questions about their coming day's activities — or on-going personal needs. Within minutes, after a summary discussion in reference to the Night-report, and the main events of this day, Vic and I made for the dormitory, depositing the tea-tray into the kitchen, and acknowledging the names of the patients we passed, en-route. Whilst Johnny and Sid continued, in serious conversation. The ward routines were underway.

Breakfast was almost over, with Vic and I assisting in offering seconds where food remained in the tins. Johnny had the Medicine trolley wheeled out into the day-room, and stationed it close by the three doors junction of kitchen, dorm, and ablutions entrance. He called me over, to assist him in special distribution to the less ambulant residents, and to anticipate my learning the medicine rounds as soon as possible — to take over in his inevitable periods of absence. And, obviously, it was an excellent way to be more closely involved with every patient on the ward. Sidney, as Charge, was already busy on the telephone. In total, there were about fifty patients on this large ward, with an almost identical number, located upstairs on E2. Ward personalities emerged from the outset; first was Martin. On arrival into the igloo like, narrow, ward passage preceding the gallery, Martin was one of the two animated patients sat down outside the kitchen entrance.

Martin

Dressed in well laundered hospital clothing, he was five-feet nothing Leprechaun tall, balding at the forehead, and boasting a contented convex waist corporation. Most attractive was his endearing, almost fixed smile; a moving cloud of ambiance, wherever he travelled. Martin was born over forty years ago with manifest febrile epileptic fits, which prevailed and developed into a full blown epilepsy but diminished, with time, medication, and good moral care — he was an orphan. In historical parlance, Martin was labelled as a child, in the 1920s, as Epileptic and Mentally Frail and Deficient — idiocy. Martin more Munchkin — than Myshkin.

Sid informed me that it was unusual, in those early days, for patients with his handicaps to live beyond forty years. And, remembering only too well my experiences on Bramber One and, so far, of Epileptic personalities, well - affable Martin did *not* fit that mould, *that* was for sure...

In his early years, Martin's behaviour was recorded as disturbed and aggressive, assertive...

I felt that I, too, would most definitely have been so too... think of his then pre-war peers ... think of the sheer numbers ... and, the then extreme paucity of resources.

God... good for him.

He was neither Saint, sinner, or *idiot-savant* but, rather, like an overgrown occasional irascible child — obviously, my own shorthand way of accepting his normality.

And so, I was introduced to Martin.

Due Medication — a small dose of stabilising Epanutin each day. Also, in the medicine queue, several people behind, was a tall, straight-backed, middle-aged man, immaculately dressed — at least, say, in comparison to Martin and most other long-term hospital, indigent residents. This was James.

Ex-RSM Jim

James, a Services Patient, on the *Ministry of Pensions* list, had been in and out of hospitals for over twenty years — since 1945. He had been badly wounded on a number of occasions, during the war in Europe; eventually, it was recorded, he was found hidden amongst a pile of dead. He survived, but with severe head-wounds, which left him brain damaged, and unable to live in the outside community. James was an ex-Regimental Sergeant Major, of the Royal Artillery. Prior to his long-ago first admission, at home, he had fallen down a steep flight of stairs... it was the last straw.

We were just handing Jim his plastic cup with orange juice and two pills with a 'Thanks John... and... eh... Nice to meet you, Barry...' from Jim, when a loud angry voice and wild shuffle occurred, at the rear of the short orderly queue.

Jim stopped his hand movements, suspending the motion of pills to mouth and drink to down them and, turning his head, said disgustingly 'Might have guessed, bloody Tusker again... who's he bullying this time?'

Staff adroitly stepped out, away from the trolley and, looking towards the source of the disturbance, spotted Charlie Red — nicknamed Tusker, for his infamous habit of brandishing, and too often attacking, with his wooden, steel tipped crutch. He had a gammy leg, and had needed a support for many years.

One of the patients, Ian, was eager to get off early to work at the IT yard, and, in his eagerness to get off to The Greenhouse and some particular plants he was nurturing, had accidentally nudged Charlie, who was only inches in front of him. And Tusker had instantly turned to threaten poor Ian, who was full of profuse apologies and some fear as he, like all the regular ward staff and patients, knew only too well of Charles Red, and his infamous bad temper. But, fortunately, one obvious look from Staff John was itself enough — and, in front of all these witnesses ...

The Medicine round continued, without further incident. Within half an' hour or so, the ward was almost emptied, as the patients went off ward to their respective Therapies — or whatever organised appointments. And, as with all ward routines, with the medicines, breakfast, washing-up completed and patients' initial needs of this day underway, came The Staff Breakfast break.

The small square-table, four chairs, white table-cloth, plates and utensils were laid in preparation by Victor, while the Nursing staff anticipated the next round of morning duties — after twenty minutes or so. The assembly was placed in the dayroom corner, against the first large window, and directly opposite the junction of the three-doors — where we had a broad view of the whole ward, and could clearly hear the ward telephone, if and when necessary. At breakfast, Sid outlined some more of my duties, and intended learning activities.

Designated duty; after every breakfast, I was to henceforth attend the small clinic room, just off of the large dormitory. One specific chore was to attend to a quiet, middle-aged Freddie, a diabetic and severe excema skin sufferer. And so, starting that very morning, I carried out a litmus test on his supplied sample. And, afterwards, dabbed on a thin layer of white, claylike Betnovate onto his angry ragged patches of affected skin tissue. Daily, I changed a number of patients' dressings, for the inevitable minor ailments — anything more serious was for England Ward, or the ward doctor. The standard long-stay ward routine duties, quickly and comfortably fell into place.

That afternoon, at the hand-over, I was introduced to Ken, our ward volunteer — a local Chichester fireman, family man and another dependable rock, for resident patients and ward nursing staff. He was in his mid-thirties, quite large in girth, and was always casual but immaculately dressed — and always in good cheer.

Ken had a wonderful wide ruddy face, long tied-back fiery-red hair, and deep-set brown-eyes, with an umbrella of thick red bushy eye-brows. Noticeable was his tree-branch moustache. I was reminded of Summersdale patient RAF Brian, a confederate of fictitious comic hero *The Champion* [54] and his Tangmere Spitfire aircraft; and of Captain W.E. Johns war-time fictional pilot, Biggles. But it was, most, as a cartoonesqe copy image of BBC radio and television endearing leaned comedian, Professor Jimmy Edwards, the comic's proud, bushy handlebar moustache, *that* with which I would most fondly remember of our humane, auxiliary staff volunteer by. 'Our Jim' (as BBC said), was a real-life wartime RAF flying officer.

Fire

It was one afternoon, several weeks later, when a dramatic incident occurred which, later, would become burned (no pun intended) into my memory. Dinner was over, and medicines just completed. Ken had just arrived, and we were congregating in the ward office, anticipating The Handover. Vic was showing the staff several of his latest pencil sketches, one of which was to be published in the near future. Suddenly, we were interrupted by Harry, a very excitable patient of ours, who burst into the office.

'Puff puff. Fire ... There's a Fire ... smoke ... in the passage ... gasp...'

No fire alarm had yet sounded.

We looked at Harry and responded.

Sid declared serenely, 'I'll ring the main office and fire brigade ...'

Ken, Vic and I agreed immediately to accompany Harry, and check it out. As we arrived on the scene,others, mostly patients, were looking anxiously up a flight of stairs and at a closed door, under which a regular spiral, of dark smoke, was indeed, clearly visible.

It was the small staff-room, where I occasionally spent time in private study. There was a small television in that room, and the possibility of someone up there was already apparent to us. Ken was our expert, and Vic and I looked to him for immediate guidance... Further down the corridor was the nearest fire-point, an enclosed red fire hose and small axe with an adjacent *Break The Glass* fire alarm.

'Yeah. Right! No time to lose...', Ken replied. 'If Vic goes back to the ward, and tells Sid where it is, Barry and I will go up there and try and investigate — in case there is someone there; where there's smoke there may be fire. First, better ring that fire alarm... would you break the glass in that box, down the corridor?', he said, to a white-coated colleague who had just arrived, and added, as he departed down the passage and Ken and I ascended the flight of stairs, up to the doorway, 'I'm surprised the alarm hasn't rung ...'

Though smoke continued from under the door, there was no sign of any flame or felt heat, as we stopped outside the door at the top of the short flight of stairs. No human sounds emanated from within. I informed Ken that I knew the layout of the room. It had little furniture. A table and chair on the right-side of the room, where I usually worked. And another small table, with a television on it, in the left hand corner. In front of which were two low armchairs... perhaps, someone could be in there, and unconscious, whatever ...?

'Barry, smoke generally rises towards the ceiling. If we go in, I suggest we get down on our bellies and crawl forward, and see if there is anyone in there. *But, be ready* to back, if we meet any fire and flame. Tie your handkerchief round your mouth, as I'm going to nudge the door open... step to the side of the doorway. Right. Now...'

Ken turned the door-knob, and pushed the door-ajar, then opened it enough for us to enter. A thick choking black mass flooded out, but there was *no* sight, or sound, of any signal flames. As we went into the smoke-filled room, the loud shrill and shriek of the hospital fire alarm went off... it was highly probable that Sid had already phoned the station before contacting the main office, and the fire brigade from Chichester were already on their way.

So, together, flat on the floor, Ken led the way in and I, holding onto his feet, arms stretched out, was close behind him. The smoke was certainly thick, but it was most dense over our heads. As we moved forward, it seemed like hours — yet, from our arrival downstairs, was only really a matter of a few minutes. And as we so slowly, gingerly groped our way onwards, there was no sign of any other person. Suddenly, I was startled, as I felt, rather than saw, someone standing in the choking smog up above me, wearing a gas-mask and holding a small-axe, and then, there was another man gesticulating for Ken and myself to withdraw, as the fire brigade formally took over.

Back in our E1 ward office, as we reported the event to Sid, Vic and John, I was silently amused in noticing, that whilst our skin and clothes were not surprisingly blackened by the clinging smoke, Ken's now black moustache was otherwise completely unaffected — all that practice I mused. I had no way of knowing the outcome of that brief adventure, though no news indicated no casualties. But, it could have anticipated my involvement, as a part-timer night Staff nurse and *rescuer* in a significant ward fire on Amberley One, some years later, in which I would play a leading role. But that event, as the cliche runs, *is* another story....

On The Carpet

Mid-morning, on E1, and we were enjoying a tea-break. The four of us were seated in the large day-room gallery; Sid, John, Vic and myself. And I had a burning question for him. I asked. ...

'Who? ... Who Sid? ...' Curious, giving him full attention, I looked across at Charge, our local COHSE (Confederate Of Health Service Employees) Union Secretary, and wondered, *what* hat he was about to wear.

'Yeah, *why,* Sid, what's this admin visit... about...?', asked Staff.

Vic, whilst equally giving Sid his undivided attention, said a meaningful nothing, at this initial response. But, did I see a slight grin, as if he already had some glimmer of what was to come. 'What I can tell you all is that it's *something* to do with *The Annual Budget,* and the possible future of the Eastergate block.', replied a very patient Sid. 'And, before you start on about a likely ward closure, forget it. That's in the future, whenever that will be, but it's impossible *at this time,* that's for sure.'

We were pacified, and any instant panic vanished, with Sid's re-assurance.

'Erm ... What time is this visit, Sid?', said a no-longer mortified Staff John.

'What's the time now?', Sid said, looking casually at his watch; 'Almost eleven... any time now — in fact I can hear voices, must be in the corridor ?'

And, sure enough, three people, two men and one woman, surfaced in our day room. The ward was, not unusually, empty of residents at this moment — though one patient was in the dorm, resting on his bed, feeling a bit out-of-sorts.

'Ah *there* you are Sidney.', called out Mrs. Vatson - the Office duty S.N.O. '*And,* good... your staff with you... excellent...'

Full of enthusiasm, she waved on her two colleagues in train, behind her, to follow.

'Stay where you are, please, Sid. We could do with a cuppa ourselves. Only good news, we think so, anyway.'

Which she gushed, uninterrupted, and made for mouths wide open and well surprised group. Oh bloody hell, I thought, hope it's not a Trojan horse, an advent bringing of Orwellian bad tidings, with just a sweetener being introduced.

Beside Office' Mrs. Vatson, other messengers, included Consultant Psychiatrist, Doctor Joyce, and, from *Patients Affairs*, Admin Baz, our Hospital Administrator. All three visitors wholly trusted and popular, amongst staff, and especially so amongst the nursing staff. If there was to be any bad tidings, they could certainly soften the blow.

Thank God, it was not to be bad-tidings, not even bad-timing, Sid and Vic, and certainly our three official visitors were, over the years, well used to such admin ward visits, pre-Annual Reports, albeit preparatory for any Enquiries for budget balancing, or anticipating *any* sort of changes (including politic) affecting patients and staff needs, and the building fabric of the ward and hospital premises in general. But, new Staff nurse John, and third-year student RMN Barry, were *not* familiar with such business.

Mrs. Vatson explained that, towards the end of each fiscal year, the accountants assessed how, during the past year, the hospital's credit, debit and merit accounts balanced. It was then politic to appreciate that, if the admin had been too frugal or over zealous in expenditure, the following year's government budget would be decided upon. The reason for this visit was if there was a surplus (due to good house-keeping) then the money must be used — or their next year's allocation would certainly be considerably reduced.

A strong influential factor was that the hospital resident population (bed state stats) was definitely on the wane, as the NHS was able to access vast scientific clinical and technology advances, following the end of the last war, and this hospital's excellent movements into its more Community services (as *The Worthing Experiment* and General hospital Psychiatric out-patient services; and greater use of MWOs and the *Social Services* et cetera, in the 1950s and 1960s, have demonstrated). Our benign visiting trio indicated that the Eastergate block, and its hundred plus long-stay beds are, and will be, needed for at least several more years — and some of this year's savings was on offer, for Eastergate One.

Dr. Joyce

'One huge Carpet... what, wall-to-wall... this *entire,* gallery-size, patients' day-room ...?'

Sid asked Basil, delighted, but still incredulous, at the probable expense, the what-what *luxury*, as Admin Baz out-lined that Patients' affairs had already provisionally agreed with Doc Joyce, and Mrs. Vatson on behalf of the PNO and Nursing body (the hospital's representatives on The Management Committee.). 'Yes. Soon. And we would like to have *your* staff, and your patients' thoughts on the matter', insisted a very sincere Mrs. Vatson — the same warm hearted Senior Nursing Officer who, in civvies, had welcomed me on my first day back in 1967, at my reception in the main office, as I had stood dripping at her feet in a pool of rain water.

'That's right.', Doc Joyce grinned, nodded, quick agreement. One of Dr. Joyce's duties was to attend Nightingale Two ward, as a Psychotherapist — his pedigree included Dr. Ernest Jones, a friend and biographer of the great Doctor Sigmund Freud. Dr. Ernest Jones had been employed at Graylingwell in the 1940s, as an Honorary Psychotherapist.[55] Our amiable quiet man, Doc Joyce, was renowned for his sense of humour as much as his enormous humanity. One favourite and true anecdote — later to be told to me by himself (and confirmed by other sources)[56] — sounded like an episode from the television series *Z Cars*.

Not long ago, during one ward based office interview *behind closed doors,* member of staff alone, Doctor Joyce had been confronted by a distressed patient who held a pistol (how) to the doctor's head, when the phone rang — the hospital exchange, informed of his whereabouts, had put his wife through to the ward (did he ever tell her?).

'Eh. Oh, hello dear ... I'll be delayed for a while - as I'm being held up ... but I'll get away as soon as I can ...' By the time the police arrived, and placed armed men in position, it was all over... our loveable Doc had talked him down, and taken the pistol off him (I never learnt whether it was loaded or not — neither did he). Our psychiatrist then persuaded the visiting officers to take no further action — as '*Everything is under control Officer!*' Oh, our quiet man had a lovely sense of wit and humour and, especially, lots of patience.

'And, yes we *have*, we believe, considered maintenance of the carpet, and its likely wear and tear...', added a delighted Admin Baz. (Both Baz and Doc Joyce would be colleagues of mine for many years ahead, but we couldn't have envisaged it at that time ...)

For all of us present on Eastergate One ward, *The Carpet* was not just about economy or its utility, we had a collective, massive repository of past-and-present experiences, easily related to the moral and cultural, and past practical implications, of carpet replacing, historical asylum house-use, of rushes, then flooring covered by cold stone-tiles; straw-wood-linoleum-rubber-and now, on offer warm-woollen, carpeting.

Staff awareness, of on-going urine soaked bedding, clothing and floors - and the health and cleaning responsibilities; for example, on the Elderly Mentally ill (EMI.) on Bramber One, and Chilgrove One wards; and the large female block of Edgworth and Fawcett, mostly for elderly and demented residents; Admin Baz informed us that some carpet was already being installed, as: '*Flooring subject to urine soaking was covered in water repellent carpeting — good in short term only.*'

But, equally, credence must be given to the clean, aired, polished and immaculate, Rehab wards; these included *both* of the two Eastergate long-stay wards. And it didn't need Vic, our ward orderly, to point all this out to us... asepsis maintained. The hospital's own managed, cleaning and portering service department, worked closely with the medical and nursing professionals, and ensured that no infestation, poisonous infections and alien viruses be allowed to grow on *their* wards.

I was much daunted, no haunted the better word, in having read the 1946 book of journalist Mary Jane Ward's *The Snake Pit* [57] and, even more so, of the later 1948 film (deemed a Horror Film) of that name, and immense public media outrage in its wake. Much of it at the audacity of showing *this* dirty linen in public, and wanting to, erm, hide it away. Under the metaphorical, *and* real carpet. Not on for public consumption.

There was a long pause following senior nurse Mrs. Vatson's question, what did we think of the suggestion — *what* did we honestly think, feel, about it? God. I thought it was bloody *marvellous*. But, cloistered, my own deep feelings stayed down, as the trumpets of Jericho (and ancient Memphis), shook the very walls of human fear and blind prejudice — yet, subdued, laconic, I replied. 'I think it's a *great* suggestion .' Quietly spoken, sussurated, me under the red rose. ... And we all agreed on the motion.

There is one iconic image, in an old Picture Post [58] graphic still photograph, culled from the movie; and a torrent of correspondence and leaders which responded to its commentary — which today I hold, in my mind. It was the *forbidden carpet* scene in *The Snake Pit,* when the horrified, agitated ward nurse tells Virginia she must *not* step on the centre ward carpet, but walk around it, like all the other patients. It was taboo... *Keep Off The Grass* outside, *Keep Off The Carpet* inside. And so, Virginia was placed on the, ironic metaphoric, *magic* carpet. Virginia had other ideas.

Resident on a 1940s American acute psychiatric ward, alike, perhaps, our Barnet Two and Bramber Two, Mrs. Virginia Cunningham, whose sanity was painfully beginning to return, *defied* the hospital rule (any piece of carpet was so *rare* it had, *had* to be for decoration only) defied *not* in malice, but in asserting her will to return to life. And so, shoeless, in bare feet, Virginia moved on, and stepped forward, *onto* the *forbidden* carpet; and, so, assumed the dignity of respecting, knowing, the fabric of the carpet, itself as, too, a part of her life, and began a full recovery.

Shortly after the new carpet had been laid down, in the large day room on Eastergate One of that time, Admin Baz recalled a telling memory; 'On the day the wards were carpeted, the ward charge nurse had to visit the admin offices and, he'd said, he *had* to tell us what he had just seen. The working patients had just returned to the ward, and stopped at the door to the day room (before access to the dormitory and ablutions) and, upon seeing the new carpet, and without *anyone* saying a word to them, they promptly took off their footwear before proceeding further. Baz said I used the argument that the mind is influenced by its immediate surroundings, and eventually got carpet laid in *our* own admin offices.'

Monday, July 21st 1969
Luna-ticks and modules

Mick, recently qualified RMN and an ardent Christian Scientist lived, with his young family, within easy walking distance from our new residence in Eastham Road in Littlehampton and had agreed, when our shifts coincided, to give me a lift, to and fro from work. He was a regular Staff up on E2 and, this morning, his Charge was off duty, and The Office had detailed me to start upstairs, and assist with breakfasts, medication and whatever tasks could be helpful to Mick's fifty plus residents before, later descending back to my base on Eastergate One ward.

This morning was very special; in its way, *special* for every living being on our planet — present and future scientific possibilities, *not* necessarily probabilities. We were five hours behind the American East Coast time line, namely the NASA rocket base at Florida, from where, on Wednesday the Sixteenth of July 1969, a large manned rocket, dubbed Apollo 11, had departed for real, aimed for *The Moon.* The broadcast *live* commentaries, out of Florida, had many of us, both staff and patients, spellbound — almost all...

My generation, born in the late 1930s and during wartime Nineteen-forties, were media fed on comics, and *Boys Own Paper* magazines [59] facts and fiction, BY ROCKET THROUGH SPACE. Seen, on the cover, a drawing-board pic of a rocket, high up in space and, in ten mins (it said) London to New York — a space hop, viewed as one easy example on the front-page, of a battered sixpenny *Practical Mechanics* magazine.[60] Such magazines were enjoyed, and hoarded, by a surprising number of our older hospital residents in the back-wards. Also to be found in the bedside lockers of some long-stay patients, were well thumbed, torn and tattered bundles, of *Meccano* mags and Science fact & fiction, among Fantasy adventure paperbacks; magazines such as *Galaxy,* and *Outstanding Science*. [61]

Eastergate Two longstay residents, Doc and Boots, were two such patients who had sat up, all the previous night, awed, watching the *Moon Landing* on the small black and white ward television, accompanied by a transistor radio, placed on a long-back by Doc's side to be played when the TV lapsed from time to time. Evidence of their vigil, the radio left on the chair and, on the vacated chairs, small debris of empty, crumbled, crisp packets and choc wraps, and several dirty cups and saucers. On my arrival, the two stalwarts had just retired for a lay down, before having their breakfast and, departing for their hospital jobs — Doc to The Printing Department, and Boots (of course) to the Boot Repairers.

Staff Nurse Mick and I had a glimpse at our respective domestic box, before our departure for work and were well focused, on the hot topicality of this *great* real life adventure, and its fact and fictional prequels. We spoke of the foundation science-fiction works, of the Victorian and early 19th century fantasy novelists, Jules Verne and Herbert. G. Wells — and their genius classic, imaginative stories of mankind's to be believed, inevitable *journeys to the moon,* and beyond. And, how our grandparents and *their* parents, and *their* forebears, anticipated the transition from Montgolphier balloons, Zeppelins, Horse-drawn coach and buses; and how, in just two generations, all of us, patients and staff, lived, existed now, in a world of flying aircraft, jets and rocket modules (including wartime V1 buzz bombs and, later, V2 rocket missiles, which I too, had personally witnessed as a child standing in awe on the playground of Reigate, Spurgeons Orphan Homes as they flew over us, and seen to fall down ahead, over London and Surrey landscape back in 1944, but twenty-five years ago).

Collecting his stabilising singular one tab a day, at after breakfast medication, Doc, who was usually mute, suddenly spoke to us in a subdued low voice, recalling a time, as a Medic Student back in the 1950s, *before* onset of his illness, and asked Mick and I if we knew writer Arthur C. Clarke's *Sentinel.* And, had we seen Robert Heinlein's film, *Destination Moon.*[62] And how very like that film rocket, on the hazy black and white ward television, it resembled the Moon Landing NASA rocket module. We nodded, said Yes, we remembered, as children, seeing that post-war landmark. I said to Doc, who still kept a number of *Astounding* Sci-fi mags from student days in his bed locker (it was the *only* time I would ever hear him in conversation) did *he* ever read Arthur. C. Clarke's book, *The Exploration Of Space.*[63] He paused, as his reading glasses shifted upon his nose, as if a definite memory gave him a fraction of old long-forgotten clarity, and stared, frozen for a moment, stared at me, and said, '*Yes.*' *Yes* he recalled the book, and especially the book's illustrations of the *Spaceship On Moon,* [64] which he too recalled, and which reminded him of the Module nose cone of The Apollo. Eastergate Two Doc departed off to work in the hospital's Printing Department, and Boots went off to the Cobblers.

An hour later, Mick and I joined Sid and Vic downstairs, for a cup of tea and elevenses. We mentioned our brief conversation with Doc on giving him his medication. Sid replied softly, 'Sad you know... Doc... he's been here over ten years now... He was a young lecturer at a University... practising Doctor once... wrote a *Medical Textbook* when he was young — sad... he had a severe schizophrenic breakdown, but he's now better than he was... I remember when he was first sectioned, he used to be *very* aggressive. Reckon he could live in the community, now though, cause, he's so damaged he'll not be able to practice medicine again, though.'

Tusk

Late morning. Quiet. Staff John was off-duty; Sid was off the ward, visiting The Office on COHSE business, and I had just arrived back with a box of refills from the pharmacy. Vic had been in the ward kitchen, but came into the office on my return, to ask if I fancied a last cuppa before we prepared for our patients mid-day return for lunch, and for a few tds medications. Of a sudden, breaking the peace, we heard an abrupt loud shriek of anger, followed by an even louder scream of fright; an echoing noise of crashing, and what sounded like objects being hurled and thrown about somewhere, and very close.

'Bloody hell! ' I exploded. 'What the hell was that?'

'Sounds like it's coming from the dorm.', replied Vic, as we both strode off in the direction of the disturbance.

As we entered through the doorway, the source was self evident; on the right side of the ward were two figures, on appearance a giant enraged Tusker, his right arm upraised and, using his metal crutch as a weapon, stood battering a terrified diminutive Martin, crouched in a foetal ball at his feet; both located at the foot of Tusker's bed, and in a pathway, between a row of unoccupied beds. They were otherwise alone, on the ward.

Unsurprising, Tusker froze his action, as he spotted us, and saw we were drawing closer to him and his prey. As appropriate, Vic dropped behind me as I, my duty of care, taking the confrontation in at a glance. We stopped, a few yards between us, and asked what did he think he was doing... and:

'*Why*... Charlie... What's Martin done to annoy *you*... ?'

Martin, although clearly hurt, we could observe markings on his face hands and arms where he had attempted to shield himself from Tusker's angry blows, looked to Vic and I, with clear relief. Oh how I dislike, no hate, bullies. Tusk Charlie, non-plussed, replied....

' Why!... *Why?*... Stupid little git annoyed me, *that's* why ...'

'What! ... Is that it ...?' Incredulous. For a second, Vic and I just stared at him.

I looked at him, into cold fish eyes, and expressed my disgust at this yet another example of his bullying, and unjustified act of aggression, against anyone appearing weak and stupidly vulnerable, in his eyes. Before I could comment further, he added, 'What's 'ee got to be so bleeding 'appy about anyway. Always grinning an *so* so nice... gets on my wick.'

'I see... So you hit him... for *that*...?', I replied. A little diffused, not deflated, and still defiant, Tusk turned his venom on me, at me now, but *not* Martin, and so taking advantage of this fact, I turned and looked behind me. 'Vic... could you help Martin up and move him behind me, and out of this man's reach.' No comment needed. But as this action took place, mammoth Tusker made it clear he wasn't beaten yet. And, as he moved slightly to one side, I realised he had, clasped in his lowered left hand, the thick neck of a jagged, broken green beer-bottle. Talk about the cavalry; as Vic held Martin, I grabbed a pillow for a shield and went to disarm the bully, as he went to attack me and, as the broken-glass and his metal crutch glanced off my pillow covered, out-thrust right arm, Tusk lost his balance and Charge Sid came striding through the doorway. It was over.

Totally deflated, a subdued Charlie threw himself down onto his low bed. Sid told him, in no uncertain manner, that he was lucky he was not being sent up to Bramber Two, or put in a side-room, to cool down. Tusk acknowledged that, perhaps, he had been a bit rough on Martin. Later on, filling in the inevitable *Incident Form,* and having addressed poor innocent Martin's wounds and such bewildered demeanour, as a further precaution, Sid gave Charlie a PRN dose of liquid largactil, which told Tusker that this event was, thank heavens, over.

Pantomime

'Have you heard when someone climbed up onto the roof, and put a chamber pot on top of the weather-vane over the front entrance ...?' Baz, from Patients Affairs, was reminiscing. He'd started work at the hospital in 1950, just after the NHS started. (Much later, Baz and I checked out this event, out of curiosity;

Roy M., a senior clerk at the time, said it was an office clerk, Barry M, who did the deed, aided by another office colleague, Arthur I., who kept watch — Roy believed it was in 1949.)

Charge Sidney — and quiet man, Doc Joyce, who'd started at the hospital in 1954 and had just finished a ward interview with one of our patients, together with Admin Baz, Staff John, Orderly Vic and myself, were enjoying a tea-break mid-morning in the dayroom. And the days of 1940s, and early 1950s, were recalled. Sid and Doc said 'Yes', they knew of it well — it was more than a prank, it was a gesture of rebellion ... and recalled other hospital family acts of rebellion. I was surprised at this friendliness and forthcoming, of one of our Senior medical staff, socialising with junior nurses (est moi), *and* auxiliary staff. But, after nearly two years, I felt I was one of a cohesed body of staff and residents, as *they* recalled those early postwar years.

'Erm ... What was *that* about then?', I boldly asked, of the two elder statesmen.

'Before television was introduced into the wards after the Coronation in 1953, off the wards, there were occasional cinema shows in the Main Hall. It was Dances, and patients singing up there, on the stage in the Hall — those weekly dances for the patients — remember, the *total* segregation of staff and patients... those dances allowed a mixing of the sexes.' Enthused, warm loquacious Baz, recalled early NHS days.

'That's right' Sid continued, and looked to Baz for confirmation. 'And the men, male staff and their patients stood on one side, and the females on the other side, the dance floor in the territory between them. And all those deft attempts to pass notes, from one side to the other, when they could... The dances were very popular, weren't they.'... 'But the chamber pot...?', I interrupted, remaining curious as to what, and why, it had occurred.

'We're coming to that', said Baz, reliving the zealous postwar Spirit of that time. '... Since The War, local voluntary organisations continued to do what they could, and had done so generously, since The Asylum first opened, to entertain or occupy the hospital patients; visiting the hall and giving shows and concerts ... The hospital staff (reps of all trades and professions) too, voluntarily, provided entertainment, athletics, sports and charabanc outings out of the hospital, for all patients wanting to, and able.'

Baz grinned, as he looked to Doc and Sid to let him know where he was at. John, Vic and I just sipped our now cold tea, and waited... We had not, after all, been around *here,* in those post-war years, with so few staff, and so many patients.

'Each month, *The Wishing Well,* our in house hospital magazine, accepted contributions from Staff and patients and gave notice of entertainment to come; and opportunities for including comments on recent events. And, well... The magazine had advertised our annual Christmas pantomime, in which staff volunteered and organised their own show, these were always hilarious... With an influx of new medical and nursing staff, including pre-war returning veterans, they started to *influence* the storylines, and topical visual jokes ...', Admin Baz reminisced. 'There was this one early Nineteen-fifties Christmas pantomime, with considerable staff satire, which was so funny, but subsequently *not* acceptable to The Management (who quickly killed of all the pantomime shows, completely). Great pity, 'cos there was a lot of real talent in the hospital, and it did unite all employees, with the patients, and their relatives and visitors to our hospital community.'

'I *happen* to know, the offender.', Doc Joyce said, slow, mischievous, eyes twinkling, talking almost at a whisper. '*The Wishing Well,* at that time, printed an anonymous critique of a decision recently made by *The Management.* I think it was something about 'replacing old red tiles' somewhere or other... and, to which, the nursing staff had voiced their reservations.'

'Anyway, the *Anonymous* contributor was known by most Junior Doctor colleagues to be *one* of them, and was known to be popular with the nursing staff, for his often outspoken views in support of specific reforms. But, The Superintendent took it personally, and was furious, as no-one would confirm it was Doctor X who was the collaborator. '

'What happened ...?', I asked.

'As you can imagine, the Medical Superintendent was furious. And absolutely *no-one,* nurse, doctor or patient, would betray the junior doctor to Dr. Carse — on this small victory. And, no-one ever did.' The hospital, an extended family.

Thursday 14th August 1969
Brighton

My alchemy weekend at The Dicker, a few weeks back, and introduction to some full-time students of *The Work* (*The Great Work*) was still fresh in memory. Whilst applauding the value of my Merry Meeting with Tolkien's cousin Marjorie, and her import on alchemical and psychological teachings, of

Gurdjieff, Ouspensky, Nicoll, et als, — I was saddened to realise I could *not* take up the Admiral's kind offer, to attend The Dicker on any regular basis. But, he relayed to Bunty that I was welcome to attend occasional lectures, held at a Georgian House flat on the Marine Parade in Brighton. And I did, for a little while.

As I travelled back home to Littlehampton, on the Brighton train, I stared our of the train window and, in the act of sitting still, as the train sped on — presenting, impossible to count innumerable separated and then joined-up panoramic, framed visual pictures and, then, applied one of the Exercises on Self-observation. I stared, fixedly, out through the clear glass of the train window, at the passing view. Next, I stopped, suspended, the automatic on-going commentary, of my so-called inner thoughts. Then, with *supreme* effort, I commenced a controlled awareness, witness, inner-self-observer: I recall, that I actually *felt* a different, physical, bringing in to focus located matrix behind my eyes (with a slight pressure in my fore-brain). And, first noticed the re-focus changed my dimensional observation, into a proper (I concluded afterwards) *three* dimensional perspective. The eyes behind the Seer were viewing this reflection from within — a Fourth Way... I suspected.

There is plenty of reading on the Fourth Dimension in other threads [65] to describe, existent terrestrial, organic plus differences between a One dimensional tunnel world (Two dimensional Flat picture world) and the visual geometric Three dimensional world of length, breadth and depth. And.... Our memory in recognizing, identifying, presented phenomena, unthinkably translates into the flat, two dimensional pics and *remembers* the Third — and, lazy, my eyes grow unused to *seeing* true depth, the unbiased, fresh, in-depth Three-dimensional terrestrial world....

In this integrated (I was in control) Self-observation Exercise, I was *momentarily,* acutely *aware,* of other possible implications. Of, *yes,* an inner-geometric-vision of the four dimensions (Graves' love) and more, *much* more. Other daytime' *unaware,* other sure, unused, conscious, labile practising *savant*: and Science-fiction multi-dimension *idiot-savant* — robot, hyperactive, hyperdrive sources of energy. *Being a Source....* and, directly, lost the vision ... lost the moment capacity ... to unite with it all. Odd. I was a little afraid rather than just surprised during this insight.

For several days afterwards, I attempted the exercises of the Gurdjieff, Nicoll and Ouspensky *self-remembering* classes, led by the learned Admiral — in acquiring a living, of the instant, consciousness. I recall making up a number of beds, on Eastergate Two ward, when I was, for awhile, alone, and it was quiet; conditions making the experiment so much easier at this time.

But, of course, I was *not* a member of an active Fourth Way School... a Mithra School of Magic, learning, and living of other greater realities; physic and psychic; about, and within us, sentient beings, as at The Dicker (my choice was made). I was working on my own, groping blind in the dark, in this field (whilst attending the Nursing School) albeit attempting the *Fourth Way* doctrine; I, one of Gurdjieff's idiots; not Yogi, Monk, or Aesthete, but, the Fourth Pathway of normal living; plus extra-mural study... viable, when I could.

So I was on a different path. But, in my own isolated, dark underground, inner mind working, thread labyrinth. Sadly, inadequate, subsequently on my own, I lost the intensity of inner-vision, that I had experienced for such a too brief period... I clearly did *not* have the needed *capacity* for this Knowledge, and application of Higher Learning; but the brief searchlight, insight and its trace would stay within me, while I lived and while I decayed... in silence.

And, with domestic and growing professional demands, these practical exercises diminished; though my two friends, Hugh and Winifred, up in London, continued to support my attempts at such 'heretical' thinking.... And doing, as I devoted a more voluntary life in service, to others, whose needs were greater than mine. (God, that sounds pompous.)

Professional

Mandatory six-months stay, on the Long-stay Eastergate Block, was almost complete, and I was asked if I would work on Bramber Two, over the Christmas 1969 holiday. Several weeks before that date, Sid informed us that a new round of Mental Health Reviews would be underway. These one to one Clinical meetings ensured *all* patients were examined, at least once per year... if practical, every six months, or so — this, of course, was separate from the regular weekly ward rounds.

Now this, to be, round of examinations purpose, was to properly gauge if any and all non-sectioned long-stay, usually over two years in the hospital, residents, could be discharged back into their pre-admission locality; much depended on the social, as well as economic, viability of an end-point decision — relatives, often and for whatever valid reasons could-not, or would-not, support the discharge of their kin, back to a previous abode.

Much was always dependent on resources; available Local Authority parish accommodation; DHSS financial support benefits; GP and tandem psychiatric clinical and social support back-up, and real resources; for those ex-patients who remained isolated, and vulnerable, to the day to day stresses of the *normal*, never ideal, existence into an often norm, no Sanctuary, hostile community; at last Free, and alone, freedom from their previous hospital home — deemed Institution.

Several days later, I learnt that Eastergate Two patients were all due to be interviewed, from the following Monday morning onwards. Early on the formal Review agenda, were Doc Boots, and young epileptic Michael. I did not learn the fate of Doc, but suspect he was discharged to a Home near relatives, when he disappeared from E2 not long afterwards.

Quiet diligent Boots, soon had fate determine his imminent discharge. There was an ongoing government policy to run-down all large State caring institutions, and replace them with *Purpose Built* smaller units *In The Community* at large; the hospital' Bakehouse, Upholsterers, Boot Repairers and The Tailors were all soon to be closed down, with their skilled craftsmen retired or otherwise moved on (the Printers would last awhile longer) but, this also meant that the patients employed on those units also lost their work — and Eastergate Two Boots was on that list. Admin Baz related that the hospital Cobbler died before the date of his retirement, poor Boots, who had happily worked alongside that hospital craftsman for many years, was so grieved that he too soon passed away.

Young epileptic Michael was offered the choice of staying in the hospital as long as possible, or be transferred to an alternative, albeit smaller deemed, more appropriate, Community Home; he declined the offer to be discharged, and would move on to other wards. As E2 closed down, I last heard of Mike on Summersdale.

Now I was only too aware, that the majority of Eastergate One's residents, and all of the E Two's patients, were resident in the hospital as Voluntary patients, and, for whom this, their long-stay residence, was a Sanctuary, Home *and* their work-place. It was thus, hardly surprising, that the ward atmosphere became taut, as many of its residents displayed their *angst* in noticeable displays of florid psychiatric symptoms, which had long since seem buried, with minimal occasional medication.

I drew this observation to NUPE Charge (Sid's opposite) Simon's attention, at one staff breakfast. I said, 'Honestly Simon... it's difficult to gauge whether they are deluded, hallucinating, or acting up... even malingering. Course, I appreciate the pressures they feel they are under, of being moved on — if they are given no choice — to stay... or be moved on — and compulsorily...' He had my drift, and replied, matter of factly, 'They're *Professional...* been here a long time... learnt to be professional... Yup, bound to be so... number of cases.'

'What *do* you mean ...?' I was puzzled, by this staunch remark. 'Well, as patients recover from their acute states... gain insight, *they know* that most of their symptoms can be contained by themselves; propped up by medication, preferably *without* unwanted pressures to live beyond their capacity.' 'Well ... yes ... but ...' I started to interrupt, he continued, 'Occasionally, p'haps inevitably, sometimes they *might* suffer an acute relapse.' Simon clearly guessed my conundrum; 'And, I reckon... only human... sometimes, *in a crisis...* out of knowing, they *can* parade bizarre symptoms; and, hopefully, get what they want *because* of their new found self-control. Whereas, for the most vulnerable, such pressures can invoke a real relapse ...'

During my last few weeks, on the long-stay block, there were an unusual amount of flare ups but, fortunately, no-one went *up-the-stick,* and into a full resumption of their earlier acute, even chronic, past illnesses. And it would soon be time to move on, after six-months mandatory time served on the long-stay Eastergate Block.

Bramber Two again

Christmas 1969 and New Year in Littlehampton — Sara and I decided we would, this coming year, subsidise our low income by taking in several lodgers... and to increase overtime at the hospital — thus the mortgage and inevitable, normal, increased economic demands on our domestic life. Life on Bramber Two was relatively uneventful; the ward ran, as with the body of the hospital, on a skeleton staff, over the whole of the mid-winter holiday period, and into the New Year of 1970. And, there were no Study Days, as the School was closed for the hols duration.

Fortunately, a number of residents were away, accepted on home leave, for the duration of the festive season. Doug was on duty throughout the holiday, but his Staff and student were on leave into the New Year. I was detailed to fill in on his shift, and much of the time we worked alone. The ward seemed quite peaceful, and it was not just a consequence of Christmas cheer, though surely it helped — no, I felt it was a direct result of fractious, moody Tall John being *away* on leave, to his devoted long suffering mum, who had other relatives staying with her over the Christmas.

Tall John's intolerance, and short-fuse, too often set off Can Terry and other disturbed patients, and this now included The Boy (what a misnomer) who, since his October admission when I was present on overtime, had quite frequently gone *up-the-stick,* too often triggered by Tall John. The lanky, muscular, Boy was, for the moment, content with a full bag of gift goodies, which he was dipping into and munching, as he sat in a longback watching the television, among a contented group of residents, sat in a crescent around the ward television and enjoying a Special Edition of the *Morecambe and Wise* comedy show — staccato bursts of group laughter bound their avid attention.

Romantic Jim and Rainbow Jill

Jim, dressed today in clean white shirt, its sleeves rolled up, grey flannels and *polished* black Oxford shoes, had a girl friend, a resident on Barnet Two, Rainbow Jill (I called her); she always arrived, dressed fresh, clean and pressed, in colourful, if oddly matched, raiment, with gaudy (always Persil white) puffed sleeve blouse (with v twin apple breasts), and a rather brief pleated skirt, like a wired lampshade, a dandelion puff; her underside a spark flashing postbox brief red pants; or, as this day (mid-winter!) a white frock, accompanied by open bright red sandals, displaying matched painted red toe-nails. Often, she wore short, white, cotton bobby socks — and, when well, oh how Jill chuckled and bubbled.

But for me, and others, it was Jill's endearing tinkling norm sing-song giggles, with a laughter and lilting voice, which gained instant attention and approval. At times, Jill would be absent for days, and we concluded it was either due to one of Jim's competitors enjoying her favours, or her own dire schizophrenic illness was in an acute episode. But, this Christmas Day, Jim was privileged, and, after the festivities of their respective ward *special* lunch was over, and before I was to go off duty to my own home fare, I greeted rainbow Jill at the ward door — open for Christmas.

'Happy Christmas Barry!', sang up Jill, as I opened the door to her. 'And to you Jill...' 'Erm... is Jim in...?' Before I had time to reply, his eager voice behind me adroitly replied. *'Happy Christmas* Jill... Come in... *Come In.*'

Now *Romantic* Jim stepped up, to give Jill a quick hello kiss on the cheek; and duly escorted her into the dayroom, with myself in train behind them. Realising the obvious, that they were not alone, together, they looked to me, and then to the Quiet Room, a, till recent, single bedroom, off the dayroom, and now with a small table, rug, and two chairs to the table, and in its corner, a singular padded long-back chair.

Most important, it had a door to closet for privacy; it was often used on visiting days, and helpful, when any patient wanted to be alone for any length of time — there was mutual unspoken agreement, with all the ward residents, to respect this facility — and it was always unlocked. I needed no prompting and, the door already ajar, I looked in, and confirmed that the Quiet Room was indeed vacant 'Erm... Barry... all right, if we go in...' Rainbow Jill unusually, quietly lisped. 'Yes... Yes, *of course* you can...' 'Eh, Barry, and could you ... if possible ... erm ... see we're *not* disturbed', Jim interjected, which was most unusual as Jill generally did all the talking for both of them. 'No problem Jim. I'll be in the dayroom, and keep an eye on your door.'

And, with my given reassurance, Rainbow Jill and Romantic Jim adroitly stepped into the room... a brief Sanctuary, and closed the door. Sad, that they were condemned like a Brecht or Wedekind [66] play, made into a silent-film, with doomed actors. Jill in an exotic and erotic, living role as *Lulu*; cast out of a 1929 *Pandora's Box*[67] with Jim, her shadow... two innocents at home?

I moved away, in the direction of the others, and seated residents, engrossed with the antics of comedians *Morecambe and Wise* on a pre-recorded TV Christmas show. Twenty years ago, the patients would have been able to laugh at the live staff pantomime, in the Main Hall; now, it was a black-and-white small raised television in the ward lounge. Moving on...

God knows... Jill and James, both in their late twenties, had precious little in life to enjoy — Jim, an ex-Merchant Navy man was mostly quite shy, whereas Jill was very active, in every way; she had been formally prescribed The Pill for sometime as an obvious, but also considerate precaution. I don't know, but as long-stay sectioned patients, it was probably the only freedom they were able, at least to *sometimes* — enjoy.

About twenty minutes later, and moments before, Dougie called me into the office to anticipate our Handover to the afternoon shift — Jill and Jim stepped out of the quiet room, looking a wee bit dishevelled, and (Good!) looking rather smug and pleased with themselves.

I was sure I overheard Jill playfully ask of Jim, 'Did you enjoy your present?' He didn't reply, just grinned, albeit looked just a wee bit sheepish. Sounds of continued laughter, still echoed from the area of the ward television, and even Can Terry appeared to be enjoying the show, his horrors, awhile, held at bay.

On my departure, I wished *A Merry Christmas* to everyone; the young, acutely ill of Bramber Two, and the long-forgotten, vacant and hollow, the disinherited, elderly men, who waited down on Bramber One for Godot.

Christmas over, and Doug's regular Staff nurse, sociable Bob, was back on duty. Big Robert had at least three other members of his family, as qualified RMN staff, employed at the hospital; his wife was recently qualified and working over at Summersdale, and would shortly be promoted to Ward Sister — his older brother was a Senior Nurse, employed in admin at The Office. I dubbed Bob, sociable, due to his own and his family's enthusiastic activities in support of the hospital Social Club.

Shortly after Sociable Bob's return, I had cause to be grateful for his robust presence. Once again we had a normal full ward, all residents who had been on leave were back on the ward. Tensions were much in evidence. The holiday period had proved to be cold, wet and miserable — and no-one wanted to go out, for any walkabout. Tall John was his usual immature, truculent self, and that afternoon did a round of his fellow patients, first asking, then demanding; '*Give me a fag.*', with his usual tact, or else...

Tall John generally avoided Can Terry, and Romantic Jim, knowing they wouldn't stand for his threatening demands but, he did *not* bargain with the explosion he received from our still recent, new admission, The Boy. The latter did not *say* anything, he just thumped and knocked down an amazed Tall John — who, deflated, quickly backed away.

The released anger and frustration of The Boy, tall strong and psychotic, he directly backed off all the other patients; initially it took three of us staff (reality, meant lucky if there were two of you — but often you were alone) to hold down his wrath ... so, Staff nurse Bob and I struggled with our enraged patient, as we walked him down the dorm to the corner padded side room to cool off.

Doug rang the Duty Consultant, and subsequently drew up a substantial dose of PRN largactil in the ward clinic; whilst we, Bob and I, sought to remove The Boy's thick soled shoes but, as I momentarily turned my back, stooping down to un-lace his shoes, The Boy, with a scream and a huge surge of strength, threw Bob backwards, and I received an almighty rabbit slice punch on the back of my neck... I fell to the floor, for a moment stunned and, as Charge Doug arrived, with Bob's assistance, he gave the tranquillising injection, though it seemed ages before Boy settled down, and was allowed to return to the dorm and dayroom.

In retro, that incident would mark the *only* time I was physically assaulted by a patient, in Graylingwell psychiatric hospital. Later on that afternoon, Bob and I, as 'witnesses', filled in the inevitable *Incident Form.* Little did I know, that it would be my *last* ever use of a Pad — as, upgraded, these side-rooms would soon become valued single bedrooms, and replace the previous isolation rooms facilities. At one time, *every* ward had its own pad, in occasional use since the Asylum's inception in 1897, and all visitors to the room had, *had* to have their names entered into the ward's *Seclusion Book* if they were in use...

It was Thursday early afternoon and dark on the ward, the lights generally left on all day, bored and often fractious residents were making frequent visits to the small ward kitchen, for gallons of tea, and numerous trips to the ward office; for fags, chocolate or *'How much have I got'* requests, to be signed for by patient and staff — this, their own pocket money float, contained in brown envelopes and kept in a locked drawer; it was, of course, separate from monies held in the Patients Affairs department.

Lunch finished, and washing up chore completed, awaiting the next duty shift to turn in, I sat down and chatted awhile with Tall John, aware he had a short attention span for any conversation... 'So you see John, apples and pears are *different* items of food; but both are called fruit ...' It was no use, he thought I was saying they were different but the same - and remained most bemused.

'Barry, I *want* to go to pictures in the hall, this afternoon. You *can* take me, if Dougie says it's all right, *can't you...?'* Daring me to say no... I was due to go off duty, and intended to do some homework over at the school... But, well, a favourite musical of mine *happened* to be showing, *Singin' in the Rain,* [68] starring fabulous dancers Gene Kelly and Donald O'Connor, and feisty Debbie Reynolds.

'You sure you don't mind, can't justify overtime, I'm afraid.' Doug confirmed when I joined the Handover. 'No, it's okay, he's not been too bad the past coupla days.' I reassured our Charge Nurse — John smiled expectedly, as he stood just outside the office.

Although he had problems with any prolonged conversation, or any demand for altruism, Tall John was at some ease in watching the television, or a large screen film show, perhaps he didn't have to think, or use his imagination, just respond; unlike fellow patient, Can Terry, who experienced enormous problems with any and all media stimulation.

And so, together, Tall John and I went to see the film in *The Hall,* that dark rainy winter afternoon of December, as 1969 drew to a close. We enjoyed the film, John as good as gold — even forgot to ask for a cigarette.

The Hall

Now, during the 1960s, it was customary, at the end of a cinema show, theatre performance, public dance and other public gatherings, for the audience to stand up, and in silence, remain so, whilst the National Anthem was played out. And, so in The Hall at the hospital, after *Singin' in the Rain* [68] and its credits finished , the lights came on and, with one or two exceptions, we, the Royal we, all stood stock still — in a complete hush, singular at oneness, within the bubble of the hall. To me, it seemed quite incredible; given the setting we were in.

Throughout the rest of the day, I reflected on a private *inner* experience, mine, in the hall at the end of that show — and, standing quiet alongside the child-like tank of Tall John during The Anthem. It *compared* strongly with the concluding scenes and play-out background of that dour, but superb, indeed authentic Asylum life of twenty-five years ago, in America, as illustrated by the black-and-white fiction... but, perhaps, too, so powerful documentary-like presentation of the black-and-white 1948 postwar film, *The Snake Pit* .

At the end of The Dance, held in the fictional hall of the American *Juniper Hill State Hospital,* a female patient stands on the hall stage, before a microphone and, with a wonderful crystal-clear *pure* from the heart voice, sings - like an angel. Everyone present unites and, in the hall bubble, the audience freeze, stop, and, as if mesmerised, revere the sad soulful lyrics of this adopted Asylum anthem. '*Going Home*, going home...'. The music score sounded like (and was) that of the Czech composer Antoin Dvorak's [69] Symphony No. 9 in E minor Opus 95, *Goin Home,* part of the classical *New World Symphony* (second Movement) though, I certainly didn't know that at the time I first heard it, in fact, I had never heard of the name Dvorak, but I was familiar with the gut stirring words of *Goin Home....* With no Home to go to.

To me, it addressed all people; patients, too many, alienated souls, who are displaced, by illness war, whatever circumstance; effectively made homeless... who know they are unable to go back to *any,* let alone forward to '*all the friends I knew.*' I felt the momentary, catharsis, much *deeper* than having, needing, somewhere, a place with people and, really being loved (and loving someone) in a place called Home. It was about an *inner,* invisible, intangible *feeling* of having been abandoned, rejected, whatever by life. God and mankind, if you must... of feeling helpless, unloved and unwanted; *The Asylum* Anthem, and its singer's vibrations, penetrating right within the marrow physic of my wilting bones, *patients* standing bones and, psychic wanting, waiting — captive souls.

And, oh yes, I too knew that emotion, of feeling alienated — emerging from an emotional sterile childhood. And of actually being, feeling *abandoned;* most probably triggered, as *just* another, ultimate, wartime casualty: one of many thousands. It was quite normal in those days. I was later cut to the quick, when attending the *North London Polytechnic* in a 1970s viewing, of a graphic documentary black-and-white film, which showed being evacuated wartime children and, as refugees being taken to a *Reception Centre* ... for a selection. I was homeless from 1939 to 1951, for twelve long years.

I'd been one of those refugees, aka evacuees (again) aged seven in 1944, who were temporarily, till early 1945, evacuated and relocated with other children of Spurgeon's Orphan Homes from Reigate. I vividly recall us, over one hundred bunch of us, walking down the crowded centre of an otherwise 'silent' Holmsdale Road, towards the Reigate railway station. We'd no idea where we were going, or why; and in one long crocodile, with thin bland cardboard boxes hiding smelly black concertina rubber gas-masks slung over thin shoulders and a few pithy belongings, packed in a minute back haversack, we Orphanage children were again being evacuated. And, so recently, I was yet again, relocated, only months before that, and since 1939. But, at seven years old, I didn't know squat what. And so, after many hours of train journeys, in one detached small group, I was taken to a *Godre'r-graig* mining community Church Hall, in the Swansea Valley of South Wales, where most locals spoke a foreign language (Welsh); and waited, for *someone* to choose and collect me. - It was a kind mining family, Mr and Mrs. Rees, with daughter Joan, who took me in. The documentary was one of a series of superbly real-life films, made by The Robertsons, and produced, I think, in the 1940s (and early '50s) for the benefit of Welfare officers, and Child Care Officers, and other, pickup, Caring agencies.

Oh, yes, I knew the subdued anguish of being long homeless, and abandoned — like so many of the residents in the hospital — and it had momentarily surfaced.... And, at one viewing of the old wartime documentary film of Receiving child Evacuees in Church halls, whilst attending a College course, I could *not* subdue, contain myself... and, quietly, exited my standing bones in the dark... stood up and, crabway, moved sideways through the substantial student audience, from that, one off, cathartic release. And, in so sharing it amongst others, that bubble burst.

After a brief Christmas and New Year stint, on the Refractory ward of Bramber Two, I returned to finish my mandatory placement on long-stay Eastergate block, which concluded at the end of January 1970. I then commenced the Community Block. Away. Out of the Main Building, to be based down the Farm Road, and located in the old Farm Yard, presently used for Industrial Therapy.

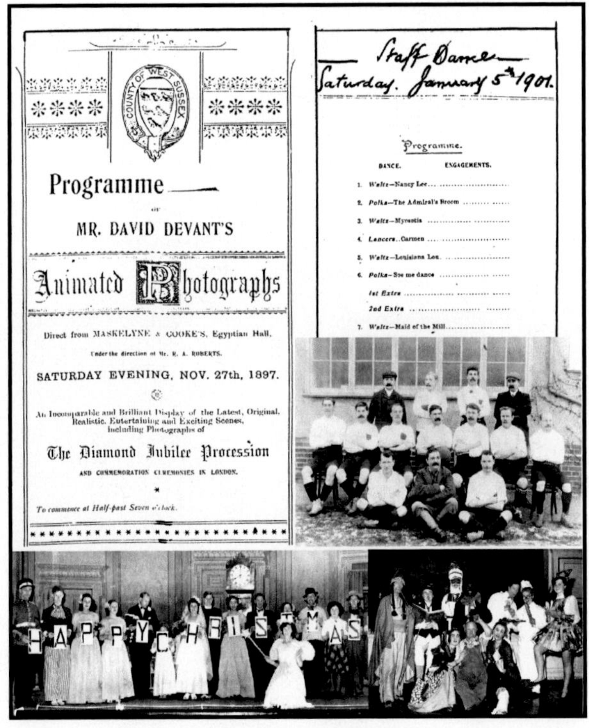

From its opening in 1897, until its Centenary, Graylingwell Hospital provided entertainment for staff — and patients — ever caring for all its charges..... Photo sources from WSCC County Archives and hospital staff.

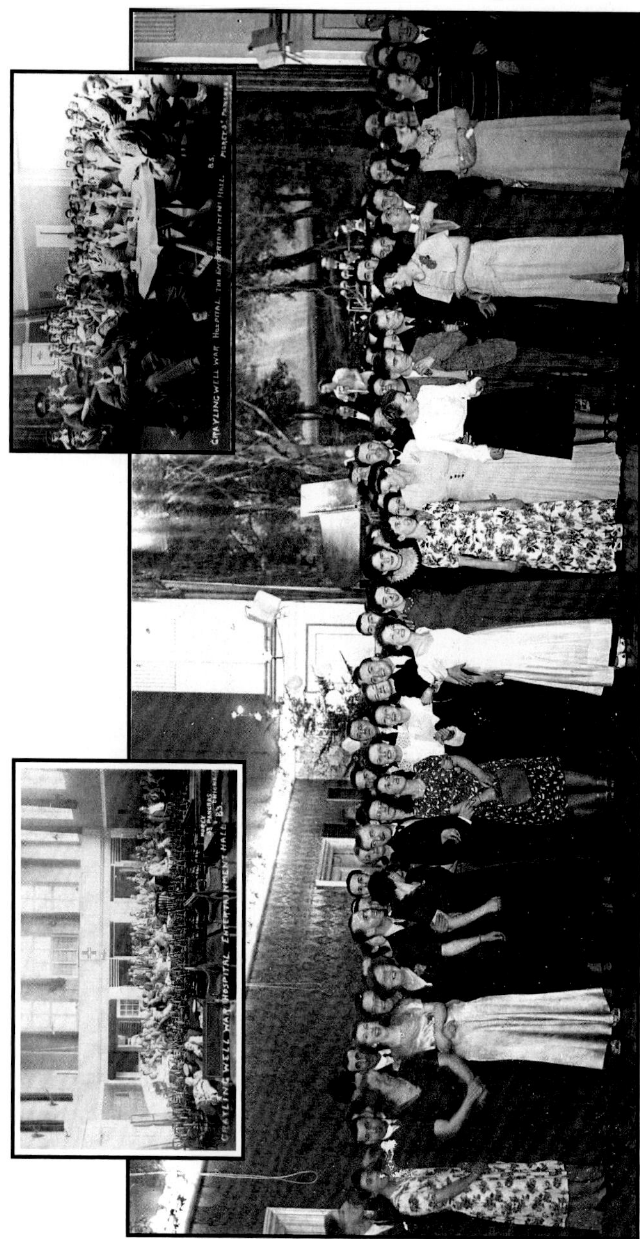

The Main Hall served many civic and entertainment uses during existence. Above, a 1950s Staff Dance. Staff and Patients held regular Dances, Cinema & Pantomimes. During WW1 (see two smaller Pics) it served many functions, incl dances & dining room. I recognise a number of (to be) charge nurses in the 1960's and seventies in the main picture.

Chapter Eleven
Community Block

'The longer I live, the more plainly I see that gentle must be the strain on fragile human nature; it will not bear much.' [1]
Charlotte Bronte. 1857.

16th February 1970 to 5th October 1970

Community Block—Industrial Therapy—The Sheds—Mrs. Maclintock—Aka The Barn—Family Affair—The Farm—Architect Milkman & The Teacher—Joker Laurie—Evil—Anti-psychiatry—Remedies—Two Hues—Acolytes—Sandown—Drying Out—Pressures—Groupwork—Homework—The Final—Postscript

16 February 1970
Community Block

Monday morning was frozen butter, a needle wind, and an umbrella of grey drizzle. It was the first day of our last RMN teaching Block, at the hospital Nursing School. And, in the run up to the Finals, two new students were with us. One candidate was an ex-Squadron Leader from Tangmere, of whom I had only met the once — at a pre Christmas study day. Richard (Dick.) had recently taken RAF retirement (he was in his late fifties), with enough relevant qualifications to enter for the Registered Mental Nurse finals this coming year. RAF Richard kept himself most private, and presented, non-smiling, a small, lean smart-dressed, intense, dignified, clean shaven gentleman who, as yet, seldom spoke in our company. An unknown.

I knew little about the second addition (new to Harry and me) — he was already double trained, both State Registered Nurse, and a recently acquired Fever Certificate. Francis wanted to qualify as an RMN, and intended to practice in this field. In his late twenties, small, dapper, self-assured Francis was a sociable, most welcome recruit from Mauritius; as Chilgrove Ahmed, lively Guitar Jacques (Jack) and other peers — young men and women from that tropical island, who joined our band of caretakers.

Professional staff colleagues and visitors included many immigrants and students from Africa, Australia, Canada, Eire, Europe, Greece, India, Italy,

New Zealand, Pakistan, South Africa, Spain and the West Indies, I *recall* hospital caring staff from *all* of those faraway places and, closer to home, Scotsman, Irish, Welsh, and from the English Counties; *no shite,* good people. I was proud to work with *all of* them, in our long stay asylum community. Mr Ammon, Principal Tutor (he'd replaced Mr Watkinson after his promotion, and move to elsewhere), accompanied by our ex- RAMC tutor, Mr Ilford, greeted us with an Ammon earnest, 'Well, let's get on with it — you've an *enormous* amount of Revision, Clinical Practice and Community Visits to achieve in these three weeks.' Mr Ilford distributed a three-page Handout, a *Mikado* list: '*I've got a little list — I've got a little list.*' [2]

Community Visits.... Week One Agenda. *Tuesday* 17th Feb.1970. *Egham Industrial Rehabilitation Unit*[3] for an afternoon's enlightenment. On *Wednesday* 18th Feb, at 2 pm, we were all present for a talk from a senior *Probation Officer*[4] at our own school. *Friday* 20th Feb, we travelled out for a formal visit to a hospital for *'Mentally Subnormal'* residents. Perhaps aptly named, *Coldeast Hospital,* with its 622 beds, was located near Southampton in Hampshire. We found the visit quite traumatic. It seemed so much more austere, compared to our Hospital with psychiatric patients (as the 1959 MHA rightly observed, *Subnormal* was *not* Psychiatric). But, its sheer size still identified it as a benign, caring institution.[5] We related to its warm beating heart, like *St. Lawrence*[6] and other institutions, despite a massive national (under the carpet) paucity of resources, merit pictured by the Court photographer, Lord Snowdon.[7]

Community Visits. Week Two Agenda. The brief one day Visits, included travel time to and fro, and left us little space, during school days, for in depth revision. But, visits were *very* effective. The four of us were most receptive, during those well planned experiences. *Monday*, 23rd February 1970; we separated, to begin a round of full working day visits, placed with four other bespoke caring specialists — *Psychiatric Social Worker, Mental Welfare Officer, Kingsmead* Day-Hospital and the role of *Health Visitor*. First, on my Mikado *list*, a day with a Psychiatric Social Worker (sometimes known as a PSW, or MWO, a Mental Welfare Officer), out on domiciliary (Home) Visits around the Petworth District (after RMN qualification I would qualify, and practice, *both* the PSW and MWO community roles). *Tuesday*, the Twenty-fourth, Harry and I were detailed to spend the day at *Sandown* Alcoholic Unit, alternating, the next day, with Francis with Richard. Whilst back at the school, Harry and I enjoyed an earnest debate, with Mr Ilford, on *The Elusive Self* — that subject which intrigues me so much . Not out of *ego,* but its incorporeal subject, much at the core of our personal and professional work. If Personality is a concrete formation of Habits — biological trace helical pathways — *what,* when, or *where*, is *The Psyche,* the inner self. Always, *what is Real Consciousness* — if it is *not* just an inverse, reflected, Asimov mechanical, bio-robotic... me... Me...ME ... but a sum of transient, halflife atomic mass' properties; independent and collective — and, and ...?

26 February 1970

Thursday 26th Feb, all four of us travelled to Southsea, Hampshire, to a specialist *Child* (and Family) *Psychiatric Unit* cluster, situated in the grounds of *St. James Psychiatric Hospital,* off Locksway Road, Milton, and called *The Wessex Unit For Children and Parents*. We, I felt, had, *had* an excellent encounter with the unit's staff, and some of its residents.[8] *Friday* 27th February 1970 (my 33rd birthday), I spent the day with a male *Health Visitor* (a then *rare* breed, it appeared), in The Chichester District. I accompanied him, on a round of home visits (his wife was also a Health Visitor!).

Community Visits. Third Week. *Monday* 2nd March, I spent the day with a *Mental Welfare Officer* (as our Graylingwell icon MWO George), based with a female colleague in Stoke Abbott Road, Worthing. In company with the MWO, we spent sometime at a Registered Rest Home, off Tarring Road, that accepted ex-Graylingwell disabled patients (paid for by the DHSS). Two other visits were somehow sandwiched during the third-year *Community Block*; one, to charity supported *Cheshire Home*[9] in Liss, Hampshire, for the extreme Physically Handicapped (amazing — one paralysed man demonstrated his ability to paint with the brush held in his mouth, and the painting was great — he also used an amplified electric voice-box to communicate). Second, an additional visit, was to a *Child Guidance Clinic* for troubled children and their parents, in Worthing, with local authority Child Care Officers (social workers); in liaison with the Education and National Health Services.

Stored-away. I recorded in my Magpie notebooks, jottings on *new* domestic routines, and ongoing enquiries; more and more droppings — *lists* and lists of want to read books; have to reads, and considerable research data. As much as possible, empirical research was executed on myself, with written up past Exam papers — marked by Mr Ammon — and encouraging results.... And, there were pages of miscellaneous hieroglyphic notes, relating to my erratic, yet consistent (obsessional) pursuit, of alone extra mural studies.... Most studies in pursuit of the vacuous conundrum, echoing (once again) Dr. Nicoll, in an enquiry into *Neurasthenia* (nervous debility, *Shell Shock),*[10] as to *what* is *Real Consciousness*. And wanting to expand it (if I could find *it).* If I could acquire the *capacity* — and for how long ... Many shaky scribbles were noted, on my Southern Railway journeys between Littlehampton and Chichester.

6th March 1970

On Friday 6th March, we sat for a routine Test, a *Community Block Exam* — mostly based on acquired accrued knowledge, from *The Community* visits; and were then briefed for our next practical assignment, down at The Farmyard, which was now converted to the site of the hospital Industrial Therapy Unit.

15th March 1970
Industrial Therapy

As Harry and I strolled *down* the slope of the Farm House Road, we passed several lone somnolent walkers, stooped, crooked particles, with slow heads up and down, and dipping largactil gait. We joined the steady flow of molecules, made up of more awake, bound, garrulous twos and threes, which mingled on the mend patients, and affable colleagues. Almost three years about the hospital, and we knew most of these ramblers. And, even if no names came to mind, we were *familiar* traces to them. Our Patients' faces, diagnostic traces — to most of us, The Professionals. All of us, at close to nine o'clock, that dull weather, Monday morning, were travelling down towards one of the buildings of the Occupational and Industrial Units; to the Gardening sheds and Greenhouses; The Farm House; Chico's chicken yards; *specifically* — to one or other meaningful destination.

There too was Ole Bill, off Duncton Ward, directing the mostly human traffic at the centre-point of the crossroads, outside the entrance to The Yard (Senior office clerk Roy M recalled numerous incidents, with Ole Bill being picked up by the police in Chichester; onetime, at a T junction outside *The Wellington* a pub situated but yards away from the Royal Military Barracks, Bill stood centrepoint in the road and sedately directed the flow of traffic... and so, he was experienced in directing human and tin traffic) leading off to scattered *Gardening* units, around and behind The Yard. Beyond *that* pathway was a closed five-barred gate, marking the western boundary of the hospital grounds, also the bottom boundary sump of the mostly shallow rill of the River Lavant, down from the chalk hills on its way to Chichester and the sea harbour waters below and round to the south-west of the estate.

To our right, at the crossroad, and South, leading out of The Yard and in front of The Farmhouse, was the curved crescent, narrow hedged in previous cattle and livestock *Drove* road — off of which was located Chico, and his noisy feathered charges. Close by, about a hundred or so yards on, lay the outlying 1932 built villas of Richmond and Kingsmead — adjacent to the green playing fields of Graylingwell. At the bottom of this probably thousand or so years old original trackway, straight ahead, was found, (surprise surprise) *The Farmhouse,* with its own enclosed grounds, pond and wells — including The Grayling well.

And so, to our immediate left we entered under a substantial archway, like the OK Corral, down into the enclosed square of the old cobbled farmyard (stable yard) slowly, its surrounding, low, buildings which, not so long ago, till 1957, had contained the hospital Dairy, and tabled substantial orchard fruits, and so many, many tonnes of farm produce, used by the Hospital since its inception — and before. The Asylum's splendid Records, held numerous dated *lists,* recorded in many books; some volumes vellum-bound for posterity, and housed within the hospital's own archives — later, possibly, to lie alongside ancient forebears' parish Manorial Records in Latin perhaps; and back in time, difficult to decipher, Museum hieroglyphics... fossilised in time *lists*... and other, detected, time-eroded surviving artifacts, and codex records.

The Sheds

Hospital farm flora and fauna produce, had previously been sold at Chichester and Barnham Markets — prepared about this old farm yard. About The Yard's site, outside it, around its perimeter, were a few ragged wooden structures where horses and carriages, and farm machines, had only a decade ago been stored. And dairy stockmen' slumbered their cattle. The farm dairy was but a short time ago active within the yard. Fowl, chickens, cows, geese sheep, turkeys; and prize winning pigs were all slaughtered here. And its carter farm-carts and horse-drawn carriages and ploughs and tractor sheds about its cobbled yard. But, *all* surviving remaining old farm structures, in the 1960s, were slowly being converted into OT and new patients *Industrial Therapy* workshops, or made redundant. The old farm buildings were being demolished — ending a site history, of almost a thousand years.

The Occupational Therapy sheds (actually brick buildings), and Industrial Therapy units, on the four sides of the farm yard, were numbered. Number One Unit (Shed), on the right as you entered *The Yard*, accommodated female OT patients, escorted by ward nursing staff. The ladies appeared to be occupied in embroidery, knitting and similar sedentary pursuits. Numbers Two and Three Shed units were located on the left (with a minute adjoining annexe containing a toilet and wash basin) — within these units, in connected rooms, male patients, mostly from Bramber Two, and always with an RMN Staff or student escort, guarding against any accident or psychiatric disturbance — *and,* unaccompanied, some Rehab residents, off Duncton or Cavell One wards.

In Two and Three, around wooden tables (with the already familiar coloured plastic chairs) sat often bored patients and staff, performing repetitive, mostly simple, albeit tedious, dis-assembly work, contract work, which allowed some payment — its workers taking apart old wireless and telephone equipment fittings, and other such bits; to be separated, and stored into marked boxes, which could be re-used in factory assembly. I thought of centuries of poor-house and workhouse inmates and day-attenders, earning their food and lodging from unpicking oakam-rope, and other contemporary dis-assembly, in (then) labour yards.

Number Four shed, on the right as you entered the yard, was sited directly opposite Two and Three — with storage, and more competent male patients doing carpentry and other such creative work. And directly ahead from The Archway entrance was Number Five shed. Known as *The Barn*, this was the main *commercial* hub of Industrial Therapy, with its workers assembling packs of DIY domestic apparatus, such as hat rack stands and kitchen sink tray sets. At one end of this substantial unit, double doors opened, onto a concrete ramp where lorries backed up to, and loaded up sealed boxes, destined for *Hago Products* at Bognor Regis. I'd already worked in sheds two and three when accompanying Bramber Two's patients — and pleased to be placed in an active role, within No.5 shed.

Mrs. Maclintock[11]

Sat at a small table just inside (Fares please!) the entrance of No. 2 shed, on the left of the yard's main entrance, sat one happy lady radiant with altruism, giving out for free, soft sparks of abundant Goodwill; of uncertain middle age, small, slim, brown hair, blue eyes — looking direct, smiling, at you, softly firmly spoken, knowing; and, instantly, *you knew* just how far you can go, with taking her kindnesses for granted; dressed in her blue Sister's nurse uniform Mrs. Maclintock, SRN, RMN, at ... *in charge* ... of The Yard IT activities — her absent boss Mrs. Plant a Senior Nursing Officer, in turn accountable to the PNO — Principal Nursing Officer.

I blame Aggie (Mrs. Maclintock — Aggie, from Haggis, her delightful Scot accent pure, Cronin '60s *Doctor Finlay's Casebook.)*[12] The wonderful warm atmosphere, down *The Yard,* was largely of *her* making. At her station was the yard telephone, adjacent filing cabinet, and, on a side table, a blue *Dansette* record player; a hospital electrician had kindly set up a tannoy and microphone system, which played into all units (with on-and-off switches) whereby the radio *Light Programme,* or requested long-playing 33 1/ 3rd rpm. records could be relayed, while the patients attempted their labours.

If Music be the ... 1960s lively whimsy rhythms of Jimmy Shand and Kenneth Mckellor, energetic bagpipes accordion foot tapping; Hank Williams and Jim Reeves (*Golden Greats*), sing along folk singing ballads; Elvis' and The Beatles classics — were all listed, and library stacked, within arms' reach of tuneful Aggie. No.1 on her play-list was, and there's no doubt, the delightful medicine of *The World of Val Doonican* — a '69 Decca L.P. This was, in particular, played By Request, over the tannoy, many times over the three months I attended the unit, and always raising a chorus, was the humorous *Delaney's Donkey,* and *Paddy McGinty's Goat* — appropriate perhaps, down in the Farm Yard. As we waited that first morning, on duty at Industrial Therapy, familiar faces began to arrive.

'Wotcha, Barry...', it was Laurie, formerly of Summersdale, back in '68. He was emerging from a long acute suicidal episode, on one of his damn so sad, manic depressive spirals. 'Are you coming over to us at The Barn?', he enquired, with a cluster of friends about him. I grinned. 'S' right Laurie ... be over shortly — after Mrs. Maclintock and I have finished our chat... 'Grr ... eat!... You *and* Aggie... terrific ...', a nice welcome.

Aka — The Barn

And Laurie and his merry little band separated, sauntering off to their respective work places. Harry stayed to work, about No. 2 and No.3 shed — those units already well known to me, when I had regularly escorted and stayed with nine or so acute patients, down from Bramber Two ward. Our other two third year colleagues were working in the Occupation Therapy pre-fab sheds — opposite the Front Entrance and adjacent to the large detached church.

Number Five shed, the semi converted old barn, was dominated by two, long, much weathered wooden (no idea *what* wood) tables, standing close, parallel in the centre of the large room. I reckoned they were still *in situ* from their previous uses, when it was functioning as a farm, even if previously placed elsewhere within this unit; all around the four sides were stacked square flat boxes, and a variety of factory wrapped black and chrome fittings, all items to be brought together in singular sets (to assemble *Hago* Hat Stands) — piles of finished work stacked at the far end of the barn. A number of smaller tables, all in use, were located around the periphery, and adjacent to the stacks of to be used materials.

Behind the wall of the finished stack, two large barn-doors opened outwards, onto a recently laid concrete ramp where, once per week, finished contract goods were collected by lorry and taken off to Bognor Regis; one old hand commented, nostalgically, that only yards away from the bottom of the ramp, two large tiered pig sties had at one time existed and, sure enough, if you looked hard along the overgrown ground, it showed stone and concrete runnel remains of its previous foundations. The central tables, where assembly took place, had a set of well oiled metal rollers placed on the end, along which each finished box was pushed and collected; the whole process manually conducted, to the often patter of the chat of the workers, and cheery music off the wall fastened tannoy; together, staff and patients willingly worked, as a team.

Family Affair

A crisp Spring morning. Entering the yard, about a quarter-to-nine, I was greeted with squeals of happy laughter and the sight of Cheshire cat — Sister Aggie standing outside her office and looking at the seeming frenetic antics of two nursing staff. Shirley, a grinning Staff Nurse down as escort from Summersdale, was attempting to clackety gallop. She was pushing a loud, shrieking, young student nurse, who, herself, was laid back in the sump of an old chipped wooden basket, her slim black stocking-clad legs akimbo, across the coarse cobbled yard in a rickety wheelbarrow — Ruth was 21 years old today.

Joker Laurie, and three or four other patients, stood outside the entrance of Number Five shed and applauded obvious pleasure, at this unusual, but happy, shared, brief festival. Staff Shirl Brown was very much at home in these grounds, especially around this part of the old Graylingwell Farm... indeed, she grew up in the hospital grounds with her parents, two sisters and her Uncle Cecil.

Cecil Brown and his wife (no children) lived in a thatched cottage at Martin's Farm, close by the main South Drive gatehouse entrance. Their neighbours were the popular hospital engineer, Mr C. and his family (firm friends for many years with all the Brown family), their children growing up alongside one another, on the hospital campus, in infancy and teens through the war and postwar years. Subsequently to their upbringing on the enclosed estate, the C's two sons would become Doctors. Years later, I had the pleasure of meeting one of the C's Doctors (and his wife), later a Professor, living in Australia.

Cecil's younger brother, *Ron Brown*[13] and his three daughters — two would graduate as RMNs. In time, I would speak at some length with two of the three as nurses; and to father Ron — and mother Nellie. The whole family, at sometime, working for the hospital patients, serving in one *capacity* or another: Truly a family affair. Cecil Brown moved from the West Country to Graylingwell Farm as a maintenance man, probably in the late Nineteen Twenties — an old photograph shows Cecil on what looks like a small tractor or mechanical grass cutter, adjacent to the newly built Richmond Villa, circa. 1931 — at his retirement, in the Nineteen-Fifties, he was the Farm Foreman.

Ron arrived at the hospital with his family in 1939, at the outbreak of war; initially employed as the hospital shepherd, on a salary of two-pound-four-shillings a week... covering night and days, with only Saturday afternoons off. Even then, he had to visit his charges every night to check they were all right. On arrival, Shepherd Ron had to care for five hundred sheep, of which he had a hundred and fifty breeding ewes, all kept on the hospital farm, located, he told me (in his retirement) about Millfield, near Saddlers Mill, and close by the Lavants and *The White Swan* inn.

The hospital's herds were kept out in the open fields — the sheep enclosed by hurdles made by himself and his assistants and fed mostly on root feed. Staff Nurse Shirley explained to me how they had had to sow a wheat field with clover, as they rotated the crops (the sheep fed on the clover), then planted a field with turnips — and the sheep were shifted to that field to feed on the turnips. Shirl recalled visiting her father, who was dressed for all weathers and holding his stout, tall crook — tool of his trade, at his Graylingwell Shepherd's hut. This hut was moved about, on four small metal wheels; Shirl recalled helping to push and pull it manually, from field to field. It had a distinctive smell of tar and linseed oil — a solution of stock, tar and linseed oil, which he put on the sheep's hooves for protection. I thought I had seen one of these huts somewhere, rusting within the orchard grounds — she said the local Chichester Museum had one, *but it didn't smell right*.[14]

Shortly after the late war, the hospital reduced their herd of sheep, and expanded their often prize-winning,[15] milk yield pedigree cows; and so, for the *next* ten years, Ron worked in the Dairy as a cowman — situated down here in The Yard and close by the Farmhouse. When the farm closed in 1956, Ron transferred to working indoors; no more always outside in all weathers, night and days.... he moved on, and was sheltered in work from the elements — former farm hand, shepherd, then cowman and dairyman, Ron accented his pleasure, as he recalled finally moving into the hospital's kitchens; and, then, also, working part time as an auxiliary nurse, on the male wards — he retired in 1968.

The Farm

In listening to the Brown family's tales, I found it easy to visualise these same hospital grounds in transition from early, low marshes into Belgic, Roman and Saxon days — to medieval chase fields, with Nobles and clerics riding in pursuit of deer and other game... with the Lavant water close by; and, latter times, into a series of settled enclosed farms — and its modern use since the late 19th century, as an Asylum and Sanctuary. I was fascinated by the Browns many anecdotes, in reference to their working with and, alongside in treating so many psychiatric residents during all those years ... The tales I heard from Ron, Shirl, and their family of the pre-war, wartime and post-war years within the hospital estate.

Shepherds, Cowmen, Pigmen, Poultrymen, Gardeners and Tradesmen — *all* had selected patients (most off the long-stay wards of E block) working with them — for a princely sum. *Ron* said, by way of an example, '*As a hospital Shepherd or Pigman, we received an* extra *Ninepence a week extra per person — to Supervise and Care for our patients... and be their friends.*' The patients, too, those classified as 'working outside', received '*extras*' — more food, tobacco, pots of jam... and friendship. During the war, Ron the shepherd had two regular patients with him (then, his only contact with the hospital wards); Bill H. and Frank R. Ron informed me, during one conversation, 'I used to have the two patients... And some patients could do the job as well as I could, you know. They had bad turns, don't they, and this Bill he'd come after you with an iron bar, sometimes.' [16]

'Really. So how did you cope with that?', I asked with considerable interest.

'All you had to say was "Bill go down and get those hurdles." And he'd go straight down and get them, you know. He was chasing the Devil or something.' 'So you had a good relationship with him?' 'Oh yes.' 'Where did he live — do you know what ward, or area?' 'I should say he came from E ward.' 'So, that would have been Eastergate?' 'Eastergate — yes ... And then I had another one — Frank R. ...'

'How old would these patients have been, when you had them? Were they getting on — or were they quite young?' 'Well, Bill would be in his fifties, I suppose. Frank R — he would be between forty and fifty, I suppose.' 'How long had they been on the farm, before your arrival ?' 'They probably had — Frank was a religious Mania.' 'But, do you reckon he *enjoyed* working with you?'

'Oh yes, Frank was very good. But there was a certain tree in Graylingwell, he would get down and pray to him (it). But, Frank was very good. And there was another one, Freddie W... If you let Freddie catch hold of you, he would nearly break your ribs.' Shirley, who was present when Ron conveyed these memories, added — 'Freddie would say, "*Come on then, Ron, let's have a laugh.*" And he proceed to tackle dad.'

Ron continued, 'When I was in the dairy, this Freddie — he came doing odd bits in the dairy, not milking or anything. Sometimes, he'd go down with you, when you took the cows out. Of course, you had to clear out the cows every day, and in the yard you had the cow manure all piled up. I was wheeling a wheelbarrow one day, and he caught me in the ribs ...' 'What — playing with you?' (boxing), I asked. 'Playing, he was... but he hit me quite hard, and put me off for about a week.' (I could not help thinking of present day Ole' Bill.)

I recalled that the Brown girls had lived their entire childhood, and early teens, about the hospital farm, and its institution. I asked Shirl, 'What was it like being brought up in a hospital. It was enough, being in wartime?' She replied, 'It was a lovely childhood.'

'What do you remember of patients alongside you... then?'

'They used to come along out of their walks, and they would look over the fence and ask us to show them our dolls and things, and the nurses used to talk to us. And Freddie, one day he decided that he would show us one of the horses out in the field, and he picks Cicely and I up, one under each arm, and carted us off down to show us the horses. Mum saw him disappear.' 'Panic?' Shirley chuckled. 'Yes — and he used to come over every Sunday, and help dad move the chicken house.' During our conversations, Shirley reiterated her love of the farm animals and the hospital farm life, patients and staff. 'We were really, *all* of us, like one big family — you know, Barry.' But, personally, she admitted, her first love, as a child, was for the horses ...

And I was reminded how a century before, in the mid-late 1850s, a girl called Anna Sewell[17], had lived awhile, in the nearby rented *Grayling Wells* Farmhouse, only yards from where we were standing in The Yard — with her Quaker parents; father a Chichester banker, and her mother a published writer, and ardent social worker.[18] Anna was, of course, the to be famous author of 1878 *'Black Beauty. The Autobiography Of A Horse.'* [19]

Why, at first glance, the opening Chapter, indeed, the first paragraph of that classic (*My Early Home*), read to me — as if — an exact description of the field and pond, located at the rear of the *Grayling Wells* Farmhouse, and its sloping meadow down to the Lavant brook at the bottom (actually, it might have been modelled on elsewhere). Anna would have prepared their horse and buggy, in this very cobbled yard, before driving her Quaker father off to work, at his Chichester bank. A real sense of history about this very spot. And a part of the history of Graylingwell.

The Architect, Milkman and The Teacher

Paul was a tall, sullen, young resident from Amberley One who had been, for some years, a high achiever, studying Architecture at University, prior to a full schizophrenic breakdown; he was reluctant (unable) to socialise with other patients, but could respond to staff requests in brief staccato exchanges — before striding off in response to the demands of his illness: however, he had admitted to me that he enjoyed being able to do something 'useful and constructive' without any pressures, down here at IT. He had experienced his first breakdown five years ago, and this was his third hospital admission.

Also, working in Number Five shed, alongside Paul on The Rollers, was Peter, presently a day attender from Chichester. Pete, an affable quiet slightly corpulent gentleman in his mid-twenties was, till a few months ago, a very active local milkman, a dedicated family man with Marion his wife and two young children; and, at work, an equally dedicated Trade Union member. His marriage was under great strain, as attrition (caused by disillusionment in his Union work — mostly out of hours) had badly affected his day to day living, inevitably bringing on an acute reactive depression. He had been admitted to Amberley while mute, almost catatonic, as I remembered, whilst working with Pete on the ward over some six weeks or so — and I shared his joy, as he went

Home On Trial with his TTOs for the first time. Now, he was discharged, continuing his recovery as a day attender and getting his self-confidence back ... and, more so, a measure of his previous competence to do things for himself — and others.

Another professional man, working within our transient group, was Jonathan, Jon as he preferred to be called. Like Pete, he was a five day a week day attender. A qualified schoolteacher, he too (like Peter) had suffered a nervous breakdown, through sheer worry and biting consistent over work; result — from a former substantial granite will, Jon had reduced, by attrition, to a sink of shifting sand — and a huge loss of confidence and self esteem at his place of work, and in his private life. In rank despair, Jon had broken off his engagement — fortunately, his fiance Jacqueline and his family continued to support him, despite the often awful verbal assaults he cast at them. Pete and Jon were on paid sick leave. Paul would never be able to resume his University life, but retained sufficient social skills to be able to occupy his time.

I enjoy working with recovering patients, in the Industrial Therapy unit. And as the daily routine kicked in, down at No. 5 shed (The Barn), I felt comfortable. Our patients, clocking in and out each working day, reminded me of my demob, and my first job post army discharge, back in December 1958. And working at Moss Bros. in Covent Garden, as a Query Clerk, in 1959, when employees had to manually clock in and, at the end of each day, manually clock out — every (non executive) time card, recording the exact minute of arrival and departure. And, if more than... say, fifteen minutes late, you *lost* that day's pay, *and* might as well go off home, or whatever. Just inside the front door, of the IT's Number Five shed, was an almost exact replica of that Moss Bros. typical clocking in card, and Clock. For all serious patient contenders, residents and day patients alike, this was Industrial Therapy; a possible gateway back into the community at large.

Joker Laurie

I knew Laurie well, from my three-month Summersdale placement, back in the autumn of 1968. Lawrence, a young man of twenty years, had been a patient, presently, for eight months, resident on the long-stay ward of Anderson Two; he suffered from diagnosed manic depression, and during episodic manic phases would be (predictably) very restless, very talkative and amiably intrusive towards others, patients and staff alike.

Lawrence was a likeable lad, always telling jokes (most risque), and gathering an audience around him. At Industrial Therapy's No.5. shed, he would, rather too frequently, stop others from working, in a compulsion to relentlessly tell one joke after another, rather like a chain smoking habit. I had no wish to stop his attendance, but had to arrest, at least temporarily, this *urge* to so frequently disgorge his jokes machine.

As an Exercise I suggested he think of and write up as many jokes as he could for posterity — and, he did. It worked. For a time after, whilst retaining his good nature, Laurie joined in, working at Industrial Therapy. The detailed jokes — thirty four of them, are, as promised, here appended for posterity (*rude* ones included).[20]

The joke material, bearing in mind Laurie was an in-patient, a resident in a long-stay psychiatric hospital, was quite revealing; it demonstrated a lack of stigma, and an ability to laugh at himself, despite the heavy Bunyan back-pack he had to bare ... to laugh and share — and stimulate others, staff and patients alike within our hospital, with his God's given gift of compensatory good humour. In fact, so successful was the jokes Exercise with Laurie, that I instigated a further learning exercise — for myself. And carried out a *Social Survey*, first clearing it with Aggie, on *all* twenty two patients then attending The Barn; to ask of them what *they* personally thought, and experienced, *whilst* attending the Industrial Therapy workshop.[21]

On a recent visit to The Yard, I'd bumped into Alternative Bob, who was coming from the other direction — he'd commenced saying his goodbyes. Colleague Bob, now qualified, decided to re-train as a chiropodist. His divorce was already underway, and both he and Jean, his wife (they had no children) who was staying on awhile as a Staff Nurse, had met alternative partners. Bob converted to being a vegan. And, one result of Bob's Erving Goffman studies, and a full conversion to Anti psychiatry and Sociological studies, meant a radical changing in his lifestyle.

Alternative Bob RMN felt he could no longer work within the profession, indeed specifically, he admitted, no longer having the *capacity* to work with and for mentally ill. During the past three years or so, we had enjoyed numerous conversations on what we perceived as Good or Bad methods of caring, for those patients suffering from any form of mental illness. And how different global, and localised UK attitudes and facilities, manifest as either, good and essentially healthy to their afflicted, or, bad. And, God knows, there was an abundance of recent witnesses, of this rank abuse, despotic and, yes, evil —

misuse of the knowledge and available treatments, for the disabled and psychiatrically ill.

As the Final exam, due October 1970, approached its zenith, I found myself at a watershed; occasional insights had changed curiosity and internalised (often hidden to others) into a growing strong desire to *want to know* — an unlimited body of Questions sans answers. And, without, found lies (learning to recognize such). I was *naked* in my Hans Christian Anderson Emperor's new clothes; myself standing to stare, from ragged, transient, bare bones and, with a considerable *capacity* of — erm, self-doubt. About moral philosophy.

I wanted (alchemy declares you are offered what *you* need, *not* what you want and what you desire) a deeper depth of understanding, as to how *and why?* How *good* can become *bad* and *mad,* then more subtle — *evil.* And *how* to define *What is Good,* and what is *'bad faith'* — as with Jean Paul Sartre. And how, presently, post-war Anti-psychiatry was coming into hospital and media politics. Certain post-war academics appeared to be reflecting the prospect that apart from outright *forensic* evidence of lunacy, as in the wake of the first world war (Dr. Kidd back in 1897 defined, as *scientific,* lunatics), all others of a nervous debility were probably malingering. Or perhaps, but misguided political dissidents.

Evil

Pre-war — when I was but six months old, an English periodical *World Film News* [22], under one subheading, *Frank Capra,* had Capra quoted by an interviewer saying: "Pictures aren't a snob business, they're entertainment... if you want to say something serious once in a while, then do it through comedy or fairy tale, anything but the pulpit attitude. Look at Disney."...' Just so, for In 1937 Walt Disney released the world's first full length animated feature film — *Snow White And The Seven Dwarfs*. There was a lot to say. Plenty going on.

The *next* paragraph under *World Film News* was about chilling *Censorship...* the interview continued — 'He', (Capra), 'began to talk about his film *Lost Horizon,* [23] ... looks upon it as an experiment and he was annoyed because the French office had cut out ten of the most important minutes; the main crux of the discussion between Conway and the Lama and also where Maria became an old woman. "*They don't think it's pretty! Well, it's the last of my pictures that'll be shown in France!"...*' From America, Capra felt his film's best bits were censored, and left on the French cutting room floor.

Unhappily, *much* worse *censorship* was already underway by France's neighbour Germany. In the same Aug. 1937 *World Film News,* found at the bottom right corner of page 23, under subheading, *Austria* — annexed by the Nazi Third Reich, it said; 'Fritz Hirt, of Berlin Tobis, after long consultations with Reich Film Chamber, obtained a permit to show Austrian films throughout Germany — *provided they comply with the German Aryan laws.'*

This would have been a reference to the recent infamous Nazi government mandate, *Nuremberg Laws...* specifically, The '*Reich Citizenship Law of September 15, 1935*' — and its supplement, *'Decree of November 14, 1935.'* This totalitarian decree, insisted, all its citizens be only of *pure* German or kindred blood; and, deliberately, excluded all those of the Jewish faith, though German born residents. The Nazis soon expanded this qualification of entry to being a member of this imaginary, *pure,* Master Race — declaring all other humans as not-so, but subhuman and, in purifying the Germanic race for their new Reichstag Europe — exterminating The Sick, Epileptic, The Weak, *Mentally Ill*, Defective and Physically Deformed; Gypsies, Slavs, Russians and begat '*The Final Solution*'; mandating *Corporate Murder as law.* To me, that's pure *evil* at work.

I researched a Mikado *list* — of contemporary propaganda, documentary war films which contributed (as a list of anti-war *books* of the Great War of 1914-1919) a *substantial* body of *forensic* evidence on the *deliberate* abuse of a 'duty of care', to *millions* of enslaved captives; demonstrating this dark *evil* at work in our — my — lifetime. Amongst (there are many more) the robust list of cameramen, are dedicated professional film makers, who provided considerable evidence, for posterity. I found; Frank Capra, Claude Chabrol, John Ford, Alfred Hitchcock, John Huston, Claude Lanzmann, Marcel Ophuls, Akira Kurosawa, Alan Resnais, Roberto Rossellini and William Wyler. Most, if not all of them had, at-the-time, documentary contributions, war work, heavily *censored* — cut removed for posterity.[24]

Huston's documentary of the 1945 Italian *Battle Of San Pietro.* was actually filmed on location. He was a dog soldier cameraman, present during the ongoing grisly battles, and *followed up* the aftermath subsequent psychotherapies — of talking, behavioural and physical therapies, of a legion of psychiatric (emotional) traumatised war casualties. Huston's highly sensitive *original* and brilliant documentary film, *Let There Be Light,* filmed in the USA military Mason Hospital, was banned from the general public for at least thirty years, as being too gruesome. In his war casualties disclosures, Huston (et als) classic documentaries witnessed so many wartime deaths and undead, dismemberment, most censored... for public consumption — for decades.

In my search for *how,* in definition, good can become bad and mad, then evil, I compiled a brief *list* of films (but a sample) of on offer, heavily censored, *forensic* evidence of *Genocide* and *Corporate Murde*r; of rank, evil abuse. I compared the Axis resources with Allied records — to a proper *duty-of-care*, using contemporary records, and personal research, from our own hospital *Annual Reports*.[25] And, from personal staff interviews, and case note records, showing proper moral use of facilities in Psychiatric and Emergency Medical Services (EMS) hospital institutions — available in wartime and post war years, in Graylingwell, Great Britain, and Allies' resources. [26]

I pondered ... You can get used to anything. To be able, to mostly 'Do as you are told'... well, within limits — trusted government, and its recorded literature... Erm!... It's called being normal. But... the domestic, normal, in an Enemy occupied, fear-ridden country. In Vichy France, its natives were force-fed by daily doses of Nazi lies and, in perpetuity, the experiences, and witness, even forced participants, to horror and murder... There is a snippet in one propaganda film clip, in *Eye of Vichy,* a woman is seen wearing a bought pair of shoes, made from cut off human hair. Ok! — if the cut hair was willingly saved by a living person at their own bequest in a climate of austerity, to make do... and mend. ... But!

Revealed, in the short list of Docs referred to above — are seen *mountains* of film footage, disclosing a hideous array of *millions* of heads of hair, taken off unwilling and murdered victims, and piled up for recycling to be woven into cloth, for clothes, sacks and shoes; to make a tidy and unstated commercial profit for the manufacturers. Nothing is to be wasted and, in those so-called labour (later extermination) camps, all became manufactories, industries of death — and all broken bodies became potentially useful to the Enemy war-machine; with piles of teeth, torn out of the unwilling alive or dead bodies; heaps of unseeing broken and unbroken spectacles; any and all personal belongings separated and anticipated for redistribution; even the cremated ashes, of the legally murdered, were attempted for fertiliser. [27]

As I watched a copy of Resnais' 1955 *Night and Fog* for the first time; seeing a flat, one dimensional, but brutalised truism, of past nightmare Nazi roundups, and *Hell-on-earth* life in the camps, paraded before me. When, *The Horror,* several freeze frames arrested my attention — and discharged a *tremendous* shock, into my otherwise zombie consciousness. Such experience described by Colin Wilson[28] *'of awakening when things somehow slip past* (his) *intellectual guard; the result is a paralysing sense of nausea.'* Wilson was referring to Sartre's *Nausea* experience... an antithesis of the poet's and, presumably, mystics who experience the *good* slippage. I saw *pure* evil, felt aberration, momentary, I *felt* what was evil wasn't involuntary, mortal mental illness. But evidence of Genocide.

Submerged. In a run of an already now too common theatrical display, of ghastly piles of emaciated corpses, skulls, ovens, brutality; and piles of human debris, awaiting *domestic* processing and *commercial* redistribution. *I saw several film frames of a row of propped up recent headless, but otherwise whole cadavers, viewed within a wooden hut. And worse, a stacked pile of adjacent complete heads, eyes wide open and fixed staring up at the cameraman — waiting, stacked within a large* domestic *bowl a few feet away ... This camp's* domestic *assembly awaiting processing — to extract their fat for soap, and whatever...*

This real life and death sequence I had *not* seen, in any previous pic — or in any fact, or fiction, form of Hammer gothic film. Such a sequence would normally have been censored out or, otherwise, certainly have ended up on the cuttings floor (just as Director Capra's pre-war 1937 *Lost Horizon's* fiction frames, to pre-war Frenchmen, and John Huston 's 1945 *Battle of San Pietro* American documentary film) as *not* acceptable.

Resnais film was *too real,* too awful, for designated wartime censors — and the French public. Such forensic evidence of evil *normally* hidden, from a general public viewing. Many of our diagnosed psychiatric patients, too, had been brutalised helpless, in their past, and realised an evil presence; herein a legacy of two recent world wars. Shell shock, a net result.

Within this thread, I considered such experience in attrition, may have had, for example, an immense Sartrean understandable *reaction,* to the evils of Nazi *Vichy,* and radical retrospect contribution to *Anti psychiatry.* In practice. *Just an opinion,* about disillusion of experiential good, *always* prevailing. Another, but bleak, existential view of reality. [29]

What then is defined, and accepted, as *Good,* and *what* is bad. Sir Richard Burton (1821-1890) the eminent explorer, (by way of an introduction) put it simply in his long poem *The Kasidah* (V verse one):

> 'There is no Good there is no Bad ; these be the whims of mortal will:
> What works me weal that I call "good," what harms and hurts I hold as "
> ill"...'

A huge body of knowledge (certainly, *one* of the good books), which espoused recognition, in the 30th chapter of the Persian Yasna, Max Muller defined[30] *Madness,* as being a thin divide between wrong as sad, and bad good — and descent into Evil. In Muller's translation of the *Zend Avesta* (Good Words Good Thoughts Good Deeds), he said:

> *'All Goodness is Reality – and called the Good Mind; whereas, the negated aspect, through Unreality, this bore the name of evil mind.'*[31]

Unreality, lazy negativity, perhaps, aka Bad Faith.

Anti-psychiatry

Recent academic references to anti-psychiatry, in the 1960s, had *suggested* to me a total rejection of the asylum patient's own experience, being diagnosed as an illness, and stated that there was no such thing as a mentally ill patient — *only* a dis-enfranchised, political person.[32] And, certainly, there was considerable postwar *forensic* evidence, on global abuse of certain countries' medical facilities; e.g. in Russia and China, where there were imprisoned politically incorrect individuals, who were *not* ill, who were maltreated behind locked doors; and detained, even liquidated; so designated *patients,* within their State psychiatric hospitals. Little difference, from not long ago Nazi concentration camps.

One RMN Worthing colleague, a Community Psychiatric Nurse, CPN John Donnabie, recalled his *Shenley Hospital* student days, working in one of psychiatrist Dr. Cooper's 1962-63 experimental hospital Villa units; and how he was shocked when, for a while, it was accepted that urinating *anywhere,* in and on the ward, was *initially* acceptable, as part of the retro-therapy. A group of psychiatrists emerged, which included clinically qualified physicians and psychologists, and peacemakers as Karl Jaspers — emerging into a *New Existential* School of *Psychotherapists,* working in the same psychiatric field. These robust, psychoanalytical orientated practitioners, worked to eliminate Sartrean Angst, and aimed to socially re-construct a Good Life. At least a better one. They said ... first 'let's look at our present hospital regime, for diagnosed, mentally ill and disabled psychiatric — disturbed patients.'

I found Colin Wilson's *Introduction to the New Existentialism* [33] a useful antidote to much of the nihilism, of the dour post war Parisian Left Bank so-called student following, *Beat* (down beat), new wave Jazz music, defined by Jack Kerouac philosophy[34] — with Sartre, its European principal icon. Colin Wilson noticed: 'There are no peak experiences', in Sartre. [35] There were no good slippages, in *Beat* or in Sartre's post-Vichy world; consequently, both good (which for years had been non-existent for a mass enslaved population) and evil appeared, to him, to be negative. In *New Existentialism*, with its focus on goodness and positive use of Psychotherapy, there was Gordon Allport, Abraham Maslow,[36] Rollo May, Carl Rogers, et al — whose work, post-qualification, I eagerly drew upon. And (in use at Sandown's alcoholic rehab *Therapeutic* Community), there was a focus on *Group* Psychotherapy as in *Family Psychiatry,* by Dr. John G. Howells. [37] I found Howells an excellent antidote to the pessimistic (with good cause, as I have drawn on) — previous nihilistic Existentialists' philosophy. But, all of this *therapeutic work* was in the near future. None of the above listed authors were to be found in *The Red Handbook,* or in any found current textbooks in *formal* use at the hospital, in the mid sixties.

Graylingwell's consultant psychiatrist Dr. Joyce agreed, when in pursuit of its origins, I asked him in 1970 , about this growing trend of American and European anti-psychiatry, in politics and literature, and of its psychiatric casualties.... He said he understood Laing's beliefs, that his military experience had taught him, and found in his books, and the need for change, that aspects of Care and Treatment, should properly be regularly examined and updated. But, to cast out untreated, uncared for, psychiatric patients — out onto the streets, to fend for themselves, *as normal* (as some media made of this approach, anyway)... No way! And Drs. Cooper, Esterton, Laing et al too, like Dr. Joyce, did *not* at all advocate such harsh political treatment. No Way!

French philosopher Sartre admitted to gross nihilist suffering; including his personal anguish, during the crisis period of his countrymen's wartime occupation, and post-war damage. Origins, perhaps in contribution, to an emerging philosophy of anti-psychiatry — *and* politic denial of collective submerged, *angst* and trauma. I read confirmation in two published answers, I thought, in two recent published interviews with *The Playboy*[38]. And, more evidence, in *another* insightful interview, titled *The Parisians and the Germans,* in the *Playboy* magazine. [39] Both copies of *Playboy* given to me, by patients on Amberley One Ward. Sartre described how terrible the four years of Nazi occupation were, and of the profound effects of the *Vichy* armistice upon his captured French nation. (Albeit all Occupied countries.) About himself, in particular; amid the helpless horrors of the concentration camps:

> 'We looked at one another we seemed to be looking at dead people. The dehumanisation, this petrification of man, became so intolerable ... the terrible thing is not to suffer or to die, but to suffer or die futilely. ... From the start of the war until the very end, we did not acknowledge our actions, we could not lay claim to their consequences. The evil was everywhere. Each choice was bad; yet we had to choose, and we were responsible. Every heartbeat plunged us into a guilt that horrified us. ... Paris was dead.'

The above words appeared to conflict (or confirm, in a specific context , surely an oxymoron, depending on which viewpoint) with one of Sartre's statements, made in 1944 (after Paris was freed?) when he remarked *'Never have we been freer, than under the German Occupation. This total responsibility in total solitude, wasn't this the revelation of our freedom?'* [40] Thinking of *Vichy,* I read of this philosophical statement that (in retrospect?) his France (as all occupied territories) was divided by a choice (he wrote), collaborate or not (with the enemy); which surely pre-supposed that *everyone* really had had a choice; if they wanted to live, or not — to be enslaved or exterminated, in a labour or concentration camp.

On night duty, alone on Bramber Two locked ward (See Chapter Five) I read of a similar philosophical statement (survival or submission) made by Arthur Koestler, [41] when retro writing of his stay in a Spanish Prison, during the Civil War, and declaring how free (his thinking at one point) he was.... And comparing my locked in, and sectioned patients, to help and contain *their* true afflictions — as apart of imprisonment, for *non compos mentis* politic crimes. But, of course, being free or not, is not all in the mind — or is it? It's a physical fact. And, as to recent pre-war roots, leading into the denials, and ways of coping; many of the world's populace had already endured the terrible years of the 1914-1919 Great War, and its terrible aftermath. The years between the wars, twenty years, being but an Interlude. State hospitals still had wartime mind and body casualties, in the 1960s.

I supported several Italian patients resident in the hospital. Gino and Dominic (not related) were schizophrenics, for a time, on Bramber Two; transferred to the Eastergate block, before being discharged into the community. Both men were from large families, with war widowed mothers (who made regular visits and sought me out — for a chat about their sons); Dominic had over indulged, albeit briefly, in LSD at University in Naples.

I have one particular memory of another Italian gentleman, a scholar, one isolated referral — living alone in the Worthing community. He was an exiled mysterious gentleman, from a noble *titled* Italian family; a black sheep, he described himself to me; a real life penniless Baron living by himself (he really was a Baron). I drew evidence of his 'distressed' circumstances from him; and saw some of his personal effects, about the humble rented terraced property. I visited him for some months as a later, Psychiatric Social Worker, in Worthing. From the late ex-officer and middle-aged Baron, I heard about what had happened to him and his family, when they sided against the Germans and the 'fascists'. Much that I heard was similar to numerous descriptions of other refugee Europeans. Also, I heard how wartime trauma and stress separated him from his family — who *ejected* rather than rejected him (his words), when he became mentally ill, towards the end of the war in 1944. Since the war, he had suffered bouts of mental illness.

The Baron was a fervent intellectual, with a passion for Italian history; and I recall, sad yet pleasant, his descriptions of existential philosophy, in early postwar academic circles. We chatted a little about recent new (to me) names, like Goffman, Laing and Sartre; and emergence of anti-psychiatry; and the Baron told me about Italian Philosophers (names I'd never heard), and of his bad experiences in being (he felt) an abandoned state patient, back home in Italy. On departure, I compared my brief *out patient,* the Italian Baron, with our unknown Colonel, who I had briefly been acquainted with — and who died on England ward (see Chapter Nine.) They were, for me, singular icons of reality; examples of the nameless many, rank and file *statistics* — certain victims, outcast by the Second world war.

One name the exiled Worthing Baron mentioned to me, was Norberto Bobbio[42] a now quite elderly Italian Political Philosopher, who, like Karl Jaspers and Jean Paul Sartre had, in his lifetime, confronted considerable corruption, poverty, *propaganda*, pollution, and *decadence* — much experienced in his political career; and finding *inevitable* destruction of blind Romanticism when facing up to the ugly realities of hideous wartime and postwar years.

Bobbio addressed the issue in the last chapter of a recent published work in 1948.[43]

For existential John — Jean Paul Sartre's wartime diary had recorded the completion of his nihilistic, monumental *Being and Nothingness,*[44] in October 1942. Bobbio's postwar requiem *The Philosophy Of Decadentism. A Study Of Existentialism* [44] — in which he answered (yet complimented) : — '*Sartre's man is the sheer antithesis of the Christian God, who creates the world out of nothingness: he creates nothingness out of the world.*' Both intellectual giants reflected *purity*, absolute integrity, in their existential philosophical writings; and their own direct experience of then seeming endless horrors, in war torn Europe. An emergence of *post-Romantic nihilism,* in Literature, Philosophy, Politics and Psychiatry, comes to no surprise; and postwar psychiatrist Dr. R.D. Laing's stance of anti-psychiatry a robust determination to rise above nihilism — and *succeeded* in abreactive psychoanalytic work, as in London, and Tavistock explorations.

Remedies

Asylums and Psychiatric hospitals, like Monasteries, were places where people looked to as Lazarettes and places of refuge, with a wish to be housed, cleansed, *purified* of bodily sins toxins and mortal distress. A pre-Johnson 1684 English Dictionary[46] (in my possession) defined:

> '*Purification.* A cleansing, purging : and more properly, the anniversary day of the blessed Virgin Mary *her* solemn purification *(according to the Law, Luke 2, etc*) and presenting of her first born, our blessed Saviour, to the Lord, in the Temple of Jerusalem.'

I noted absolute religious sanction as its provenance .... Other faiths have a similar legal definition of purification.

Close to that time of 1684, I had a maternal ancestor (in my cocktail of genes). He was a non-conformist Protestant *Puritan Divine;* Dr. Thomas Manton DD (1620 — 1677) Oxford Doctor Of Divinity, no less. He was a devout cleric, who served and spoke with Oliver Cromwell, who was *persuaded* to open the rebel 1653 Parliament in prayer. This event lists him in Cromwell's letters as *Mr Manton.* [47] Then, having survived the Commonwealth, Manton briefly served King Charles the second who, through The Establishment, offered Dr. Manton a Bishopric, with its attendant wealth and status, but Manton declined the offer, believing it but a bribe, and stating (other sources suggested), he thought the Restoration elite (in turn) too, was in excess and polluted. For a while, in 1670, he was imprisoned for his dissent[48].

What of *everyone's* forefathers, and blood relations; who or what do to others believe to be submerged, in albeit, invisible molecular genes. But... *So What?*... Diary considered. I've *no* conscious memories of *any* ancestral icon... All role models, of *good* and more, of excellence, are internalised from my lifeline experience — including current human figures. As, too, its opposite. I internalise role models of good and *bad*, wilful and harmful icons included. The body has its own memories, latitutes and limitations — impurity, the norm.

That 1684 definition of *Purity,* identified a *historic* religious figure, an icon, as the fossilised, *ideal* image, of human goodness. What is *pure* — by cleansing and purging (politic sin; viz hearsay *as a lunacy* / treason!), as legal method, to pristine status. All human world religions' practices and faiths, appear to concur with their own named images of purity; and sustain a civil (or military) administration, to serve and uphold named Prophets and priests (who often identify themselves as of God) and scientists ... to measure humanity in its name. Use or abuse: good and evil; human ethics decided what the word purity infers.

Thus... but a word for abstract and anthropomorphised God, only one *unified* God (God is Go'od) who has no name, no Pronoun except what man designates — yet allocated an *infinite* number of names.[49] *The Pure* being of which *everything* originates from, and is a part of. Human beings assert their own, selfish interpretations, to often commit rank abuse — cause multiple deaths and destruction... *God is with us,* (only us) so to purge and purify a race, or individual. Genocide, utter corruption, on a human whim. Propaganda.... Our God is better than your god. Ugh!... Much mental illness has such ambiguities, in its presenting aetiology.

On Bramber two, in May 1968, I studied a *glossary* of psychiatric reference terms; which prescribed treatment, essentially, custodial and out-patient, traditionally of *Kraepelin* [50] Origins, dating back to the early Twentieth century, aided greatly by behaviour controlling, prescribed drugs. And, moving on, on England Ward, Dec. 1968 I expanded (motivated) my glossary focus, specifically on other *different* forms of treatment in use through the decades, since the hospital opened in 1897 — till now, in the early 1970s; information came from

Case notes and numerous interviews, with patients and staff about, during many of those years.

I read, discussed, marginal, alternative, often *complimentary* forms of therapy... *not* obtainable under Poor Law, Charity or NHS on general prescription: homeopathy, meditation, yogas and robust alternatives (as well as) as being developed presently, by Doctor Laing and his august colleagues up in London, at Kingsley Hall, and Households, under the aegis of his privately funded *Philadelphia Association*; and the *Tavistock Clinic.*[51] Notably, charismatic Laing published a review, of Karl Jaspers *General Psychopathology,* in the *International Journal of Psycho-Analysis,* in 1964.[52]

The effect of 'Shell Shock' and *Shock* in general, to the mind and body of an individual, through trauma, was a principle used in cause and in treatment of an disordered person; Kraepelin's philosophy diagnosed most afflicted by shell shock as either malingerers, weak-willed, and or lacking in moral-fibre as untreatable, those unable to return to the hell of the trenches to be put into an asylum, or workhouse.[53] But, Psycho-analysis, and Jamesian New Psychology[54] were well underway, thanks to Freud, Jaspers, Jung, Nicholl, Rivers and like minded, as R.D. Laing. Stating the obvious, perhaps, but logistics and economy would *not* have been able to provide the one to one debriefing that every casualty deserved, even if admitted to. General Petain had sufficient insight, during the Great War, to arrest a general strike, by recognising his *exhausted* (at death's door) shell-shocked troops, and provided much needed relief for those troops in his charge.

I attempted *yogic* meditation *many* times, over the years, alone and or in organised Groups, but always without success (which clearly is my loss). I just could *not* empty my mind of its clutter, as thoughts and memories would always fill my inverted cup. I just couldn't empty my head (as instructed) into Nothingness, and obtain some purity. But life, fate, experiential, synchronicity — whatever occasionally crossed what Colin Wilson calls St. Neot's margin.[55] Back in 1957, whilst a squaddie on Christmas Island in the Pacific, I recall a beach tragedy, off the Main Camp area. This was at one location, off *The Wreck* (a line of American abandoned American vehicles, 1945 wartime transport, driven into the sea to rust away — too expensive to take back to the states).

I was one of a number bathing in the sea, close to shore, as the coral reef was only a hundred or so yards off (where the deep Pacific Ocean shelf dropped and dropped into thousands of feet). But, most, because there was a fierce death clutching undercurrent to be aware of ... *suddenly,* one of the other bathers had been snatched away and was nearing the reef. Myself and others saw his distress, and the alarm went out. Initially I was only (it seemed) a few yards away from him — and, yes, I started swimming towards him and, with horror, realised I was, too, losing self control, and the beach was already a narrow horizon line behind me. I was *not* at all a strong swimmer, and tried returning to the shore. And, for a split second, much of my proverbial life made a fast passage through my mind. But, Thank God, a human chain had already reached out into the receding tide; and I was saved; *not* so the other poor man, who had already fast disappeared out into the shark infested ocean, and not found for several days. The intense fear, of my near death *shock* encounter, stayed with me.

Most relevant — dipping into the *General Index* under 'Shock', of Karl Jasper's *General Psychopathology,* [56] I found the following two helpful anecdotes, on an involuntary emptied mind, phenomenal:

> 'Belz describes his own experience of a Japanese earthquake : 'There was a sudden, lightning change in me. All of my better feelings were extinguished, all sympathy and possible participation in others' misfortunes, even interest in my threatened relatives and my own life disappeared, while mentally I remained quite clear and I seemed to be thinking much more easily, freely and quicker than ever. Some earlier inhibition seemed to have been suddenly removed and I felt responsible for no one, like Nietzsche's superman. I was beyond good and evil ... I stood there and looked on all the ghastly events around me with the same detached attention with which one follows an interesting experiment ... then, just as suddenly as it came, the abnormal state vanished and gave way to my old self. As I came to, I found my driver tugging at my sleeve and begging me to get out of the danger from the nearby buildings.'

And reality, stunned from a South American earthquake[57]:

> 'Nobody tried to save their relations. I was told it was always like this. ... The first shock paralysed all the instincts save that of self-preservation. Once real misfortune happens, many regain their senses and one sees miracles of self-sacrifice.'

Sudden involuntary nervous shock *and* or voluntary meditation — both actions *appear* to arrest the functional brain, for a length of time. Surely, such nervous trauma may reveal *insight,* or foreign *invasion,* whilst so vulnerable at such a time?

After completion of the 1970 *Industrial Therapy* workshop *Survey* [58], I enjoyed an unusual conversation with Jean (No.18), and husband Mark (No.19). A likeable young couple, about Joker Laurie's age — twenty years old. Mark had acknowledged their *Dependence on Drugs,* as reason for attending the hospital, and Jean 'a singular Lack of Concentration and no place to live.' I knew nothing of their family history, or hospital case notes. It was not where I was at.

Prior to admission over five months ago, he was now an out-patient, Mark had used unprescribed drugs to dabble in Crowley *Magick,*[59] tempered by topical readings of Dennis Wheatley novels and Aldous Huxley's *Doors Of Perception* [60] experiments (Huxley under supervision), with mescaline and LSD. And topical readings, abetted by 1960s and early '70s magazines of *Playboy*; the *International Times* and *OZ.* Another underground magazine, *Spare Rib,* was an insightful Feminist mag, but I read *no* advocate on hallucinogenic drugs material, within the few copies of SR. that I had read — loaned by Jean. Most underground (but legal) magazine titles could be sent on request, free, to young psychiatric ward patients; especially if they were undergoing *treatment* under any Section of the 1959 Mental Health Act. Mark, Jean, Julie, Laurie, Spider, and other patients I knew, all qualified for these freebies.

IT and *OZ*[61] qualified the sanction of using recreational drugs, in its captions, adopted from American Beat drop-out and back-packer college students sub-culture, with Zen, Buddhist and Yogic mantras (Beatles' Maharishi on *Bliss Consciousness*) and other religious text — aided by oft quoted, domestic and psychiatric use of so-called 'mind-blowing' food, like Hash, LSD, Magic Mushrooms (psilocybin), plant and synthetic alkaloids (e.g.; Morphines). Mark and Jean insisted they had *not* used any hard drugs — mostly, it was hash, LSD, and buzz stuff, with never any intention to wilfully harm anyone, taken out of curiosity and attempts of self-discovery. Erm... just like Huxley, Ouspensky, and other notables. I had no reason to doubt their innocent intensions.... but they broke The Law. And suffered overdosing.

'How are things ?', I asked Jean and Mark, as we sat down on the slatted green metal and wood garden seat, located in the corner of The Yard outside number five shed. It was early afternoon, after lunch, and about ten minutes before our work was due to begin.

'Not bad... getting better...', Mark replied amiably. 'You know... *why*... we are here, don't you. I don't mean on probation, for taking stuff.' added Jean, with a touch of enthusiasm. I was sat in the middle, between them, as they looked to me, speaking in confidence, as out-patients, but, also as searchers. Qucstors, in sub-rosa earnest — 'Can you help us', chats. 'Do you mean *your* attempts at Magick, under the influence of stuff, that got out of control?', I asked... More in enquiry, than in an assumption of *what* they had been doing. I was curious of their original motives.

'Well, yes... but more than that. Huxley wrote, of first *cleansing* perceptions ...we *did* that ... we thought.' Mark said, subdued in his reply. I remembered reading Huxley's *The Doors of Perception,* [62] and his early remark, which said: '*I am and, for as long as I can remember, I have always been a poor visualiser ...* ' If wishing or attempting to *wilfully* conjure up images, from the vault of thoughts and desires. Like scientist Huxley, I too found this profound inability (always without any drugs or other physical stimulus), to *deliberately* be wilful, and internally visualise *something* on command (in day and night-dreams) a frequent problem. But, I decided *not* to interrupt Mark and Jean's flow.

'And... Well, it was *great* at first... terrific buzz... unexpected euphoric... um, but, erm...' Jean completed her testimony and, with a slight confessional flush, whispered: 'It was the *sexual* buzz... you know, the *energy* of sudden orgasms we, *at first,* experienced; but, as Mark said, it *then* went *all wrong,* all pleasure disappeared, and was replaced by more and more fear, and a terrible revulsion... out of our depth.'

Mark continued his commentary, in support of his wife — who he clearly adored, and reciprocated. 'We were unable to stop the after effects... friends only wanted into buzzes, and freebies, and left us. Alone, we drew the 'grams and *summoned* the names, from the other side... to serve us... huh!' He paused. Whispered. 'Like Faust (and Crowley) I guess...', I replied. 'Did you know Crowley was once compulsorily admitted into a Paris Lunatic Asylum, as a result of having tried to invoke an apparition of Pan.' (What hypnagogic horrors did *he,* Crowley, manifest.) I interrupted, to reinforce the weight of their testimony.

Mark took the point, and continued. 'We thought, cleansing ourselves to be purified, as the rituals prescribed. And took stuff...' (Some purification, I thought.) Mark continued his litany. 'Do you know *The Banishing Ritual,* the props, and so on? Jeez... *everything* went wrong; didn't know who to turn to... no teacher, only books to go by. But, someone had already given our names to the fuzz, cos of the stuff, and we were arrested, for having bought off a dealer we knew. But, like, the flashbacks continued...'

'How so? '

The look on their faces said it all, as — now feeling much better (off the stuff) and feeling safe, they recalled the horrors they had experienced, before Court, and Medic, directed them into hospital for treatment. 'Were you *always* alone in your experiments. And, erm, what did you hope to achieve... Surely it wasn't just ecstasy — the drugs buzz?', I asked. Held in suspense. They looked as if I would, eventually, deliver a Do it Yourself *Holy Grail.*

'Erm... If you can... your opinion of *What is Magic...?*', Mark requested of me. And I thought of Fotheringay, in the rural English Pub, who unexpectedly got what he wished for, in H.G. Wells book and Film — *The Man Who Could Work Miracles.* [63] And, of poor Mickey Mouse, as Dukas' *Sorcerer's Apprentice* in Disney's *Fantasia...* And, wise-man Gandalf, in Tolkien's *Lord of the Rings*; and what happened to them — *saved* them from oblivion. Fotheringay, by playful, Cocteau like, mythic, Ancient Greek gods... acolyte Mickey, by his Master (a cunning man, a Wise Man) the wizard? The hobbits, saved by Gandalf's magic — Gandalf himself saved, by the immortality of his hidden occult art. I recollect my so recent visits, to The Upper Dicker school in East Sussex, and, too briefly, well met JRRT's cousin. Magic in-deed — fact and fiction.[64]

'Look, Mark... Jean... I don't know...You could attend school lessons, and be *opened*, but probably get closer if you first studied quantum physics. However, as an introduction, you could read people like Mary Anne Attwood, [65] Budge, Butler and Firth, who experienced and also wrote on this alchemic art (Magick).... But, be aware, both of you, that alchemy and commentary on magical writings often refer to ancient sciences translated god knows how many times, down the centuries. And even to start, you need a good deal of respect and first hand knowledge and praxis; in astronomy, biology, botany, chemistry, geometry, maths, and physics ...' And I confessed, insisted, myself, to knowing *nothing by experience* — of the so-called magical arts. And I paused, as Mark and Jean loudly drew a deep breath, and exhaled with a loud... 'Oh!'. I had my reservations.

Intellectually, I would, in time, believe to comprehend PURITY as an exact measure of whatever; and its implication, that's WHY all and everything is imperfect, and must forever be changing to harmonise (or Not) with its neighbours... BUT, so what? That is life.

I continued, ' As to your original question, *What is Magic*? The adept White Magician, Butler, said: — '*Magic is an Art of causing changes in Consciousness, at will...* Make of that, what you will.' They still stared, as if mesmerised by me, as if I was about to present a replica icon key of the mythical Holy Grail; as we three ignored all the noise about us created by other patients also out of the shed — and on their break.

'Remember, both of you. Memories are past time recordings; *glyphs* cast into each living body cell tissue.... You can be trained by Masters and Teachers — in a school, in a trance, in chant, rhythm and dance. To conjure up dreams and project them. No such thing, *really,* as Supernatural — only of that which is unknown to us.' 'You mean... like alchemists, and eh, members of the Golden Dawn?', asked Mark. I paused for emphasis. 'Yeats *was* a member; 'equated magic with imagination'. And *imagination* is real enough, however fleeting — however *you* use it, eh?'

But it was time to get up, re-enter The Barn and go back to work, on the promise we would talk a little more in the days ahead — down in The Yard.

Two Hues.

It was back in the early Nineteen-sixties. I recall, with pleasure and tenderness, my good elderly friends and mentors, (alchemist) bio-chemist Hugh, and his wife, artist and retired maths school teacher Winifred — their powerful, yet soft, influence upon my extra-mural education; both vegetarians and active humanists. They were *true* advocates and fund raisers, on behalf of the *Beauty Without Cruelty* charity founded by Muriel The Lady Dowding.[66] And in common with their friends, Lord and Lady Dowding (who, whilst I knew of them from Winifred, I never had the pleasure, of meeting those good souls). Lord Dowding [67] died earlier this year, on Sunday Feb.15th. 1970. Winifred would die of cancer, in 1975. And I was to lose two highly valued friends and mentors.

In Lord Dowding's *Preface*[68] to a book, *Leader Of The Few,* by Basil Collier, Dowding said:

> 'The evidence for the possibility of intelligent communication between the quick and the dead, is in my opinion quite convincing to the open mind ... I confidently predict that all these ideas will be commonly accepted in a hundred years time, when those who reject them will be classed with those who now believe that the earth is flat. ... Faith without works is sterile.'

But, humankind is so slow to learn.

Even as I had spoken, with wannabe acolytes Mark and Jean, I recalled reading of a Greek philosopher, called *Arisleus,*[69] in an ancient alchemical treatise, preserved in Arabic, and first written down almost two thousand years ago, which said:

> 'Know that the earth is a hill and not a plain, for which reason the Sun does not ascend over all zones of the earth in a single hour ; but if it were flat, the sun would rise in a moment over the whole earth...'

The world, mortal Arisleus inferred, is not flat. Many of us human, biological robots, have *yet* to discover the other New World *within* and about us, both on earth and abroad, out in space.

In the early Nineteen-Sixties, at a Lyons Cornerhouse first floor restaurant, adjacent to Piccadilly Circus... over a pot of tea and pastries, set in a Bill Brandt photo tableaux; served by cheerful Lyons' nippies, in frilled white aprons over black dress uniforms, and white cotton tiara like headgear. My former Arthur Murray dance student and friend, retired teacher and artist Winifred, described to me a treasured memory. In a profound testimony, she recalled her dreamlike, actual *retrieval* of Hugh, her frail scientist husband — when he was very ill. And what, she said, would otherwise have been his death (years later, I thought of Jean Cocteau's *Orphee*[70] and other iconic journeys into the underworld — but *should* that read inner world?) And, I recalled other tea-time table talk, in another London restaurant, when we were chatting about a recent television play on the psychology used in a black magic Dennis Wheatley type storyline... Winifred suggested as a first aid, should I feel alone and in trouble, 'Barry, if ever, however, you come by it, you are experiencing horrible visions or hostile voices; close your eyes and imagine, visualise a white cross (no, no, no — *nothing* whatever to do, with the infamous Ku Klux Klan icon) — and negative dark illusions should disappear. At least, the very thought will help.'

Several days on, it was lunchtime, down at IT; under a dour, chill grey patched overcast sky, and a shifting light breeze, Mark, Jean and I again sat down outside number five shed (The Barn); a small group of patients waiting to go back in, standing a few yards distant, with an unusually quiet Joker Laurie at their centre. If I didn't know better, I'd have said they were being respectful of our trio — I knew of Laurie's hospital friendship, with Mark and Jean... perhaps 'there had been talk' (chuckle).

'We have something for you, Barry ...', said young Jean, as they smiled in unison... and, across my vision, I saw friend Laurie nod his head in obvious approval, as he, too, produced a warm smile, as Mark brought out a large buff envelope, from its previous concealment behind his back... and handed it across to me — a gift from the clearly delighted young couple.

'Allo, 'allo... what have we here, then...', I jested, as I opened the package up, and extracted three, foolscap, well drawn illustrations. Evidence of their recent unfortunate experiments — and expiation. The first drawing was of a familiar goatheaded icon, an illusion purported to be invoked by Crowley's acolytes (*Magic in Theory and Practice*), and brought into vision by group devotees during a ritual assembly. Second, was an equally familiar drawing, of the Indian God Shiva — with its many arms — both of these pics, I recognised, as frequently published in popular books on Magic — including an edition by Dennis Wheatley; but the third was clearly an original, drawn by and signed by Marc — it was an ampoule of a prescribed drug, Amphetamine, his own icon on addiction. I felt honoured.

' What can I say...?', I looked at them. 'Obviously, this third one is all your own work, Mark. I must say you have talent in your drawing, I reckon. Thank you, I appreciate the gesture. But tell me, Mark, why Amphetamine?' 'Well, I thought about what to illustrate, and thought the hospital and fuzz seem to think that prescribed drugs aren't an addiction.' (I knew that for decades Amphetamines, The Benz, had been used as illegal uppers and downers, for anyone wanting or needing to stay awake for prolonged periods.)

'Do you know, Barry, that there's a *huge* market, for example, on Mandrax, and Mogadon tabs', (a nocte prescription for sedation). 'If you take it with alcohol, you can get a *terrific* high; *but* it can *kill* you, with the inevitable, down, *after effects...*' 'In other words, Mark, if any drug substance is not taken in controlled doses, the imbalance pollutes your system... And, as a poison, the buzz may kill you, eh ? 'Got it...', confirmed Mike, with a grim nodding by Jean... Too many memories of bad trips, perhaps.

Nurse talking. 'You seem to have learnt that lesson well enough, you two...' 'Drugs apart, Barry, we want to learn more of the unknown — that is, of course, unknown in our experience...' Mark attempting some clarity, in future intentions. 'And. Tell me again. What, or rather *why,* did you try *Magick* — what do you think now?' I asked, rather pointedly. 'Well... As a method — short cut, I guess... into the unknown.', Mark tailed off...

Back in Nineteen sixty-four, I'd known Hugh and Winifred about four years, and was newly married, (I was several years older, than Mark and Jean) and employed at *Agfacolor Processing,* in the film laboratory at Wimbledon. As a break, though unqualified as a chemist, I was asked to work awhile upstairs (as a *factotum*) in the chemists lab, helping three graduates in their daily analytical work on the correct quality (especially its reds) of the chemicals used in the film processing. Two of the BSc. graduate chemists were orthodox Islam, from Pakistan. And the third, their boss, a Scot PhD. about ten years their senior. On the office wall was a chart, of the periodical table of elements. And held in the Manager's office, always accessible, were two thick reference books, on Bio-chemistry and Physics, published by Yale University.

We got on well but, one lunchtime, I forgot that their faith *insisted* on a special diet, and I offered several packets of flavoured potato crisps to my two lab colleagues, and oops!, I'd made a *faux-pas*. My colleagues grinned, and reminded me that anything cooked in pigs' fat (shades of the Indian Mutiny and Black Hole of Calcutta — thankfully over a hundred years ago), was *not* allowed in their diet, it was considered polluted. I was used to knowing of *Kosher* food for orthodox Jews and, of course, of the differences between a vegetarian — and a vegan ...

It's common for a *Questor* to reach a phase in life when, as a student, they feel they ought to be vegetarians — just as to meet the requirements of certain training courses in life, a man or woman may *need* to abstain, fast, and be celibate; this would demonstrate that they can control their physical nature — and its *capacity.* It does *not* infer that the candidate *must* always remain so (*unless the rules of their voluntary faith demanded it*), only that they have learnt this self discipline, if called upon to do so. Well, it happened that whilst at Wimbledon *Agfacolor Processing,* I had faced such a watershed...

Bob, my Manager and *Agfacolor* chemist, treated me kindly, as odd but harmless. I'd been debating my Ignorance of a recent read Buddhist reality, that forbade consuming animal flesh — and *how to avoid pollution* — and the killing *any* form of life, however small or microscopic. Since I knew the human body is comprised of living micro-organisms, in need of food, whilst I can't express a math equation on the premise, do *all* living cells own a quantum of invisible psychic energy — is that an attribute of the Fechner psychophysic. I still have to Work that out. And, surely, if my body was pure, I couldn't survive in an impure world.

What is it like to be Pure ? And pure of what,...?

Myths and facts. Past fairy stories abound, of black witches, and other nether creatures, being vulnerable to water — crossing water et cetera; and lately, I became much mystified on reading that *pure* water (not salt water) our H2O (uncontaminated), is a protective mantle against nuclear radiation.... Erm! Well, Mark and Jean were now off illegal drugs, for a considerable time, and continued attendance at the hospital, to remove all previous unwanted toxins. I said in parting, in answer to their enquiry, 'I suggest you select one pathway (a body of work teachings) as a method; if possible, definitely under a School... and increase your *Capacity. But, whatever you do,...* please stay well away from the horror and lunacy, in practising black magic, which will probably lead to madness, and an early death... And, think for yourselves.' On leaving my three month placement, at No. 5 shed, I never saw Jean and Mark again — though I was later pleased to hear they were staying awhile with relatives, in West Sussex, who were qualified homeopathic medicine practitioners.

28 July 1970
Sandown Alcoholic Unit

Almost three years since tutor Mr Watkinson introduced our intake to the new *Therapeutic Community* project, based at Sandown. This was, originally, the Isolation Hospital block building, of the 1897 West Sussex County Asylum... its small square front grass lawn surrounded on three sides by a well tended thick green hedge.

In 1967, it had a small croquet course in use with its tall thin iron staple hoops, long-handled smooth, brown wood mallets, and fist-sized coloured wooden balls. I visualised ghost images, animated by Tenniel, for Lewis Carroll's 1865 *Alice In Wonderland* — and at Sandown, in survival of that pre-war, long established, genteel Graylingwell recreation, dating back as early as prewar Hospital days of 1914, or so... I have seen pictures of long-skirted nurses and young children at play on this site, in a prospectus dated 1912; it was now, in 1970, converted to a miniature golf course for staff and the unit's residents, recovering alcoholic patients, in therapy out at Sandown — this island Sanctuary some distance from the Main Building.

It was my last formal placement before the RMN final examinations, and I was there for six-weeks — the unit's first attending student. It was not easy to be accepted as a student on the unit, as both residents and staff had previously declined the option of a student since its inception, although occasional pre-arranged visitors were not at all discouraged; what was of paramount importance was that nothing was allowed to interfere with the Groupwork (the most vital facet of the treatment regime) and unwelcome unsettling intruders were actively discouraged — patients ... and staff.

Generally, *only* kitchen meals delivery, medical, nursing and portering staff, were sanctioned visitors to Sandown. Permanent RMN ward staff included — Charge Nurse, Sister and Staff Nurse. Their backup line managers and support-staff, located over the main building, comprised a Senior Nursing Officer, ward Psychiatrist and a senior Consultant.

The optimum number of patients accepted in residence at Sandown, was limited to the deemed maximum psychotherapeutic latitude of the Group numbers effectiveness. *Too many* patients and staff would prove cumbersome in Group Therapy — and, inevitably, divide the ambiance of the whole body into subgroups within the unit, and destroy its purpose. The average quota of patients accepted was nine men and five women, this being the maximum admitted into the resident open-ended group — the intense, closed, group meeting for a set period (no other persons would be accepted during its existence, even if any of its members subsequently withdrew). The open group, however, admitted and discharged members during the group's existence — viz as long as Sandown Unit remained open. On my date of brief attendance, it had existed for fifty months.

It was a warm mid-summer's day, as I joined with Sandown. Behind me, I could see the water tower of the main building to the South, looming up into an unclouded blue sky, above the border green hedgerows; and an abundance of multi-coloured trees and shrubs, their thick foliage and variant rainbows ranged flowers, in full bloom. At the rear and to the Northwest of Sandown, covering a large area, enclosed by substantial hedgerows and iron palings (and fronted like a Monet painting) stood an orderly queue, on guard, a sublime tall row of poplars. This was the symmetrical laid, and beautifully maintained, hospital orchard, also in full bloom, rich in its fruit of apples, pears, plums et cetera... green fields, then, marking its periphery. Directly to the front, and behind Sandown's South hedgerow surround, sunk several large Greenhouses, with adjacent colourful vegetable and various painted flower beds.

In plain vision to the East, halfway down its concave slope (the meandering Lavant watercourse at the bottom) was the Farmhouse, with its out buildings and The Yard where, so recently, I had enjoyed an three months stay, working in Number Five Shed facility, for Industrial Therapy. As I climbed its three steps up into Sandown, and turned left into the office off the short corridor, I sensed that there was an ongoing *frisson* about the unit that was *not* to be found on the acute wards and long-stay blocks, in the Main Building; I later identified it as an air of normalcy — the patients' tensions emotionally subdued or charged, but certainly contained by Sandown residents. Yes; it was different, a different milieu to any of the wards I had previously experienced, in the hospital... there were no prevailing antiseptic odours; I could smell the evidence of a recently cooked fried breakfast, and observed a number of the residents leisurely moving about — most persons heading for the multi-purpose lounge.

Two of the permanent staff, dressed in civvies; Martin, the Charge, a slightly stout smart man in his mid-thirties or so; Beryl, the ward Sister, slightly older, perhaps around early forties — also well turned out, pleasant and homely; and third was John (surely the most common name then, about the hospital) their Staff Nurse the youngest, in his mid-twenties, lean, athletic and visibly keen — John kept his dark hair quite long, but well kept and, as I came to notice, he appeared to wash and dress it every single day, and he wore a white coat. I, too, was expected to appear in my hospital grey suit, and uniform white coat; our appearance instantly identified John and I, as nursing staff — we were mostly general factotums, though John would sometimes deputise for Martin or Beryl, in their absence.

Martin and Beryl were the key anchor, Group facilitators. The three nursing staff sat in the office, preparing for a Monday morning house meeting. They looked up as I entered the small room, and sat down adjacent to the corner secured medicine trolley — in essence, no different than all other ward offices in its furniture fittings and ward board. This board listed all named present residents, their locations and basic known at-a-glance details, such as date of admission, home GP, and Consultant. A separate last column indicated whether they were In, Out (off the unit), or were on home leave. And, there, the semblance to all of the other wards I had experienced ended.

'Morning, Beryl... Martin... John', I almost whispered, not wishing to interrupt the flow whilst Charge continued his update. He smiled, and then replied 'Sit down, Barry. I'll chat with you after this meeting. We've almost finished.' Of course I had already made their acquaintance, over a number of visits (indeed, interviews) as staff and a rep of the resident group confirmed, or refused, my Sandown placement. And as Beryl and John left the office, Martin outlined the week's regular planned routines for me, and I duly entered the details, in my proverbial notebook.

Specific chores were given to every resident (facilitated by staff), a new list each week, which the Sandown community group (with no abstainers) had democratically agreed upon.

And so, another of my *little lists (*which I'd started to refer to as *Mikado* lists*)* came together, as the week's work was structured, written-up and placed on the cork Notice board, located in the lounge. In addition to essential chores, there were other Unit routines.

Monday morning was strictly domestic — cleaning, washing-up and generally tidying up their rooms, with all individuals, after ablutions, preparing themselves for another intense working week — on themselves. Mid-day, weekenders were due back at the unit; and, after lunch (delivered by electric trolley from the main hospital kitchens), the first Group Psychotherapy Group meeting would take place. This was an Open group, which meant everyone attended — staff and residents, including myself.

Tuesday morning Group Meeting; afternoon Social Therapy; evening AA meeting.

Wednesday, morning Group Meeting, afternoon social therapy or visitors.

Thursday, morning Group meeting; afternoon Occupational Therapy — evening AA meeting.

Friday, morning Group meeting, afternoon — occupational therapy; evening optional AA meeting.

Saturday, morning Group meeting; midday those proceeding on weekend leave with TTOs where prescribed.

The remainder of residents were able to relax, through till Monday midday — though on Sunday afternoon, the unit usually organised an AA meeting at Sandown.

But, from the outset, what was most unclear was what was *my role* (other than obvious student). What , even as a *factotum*, was I expected to do, or not do, amongst these daily routines. The residents filled, it seemed, all aspects of deemed domestic tasks, in therapeutic ascribed roles. I was easily reminded of my not so long ago, in-search-of Gurdjieff and alchemic skills, visits to The Dicker, in company with Bunty, and how all allocated tasks had an *added,* not so hidden, invisible agenda, as vital towards self-purification and better self-development.

So Martin as Charge, too, began to give me things to do — initially, office bound. It soon became rather obvious that I was there to watch and learn from the staff as Facilitators in support of The Group members in therapy; after all, the unit had not experienced a staff member as a student before but, thankfully, I was soon accepted, as a to be trusted additional member of staff.

I was not a total unknown stranger to the needs of acute (on the drink), and recovering (off the drink) alcoholic patients; drink, in moderation, as so-called Social Drinking. is a good ice-breaker and inhibition release (truism of course) *but* heavy drinking and in particular, alcohol dependency, is too often media trivialised, or worse romanticised — *yet* anyone who is aware through real experience from indulgence; a close family friend or helpless child who experiences the horrific demise of an chronic alcoholic, and degradation its compulsive sick-cravings lead down into. A habit which is a source of hell on earth; abject misery for those about them, as well the addict; the constant violence to self and others, and the inevitable poverty it propagates; the inevitable ill-health it guarantees; crime it instigates and perpetual self-abuse and chronic abuse of all others about them. In the past few years, I had met a large number of such sick people, resident on our different wards...

In 1967 Amberley reception I acquainted several drying-out alcoholics. Most had been interviewed on the ward, by visiting members of then current Sandown group — as potential new members... and, on that ward, I experienced, as a first-year-student with an Experimental young drug dependants' group, meeting up with an older group of alcoholic dependants, over at Sandown. Current clinical Aversion Therapy was a form of medical treatment using antibuse and apomorphine — neither experiment appeared very successful, *but* were surely worthy in their honesty of exploration, to support both groups — alcohol, and drug dependants approved the effort.

And there was a sad brief experience at the impending death, and delirium tremens; the bed cradle sides, up for our unknown warrior, a wartime Colonel with so many invisible horrors locked within his mortal frame — on 1968 England sick ward... and, of an RAF moustached Brian, over at 1968 Summersdale — awaiting an interview from The Group representatives of Sandown. I thought he was highly motivated and an excellent candidate.

But, sadly, other hospitalised alcoholics had, like the Colonel, been addicted too long, and survived, in time, with their internal organs decaying through rotting pollution, and nutrient starvation — evidence becoming progressively more and more self evident.

Another 1968 Summersdale patient, admitted with chronic alcoholism, was diagnosed with Korsakoff's Psychosis (in lexicon, linked with Werncke's syndrome), a direct result of starvation, too much alcohol and too little of essential food, vitamins, et cetera. Mostly, I recall *his* premature dementia (in age), a total loss of short-term memory (amnesia), and delusional fictitious confabulation, in filling that gap. And other more visible visceral signs of his body's pollution; part of his crucial medical treatment was intra-muscular injections of thiamine, for three days or so; he had a poor diagnosis — treatment reduced his suffering and, rightly, the hospital staff administered their implicit Duty Of Care. As an human being, his life history (despite his Case Notes), emotions and whatever thoughts, would remain invisible, and only his body tissues remember his sufferings — so-called conscious memories had already departed. Fortunately, all our present Sandown residents had a good prognosis.

Drying Out

I had considerable respect for patients resident at Sandown; for most of them it had meant months of preparation. hard work and good faith — and not without considerable courage; all residents had had to willingly, albeit painfully, discard the Mask (behind which lay denial of alcohol dependence, and legion reasons that it came into being — and concretised); I learnt of the oft quoted maxim — a truism... most alcoholics hated alcohol dependency, but, hated their life more so. Such was their denial and rationale behind their 'alcohol reasoning', as I heard it sometimes referred to in conversation.

Before any diagnosed alcoholic was admitted to The Group, it was imperative they were 'dried out', i.e. off the drink; interviewed by the ward doctor and Sandown nursing staff, and vetted by the present Group members. The express reason for these interviews and preparation was to assess integrity of the alcoholic, who had admitted evidence of dependency, to give up the drink. And, more so, to work on dealing with their underlying reasons for drink. If *any* suspect reason was realised — i.e. they intended to save up money whilst in residence — for drink; avoid police action; or only forced by relatives or other pressure groups, to attend the unit — then the alcoholic would be ill-advised and entry to the unit refused, at that present time.

I entered the lounge, to help John assemble a Faustian circle of chairs; assisted by two silent residents (who smiled, and nodded a hello to me). I observed one other patient sat in a corner, where he could look out through the net curtains and see the rear of The Yard buildings on the right of the narrow road around its back; and, on the left side, could see the former Stockman's Cottage, presently in use as a rented family house for a nurse and his family... I had already enjoyed several energetic games of Table Tennis and Darts with newcomer Jim, who had been admitted the previous Monday, only a week before — he was, this moment, head down in concentration, working hard at his *Thumbnail* life-history notes, which he was expected to present at an Open Group meeting later this week, probably during Saturday morning — Jim had no time to stop and stare out of the window at any sunlit landscape — not yet.

Acknowledging Jim's task, Staff John looked across, and sussurated said 'Hi Jim ... busy eh ... Meeting in ten minutes or so ... ' Slim Jim looked up acknowledged cause for the remark and replied 'Thanks John — be with you in a minute.' I'd started on The Unit this day — Jim had been admitted a week ago — so we were both new to vicissitudes, offered by the Sandown unit... And I found this first group meeting was indeed strictly who was to do what domestic chores, and errands — whereas, in the afternoon, everyone should be present at the full open Group Psychotherapy meeting — and perhaps suggest any weekend incidents that would need some discussion.

During the lunch break, Martin and Beryl elucidated what to expect, during my attendance at various Open Group and other anticipated meetings, and what was deemed likely to be a Good session — and what deemed a Bad group meeting; but added a rider that it would not be possible for me to enter a Closed Group session, during my six short weeks. I accepted a Bob Dylan[71] service role... *Everybody has to serve somebody* — acting as a professional go-between, in a myriad of support actions, anticipating the biological adjustments vital to a recovery, *and* the psychological and social tools in an individual's *holistic* — albeit equally essential spiritual, cum Mental (complementing bio-brain demands) needs — as they routinely arose.

Following initial admission to dry-out, and cessation of any and all forms of alcohol, it would be dangerous to have stopped drinking and *immediately* expect the bio-body systems to adjust to the lack of alcohol in the bloodstream — the balance, homeostatic tolerance, must therefore be biochemically adjusted to prevent inevitable somatic traumas — *and* the enormous effect in the abreactive removal of their alcoholic mask, with hitherto multiple veils keeping invisible, too awesome horrors anger and fears hidden within (compare withdrawal symptoms of drug addiction, and going cold turkey).

With the foregoing in view, a 1970 Chemotherapy list was written up — and so, *I've got a little list, I've got* another *little list* — naming treatment, dependent on the state *capacity* of the body-systems and degree of the patient's chronicity... A typical very depressed suicidal, physically rundown alcoholic, would have been clinically recommended the following: *Heminevrin,* QDS (Four times daily) for nine days — this was both a sedative hypnotic and anti-convulsant, used to control the onset of parkinsonian symptoms (The Shakes — DT's — delirium tremens) — and, additionally aid as an anti-depressant and night-time sedative. Each capsule contained 192 mg powder and was soft, yellow and egg-shaped in appearance.

Cellular starvation introduced *Parentrovite*. I gave a number of those injections — it was a liquid form of vitamin B complex, applied once daily; however, 10 cc was given immediately — stat — on prescription, intravenously, to direct the vitamin B food *direct* into the blood stream — the balance given intramuscularly for four days. *Pabrinex* gave a compound of vitamins introduced intramuscularly, never intravenous — the medication extracted from two ampoules; the first 5 cc ampoule contained largely vitamin B: thiamine hydrochloride, nicotinamide, riboflavine, pyridoxine hydrochloride, benzyl alcohol B.P.; the second ampoule held 500 mg of ascorbic acid (vitamin C), also given intramuscularly.

It was noticeable biscuits, breakfast cereals (containing thiamine, etc; — Vits B and C), chocolates, fruit juices, sweets — sugar, and *many* numerous cups of cha — all legitimately helped replace still cravings for alcohol. Tensions, emotional and vascular, were inevitable, as the abreactions and evolving New men and women were being vigorously reborn, as it were. They experienced invisible tingling mixtures of *angst* and excitement in the growth of potential better and better prognosis — *but* first, those anxieties, too, needed treatment. *Amitryptiline,* an antidepressant given as a 25 mg small yellow tab in appearance — given tds (three times daily), and three tabs initially, nocte — at night.

Due to excitement, fears and added anxiety, the depression that accompanied drying out and early admission residence in the unit — restlessness at nights prescribed *Mogadon,* 5 mg, a large white line-marked Roche tab — one or two nocte PRN (if and when necessary). This medication was discarded as soon as possible — after all, there was no point in replacing one addiction with another. Some *Physiotherapy* was often needed, where muscles had wasted and, aided by the vitamins, allowed re-training in lots of exercise and social interactions — both needs well planned for, by the weekly roster of listed Sandown activities.

11th August 1970
Home Pressures

The past few Summer months I had not seen much of my student colleagues... I would leave straight for work, early in the morning by train — with numerous delaying rail-strikes and times, I was left stranded on Barnham, or Ford station hoping for a link. Fortunately, my Staff nurse colleague occasionally supplied a car lift. On these tedious journeys, my pocket notebooks became replete with numerous Mikado lists, *lists* of student references, and lists of wanted books and magazine articles — relevant, and extramural.

A little cryptic perhaps — and hinting at the mood, on 8th August 1970 I wrote, *How do you see a grain of wheat amongst a field of corn*? Conversely, how to visualise a field of corn from a grain of wheat... cosmology and alchemy. Three days later, on the 11th August, I noted down in my diary notes, a personal list, headed *Problems*. 1. Approaching RMN finals work. 2. Sara, her needs. 3. Money. Bank overdraft amount. 4. Decisions — as to future. 5. From above's inability to function well. 6. Check bills outstanding. 7. Sara's housekeeping.... At this time, I had little insight, into Sara's probable, invisible postpartum depression, which had appeared for a while after our second born — or lingered from our first born.

Even more so — emotionally and intellectually — at work I was doing great. I had a structure — a school of professionalism which during the past three years I had — invisibly — internalised. *But,* outside the work role, I was still prone to latent mood swings and gross fatigue: it would be years before I realised — there were times I had had great trouble, coping at home — *compared*, to the work milieu, where I continued to feel capable, content and quite comfortable ... It was *not* a question of a Dr. Jekyll and Mr Hyde syndrome, rather I felt secure and mature in my new profession — *but* remained insecure and immature (despite I was thirty-three years old) at home — historically, I had had no personal early nuclear family experience to model on — Freud, I'm sure, would have easily diagnosed such being but norm responses to our childhood experiences.

Our boys were now attending nursery groups, and we were contemplating lodgers. During the past four years, I lost two maternal grandparents; and, more recently, Sara's grandparents, too, had passed away — though, for a time, her grandmother had lived with us before she died. This was all quite normal — extended family life; comings and goings — more of life's inevitable partings.

Groupwork

Almost two weeks on, and I attended an afternoon Open Group Meeting at Sandown. I had already attended a fair number of meetings, and exchanged plenty of conversation with the residents. Outside any formal groups, I learnt most of the residents names, and something about them. In turn, they knew a little about me, other that being a mature student; married with two infant sons; and I appeared to be often making student jottings, sat in the office or in the lounge. On several occasions, I reassured residents that, like their Closed Group, I kept all my notes as confidential but, mostly, reassured them that no personal details about them — by name — were ever written down by me (Case notes, I shared with Martin and Beryl). One morning, I wanted to record a sketch of negative and positive exchanges between people at that meeting — no objection was made, and I sat and began my observations.

At first I thought the mickey was being taken of Martin and Beryl, albeit good natured — but it was a norm lexicon, adopted by dried out, committed Group Members... in affable conversation, Sandown's two anchor staff were adopted as the residents' foster parents, and referred to as *Mum and Dad !* — at least whilst in the building. I never talked about it, to residents or staff — but invisible, emotionally, I felt privileged; indeed, as the masks of denial were discarded, and fears and ignorance about themselves admitted — the average alcoholic became almost *childlike,* as they presented for treatment in this *Therapeutic Community* — minus alcohol, and honesty disclosed — their healing meant that, at the time, there was indeed the prospect of a rebirth — much dependent on their *capacity*. At the other end of the scale, I was already well acquainted with the burnt out, real and dependent demented elderly, on the long-stay ward blocks of the main building; lovingly cared for by a nucleus of staff. who treated their charges in lexicon as their *babies*.

During that in-between period of drying-out, and early days of admission and chemotherapy, before qualifying for a *Closed Group* after six weeks — other routine diagnostic investigations were carried out, blood and other somatic anatomical checks, including neurological, x-rays, liver-function-tests. There were also psychological[72] (See *Appendix*) landmark tests — Krouts psychogram — which indicated certain personality traits (attitudes); the Eysenck Personality Inventory and Mill Hill Matrices — to gauge an present intelligence quotient (in mind that the affect of a previous and recent heavy alcohol content had *not* encouraged use of this *capacity*): these tests completed, during the first week on the unit — and, again repeated, shortly before leaving after thirteen weeks.

In all this preparation work, I played an active support role — accompanying our newer residents to and fro, on numerous visits to the Path Lab. And visits to Dr. Harrod our Clinical Psychologist, based on Summersdale Four ward (chuckle! our own amiable BBC *Doctor Who*); who also routinely applied a sensitivity skin test, for possible psychopathic, or other hidden inhibitory tendencies, which could suggest an inability to show emotion — reflected by excessive perspiration in hand palms. I wondered what psychiatrist Dr. Joyce — experienced in Sodium amytal and LSD abreaction *(treated amnesia)* traumas, would debate on this forensic test? Such routine visits provided plenty of valuable opportunities for me, to exchange conversation with the residents, and learned professionals — no masks in situ.

There were thirteen people, presented in a closed circle — seven male residents; Stan, Sid, Paul, Billy, Jim, Jock and Bert; and two female residents, Hillary and Wendy. There was also five staff present, comprising, at the head of The Group — Sister Beryl, Charge Martin and our Ward Doctor — the facilitators, who were expected to ideally remain silent throughout — to only intervene if an emergency was instigated ... Staff John and myself were placed within the horseshoe — between Jim and Jock — and had to remain quiet, unless given stick by any of the residents and forced to respond; it was, of course, a structured group. Notably, Paul was the elected resident Group Leader and Wendy his Deputy. After sketching the layout of all members and staff location within the group, I put a plus(+) icon or a minus(-) icon against each name, as a verbal communication took place — giving support as a plus ... and an minus for giving an attack.

At the conclusion of this Group Meeting, two names sustained a minus, Billy and Stan for their — in context — outbursts, towards other members within the group. Issues became ready to be abreacted — liberated — during a Group Meeting; such as a domestic problem where previously two or more members had a set-to — displaying features of their personality, and its offences; members were thus prepared for such action. Of interest, I had registered a plus signal from Jim towards myself, when he had needed a confirmation and support on a point of issue — and where mutual integrity deserved an appropriate positive response.

Staff returned to the office, whilst the residents split up into twos and threes — complementing a conclusion of the experienced staff, who decided, it had been a very good Group Meeting. In particular, there was a recognition that both Billy (who was twenty years at least Stan's junior) — and Stan, had done *really* well. Both ex-naval men from Portsmouth, Stan had been a Chief Petty Officer at the end of the war; both residents (like father and son) had experienced, the in-common legacy of broken marriages and painful trail of unsuccessful personal relationships — compounded by, in attrition, tragic childhood experiences — and, with their previous Rockville of guilt and muted anger being expiated within the safety of the Sandown Therapeutic Community. And, for me, a small bonus — with a warm smile from slim Jim, as he said in passing me by, on my way to the office, 'Cheers Barry...'

I felt it had been a good experience for me, too.

'So what *does* constitute a *Good* Group meeting, then ?', I asked the small gathering of staff, and residents — Paul, Leader, and Deputy Wendy. I was fortunate they'd agreed to give me a quarter of an hour or so, on their collective experience of Groupwork. 'It's easier if we consider a typical *Bad* Group, first, Barry...', Paul began. 'As *you* know — if sudden visitors or unknowns — sit in The Group, we find it *at least* produces an uncomfortable atmosphere. As you have seen, we exist as a cohesive group *because* we have learnt to know and trust each other.' There was a distinct nod of approval from everyone at this preface.

'S' right ... A Good working Group has a number of elements — members well motivated, long-prepared — especially when they are able to enter the *Closed Group,* after sustaining six hard weeks at Sandown.', Martin agreed. 'You have six weeks, to prepare for the intense Closed Group. At the end of the first week, you present a *Thumbnail* outline, of your past life-story And, after six weeks, you are expected to present to *everybody* in The Unit, a typed Life Story — this is *The* emotional apex of our whole thirteen weeks stay here at Sandown.' Wendy interjected. 'Back to your question about what is *not* on. Any staff participant who arrives with a holier than thou attitude, autocratic air, using a white coat or other masked, professional, assertive role — as opposed to being sincere ...', said Beryl. 'Well... no way!' And almost, in chorus, all nodded agreement... 'Any condescension will lead into a Bad Group session.', concluded Martin.

It was early on a Monday morning, near the end of my final placement — and ten minutes or so before Beryl and Martin were due on duty — John was off, on a few days leave. As I entered the short crescent shaped gravel drive, in front of Sandown entrance, I was presented with an obvious altercation. Two of the residents, Wendy and Jim, were struggling with and trying to reason with a middle-aged man — a stranger to me, but clearly known to our residents.

'Now come on Neil — you don't want Mum or Dad to see you like this, do you?', Wendy patiently pleading with a well inebriated ex-resident who, having experienced a blackout shattering his last weekend at home, had then fled — or rather staggered, over to the sanctuary of Sandown The previous day, Sunday, he'd attended an AA meeting at the unit, but *not* returned home. The situation was self-evident, and as I approached Jim, who was trying to hold Neil up on the steps, they looked across at me, and said 'Hi Barry. We have a problem — as you can see ...'

'It's okay, take him into the office. One of us can make him a cup of coffee, while we wait for Martin and Beryl...', I suggested to Jim and Wendy. Neil stopped struggling at this suggestion, clearly he liked the proposal, and, as we escorted him into the building, I heard, then saw Sister Beryl's (their Mum's) car, entering the drive. It would be all right whatever the *gravitas* stasis — at this time.

August. 1970
Revision

I encountered many gravely ill, young, and aged persons, under *extreme* attrition — their *incapacity* to function their limbs, and focus their mind — a dark Kaftaesque existence; due to *inhibited* or fragmented, invisible, decaying brain tissue: and, having their receding, consciousness, only a limited access to shrinking islets of vital memories. Incapacity rendered them helpless, and *not* able to attend of their own volition, even their most basic needs. These persons were diagnosed as in constant need for holistic medical *and* nursing attention — both physic and psychic. This lesson I learnt well, during RMN training in Graylingwell Hospital; and practised its doctrine for many years to come — both in hospitals, and serving in the community. But I would be often confounded by the rigid fiscal politics of separating the *Nursing* care into on-going social and / or medical needs — for strictly financial savings — due accounts before patients care.

If the patient does not have the capacity to walk dress feed or be able to action from their own will their bodily needs and functions — then such help they require to be mobile and survive is properly called Nursing. This lesson I learnt well, during RMN training on the hospital estate.

To my surprise, in the midst of gross fever or psychiatric confusion, or and despite evidence of advancing dementia, in a disabled patient — I observed, there are rare recorded events when despite their in-extremis condition, and diminished capacity, a much disorientated, confused person (a wounded soul?), would suddenly sussurate — be still — then with an absolute clarity, ghost-like say — '*I want to do the right thing.*' From an old file (the patient long dead), ' Nancy. Recovered and discharged 25 May 1933.' (and a Social Report.) ' *Intellectual... Consciousness / Confused ... Attention / Distracted ... Train of thought / I want to do the right thing ... Orientation / Disorientated from time and place ...'*

I found this statement, and similar, in a number of 1930s to '60s nursing case notes when, *despite* the gravitas of an illness, a nurse or doctor, would suddenly witness, hear and then record those same words, in their notes. And I too, during my three years training, heard these seeming miraculous utterings, in the midst of a patient's infirmities and sufferings — and God, the intense emotion, respect, I felt... well, I guess these inadequate words disclose a faint trace of those memories.

It was a warm, lovely, early autumn day; I felt good, confident and unstressed — at the time — despite the hospital final, due *only* days away. I had seen Ghananian Harry, if only briefly, the day before — he was feeling rather stressed out, he admitted, in his controlled laconic way (which I rather admired — though I never embarrassed him on this feeling). Francis and the retired Squadron Leader too, would be sitting with us — though it was uncertain whether they would sit with Harry and I for the GNC Final, in October.

At first, I thought I was alone in the Nissan hut hospital nursing school, as I started to load up my first Trolley — for ward dressing... on the top and cleaned glass surface, I selected essential instruments; and, on the bottom shelf, I laid out the CSSD sterile packs of cotton-wool balls, gauze-swabs, linen-pads, and small galley-pots, and other mixed packs, anticipating a patient's possible needs — this shelf, with lotions and other stock for closure — the whole trolley preparatory for asepsis.

But, as I started to arrange my second trolley, towards the practical, I heard the muted chatter of two men's voices and, sure enough — it was, erm, of course, *pure* coincidence — Mr Watkinson and Mr Ilford happened to be working this very morning at the school; and so, after a brief hello, they both offered to be on call if they could be of any help in checking anything, after I had completed any piece of revision — and, after they departed to their office, I returned to my exercises.

The *little list* of self chosen revision tasks, selected for this morning, I had extracted from two years past Examination papers — provided by our tutors.

And so, in turn, I made up a Catheterisation; a Self-retaining trolley; a Lumbar Puncture tray; a Suture Set and an ECT Drug Tray — checking afterwards from the standard textbook and my notes. All very basic, of course. Mr Ilford, thoughtfully, came out to do a random check on several of my completed written up Questions and Answers pieces of work; and, at one point, examined my drawing up and written down answer, to a particular question on a calculation of insulin.

The syringe lay in the tray, ready to be checked by him, innocent in a shining sterile, chrome metal kidney dish... laid on the top of a ward trolley. In my limited experience, I easily recalled daily urine specimen litmus checks, and my marking up a graph-chart, watching out for an increase or decrease — beyond the allotted 2% margin, with diabetic Freddie resident on Eastergate One ward, last winter... and my only previous involvement with insulin. And so, I presented my written answer and the dummy tray — for Mr Ilford's routine inspection. 'Erm, Barry, did you check the dosage?'

My tutor looked gravitas at me — he was holding the almost — imagined — filled small CSSD syringe ... and looked *very* concerned. And the sunny day fell, darkened into a thick glutinous shadow, as dread overtook me, and my previous rank confidence completely disintegrated. 'Eh... well, I *thought* I had.' An inadequate answer stumbled out of me... almost a whisper. 'Erm... it's a wrong dosage — is it ?' 'Well — to be blunt — you would *certainly* have *killed* your patient.' Mr Ilford spoke kindly... not at all in condemnation; indeed, over the past year, he had come to know me quite well.

Sometime back, a year or more, after one of our many Question and Answer sessions, with me asking, and he in the chair answering — he remarked (and sounded so sad at the time, as he and I were alone, like now, here in the school)... I remember those very words... 'You know, Barry — I *do* listen, more than you might think.' (He'd reminded me, that time, of my learned friend Winifred.) '*You know and have plenty to say, yet hold back an awful lot — don't you* ?'

He observed how crestfallen I became at this moment, sagged shabby, a punctured balloon — after this current *cardinal* error of wrong dosage. God, *I'd have killed someone,* if I hadn't had it *checked* first — echoed my thoughts. And, ex-RAMC tutor Mr Ilford, I recall, said a year ago, 'You have learnt how to say a lot, but really say very little — of what you think and feel? An oxymoron, eh?...' Ouch! What's the opposite of being — laconic — loquacious.

But at this time, so close to the finals, I was very short of words to say. As my tutor explained in detail, the proper answer to the question — on calculating insulin dosage. And, I can *read* English; no matter how honest or sincere a person in caring might be, if you *cannot interpret* any written instructions, one might too easily abuse, or poison the patient... no matter how honest and sincere one might be. Morality. What price Integrity?

'Mr Ilford... erm — I only want... erm to... *I want to do what is right...*'

'That's all right, Barry. Glad to be able to help. And don't take it too much to heart. You will do well, despite your slow math calculations. These three years... your good track record of ward reports has moved on with you, as you moved from ward to ward — a real professional.' As he started to move off, I again thanked him. He stopped, looked at me, straight into my somewhat misted eyes, and paused, to conclude the session. 'Barry. Do you mind if I say something — a bit personal — to you ?' Oh, now what — but , though the given previous confidence was shaken, hurt — I knew it would prove so in my professional life — and even more so — in private and domestic life — in the years ahead. My weakness.

'You are, I know, a caring man — and whatever profession you practice, you'll do a good job — but, there will be times when your eagerness to share your emotions will put others, and in reciprocity, yourself, on the defensive... Try and restrain those thoughts, words and emotions — when you can observe what is happening; *Individual* Integrity often wears a thorny crown, you know... Hope you don't mind my saying this to you at this time, Barry.' 'Not at all, Mr Ilford — I know you're right. *Thank you* once again.' Gurdjieff's Self-remembering.

Homework

Work, homework — in a different format, seemed to follow me home — though no way was it planned as such. Having advertised in the local press, and *Dalton's Weekly,* Sara and I had taken in a small number of lodgers — having previously, albeit rather briefly, tried to sustain short-stay holiday B & Bs — but soon decided that that commitment was not what we wanted, in order to subsidise our low income.

Our home was a large, end of terrace, two storey house — the top floor was, in fact, a partially converted attic. The building was separated, by a narrow pavement and equally narrow access road, from an substantial green wasteland (several times a year, a Fair would materialise for a week, to the delight of our infants, Kit and Paul); enclosed on three sides by houses, one side — opposite our house — was an Industrial estate; the High Street shops, and Beach Road, led on down to the Sea, a mile or so from our house, and The Promenade; a bus station, and the Littlehampton railway terminus were all within an easy walking distance.

On the first floor were six rooms, including a separate toilet and separate bathroom. We then converted the smallest one of the four bedrooms to a kitchen. These arrangements then enabled us to rent out the three bedsitting rooms with their own communal facilities — at a later date, we would also rent out the top room too, as a bedsitter. As to our own living quarters, we lived on the ground floor, with our separate entrance and facilities — including a minute back garden.

The mortgaged home, at the top of Eastham Road, was our first — previously, separate as individuals, now together — we'd been tenants, in rented accommodation, in London and down here in the South. And now as landlord / lady we soon found out how realistic were the numerous, sometimes sad, but more often hilarious 1970s radio and television sitcom episodes; the reluctant Blood Donor in *Hancock's Half hour* ; two Scouce *Liver Birds* and the two Geordie rascals in *The Likely Lads*; and the domesticity of *Rising Damp*.

Our first two lodgers were youngsters, who knocked on our door in response to the local paper advertisements. Geoffrey was about twenty-two, round faced, a student, he said, but we never found out what of — we concluded he *wanted* to become a student but had not yet decided on a course, or qualified for entry. Geof was clean, and always immaculately dressed, in what looked to be quite expensive and fashionable early Seventies gear; and, although quite sociable, he had no visitors or phone calls; however, he said he enjoyed athletics and sports, and certainly had a muscled healthy looking body, to confirm those natural interests. Only days later, he came down with his rent book and insisted on showing Sara and I the kneecap of his right leg, which he described as 'foaming on the knee' — reasonable, perhaps an athletic injury — but it was his accompanying commentary which, at first puzzled — he said it, the offending knee, was *talking* to him — joking or a metaphor we thought — he was deadly serious; and his talking limbs became a regular topic — until he left, after a short stay — to an Arts Course, that he said he was to attend, in Brighton.

Not surprisingly I compared Geof, and his talking limbs, to patients I knew at the psychiatric hospital — especially those I knew of, with similar schizoid symptomatology... About the same time as Geoffrey's short stay, while I was away at work, and the children were that morning at Play School, Sara answered the door to a somewhat distressed seventeen year old youth, called David, in urgent need of a room to stay. He had no money, but was to register this day at the Labour Exchange (he said); she took pity on him and, having adopted the role of Good Samaritan, she fed and watered him, as she listened to a rank tale of neglect and woe — and his delight in noting our range of books, and long playing records.

But, only days later, the youth disappeared — with the whole of his first welfare payment — having registered this address at the Labour and DHSS. No rent paid, of course; but what really upset us was, more than money, he had stolen a collection of books, and records Jazz Satch, Folk Donovan, Holst and Rachmaninov, Sara's Shadows, Presley and Sibelius, all of which he sold to a local dealer. He even stole her small supply of cigarettes. I happened to spot some of these treasures on sale, on a regular visit to the Littlehampton *Arcade* shop. The find was confirmed, with my name written on a number of items, among his new stock. The dealer remembered David bringing them in, and matched my description of the pleasant youth.

Another early, but to be a short-stay; a middle-aged lady who had answered the *Dalton's Weekly* advert, but actually (while I was at work) had been accompanied by a social worker, from London. Miss Flowers (not of course her real name) took up the end first floor bedsitter — adjacent to the shared kitchen. And, from the outset, appeared to be a little eccentric.

A retired mid-to late fifties year old, plain, genteel Miss Flowers — amiable, she would come downstairs to confidentially inform in a hush to Sara or myself — 'Please. I'm not complaining, but are *you* aware that electricity is coming *down* through my ceiling (from another lodger's bed-sitting-room) and coming through the walls' — and she did *not* mean through the normal light fittings, or wall plugs. But dear Miss Flowers was a recluse, and otherwise kept to herself — and we respected her sanctuary, at first. But awhile later (Sara recalls the event and years later, still refers to this event, and others to soon follow), she came downstairs in a terrible state, with a saucepan firmly placed on her head to keep the continuing alien rays at bay. She then sat herself down at the foot of the stairs. It transpired that the *Dalton's Weekly* (London Edition) was being used by a number of London, Psychiatric Hospital, Social Workers, to find Community Placements for a number of their patients. Poor Miss Flowers relapsed, and went back up to London with her social worker. Other lodgers too, answering the advertisements, arrived from London, Brighton, and other places outside Littlehampton.

Along the first floor passage, half-way, *at the top of the stairs* from the front door, and next to the loo and adjacent bathroom, in what had previously, briefly, been young Geoffrey's small bed-sitting-room — now resided another, late middle-aged person, a retired civil servant who had been escorted down from London, to The Seaside, by his niece (actually another social worker, who would visit him from time-to-time). Mr Stoker was a very heavy smoker and, in a short time, his room's previously bright coloured wallpaper, and onetime white ceiling, became camouflaged when it developed a thick brown sticky mucus (he refused to ever open the windows; he suffered the cold, even midsummer) — and his eiderdown and bed linen displayed, like a pepperpot, an array of holes, from dropped cigarette ends and ash droppings.

Mr Stoker's health was poor, not surprising, his lungs gave him considerable bronchial despair — this complaint was to kill him. He was always untidy, not able to look after himself too well, as his relative was only too aware, polite and no trouble — though other people in the house occasionally passed him leaving the toilet, with it hanging out, as he left the little room, his trouser fly left undone to return to his room, only next door — but, we soon knew him enough to realise he would be mortified, if he thought — we thought — he intended any offence.

Both Miss Flowers and Mr Stoker had been lonely souls, who had arrived separately, on different days, and lived as close neighbours, only yards away from each other, but, to our knowledge, they remained total strangers, and never engaged in *any* conversation with each other — preferring their life-made rented prison cell — and its deemed safe seclusion. This is, was, of course, an aspect of normal community life.

Several months after quiet but otherwise, electrified Miss Flowers moved on, her room was taken by Yvonne, a single young woman who had recently moved away from her parents in order to take up a job as a shop assistant in The High Street; she proved to be a delightful normal, vivacious, happy-go-lucky tenant, with oodles of friends and often monopolised the residents installed pay phone.

While Yvonne was settling in, a few days later, we had an interesting grey suited clipboard American visitor, of forty summers or so; Mr Saltlake produced a printed card which formally introduced him as a missionary, a *Mormon* administrator; on behalf of this religious organisation, he was searching for lodgings for two young USA trainee Mormons, due in the country the following week.... the first of many to follow.

We hesitated, at first, as only the day before we had had two similarly suited religious visitors — *not* in pursuit of a room to let, but as formal reps of *The Jehovah's Witnesses* (they were always in pairs), determined to convert us to their own particular brand of Christianity; now, Sara was a baptised Roman Catholic, and I as C of E, both of us non-church going — but, fervently A.C. Bouquet, like *Comparative Religion* faith practitioners ... And so, the English missionaries went on their way, about their allocated sector.

Peter and Dudley moved in the following weekend, two young immature, well dressed student, Mormon... eh — gentlemen; grey (not grave) when dressed out and about, in their duties to convert, erm, to Christianity, us among the heathen hordes of Southern Britain... But, soon to be seen, at home — behind closed doors — in bright flowery vestments, and with plenty of energy engaging mainstream Jazz, and current pop chart music. Pete and Dud quickly befriended their neighbours Mr Stoker (in the communal kitchen), and, especially, a delighted Yvonne, who would often be regularly, and yes innocently, socialising, with the Mormons and herself, in and out of each others rooms.

Sara and I chuckled when, several weeks later, The Administrator called on us to see how his protégés were doing — and expressed his growing concern at their enthusiastic friendship with the young lady at the other end of the passage. He felt compelled to confide that his 'students' were considered delinquents by their wealthy Mormon parents — and Church fathers — who were paying for them to be straightened out, in their Missionary work overseas. We reassured him that all was well...

It had been a long hot summer's day, and I was delighted to be home this early evening.

'Where are the boys, Sara? ..' I asked, matter of factly, as I kissed her on her cheeks. 'They're in bed asleep... been a *horrible* day... ambulance... A & E... hospital... And, and...' As we sat down on the sofa, she burst into tears. And, after I insisted on making us both a cuppa of hot sweet (normally she would not take sugar) tea, I coaxed her to take her time, and give me a full account of the day's drama. She then gave me blow by blow description, from after collecting them from Play School.

It was about midday. It being such a warm sunny day, she let them, as normal, go off to play on the wasteland — and always in her full sight, at play on the green; well, at some point they were across, at the opposite side, and playing, adjacent to the fence bordering the industrial estate — when they found some juicy red berries, and thinking them probably as strawberries, which they adored, they ate some...

Soon, they started feeling ill, and being sick, but, fortunately, managed to stagger home ... Sara, realising the gravity of the situation, immediately phoned for an ambulance, which fortunately arrived within minutes, and dashed the three of them off to A & E at Worthing hospital, where they had their little stomachs pumped out, purging them of the poison berries — deadly nightshade, we thought (we went over there, later on, and removed all the wild fruit in sight — as a precaution).

The boys appeared to recover quite quickly — but, for many years, they could not touch any food with pips or seeds therein.

October 1970
The Final

The three year foundation course was up. Much bruised by my recent pre-Exam revision cock-up, during the practical exercise on gauging the correct measure of insulin, I read up and imaged, again and again, any possible questions related to its application — just in case. But most — any minute smugness that I had previously felt in my level of confidence I now eschewed.

Recent events on the home-front had kept aspects of *Care in The Community* on an agenda of possible Questions to be presented, at the hospital final — and RMN Final — and Professional qualification.

On the 3rd September, Richard, ex-RAF recluse, Mauritian Francis, Ghananian Harry, and cautious Barry, attended the hospital nursing school, where, having already taken the oral and practical elements of the internal (all four of us had passed the exercises set by Mr Ammon and Mr Ilford) together, we sat for the three hour internal written exam, compulsorily to attempt and answer all six questions. I was delighted with the last question, on an hospital *Therapeutic Community;* the recent placement at Sandown, for recovering alcoholics, paid off.

Monday, October 5th 1970

Thus, the day arrived, it was *Monday October 5th 1970*, and the due Examination final for the Registered Mental Nurse qualification... I had taken numerous formal academic examinations, as child and adult, in the past; perhaps the most embarrassing, was failing an elementary formal civil service Clerical Officer exam, whilst working as a civvie Clerical Assistant at the New Scotland Yard at the Press and Information Department (nearby the Black Museum). I recalled this day, assisting the Met in packing up to remove from the old Thames-side *Scotland Yard* to its new Victoria site, and being in its deep cellars, amongst so many past Press card applications and photos of so many of well known famous, and the insignificant (I even found a temporary Press card of myself, as issued to a round faced, innocent, sixteen year old youth as a Fleet Street Central Press Photos, Gough Square, runner — in my first job, on leaving school) I failed the CO exam, due to my inability to do the Maths paper, and the mental block which instigated that unforgettable failure... most people have such memories.

Autumn was drawing to a close. October trees, now thin and bare of leaf, lined both sides of the hospital drive, and out of the grounds, left with a running stream close to the edge of the narrow road; mostly in shadow, cold wet naked branches — though it had stopped raining — high above displayed, beneath the dark and cloudy sky, arched shaking Shiva arms, hands and finger tips — linking the left and the right, beckoned me on along the pathway.

For an umpteenth time, I strolled down the slope of (Bishop Otter) College Lane, formerly Love Lane, to its end, into Spitalfields Lane, and Eastwards. I crossed the Road, turning left, and, just a few yards on, entered a location marked on an OS Map as City Hospital (one of a collection of low buildings, a recent TB and Fever *Isolation Hospital* which, historically, possibly in the 1920s, itself replaced the old Pest House), formerly, a matter of a few hundred or so yards, in Love Lane. History, moving on, would again, soon, replace these buildings too, where I was to sit my Final — another Chichester site for its housing needs.

Together, we sat our Final, Ghananian Harry and I (RAF Richard and Mauritian Francis were not present — different agenda), and applicants directed from other district hospitals — including a number of first and second retakes — it was not a large gathering. As with the hospital final, it was a three-hour paper — there were six questions, all of which had to be attempted. Having learnt to pace myself, I allocated so much for each question, and then padded out where I could.

To my pleasant surprise, Q5 was on ... diabetes — and, of course, about insulin. In conclusion, I knew I had written many pages and, initially, felt quite pleased, but.... but, I was under no illusion, like all exam work, that quantity equalled quality; and so, Harry and I had no idea what the outcome would be... at least six weeks, we thought, till we received our results — in the post. We would not have to wait very long. There would be no grading — just a Pass or Fail. ... I Passed.

And, a newly appointed Staff Nurse, I was immediately placed on Bramber Two ward; with Dougie, Tall John, Sailor Jim , Can Terry and The Boy...

Postscript

Mental Welfare Officer humanitarian and raconteur George Pople (b.1906 — d.1989), in his *Forty Years On The Parish* (Unpublished Oral History, 1980), told me that he was, in 1948, the last Relieving Officer of Bognor Regis in West Sussex — enrolled in a formal office that had had a pedigree since the English Statute of 43rd Elizabeth, dated 1603 — when the first legal directive was issued, to local church parishes, to administer and raise money by means of a poor-rate for poor relief; to give succour and well being for the poor, sick and needy ... This mandatory Poor Law Act was how the term *On The Parish* originated. George was appointed, in the early 1930s, as Relieving Officer, and represented, in the field, an unbroken line since that inception — in work so often hidden in dangerous tasks, alongside the delivery of charity, in pursuit of his duties, and including much of the work which today is executed by the Police Force, Health and Social Services.

As the 1948 Mental Health Act came into practice, its new lexicon required a formal term to replace the name The Relieving Officer, in their Mental Health duties; George had a delightful anecdote about this important, and vital grossly under-estimated *politic* role — in connection with compulsory admissions, to be detained — or not, into hospital or other designated Place of Safety — for therapeutic treatment.

R.O. George related the following to me in his personally, recorded oral history (in transcript) — : 'I was attending my usual Rotary meeting, and sitting opposite me was a visiting Rotarian from London. Somebody told him my job, and he said — "Oh, you'd be rather interested as the new Act renamed the old Relieving Officer as the Duly Authorised Officer." He said, "The man who was responsible for drafting these laws, when it came to the Relieving Officer's part of it, said, "We'll have to find another term for this chap because he no longer exists legally and, I know, he's duly authorised under The Act, so for the time being, we'll call him Duly Authorised Officer."

'Unfortunately, he was taken ill and, to his horror, by the time he got back into the service, he found that his temporary description had become law. And the term which he had put down, for reference use only, had become the legal term, and therefore for the next six years the Relieving Officer became the Duly Authorised Officer.'

Later, followed the 1959 Mental Health Act, which repealed the 14th Century Royal Prerogative statute — and George became one of the new Mental Welfare Officers, in that role, I first became acquainted with him in execution of his duties whilst he was admitting compulsory psychiatric patients into Graylingwell Hospital, in the late 1960s and early 70s.

A decade on, after attaining RMN, and additional professional qualifications, I was issued with a formal 1976 warrant card, which empowered me to act on behalf of The West Sussex County Council as a Senior Social Worker — just as a student RMN in the Nineteen sixties I had met good icon, ex-Relieving Officer — Mental Welfare Officer George Pople. (aka Workhouse, MWO George). I, too, would come to wear the same worthy hats of Child Care Officer *and,* Mental Welfare Officer. In this *capacity*, for some years, I regularly attended ward rounds at Graylingwell in a formal link between hospital and community as qualified Approved Social Worker (Duly Authorised Officer)... into the late 1990s.

On one occasion, attending a Ward Round with Nursing Staff and Ward Psychiatrist in attendance — an unusual conundrum was presented by the doctor to our gathering, sat in a small enclosed circle within what was an updated, and well partitioned, Chilgrove One ward, in the mid 1980s.

Mrs. Wilkins, the ward Consultant, looked around our small circle and stopped, then with a sweet smile fixed her gaze on myself, as Approved Social Worker. 'Bit of a conundrum, Barry — be glad of your feelings on this matter... You all know Gladys, on Barnet Two, — been here for quite sometime. She can still be rather aggressive at times — incident early last week as I recall — Anyway, there has been no need for her to be on a Section for quite sometime ... no relatives — and, Glad continues to want to stay where she is... 'Its here, me mates are', she says — and, though she will obviously have to move on in the near future as her ward is closed down...'

'What's the problem, Mrs. Wilkins?', I interrupted.

'She needs an operation and, without it, is putting her life at risk — the longer the delay.'

Our Consultant Psychiatrist proceeded to give details, of the need for Gladys to go down the road to St. Richard's General Hospital, for this apparently routine op.

'The problem is Barry, she is adamant she will *not* go to St. Richard's and have the op, and I am very concerned for her. After all, we *do* have a responsibility for her well being, even if because, as she insists, *"I'm Voluntary, Doctor."*... We are responsible while she is in our care — and will be negligent if we do nothing... and allow Glad to just die...'

'Ah! — I see your dilemma.'

'Thought you would. As you and I know, we — the Royal we — The Hospital and the NHS, have a Duty Of Care to our patient...'

And together we assumed *The Prerogative* — now *sans* the Royal mantle.

'I agree', And added. 'If necessary — you suggest she might accept the op if she is placed on a temporary section... Have you put this possibility to her? Guess in one sense it's a bit like blackmail — though the rationale is a genuine one of concern — not politics.' 'That's about it, I reckon, its down to a Duty Of Care.' Compassionate, Professional, Dr. aka Mrs. Wilkins smiling, concurred.

Gladys had her operation, and made a good recovery. Following the possibility of the need for *The Section*; I'd agreed to the possibility — anticipated it, as a *protective* life-or-death issue. Together, we *had* had, a responsible *duty of care* to our hospitalised patient; and so, echoing Graylingwell's Admin Baz on life or death issues: *Better Court than Coroner.* Our long-term patient, Gladys, had made her point, and said, she felt, in retrospect... 'Okay!' and retained her liberty; to come and go safely, about *her* sanctuary, *and* in the community.

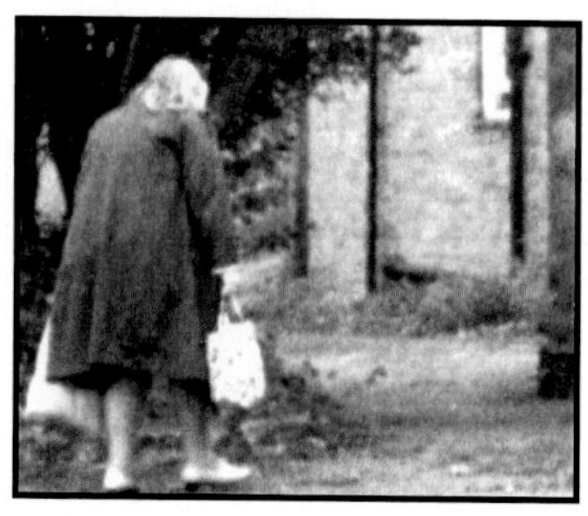

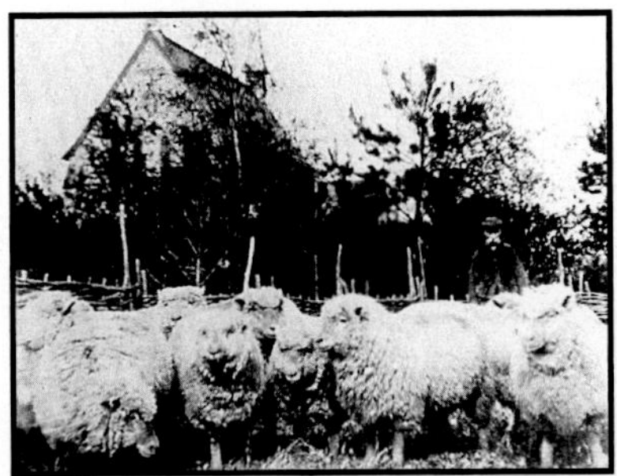

1930s. Between the wars. Undated. Graylingwell Hospital shepherd with some of his sheep. In 1940 Mr Ronald Green took up this post of shepherd, with over 500 sheep in his charge.

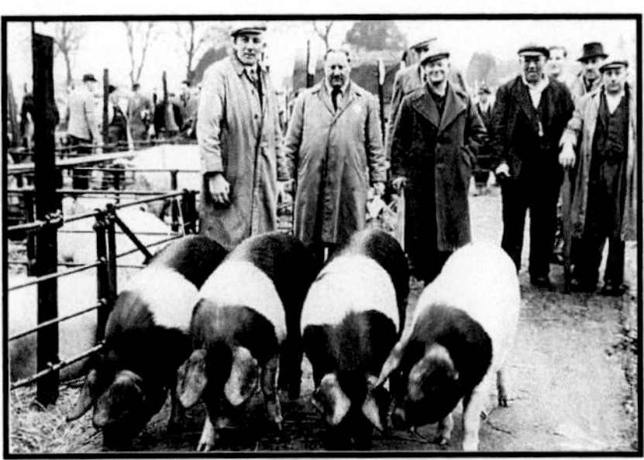

1957. Graylingwell pigs to Chichester market. Staff L To R : Cecil Green farm foreman, Harry Higgott farm bailiff, front & middle third left Fred Strudwick, tractor driver ... far right pigman Fred Hancock.

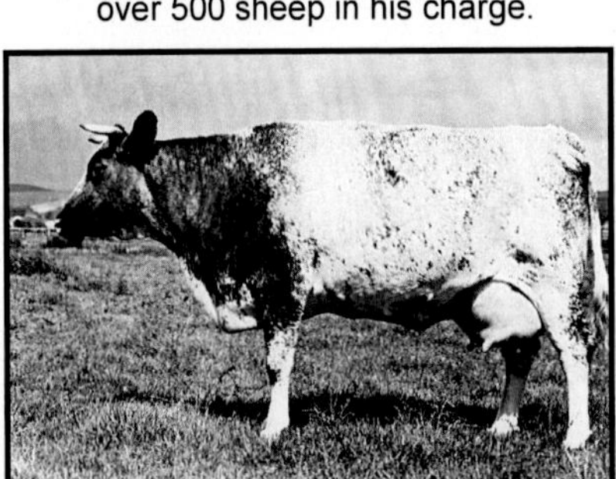

1954-7. *Gracie*. Annual reports recorded in Milk Yield Competiton this cow placed third (the breed) in National Milk Records in 1954, and won numerous other Gold awards - till sold off with all livestock on farm closure in 1957.

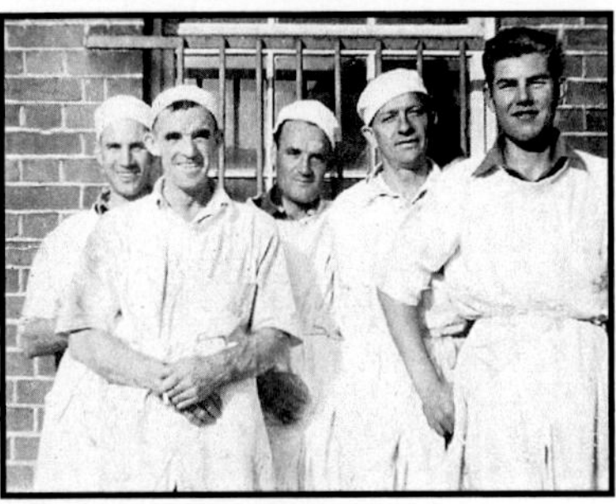

1949. Graylingwell dairy men. **Back. L to R** : Bill Oliver stockman, Bill Baldwin head stockman (lived in Stockman's cottage), **middle** George Philips stockman, **2nd R,** Ron Green stockman. Ron worked 8 years from 1940 as shepherd - then, ten years as dairyman & after farm closure 1957 and, ten years in the kitchens - assisted on the wards as Ass't nurse, until retirement in 1968. **Far right** 17yr old John King who ret'd 1995.

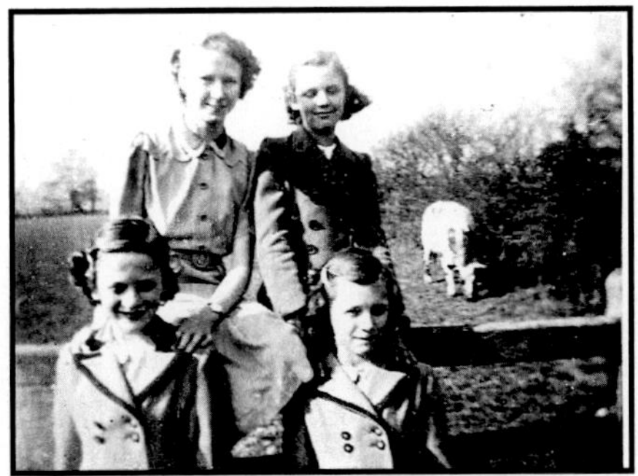

Left. 1948. Children living on the hospital farm. Three are Ron & Molly (Snr) Green's girls. **Top left** friend Brenda Twine, **top right** Molly Green (m. Hunt): **front left** Cicely Green (m. Glover), and **front right** Shirley Green (m.Wingham). Molly (Jnr) & Shirley would qualify as Graylingwell Registed Mental Nurses.

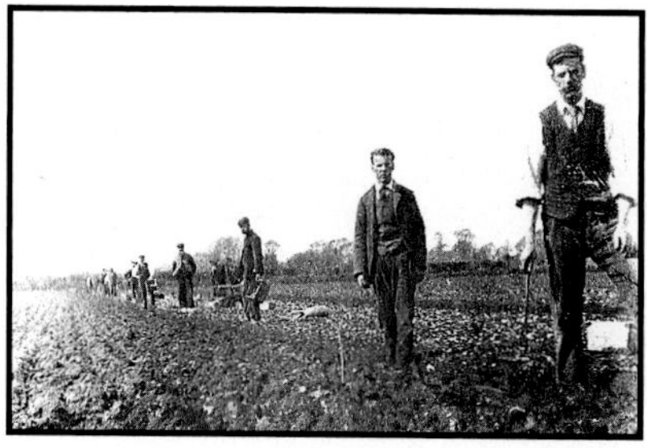

1940s Graylingwell staff and line of recovering patients, in his charge, planting potatoes.

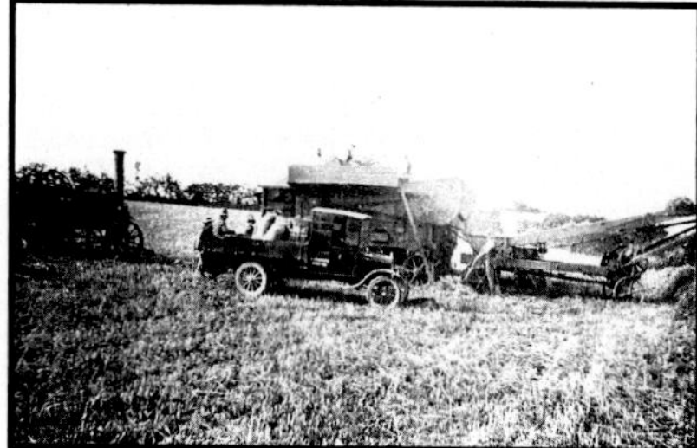

1940s photo of staff and patients harvesting on Graylingwell Farm. Is that an old 1920s model T Ford. ...

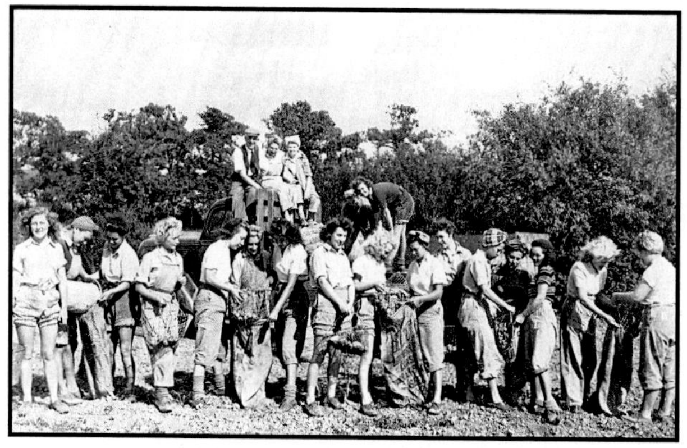

Wartime on Graylingwell Farm. Land army girls assisting in the harvest. They also had Italian prisoners of war to assist them in their work. On top of the lorry stacking the filled sacks is i / c foreman Mr Cecil Green.

Graylingwell Hospital Farm (1897-1957), hugely successful throughout its existence, benefiting hospital patients : and made possible by excellent stewardship by *'contracts'* with the outside community (as Barnham & Chichester Markets). This included its existence during the years as a War Hospital (1915-1919), and, included support of Summersdale Villa in EMS military occupation (1940-1945). Abundant records - now in Chichester Archives - support this fact.

Notes, References and Sources — Chapter One

1. Charles Dickens (1812-1870). *Great Expectations.* Joe to Pip. Ch. XXVII. 1861.
2. Rev C.H.Spurgeon (1834-1892).... *Autobiography.* Vol 1, *The Early Years.* 1834-1859. And. Vol 2, *The Full Harvest.* 1860-1892. Published. The Banner of Truth Trust (Reprint) 1976. See. Vol 2 C.10 *A Home for the Fatherless* (thinking back, at Reigate, almost 80 years later — I agree):

   > 'We have heard it objected to Orphanages that the children are dressed uniformly, and in other ways are made to look like paupers. This is earnestly avoided at the Stockwell Orphanage, and if any friend will step in and look at the boys and girls, he will have to put on peculiar spectacles to be able to detect a shade of the pauper look in countenance, garments, speech, limb, or movement.' (Vol 1 p.171)

3. *Spurgeons Child Care* aka *Stockwell Orphanage.* London. 1867-1939. *Spurgeon's Orphan Homes.* Reigate. (Surrey) 1939-1953. *S.O.H.* Birchington. (Kent) 1953-1979. *Spurgeon's Child Care* subseqently world wide registered Charity its Headquarters, based in England, with Regional Managers in charge of fund-raising, and work with families, children and young people — at home in UK, and overseas.
4. *The Illustrated London News* Nov. 12, 1859 p.474-476. And. *Spike Island. The Memory of a Military Hospital* by Philip Hoare. Fourth Estate. 2001.
5. *West Sussex Gazette.* July 13th 1899.
6. Ibid.
7. Sigmund Freud (1856-1939). Freud's *Interpretation of Dreams* was ready in 1899, but post-dated a First Edition, in German, printed in 1900 and giving birth to the modern concept of Psychoanalysis. His first full English translation of the original book appeared in 1913 (with additions to each subsequent edition). The subject of interpreting peoples' dreams has, of course, been practised by artists, poets, tribal medicine soothsayers and religious prophets, throughout the history of mankind. Often interpreted as a source of divine communication. I discovered a revealing, but lesser known, scientific investigation on The Study Of Dreams, in *A New Model of The*

Universe by Russian P.D.Ouspensky. (Translated by R.R.Merton. Published. Kegan Paul, Trench, Trubner & Co . London 1931. See Chapter VII *On the Study of Dreams And On Hypnotism.*) O insisted his interest in Dreams existed *long* before he'd heard of Freud & his Studies. Another work on *Dream Psychology*, specifically on treatment of *shell shock* as opposed to generic psychiatry (aka Mentals in 1918), was to occupy much of my 'spare time' in the years ahead. This was *Dream Psychology* (1917), one of two books by Dr. Maurice Nicoll (1884-1953) written when a Captain in the RAMC. Viz. *Dream Psychology.* Oxford Medical Publications. London. Hodder & Stoughton 1917. Second Edition 1920. And, *In Mesopotamia* by Martin Swayne (pseudonym), Hodder & Stoughton 1917. On returning from the Mesoptanian war zone (1914-1917), he was later transferred to the *Empire Hospital for Officers,* in Vincent Square, Westminster, SW1 in London, where Nicoll continued his work, with servicemen in shell shock. *In a letter* to his father, he said:

> 'Our lot is composed of Dr. Maurice Craig, Henry Head, Farquar-Buzzard, Rivers, McDougall, Fernside, Professor Elliott Smith, Branwell, MacNamara, Miller, Riddoch and myself and they are, thank the Lord, all as keen as mustard ...'

(See *Maurice Nicoll. A Portrait* by Beryl Pogson. (1961). Published. Fourth Way Books. New York.1987 ed. pb. See, *Empire Hospital* 1917-1918 pp. 50-66.) One question, subject of an October 1918 *Symposium,* (*Dream Psychology* 1920 ed. p.ix) of Dr. Nicoll's — with immense implications — was to intrigue me for my lifetime until, myself already in decay, it clicked. "Why is the' Unconscious' Unconscious?" (See. *Better Court Than Coroners.* Chapter Eleven. Notes & refs. No.10.)

8. *West Sussex Gazette* served Sussex, Surrey, Kent and Hampshire. See. Ju13th 1899. Page two. *Jotting For Sussex Readers.*
9. *Moodie's Zulu War.* By D.C.F.Moodie. With an introduction by John Laband. Published. N & S Press. Cape Town. 1988. Ref. *Appendices. B. ... Men present at the Defence of Rorke's Drift, 22nd January, 1879.* (See pp 249-250.)

10. *The Terrible Night at Rorke's Drift. The Zulu War, 1879.* By James W. Bancroft. Published. Spellmount Ltd in 1988. p159. *Appendix B. Casualties at Rorke's Drift.*
11. See, *Laws of England* by Sir William Blackstone. London, Strahan. 1809. Vol One. Chapt VII. *Of the King's Prerogative*, pp.237-280.
12. *Mental Health Act. 1959.* 7 & 8 Eliz.2. Ch.72.

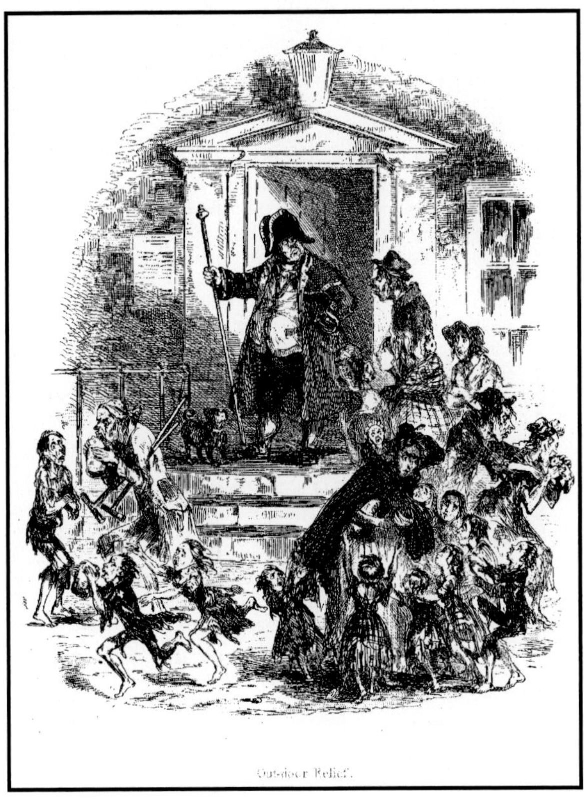

1840. Outdoor Relief. After the 1834 New Poor Law Act, The Beadle became a most important local authority, semi-police officer; dealing with paupers, disabled, numerous orphans, homeless and other 'nuisances'. (*Sketches of Boz,* 1836, and *Oliver Twist, 1838,* by Charles Dickens: Picture by Phiz-Hablot Knight Browne (1815-82), from *Sketches of London* by James Grant, 1840 ed. — workhouses: See also C5. BCTC, notes 24 & 25.)

Laws of England,

IN FOUR BOOKS.

BY

Sir WILLIAM BLACKSTONE, Knt.

CHAPTER THE SEVENTH.

OF THE KING'S PREROGATIVE.

IT was obferved in a former chapter[a], that one of the principal bulwarks of civil liberty, or (in other words) of the Britifh conftitution, was the limitation of the king's prerogative by bounds fo certain and notorious, that it is impoffible he fhould ever exceed them, without the confent of the people, on the one hand; or without, on the other, a violation of that original contract, which in all ftates impliedly, and in ours moft exprefsly, fubfifts between the prince and the fubject. It will now be our bufinefs to confider this prerogative minutely; to demonftrate it's neceffity in general; and to mark out in the moft important inftances it's particular extent and reftrictions: from which confiderations this conclufion will evidently follow, that the powers, which are vefted in the crown by the laws of England, are neceffary for the purpofe of fociety; and do not intrench any farther on our *natural* liberties, than is expedient for the maintenance of our *civil*.

THERE cannot be a ftronger proof of that genuine freedom, which is the boaft of this age and country, than the power of difcuffing and examining, with decency and refpect, the limits of the king's prerogative. A topic, that in fome former ages was thought too delicate and facred to be profaned by the pen of a fubject. It was ranked among the *arcana imperii:* and, like the myfteries of the *bona dea*, was

[a] chap. 1. page 141.

Y 3 not

The English Royal Prerogative was introduced in the 14th Century — The Monarch, then, a divine ruler. In the 18th Century, The King's Prerogative still mostly only protected the wealthy upper classes, but gave little support to those dependent on the cupidity of the Parish Poor Law. (Source. Blackstone, *Laws of England,* Volume 1, 1809.)

Notes, References and Sources — Chapter Two

1. Philip.D.S. Chesterfield, 4th Earl of Chesterfield (1694-1773).... Politician. See *Lord Chesterfield's Letters To His Son*. Letter XXXIV. Isleworth, September.15th.1739. *Chesterfield's Letters To His Son,* By Oliver H.G.Leigh. Published. London. The Navarre Society. MCMXXVI. In Two Volumes. (See) Vol.2. Appendix. Juvenile Section (1732-1741). p.369.
2. *The River Lavant* by Ken Newbury. Published. Phillimore.1987.
3. *Forgotten Lunatics of the Great War*. By Peter Barham. Published. Yale. 2004.
4. Robert Noonan (1868-1911), aka Robert Tressell. See *The Ragged Trousered Philanthropists.* By Robert Tressall (correct spelling). Published. London. Grant Richards Ltd. 1914. *Tressell Of Mugsborough.* (aka *One Of The Damned*) By F.C.Ball, Published London. Lawrence And Wishart Ltd. 1951. *The Ragged Trousered Philanthropists.* By Robert Tressell. Published. Lawrence & Wishart. London. pb.1955 first complete edition. Reprinted as *The Ragged Trousered Philanthropists.* By Robert Tressell. Published. Lawrence And Wishart. London.1989.
5. *War Gossip* in *The Family Economist*. Volume Third. p.142. London. 1855.
6. H.G. Wells (1866-1946). See *The War That Will End War.* Published by Frank & Palmer, Sept. 1914. Wells complimented his Nineteen fourteen missive in 1940 in 'A Penguin Special' a thin paperback titled — *The Common Sense of War And Peace. World Revolution or War Unending*.
7. H.G.Wells. Published on the 7th August 1914 in *The Daily Chronicle* — only days into the conflict.
8. Jean-Paul Sartre (1905-1980). See *The Age of Reason*, *The Reprieve*, and *Troubled Sleep* (aka *Iron in The Soul).* Confirmed in an article in *Playboy* magazine (USA ed). May 1965. Playboy Interview p.69 - 234.
9. Jean Cocteau (1889-1963). See *A Call to Order,* by Jean Cocteau. Translated by Rollo Myers. Published. London. Faber and Gwyer. 1926.
10. *The Language of Flowers. A Collection of Poems* by Gerald Le Blount Kidd. Publ. Millstream. 1991.

11. Major-general John Hay Beith (1876-1952) aka *Ian Hay,* author of fiction and non-fiction. See. Early Great war novel *The First Hundred Thousand by The Junior Sub.* (Aka Ian Hay.) Published. London. Blackwood.1916.
12. Non-fiction. *One Hundred Years Of Army Nursing,* by Major-general John Hay Beith, C.B.E., M.C. Publ. Cassell.1953. p.314-5. (Major John H. Beith, 1931. Late Argyll and Sutherland Highlanders in WW1.) Due to its close proximity to hospitals close to the coast of the South of England (compared to Scotland), it's probable, among the influx of other ranks were included soldiers of the Highland Regiments arriving at D Block, Netley at Southampton, as war casualties. Many trench wounded were then transferred to *Graylingwell War Hospital,* Chichester. Casualties would certainly have included soldiers Beith (Ian Hay) as a Junior Sub had viewed, waiting in *The Shed* at Netley, Southampton Dock, and newly arrived from the Somme battlefield.
13. *Legacy Of The Somme,* 1916 by Gerald Gliddon. Published Sutton 1996 p.vii.
14. *Statistics.* In one day, on August 6th 1945, Hiroshima, Japan, was decimated (some 60,000 Japanese men women and children (were) killed, and 100,000 injured) by an atomic bomb which, in size, dwarfed the largest of any previous bomb or artillery shell. Source. *Hiroshima,* by John Hersey. Penguin Books pb. Nov.1946.)
15. Henry Williamson (1895-1977). See *Genius of Friendship*, By Henry Williamson. Published. Faber and Faber. 1941, see p26. The friendship was between Henry Williamson and T.E. Lawrence (aka T.E.Shaw) — both veterans of the Great War. In my preliminary research for *authentic* (viz witnesses and identified participants) written records, relating to psychiatric origins of first world war's survivors, who were diagnosed with a form of shell-shock, or war-neuroses and latterly NYD (Not Yet Diagnosed) post-war labels of anxiety-neuroses, I subsequently followed the advice of our ex-RAMC tutor, and looked to art and extant published literature, of the then recent 1914-1918 Great War — and its aftermath. Williamson noted, in 1936, a total absence of other-rank contributors:

'A regret to me - the absence of the other ranks; but of course an officer never sees them.' (*Genius of Friendship* p.65).

See, also, *The Linhay on the Downs,* By Henry Williamson. Published. London. Jonathan Cape.1934. *Reality in War Literature,* pp.224-262. My literary (and clinical) searches, certainly confirmed Williamson's observation. But, after the second world war, there emerged an abundance of all ranks, and civilian recorded witnesses, using a plethora of media resources.

16. See *Forgotten Lunatics of The Great War,* by Peter Barham. Yale 2004, and *For The Sake Of Example. Capital Courts Martial 1914-18. The Truth,* By Anthony Babington 1983. (Reprint. Published. Leo Cooper. 1999.)
17. *British army General Routine. Order* No.2384, issued 7 June 1917, in France.
18. Robert Graves (1895-1985). See *Goodbye To All That*. Published. Cape.1929. Cassell.1957. Penguin 1960 p.b. *and.*Folio ed, 1980 see (Chapter) 15.
19. Evidence. In an ongoing search for relevant non-fiction *witness* books and documentary films, prompted by our ex-RAMC school tutor, in time, over the forthcoming years, I assembled the following *introductory* list:

(i) Documentary Film and Essay. *Shoah.* by Claude Lanzmann. Film.1985.
(ii) Book. *Is This a Man* (The Journey); and, *The Truce*. By Primo Levi. (1919-1987.) The Italian chemist was one of *'six hundred 'pieces'* reported by a corporal to the German gestapo officer in charge of Levi's train transport. Primo Levi was an halfling in Monowitz one of the forty or so Auschwitz concentration camps, for eleven months, 1944 till 1945.
(iii) Books by Bruno Bettelheim (1903-1990), a survivor of concentration Camps Dachau and Buchenwald, 1938 to 1939.
(iv) Both, Levi (d.1987), and Bettelheim (d.1990) after surviving the camps, and suffering from rank clinical depression (not surprising) would eventually, commit suicide.
(v) But, a few years on, a little de-classified 21st century Google released data revealed an unburied past; an uncounted total of A Bomb and H Bomb (are there others!) global thermonuclear *test* casualties.

During the early days of the USA wartime A bomb *Manhattan Project* (c.1942):

'Early on, the scientists adopted the nickname "gadget" for the bomb that would dominate all of their lives for the duration of the project and, for some, through many years to come.' (*Picturing The Bomb*. Introduction by Richard Rhodes. Rachel Fermi and Esther Samra. Published. Harry N.Abrams, Inc.,1995. See p.96.)

20. Andre Gide (1869-1951). See. *The Journals Of Andre Gide*. Volume. IV. 1939-1949. Transl. from French by Justin O'Brian. Publ.Secker & Warburg.1951. p.136.
21. Malingerers and Conscientious Objectors. *Not a* coward, no white feather, as in Mason's *Four Feathers* Faversham (who, in the novel, after unjustly being branded a coward, spent six-years self-exile in The Sudan — in redemption). See *Four Feathers,* by A.E.Mason. Published in 1902. Faversham was a Conscientious Objector. Persons of age, rejected by the authorities on health grounds, like Jean Cocteau and Ernest Hemingway in WW1, and Julian Bell, in the Spanish Civil War, 1937. Some chose to serve as ambulance drivers — in a battle Front Line, like Cocteau and Hemingway.
22. Eric Maria Remarque (1898-1970). See *All Quiet On The Western Front,* by Eric Maria Remarque. Published. Boston Little, Brown, And Company.1929. Transl. A.W.Wheen. p.135.
23. Henri Barbusse (1873-1935). See *Under Fire,* by Henri Barbusse. Published 1917. Chapter 12. *The Doorway.*
24. Fritz Lang. (1890-1976.) *Dr. Mabuse the Gambler* (aka *The Fatal Passions*), a silent film out in 1922, was one of three 'Mabusse' films. The second, *The Testament of Dr. Mabuse*, a talkie, was released in 1933, but reported as banned by Nazi Germany's propaganda minister Goebbels on 29.3.1933, 'for legal reasons of endangering public order and security ...'. The third Mabuse film was made back in Germany, (he'd emigrated to America in 1934), called *The Thousand Eyes of Dr. Mabuse*, released in 1960.
25. *A Message To The Neurotic World,* By Dr. Francis Volgyesi. Published. Hutchison. 1935.Chapter One. p10-11.
26. Graylingwell (retrospect) *Annual Report*.1920.

27. *A Brief Review of the Cases Treated in the King's Section of Graylingwell War Hospital. 1915-19. By Major James I Maxwell. (Annual Report 1920.)*
28. Ibid. 1920 p.*42* . Report by Major William Pearson; a subsection '*Operations on Nerves* ' (Total 92 cases), included one salutory fact:

> 'Unfortunately, owing to the neccessity for transferring convalescent cases, and maintaining empty beds in the Hospital, it is not possible to speak with any certainty of the final results in these cases as a whole. During the closing period of the work. however, a special Army Order ...' (and there the fragment on treatment On Nerves ends, as p43 was missing.)

29. Bruce Bairnsfather (1887-1959). See *Bullets and Billets,* by Bruce Bairnsfather. Published by Garden Press Ltd., December, 1916.
30. Lt. Ernst Junger (1895-1998). See *Storm Of Steel,* by Ernst Junger. Published in Germany 1920. English translation 1929.
31. The 47th (London) Division.1914-1919. Edited by Alan H. Maude. Published in London Amalgamated Press (1922). My maternal grandfather, James Walter Manton, served in the 47th as a rifleman in the trenches, from 1916-1918.
32. Siegfried Sassoon (1886-1967). See *Collected Poems.* by Siegfried Sassoon. Published. Faber & Faber. 1947. p.73. Poem *The Effect.*
33. *The Divining Rod: its History, Truthfulness & Practical Utility,* 1914 edition (it went through numerous editions). By John Mullins and Sons, Bath. Where there is *water,* there is life and, without it, terrestrial visceral existence — AS WE KNOW IT — would cease to survive. A typical human *body* consists of:

> 'Enough water to fill a ten-gallon barrel. Enough fat for seven bars of soap. Carbon for 9,000 lead pencils. Iron for a medium sized nail. Lime enough to whitewash a chicken coop. And small quantities of Sulphur.'

(Source. Dr. Kenneth Walker. How man became his own worst enemy. *Picture Post*, 17 July, 1954. p.38.) And a *human* ingredient.

34. *Wells and Springs of Sussex* By F.H.Edmunds Publ London 1928. p.74.

35. Glover J. *Place Names Of Sussex* 1975. And *The Lands Of Graylingwell,* by Barone.C.Hopper. Publ *West Sussex History* Jan, May and Aug. 1988.
36. Dr. A.J.Cronin (1896-1981). See *Adventure In Two Worlds. An Autobiography* By A.J.Cronin. 1952.
37. *Johnson's Dictionary. A Modern Selection,* By E.L.McAdam, Jr. & George Milne. Gollancz. 1963. Introduction p.xii.
38. Dr. Samuel Johnson (1709-1784). See *A Dictionary of the English Language*. By The Author, Samuel Johnson, LL.D. The Twelfth Edition. Published. London, 1807.
39. Plato (c.427-347BC). *The Collected Dialogues of Plato*. Edited by Edith Hamilton and Huntington Cairns. Bolligton Series LXXI. Published. Princeton University Press. 1973. *Phaedrus*. p.510-11. And, Of the Greek Divine aspect on Philosophy of Parmenides & Empedocles, *Reality,* By Peter Kingsley. Published By The Sufi Center. 2003.
40. William James (1842-1916). See *Brief Course of Psychology,* By William James. Published. Holt. (USA) 1892. See last chapter. (This one volume was an abridged version of the two vols *Textbook of Psychology*. Published.1890 ed.)
41. 43 Elizabeth, c.2 1601 Poor Law Act. Cap.II. *An Act for the Relief of the Poor.*
42. *4 and 5 William 4, c.76 1834 Poor Law Amendment Act.*
43. *Report of Westhampnett Union*, March 14th, 1836. In *House of Commons Pape*r No.108 of 1838. Data taken from *The Last Hundred Years* (p130) by Sidney & Beatrice Webb.
44. *Classification In Poor-Law Institutions. By Or In The Buildings.* Issued by The Poor-Law Officers' Journal. London.1914. p24-25.
45. Sir George Nicholls K.C.B. *A History of the English Poor Law.* Published. P.S.King.1904. See Vol 2, Chap.XV. p248.
46. *Manual of Military Law*. Published by War Office 1914. HMSO pp.468-469.
47. Echoing, colleagues, Drs Brock, Freud, Jones, Jung, Kidd, Myers, Nicoll, Pierce, Rivers, and many others, on lack of facilities for treating war casualties. And in particular long-term, over two weeks, shell-shock wounded.

48. *Shell Shock And Its Lessons*, By Grafton.E.Smith. Published 1917. Chapter IV. Some General Considerations..
49. *The Story of England's Hospitals*, By Courtney Dainton. London Museum Press, 1961 p9.
50. Poor Law before 1946. See, *The Poor Law Code, And the Law of Unemployed Assistance,* By W. Ivor Jennings, M.A., LL.D., Published London. Charles Knight & Co., Ltd., Second Edition. 1936. p204-205. (The hospital, pre-1946, as a formal asylum was, under the extant Poor Law, classed as a *special* workhouse.)
51. W.H.Ainsworth (1805-1882). See the Novel *Jack Shepherd,* by W.H.Ainsworth. Published. 1839. (See. George Cruickshank's cartoon in Chapt.VIII, *Old Bedlam.*)
52. *On the Road. A Description of some Casual Wards by the South-Western Counties.* A Series of Articles reprinted from The Western Gazette, January-May, 1928. Balcombe. (Sussex.)
53. *Three Hundred Years of Psychiatry 1535-1860.* By Richard Hunter M.D., M.R.C.P., D.P.M. And Ida Macalpine M.D., M.R.C.P. Published Oxford University Press.1963. p.vii.
54. *Handbook for Psychiatric Nurses* (Ninth edition. The red book was a compilation .Edited by a physician (Dr.) Brian Ackner. Published in 1964 by London. Balliere, Tindall & Cox. The textbook's content was approved by the Royal Medico-Psychological Association (aka RMPA). Noticeable from the outset there were Sixteen different professional Contributors to Ackner's work.
55. E.g., *A Handbook For Psychiatric Nurses.* By Sugden, Bessant, Eastland, and Field. Published. Lippincott. 1986. And: *A History of Mental Health Nursing*, by Peter Nolan. (later Professor). Published by Chapman & Hall. 1993.
56. *Handbook for Psychiatric Nurses*. Chapter Six .*Terminology and Classification.*
57. The post-war *Watershed* of 1946 presented me with numerous sources: *Psychiatry. Theory and Practice for Nurses,* by (Dr.) H.C.Beccle MB.,MRCP., DPM. Specialist in Neuropsychiatry. RAFVR. Deputy Medical Superintendent, Springfield Mental Hospital. Psychiatrist, West Middlesex County Hospital, etc. Published. Faber and Faber Ltd. London.1946....

Frank Capra's USA film, *It's a Wonderful Life,* was released in 1946. In contrast to Capra was Mary Jane Ward's 1946 book, based on her own experience of 1940s American state-hospital asylum treatment of Mental Illness, in her book *The Snake Pit* (which was later made into a 1948 film). The film received considerable attention in the British Media. Not till fifty years (1990s) on would I learn, through *Google* & The Web, of written past contemporary *real life* hidden horrors (with considerable photographic and clinical (aka forensic) evidence, presented to the USA media — *at that time*). Of America's admitted *gross neglect* in an owed duty of care, to its own disabled and mentally ill citizens.

The USA media's statistics included *thousands* of abused Asylum patients, locked away, and mostly abandoned, in American State institutions. For example, *Byberry Hospital* was known as Philadelphia's Bedlam.

A major pre-war USA source. *The Mentally Ill In America.* By Albert Deutsch (Intro by William.A.White). Published. Doubleday, Doran & Co. New York 1938. A recently purchased, second-hand presentation copy says:

> 'To Stanley. T. Buggess with the compliments of Clifford. W. Beers. Founder of the Mental Hygiene Movement; (and), Founder and Secretary of The National Committee and American Foundation for Mental Hygiene. 50 west 50 Street, New York City ... April 16, 1939.'

Deutsch & White's books, published in 1938, on social history, spelt out a warning of extreme shortcomings *if* a substantial lack of funding (by attrition) and paucity of investment in Mental Health continued. It meant patients, as prisoners, incarcerated, as statistics, being kept in custody, or left *untreated,* in the community, *if* there were inadequate allocated funds, even for food and medicines.

And *if* there would be insufficient funding — for even a minimum of *Qualified Caring Staff* (Duty of Care). And *if* too little ongoing funding for any Social and Clinical Treatment state facilities — for its collective *many* thousands of gross neglected, hospitalised sick. Wilful *neglect* of duty of care, using (abusing) people instead of statistics and chart algorithms justifications could, possibly, lead on to responsible authority heads being later indicted in legal Corporate Murder of their charges (*not* escape by calling it *shroud* waving).

The 1938 early watershed warned society, but *Immediate* forthcoming war years, and early postwar years, would prove a worse case scenario, yet to be experienced in the USA State Lunatic Asylums. (Source. *The Shame of The States,* By Albert Deutsch. Published. New York.. Harcourt, Brace and Co. 1948. - *See* esp., Chapter Four pp. 40-57 and published pics.). Thankfully, the government in power did respond. (See also C.7 Ref 76)

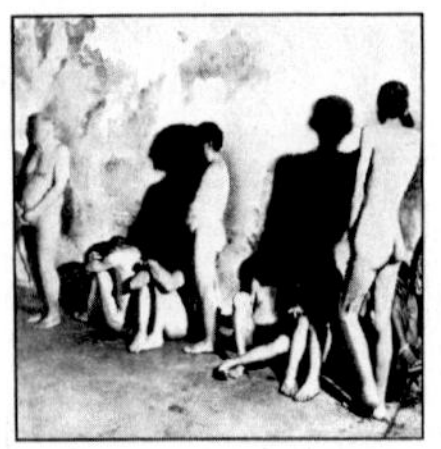

BYBERRY: The male "incontinent ward' was like a scene out of Dante's inferno. Three hundred nude men stood, squatted and sprawled in this bare room, amid shrieks, groans, and unearthly laughter. These represented the most deteriorated patients. Winter or Summer, these creatures never were given any clothing at all. Some lay about on the bare floor in their own excreta. The filth-covered walls were rotting away. Could a truly civilized community permit humans to be reduced to such animal-like level?

(Taken from *The Shame of the States* by Albert Deutsch, p.49.
Publ. New York by Harcourt, Brace and Company, 1948)

Extant additional sources: *Life* Magazine (American) May 6, 1946. Article. (*with graphic photos*) pp.102-118. *Bedlam 1946. Most US Mental Hospitals Are A Shame And A Disgrace*. by Albert Q. Maisel:

> '*... beatings and murders are hardly the most significent of the indignities we have heaped upon most of the 400,000 guiltless patient-prisoners of over 180 state mental institutions. ...*'

In war-torn Europe, most of the previous occupied countries Lunatic Asylums inmates had been exterminated, in the Nazi concentration camps Final Solution.

Thankfully, in post-war Britain, *despite* austerity, food rationing, bomb ruins and housing shortages, and staff shortages, with many associated problems, evidence of relative, *good* quality of duty of care, could be found in abundance. Graylingwell (and other U.K.) Hospital *Annual Reports* (and my own researches) indicate the comparative superb quality of care (there are inevitably rotten apples in every barrel), located in the Long-stay psychiatric *and* extant Military hospitals population, based in Britain during the war.

In 1946, Great Britain passed the *National Health Service Act* (9+10 George 6, c.81). Graylingwell's then *Annual Report* (always one year in arrears) recorded in *5.7.1948*:

> 'Entire resources of the Hospital transferred from County Council to Minister of Health. Management Committee appointed in persuance of the provision of the National Health Service Act. All patients to be treated for under under the National Health Service.'

Graylingwell, *March 1947*, recorded the recruitment of *Dr. Ernest Jones*, psychoanalyst, biographer and personal friend of Dr. Sigmund Freud, who joined the staff as Consulting Psycho-analyst: Dr. Joshua Carse, the Hospital's Superintendent, declared to the public media:

> '... three aspects of psychiatry ... *Prevention, Treatment and Aftercare.*' ...

Throughout Britain, major enquiries were well underway as to what when and how postwar help *could be* funded for its patients in care. See, for example, *Picture Post* (British Weekly Magazine), November 23, 1946. (Article with numerous photos) *Life In A Mental Hospital*, by Fyfe Robertson. pp 9-17. Subsequent readers published letters, from patients and relatives, in *Picture Post* December 7, 1946 (p35), and December 14, 1946 (p31) *'Demand For A National Inquiry'*... All P.P. contributors, were asking for funds to improve facilities for the mentally ill, in British hospitals.

Clearly, British media seemed wholly, understandably, uncomfortable, perhaps unaware of the *in extremis* comparison of American and European cousins, *in gravitas* needs overseas. And, soon enough, there were numerous outraged published articles, and photographs, of the neglected plight of patients in the forbidden buildings housing the long-stay psychiatric population. Source. *Illustrated* October 24 1953, *Inside A Mental Hospital.* Pictures that will shock Britain (pp.15-21). Patients curable and incurable (some of them criminal lunatics) crowded together, in Winson Green Birmingham Hospital — built in 1847, condemned in 1893, but still a hospital. But... *that* British *inquiry* was about decrepit buildings, underfunding, and gross overcrowding. It was *not* attacking the quality (pleading, as USA, a gross underfunding) of staff and residents. But acknowleging what constitutes ongoing good duty of care and, kindly, trained staff in attendance, within the cash-starved British hospitals.

The new British 1959 Mental Health Act, was on the horizon. On initiation into our Graylingwell Hospital wards in 1967, I was unaware of the foregoing American social histories — and the psychiatric watershed of circa 1946 with the end of the old English Poor Laws. Also see, esp. *Asylums and After,* by (Prof.) Kathleen Jones. Publ. The Athlone Press. London & Atlantic Highlands, NJ (1993) Chapter 9, p153. (See Also Ch. 8, Note 5.)

58. Satirised in 1970s, MASH, an American Army Korean war hospital, featuring Corporal Klinger in a superb long running television antiwar film series.
59. *Handbook of the Royal Naval Sick Berth Staff.* HMSO 1944. see pp.220-221.
60. Dr. R.D. Laing (1927-1989). Laing had several good non-fiction books, already in circulation in the early sixties, published by the London Tavistock Clinic: *The Divided Self,* in 1960, and *The Self & Others,* in 1961.
61. *Wisdom, Madness & Folly. The Making of a Psychiatrist.* by R.D.Laing. Published. Macmillan. 1985. Chapter Four. The Army.
62. *Under Fire,* by Henri Barbusse. First Published in French in 1916. Penguin ediition. 2003. See. Chapter Nine, *Mighty Anger.*

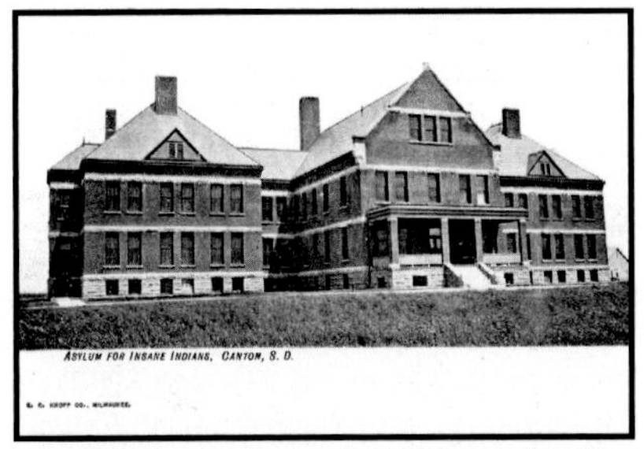

Hiawatha Insane Asylum for Indians, in Canton, South Dakota. Photo from postcard, c1908.

Canton Asylum,1899-1933. Early 20th Century USA, Snake Pit: specifically for indigenous native American Indians; the hospital windows all barred, chained residents (including children); no relatives or visitors allowed. Included on the reverse of the card: Easter Monday '08 '... The Asylum has 60 Indians from 35 different tribes...'

Each tribe had different dialects — and couldn't understand their fellow Indians — for this, too, they were branded insane, as their white staff couldn't understand them either. (Source: Wild Indians, Google, 22/02/2006)

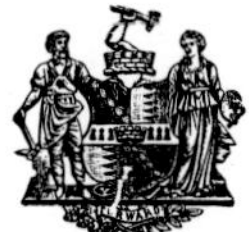

City of Birmingham.

Asylums Department,
The Council House,
28th February, 1912.

Dear Sir,

LEGISLATION FOR THE FEEBLE-MINDED.

I am desired by the Asylums Committee of Visitors of this City to forward to you the following copy of a Resolution passed by them at their Meeting on the 26th inst., viz.:—

Resolved—That, with reference to the Report of the Royal Commission on the Care and Control of the Feeble-minded, issued as long ago as July, 1908, this Committee desire respectfully to urge upon the Government the pressing necessity that exists for promoting in the ensuing Session of Parliament a Bill for giving effect to the recommendations therein contained; they believe that, owing to the lack of powers of control and segregation, the evils attendant upon the present system are increasing, that as a consequence race deterioration is threatened, and that very considerable expenditure is being incurred which might be avoided; for these reasons they feel very strongly that remedial legislation in the direction indicated in the Report of the Royal Commission is greatly needed, and should be no longer delayed.

My Committee regard the matter as one of considerable importance. A copy of the foregoing Resolution has been forwarded to the Home Secretary, the Lunacy Commissioners, and our local Members of Parliament. If you have not already taken action, I shall be glad if you will give the matter your consideration, in the hope that your Committee will be able to see their way to passing a similar Resolution, and sending copies thereof to the same authorities and persons as my Committee have done, as we are assured that it is only constant pressure in this direction that can give any hope of early legislation.

Yours faithfully,

David Davis.

Chairman, Asylums Committee of Visitors.

The Chairman of the
Asylums Visiting Committee,
Chichester.

UK public County Asylums, vigilant in being just, to its sparce, resource starved and little understood 'feeble minded' needs. The above, widely distributed, UK circular innocently (in 1912) unaware of the inhuman purgatory yet, in the 1920s to 1960s, to be experienced in the so-called, science of Eugenics in, for example, racist America, Germany and South Africa; their *subsequent* race laws — awful neglect, and abuse, of lunatics and feeble minded, including people with learning difficulties... See: *In The Name Of Eugenics,* by Daniel J. Kevles — Harvard, USA. 1997 (1985).

Notes, References and Sources. Chapter Three.

1. *The Giant Book Of Facts & Trivia,* Edited by Isaac Asimov. Published. Parragon. in 1994 ed. (Magpie Books N.Y. 1979). *Our Bodies,* p320-325. About *one* human being.
2. Of *West Sussex County Asylum,* Chichester.
3. *West Sussex County Asylum, Regulations.*1897.
4. Statute of The King's — *Royal Prerogerative,* c.1255 and 1290.
5. *The Statutes at Large. From the first year of King Edward the Fourth. To the End of the Reign of Queen Elizabeth.* Volume The Second. Published. London. MDCCLXXXVI (1786). See pp.306 — 308. Cap.XX. (Henry VIII) *How Treason committed by a Lunatick shall be punished, and in what Manner he shall be tried.* (1541 A.D.) Cap. XXI then followed... *Queen Katherine and her Complices attained of Treason.* (*This Act is not on the roll.*)... They were all subsequently beheaded in execution, *not* being judged lunatick in retrospect at the time of their guilty acts of treason towards The King.
6. *The Statutes at Large*, 1786. p.291. Cap. XLVI. (32 Henry 8 c.46 1540.) Notably, Sir William Stanford (1509-1558) English Judge and prominent legal writer described the *Royal Prerogative* in 1567 — Shakespeare was born in 1564. ...
7. The Statutes at Large, Ibid,1786.
8. Statute, 12 Charles 2, c.24. 1661.
9. This frequently meant death.
10. *Crime and insanity in England,* by Nigel Walker. Published. Edinburgh paperbcks. Edinburgh University Press.1968. p25.
11. Roy Porter (1946-2002). Prolific writer, and doyen scholar. See *A Social History of Madness. Stories of the Insane*, By Roy Porter. Published Weidenfeld and Nicholson. London. 1987... *Madmen. A Social History Of Madhouses, Mad-Doctors & Lunatics*. Tempus. 2004 p.8: also first published as *Mind Forg'd Manacles*, Athlone Press. 1987.... *The Poor Laws* existed between 1601 and 1948 — when the present *National Health Service* came into fruition. Professor Porter in his *Introduction* to *Madmen. A Social History* 2004, said:

> 'I am acutely aware that this book does little more than skim the surface of many critical topics. No substantial body of research has yet been

produced on numerous fundamental issues , such as how mad people were treated by the parochial Poor Law system during this period, or upon basic source materials, such as patient's case books as kept by mad doctors ...'

I'd never heard of Dr. Roy Porter during the 1960s and Seventies.

12. See Chapter Five, *Bramber Two* ward.
13. Clothing Card. See. *Better Court Than Coroners.* Volume Two, Forms & Lists.
14. Physical Tests. See. *Better Court Than Coroners.* Volume Two, Forms & Lists.
15. Bath time Regulations. Pursuant to the 275th Section of *The Lunacy Act, 1890.*
16. Statutory Regulations. See. *Better Court Than Coroners.* Volume Two.
17. *King's* (Queen's) *Regulations* extant in the armed forces.
18. Speller. *Law Relating to Hospitals And Kindred Institutions (Incorporating Law for Nurses).* By S.R.Spellar, LL.B., Published by London. H.K.Lewis & Co. Ltd. 1947. Refer Chapter VIII. *Injuries To Patients And Others.* (pp. 83-117). And specifically to p. 87 (D) 2.... *a duty of care to all patients...* contained within C. VIII., heading *General Principles for Deciding Liability.* pp 83-117.
19. A.Wood.Renton (1861-1933). (Sir Alexander Wood Renton KCMG.) See *The Law And Practice In Lunacy,* By A.Wood Renton, M.A. LL.B. Published by Edinburgh. W.H.Green & Sons. (And.) London. Stevens & Haynes. 1896. (With pp.1151, and regular updated laws and necessary alterations). Original source of *The* Principal Lunacy Laws, in frequent use, extant from 1897-1948 and needed, for years afterwards, in *Patients Affairs,* office administration. My copy of this copious work was used and owned (donated) by my colleague Admin Baz, Mr Basil John Boxall, and given to him by his predecessor, Felix Cassel, in 1948 — both of Graylingwell Hospital's Patients Affairs Office. Renton was in use since 1897, replete with all relevant *Poor Laws* in use during those years (1893-1948).
20. Gattie.... *Legal Aspects Of Mental Illness. Procedure.* By William H. Gattie, Published. London. Shaw & Sons. Third Edition. (1933.)

21. Jennings... *The Poor Law Code, And The Law Of Unemployment Assistance*, By W. Ivor Jennings, M.A., LL.D., Published. London. Charles Knight. & Co.1930 (1936 ed).
22. Sutton... *Chalmers Sale Of Goods, 1893, Including The Factor Acts 1889 & 1890.* By Ralph Sutton, M.A.. And N.P.Shannon. Published. London. Butterworth & Co. 1894. Twelfth Edition. 1945.
23. Spelling... Ibid.
24. Matthews.... *A Handbook on Lunacy and Mental Treatment and Mental Defiiciency.* By F.B.Matthews. 1950
25. Burdett. ... *Burdett's Hospitals and Charities*, founded 1889. *The Hospitals Year Book.* An Annual publication, which listed location Beds and Senior administration, incorporating Burdett's original listings of extant Hospitals in England, Ireland, Scotland and Wales. Editor (1967) J.F.Milne.
26. Community Care... *not* the same as duty of care — but 'negligence' the key *forensic* term *monitoring* factor used, in assessing proper standards of care in the community.
27. E.g. powerful *Duty of Care* episode of British television's *Judge John Deed,* from series One in 2001, on wilful abuse of statutory Health & Welfare Regulations and *Corporate Manslaughter*.
28. *Corporate murder bill faces new threat.* Observer. 4th February 2007. p20.
29. *Manslaughter By Superbug.* Daily Mail. Thursday, October 11, 2007, p.1.
30. *Criminal Law* by Russell Heaton, LL, Solicitor. Principal Lecturer in Law, Nottingham Law School. Published. Blackstone Press Limited.1996. See. p122. *Homicide*. Ref. case law, Adomako (1994) 3 All ER 79.... also, Google *Internet data* on 3.7.2005; Search heading — *Common Law, Duty Of Care & Negligence Law.*
31. *Pupils, The Law And A Duty Of Care*. Daily Mail. January 31st 2006. p6.
32. Gleddal...*Legal Guide*. Vol.1. From Dec.. 1, 1838, To April 27, 1839, inclusive. Published. London. John Richards & Co. 1839. See. p. 365. (Law reports) Spring Assizes, Norfolk Circuit. ... Bury St. Edmunds, April 2nd. Before Mr Baron Vaughan. Mary Glendall, By her Next Friend v. Steggall. *Medical Men — Their Liability for*

Negligence and Want of Skill. This action was brought by the surgeon of the parish of Gedding ...'

33. Spellar. ... Ibid. 1947.
34. Speller. ... Ibid. 1947. p87.
35. Chalmers ... Ibid. *Sutton.*1945.
36. Donaghue ... *Donaghue v Stevenson.* 1934. (Informant Admin Mr Basil Boxall).
37. *Collins English Dictionary.* 1979 edition p.557.
38. *The Great Plague,* in Dec..1664, and *The Great Fire* of London, in Sept. 1666.
39. *History Of Crime in England*, By Luke Owen Pike M.A. Second Series. Published Smith & Elder. 1876. Chapter VIII Suicide and Insanity. p195-p.198. And Chapter XIII. Doctrine of Insanity p.581 & p.582.
40. Suicide Caution Card. See *Better Court Than Coroners.* Volume Two.
41. Aversion Therapy. ... See. *Sunday Times Magazine* supplement. March 19th,1967 p.20 — *Your Health & The Mind.* Our Psychology induction lecturer, Dr. Harrod, had recently introduced us to Russian Pavlov (after learning of Freud Jung and William McDougall). Dr. Ivan Pavlov (1849-1946) had experimented specifically with animals, like dog's salivation, on presentation of a specific trigger — like a bell ringing, or other such preface, before its meal (or other trained responses). But, our lecturer elaborated, if an *exact* symbol, i.e. an *exact* circle, represented clarity, the anticipated trigger in human terms, what if, very *subtly,* the symbol (of truth - what's experienced) is sometimes changed or absent. And, with this inconstancy in mind, Dr. Harrod told us, briefly, of another Russian psychologist Dr. Vladimir *Bekhterev* (1857-1927), whose brain experiments applied to humans rather than dogs; Bekhterev introduced a slight and *undetected* ellipse, in the expected circle and, from this analogy, we realised a primary cause of a Neuroses. But I soon realised it was *Pavlov* who was most remembered, and Bekhterev was forgotten.
42. *Sunday Mirror*, Front Page. March 1966.
43. George I. Gurdjieff (1877-1949) was a leading light in a *New Age* Movement which, in theory and practice, examined expansion of human consciousness, both potential and actual. The generic label

of *New Age* was the title of a published Journal (1907-1922), edited by writer Alfred A. Orage (1873-1934), when he left London in 1922 and met with Gurdieff at Fontainebleu in France, and joined a new school of learning on the subject.

44. *Fifth Column At Work,* By B.Bilek. p.24. Published. Trinity Press. London.1945.
45. *Operation Grapple...* H bomb tests on Christmas Island, 1956-1957. As a sapper, I was stationed on the island from July 1956 until late July 1957 (thirteen months).

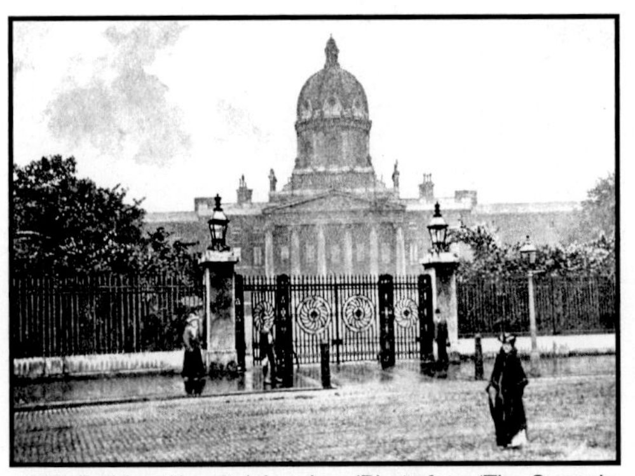

1897. Bethlem Hospital, London. (Photo from 'The Queen's London', Pub. Cassell and Co. Ltd., 1897, p.72.)

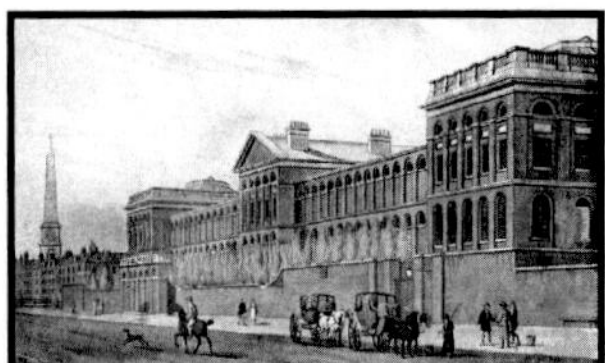

Above: 1751.St Lukes Hospital, Old Street, London. (*The Story of St. Luke's Hospital. 1750-1948.* by C.N.French. Heinmann. Medical Books 1951)

The first Bethlem hospital was established in the 13th Century, on the present site of the Liverpool St. Railway Station; later rebuilt, moved to Moorfields and, in 1815, moved to south London, where it remained until 1930, when the hospital moved to Kent. At one stage, it had accommodation for four hundred patients of both sexes. At Lambeth Road, the enlarged Dome was prominent in 1897, but later removed. The two outer wings were also removed. The centre section is now the Imperial War Museum.

Until the construction of the County Asylums — in the 19th and 20th Century — a number of pauper patients, if deemed curable (up to 2 years) were accepted at Bethlem, St Lukes — or private madhouses, but, if chronic, removed back to their local parish workhouses, or discharged to an alternative facility.

A. D. 1593. Anno tricesimo quinto Reginæ ELIZABETHÆ. C. 3--7. 663

CAP IV.

Every Parish shall be charged with a Sum weekly towards the Relief of sick, hurt and maimed Soldiers and EXP. Mariners. Continued to the End of the first Session of the next Parliament, by 43 El. c. 9. §. 29.

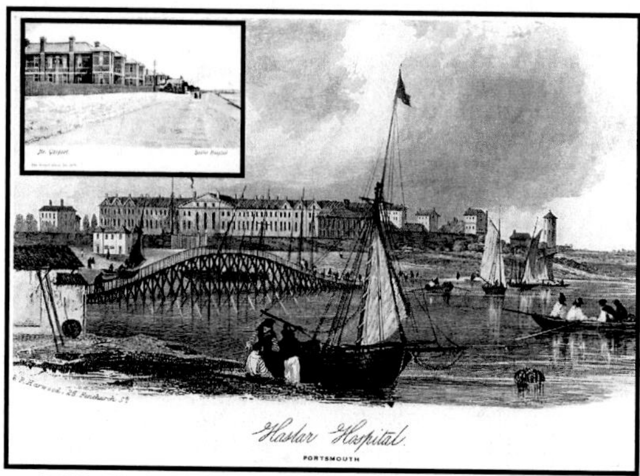

1753. Haslar Naval Military Hospital. 1753-2007. 2008-2010 a NHS Portsmouth Hospital facility. ... Now closed.

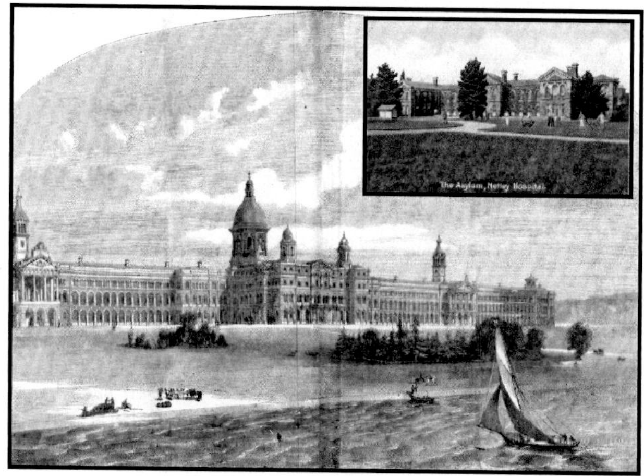

1593. The quote, at top, reads *"Every Parish shall be charged with a Sum weekly towards the Relief of sick, hurt and maimed Soldiers and exp. Mariners. Continued to the end of the first Session of the next Parliament, by 43 El. c.9 s.29"*... **1863**. The pictures above show The Royal Victoria Hospital (Netley Hospital) Southampton, Hampshire. 1863-1958. Demolished 1966. D Psychiatric Wing (Asylum at rear), 1870-1978. Netley site, now a public park.

Notes, References and Sources. Chapter Four.

1. William James (1842-1910), '*The Principles of Psychology*.' Two Vols. 1890. (c.1914 ed) Publ. New York. Henry Holt. See Vol 1. Chapter XVI. *Memory*. p683.
2. Perhaps after the 1949 G.B. post-war film, *Blue Lagoon*.
3. Norman Longmate (b.1925). *King Cholera: the biography of a disease* by Norman Longmate. Published. London. Hamish Hamilton. 1966.
4. Arthur Murray (1895-1991) — *Teach You Dancing In A Hurry*. I worked at an Arthur Murray Dance School, situated on the corner of Poland Street and Oxford St, at 167 Oxford Street in London. Our dance studio was located on two floors, upstairs and over a modern Jazz club, *The Marquee* — situated next door to the chic continental *Academy Cinema*. This was during the *early* Nineteen Sixties. At the time, there was also a kindred franchise Arthur Murray Studio in Leicester Square. A Fred Astaire dance studio existed, around this time, supported by the film actress Anna Neagle and situated in Mayfair, which attracted several of our teachers — I was asked, but declined to make the move. I recall visiting their Mayfair studio for an interview. I also recall a visit from The States, by Arthur & Kathryn Murray, to The Leicester Square studio, and my dancing with tall slim Kathryn Murray, on the pine floor.

   Shortly after I left Arthur Murray's, I did considerable work on a book for New English Library (NEL), but the project was eventually shelved in March 1963. It was to have been an adaption of the published *American* Murrays' Dancing textbook, which included; Foxtrot, Waltz, Rumba, Samba, Merengue, Cha-Cha, Mambo, Tango, Swing, Rock'n'Roll, (*How to become a Good Dancer,* by Arthur Murray. Published by Angus and Robertson. London.1959. (Prev eds from 1938.) I added, and helped to introduce, Chubby Checker's *Twist*, by using a half-cuban roll, in this new book — which was to be for *English* enthusiasts. My book then included graphics on Teach Yourself 16 Dance Rhythms — with an introduction on How To Teach Yourself for English social dancing for clubbing and parties, et cetera, and especially jiving (alternative to American *Swing*), with variants of *Mod,Trad & Latin Jazz jives* (slow stomp kick — and, fast, et cetera) — which I loved. All rhythms which I found easy (then). To jazz jive with three ladies at one time (two in front, one to each hand and spin and, one behind me to catch and spin — as I turned around) — provided, of course, that *they* too could jive.

My bro and I jived at Humphs, Humphrey Lyttelton's 100 Jazz Club in Oxford Street, and downstairs in the cellar of Ken Colyer's, at 59 Great Newport Street, just off Leicester Square. I also followed Trad gigs about London, and worked part-time at a Night-club in Greek Street, (Tropicana, to be *The Establishment.*) Jiving was sitll banned in some orthodox London dancehalls (e.g. Tottenham Royal), and I was often shown off the floor... Balmy happy days of Music and Dance, in Bill Hayly Rock'n Roll, Jazz & real taught Latin (not just square Vic Sylvester Ballroom — the real small steps, swivel & *hip*), 1950s and 1960s freestyle. Days of the truly early Swinging Sixties.

5. Colloquial 'up the stick', being insane, also known as '*up the pole*' (in the USA, being teetotal). Which may suggest an illusion to the Indian Rope Trick — out of sight and out of control. Ref. novel *Her Privates We* by Private 19022. Published. Peter Davies. 1930. See p350.... an abridged version of Australian Frederic Manning's *The Middle Path Of Fortune,* published in 1929.
6. Mensa Charles abandoned book. See *Introduction To Logic. And to the Methodology of Deductive Sciences*, By Alfred Tarski. Translated by Olaf Helmer. Published by Oxford University Press. New York. First ed 1941. Second Edition. 1946.
7. Charles L. Dodgson (Lewis Carroll), 1832-1898. *Alice in Wonderland...* published in 1865. Contrast that graphic children's tale, with his *Symbolic Logic. Part 1. Elementary.* Published London. Macmillan And Co. And New York 1896. Also purported to be written for children, but way (weigh) over my head.... To me, all — unfortunately for me — but an algebra in riddle words, metaphor, pure humour and poetry in pi. Pi — method, how to measure — eternity?
8. Not listed in Dr. Brian Ackner's *Handbook for Psychiatric Nurses,* rear Glossary.... Refer to the Ninth Edition. Published. London. Balliere, Tindall & Cox. 1964. See *autistic* singularly mentioned on p141:

> ' He may withdraw his interest from life around him and appear to be preoccupied. This inward attitude and change in relationship to the outside world has been named *autism*.'

9. Leo Kanner (1894-1981). An article, titled *Autistic disturbances of affective contact,* was published by Dr. Leo Kanner in *Nervous Child,* 1943 2: p217-250. 'Since 1938, there have come to our attention a number of ...'. In the 1960s, autism was referred (at our level) to as a feature of *Child Psychosis*. In 1971, I started as an RMN, working for several years with autistic children, and their families, at the *Wessex Unit for Children & Parents,* in the grounds of *St James* Psychiatric Hospital in Southsea Hampshire. Almost twenty years on, in Worthing, as a Mental Health Social Worker (and an Approved Social Worker), I learned of, and worked with, several *Aspergers* teenagers, with psychiatric problems, who were living in the community.
10. Idiot-savant (an oxy-moron). The Greek root of idiot, a:

> 'private person (who) see the world as if by moonlight, which shows the outlines of every object but not the details indicative of their nature.'

(quoted by Rebecca West); and Dostoevsky's epileptic Myshkin 1868 *The Idiot*, 'blessed innocent'. ... And see *The Borderlands of Insanity and Allied Papers*, by (Dr.) Andrew Wynter, MD., Published. London, Robert Hardwicke. 1875. About, Dr. Down (of Down's Syndrome) English, Medical Superintendent of 1855 *Earlswood Asylum* in Surrey, who declared:

> 'This Asylum was built for those whose brains are sufficiently well formed to be capable of receiving instruction.'

(p.166.) Ref. see, Chapter (Three), *The Training of Imbecile Children, pp.164-188)*. Dr. Down added: 'There is a lad here, however, who shows no mean constructive ability. (p.173). For savant, see *Extraordinary People. Understanding Savant Syndrome*. Updated Version, By (Dr.) Darold A.Treffert, M.D. Published by An Authors Guild back in print Edition. USA. pb.2006.

11. The Red Handbook. The first edition of this *Handbook for Attendants Of The Insane* was published in 1885 by a select committee of Scottish members of the Medico-Psychological Association, and consisted of 64 pages. After the Great War, the Seventh Edition, in 1923, of the mandatory red *Handbook for Mental Nurses* (for Attendents on the Insane), had swollen to 615pp. Our present introductory textbook, *Handbook for Psychiatric Nurses* (ninth edition), dated 1964, was reduced to 368pp.
12. *The Worthing Experiment.*1957-1958. See. Appendix One. *Social History.* Abstracts. ... *The Acres.*

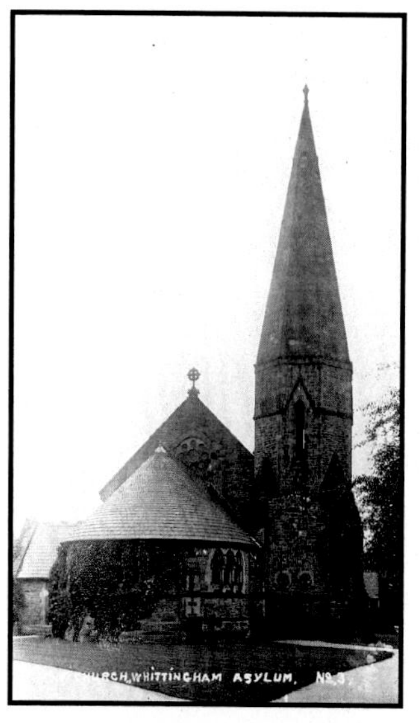

1869 - 1995. Whittingham Asylum, Lancashire, UK. 3,533 beds (1939), with qualified staff of 548 for all hours and duties; Staff numbers, as all asylums, always a problem. See also BCTC C.7 Note 78. (Photo postcard, c.1910)

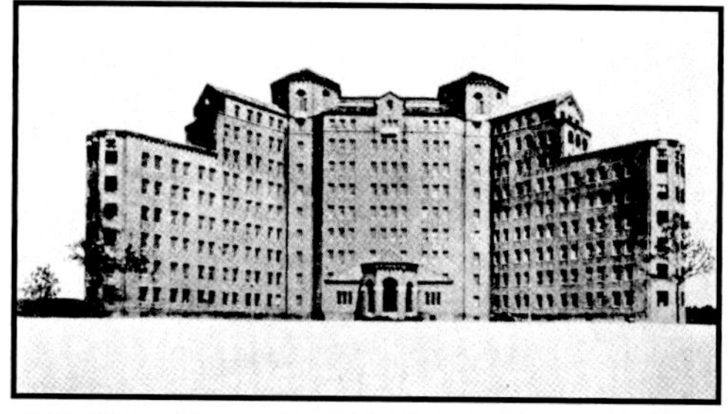

1948. Mason General Hospital, USA, also known as Pilgrim State Hospital. The largest mental institution of the time, with 10,000 beds. Now Closed and demolished. (Photo from *The Shame of The States*, by Albert Deutsch, Pub. Harcourt, Brace and Co., p.153). See, also, BCTC C.7 Note 76, and C.11 Note 24.

See: *But for the Grace of God. Milledgeville. Inside story of the World's largest Insane Asylum*; by Dr. Peter G Cranford, 1952 — but not to be published for many years. A compassionate, honest account of one of the USA's historic asylum struggles, in Georgia, to care for its insane and disabled residents. It explains the Asylum's use and abuse of 19th century slaves (afro-american), and 'coloureds', as patients, and as low or unpaid, valued, staff attendants, up to the 1950s. An excellent memoir.

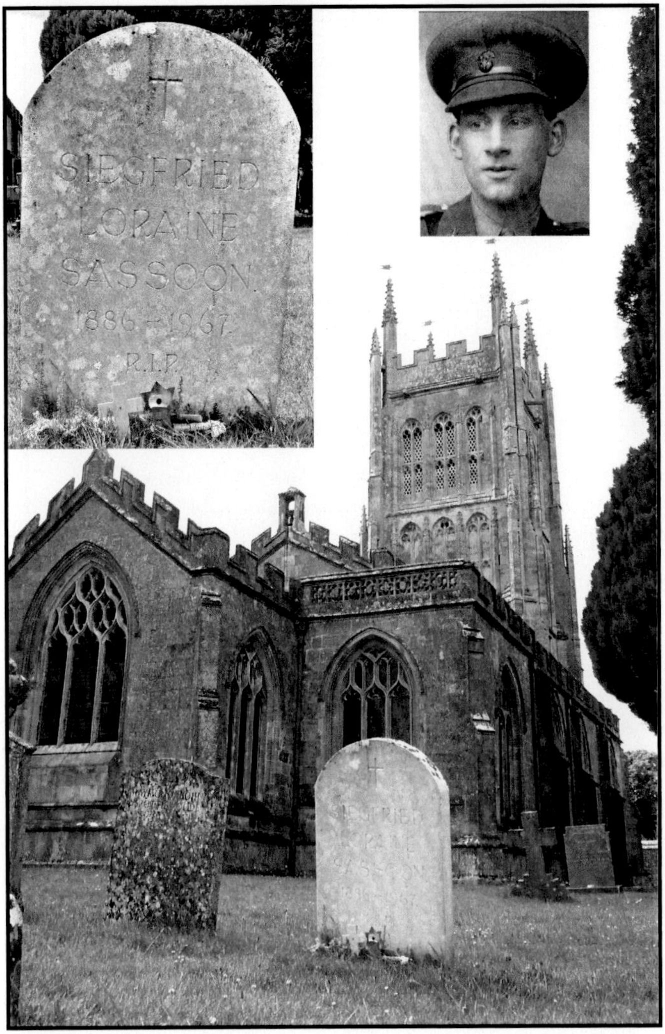

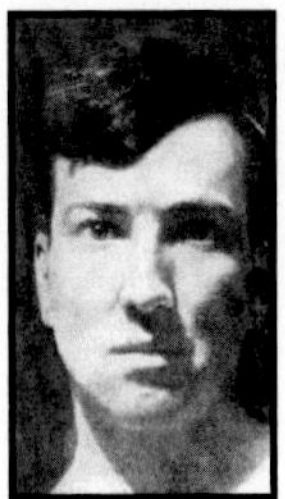
Robert von Ranke Graves. (1895-1985)

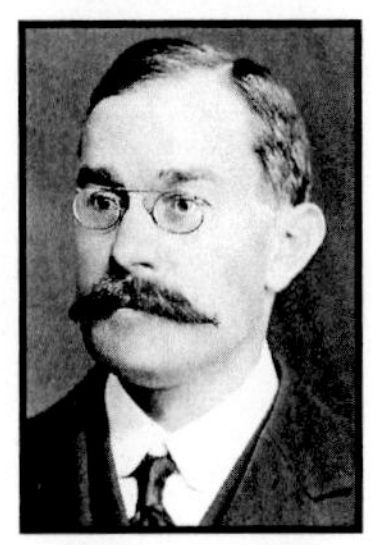
Dr William Halse Rivers (1864-1922)

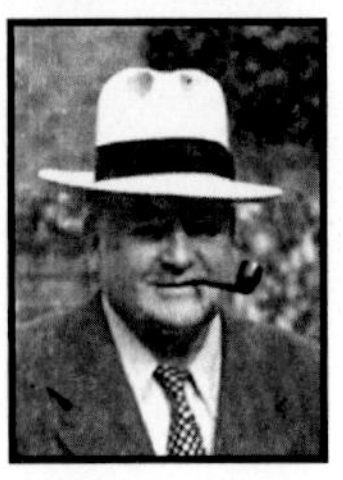
Dr Maurice Nicholl (1884-1953).

Siegfried Loraine Sassoon. (1886-1967). Buried (above centre) in the cemetary of St Andrew's, Mells, Somerset. Photo. Author. 2010 .

In the 1920 retro, *Graylingwell War Hospital* Annual Report; Lt Col. Dr Harold A Kidd, Commanding Officer, and resident Medical Superintentent of the *West Sussex County Asylum* (Graylingwell), entered: '*date, 27/05/19. As from this date, Committee appointed a Senior assistant Medical Officer, Captain Sidney Nix, RAMC, MD, BS (Durham) LRCP, LRCS (Edinboro) LRFPS (Glasgow) who had aquired considerable experience of mental diseases at Bethlem Royal Hospital and elsewhere and, during the war, had been mental specialist in charge of the Shell Shock and Mental Cases at the General Military Hospital, Colchester and Dykebar War Hospital, Paisley.*' Lt's Sassoon and Graves experienced shell shock; Drs. Rivers and Nicholl treated the malady — in treating officers of the Armed Forces by talking out therapies; one name for shell shock was neurasthenia.

204.

TOWN HALL, LEICESTER,
3rd May, 1912.

Asylum Accommodation.

Sir,

The attention of the Visiting Committee of the Leicester Borough Mental Hospital has been directed to the Annual Return of the number of patients, accommodation, &c., of Asylums and Mental Hospitals, by which the Commissioners in Lunacy require the day accommodation for noisy and turbulent patients to be increased from 40 to 50 superficial feet per patient.

This alteration is of considerable importance to Asylum Authorities in that it may necessitate the provision of additional accommodation earlier than would have otherwise been necessary.

My Committee desire me to ascertain the views of other Asylum Authorities, and to obtain their opinion as to whether the Commissioners should be approached on the matter.

I should be much obliged, therefore, if you would kindly let me know if your Committee have considered the question, and if so what decision they have come to.

I remain,

Yours faithfully,

H. A. PRITCHARD,

Town Clerk and Clerk to the Visiting Committee.

E. H. Blaker, Esq.,

Clerk to the Visiting Committee

of the Sussex *Asylum.*

CHICHESTER.

One of many distributed circulars to public Asylums and Poor Law Institutions — in 1912. (The First World War was but two years ahead...)

Notes, References and Sources. Chapter Five.

1. Henry Maudsley, M.D. *'Natural Causes & Supernatural Seemings.'*, The Thinker's Library ed., 1939. London. Part Two. Chapt.1. p79.
2. Incidents .... See *Regulations, 1897* in *Better Court Than Coroners,* Volume Two. Forms & Lists.
3. As Pursuant to the 275th Section of the Lunacy Act, 1890. Under, *Bath Rules* p.26.... See *Better Court Than Coroners,* Volume Two. Forms & Lists.
4. *To Kill A Mockingbird,* By Harper Lee. Published by Lippincott. (Philadelphia. USA) 1960. And by Heinmann. London.1963. (About the time of the Civil Rights movement). A film of the same title came out in 1962, starring Gregory Peck.
5. Russian hospitals... I was an avid reader of Solzhenitsyn, Tolstoy and other giants, in Russian literature; and could hardly ignore the frequent 1960s press reports, on so-called dissident scientists, like Andrei Sakharov. On Bramber Two ward, Dougie and I often chatted about the Russian philosophers, P.D.Ouspensky and G.I. Gurdjieff. But we also discussed the quoted misuse, of Russian Psychiatric Hospitals, by the Russian government in power; and their reported misuse of anti-psychotic drugs. (*Russia's Political Hospitals. The Abuse of Psychiatry in the Soviet Union*, by Sidney Bloch and Peter Reddaway. Published by Futura Publications Limited . Gollancz. 1977. See. 1978 pb....). Stigma will always prevail in human society; sadly. As a Mental Health professional practioner, with a duty of care, working within the UK NHS system, I have *frequently* assisted in admitting, and advised the discharge, of many sectioned patients in and out of hospital, but have NEVER admitted any patient for purely political reasons. *That* would be, is, abuse of power. In a later update, *The Sunday Observer* magazine supplement (*Observer Magazine*. 28th June.1992) summed up those years of systematic *abuse* — before Glasnost, in an illustrated article, *A Russian Madness* by John Collee:

   > 'A Change Of Mind. In the old-style Soviet Union the psychiatric establishment was seen as an extension of the legal system: to be diagnosed as mentally ill was tantamount to receiving a criminal sentence.'

Valery Tarsis autobiographical novel, *Ward 7,* is about a Soviet writer dissident Valentine Almazov who is wrongfully admitted under a Section 39 (presumably as our Section 26 of the 1959 MHA) into a Moscow psychiatric hospital. (*Ward 7*, By Valery Tarsis. Translated by Katya Brown. Published. Collins and Harvill Press. London and Glasgow. 1965). Tarsis paid tribute to his literary forebear Dr. Anton Chekov's; *Ward No.6. Anonymous Story,* published in 1892.... The Ward 6 Doctor replies why a particular patient was admitted, and cannot be discharged by him:

> 'Morals and logic have nothing to do with it. It all depends on chance. Those who are put here, and those who aren't are free. That's all there is to it. There's no morality or logic in the fact that I'm a doctor and you're mentally ill - it's pure chance.' (*Ward No. 6 and other Stories, 1892 - 1895*. Penguin pb Books. 2002 . p54.)

I was impressed, reading a biography of Dr. Chekov, and his huge efforts to administer to the physicially ill and, especially, to his diagnosed mentaly ill — with little to zero resources. And, of his iron effort, in part-time writing of brilliant plays and short stories — *whilst* he was dying of tuberculosis. (*Doctor Chekov. A Study in Literature and Medicine,* By John Coope. Published By Cross Publishing. Chale Isle of Wight. 1997.)

6. Blake.... Writings on William Blake (1757-1827), were prolific. He'd lived awhile at nearby Felpham, in Bognor Regis, West Sussex. On several occasions, I'd had the pleasure of viewing some of his original muscular red veined paintings, on public display in the Petworth Estate's main building.
7. See my pics in *The Illustrated London News,* p.761, May 11th 1957. Taken *before* the first Grapple H bomb was exploded, only days later. Other *later* colleagues were *exposed* to atomic radiation, and net results of fallout, and were not so fortunate. Section 10 of the 1947 *Crown Proceedings Act*, at that time, forbade any member of the armed forces from bringing legal actions of wanton neglect against *The Crown* — or AWRE — this aspect of the total ban, on *aftermath* information, was not repealed till May, 1983. As I recall there was, in those years, zero media knowledge expounded, on

latent genetic mutation in man, beast, polluted earth and sealife. Authority would remain in denial.... Still does.

8. The Lance- corporal from Bristol was represented, in this Test case in High Court, by Solicitor Mr Mark Mildred who claimed that, at the time of the bomb tests, he (the soldier) was *owed a duty of care....* not by his army employers, but by the now defunct Atomic Energy Authority. The Authority was not a Crown body, but its military functions came under the control of the ministry of defence, in 1973.
9. See *A-bomb test soldier wins High Court Ruling*, Guardian. p5. 18.12.1986. Also. *Evening Argus* - Brighton ed. p6. 20.12.1986. ... And see. 'Atom test claim case adjourned (Lance Corporal) was *not* prevented by *Crown Immunity* (in theory) from suing the Ministry of Defence.' *Guardian,* June 25 1987. (See) News in Brief. *Atom test claim adjourned (*my use of italics).
10. *John Wayne. The Man Behind The Myth,* By Michael Munn. Published. Robsons Books. 2003 p172 - 173.
11. Idiot Savants. Facts & Science Fiction. See for E.g.., *Day of the Moron* by H.Beam Piper and *The Universe Between* by Alan E. Nourse. Publ. *Astounding Science Fiction*. Vol. VIII, No.3 British Edition. March 1952. As authors Arthur C. Clarke & Issac Asimov have demonstrated, Science Fiction often precludes becoming Science Matter of Fact. In the 1960s and Seventies, to my frequent surprise, much media, medics and nurses, *not* trained in Psychiatry or working with classified Mentally Handicapped, knew *no* difference between the diagnosed Idiot Moron, or forever Lunatic — a fact which both generally annoyed and perplexed me, in this immutability. Twenty years on... The 1988 film, *The Rain Man,* based on the real life personality of Raymond Babitt and, especially, the ground breaking publication (c1989) of Dr. Darold A. Treffert, M.D.'s book *'Extraordinary People. Understanding Savant Syndrome.'* which broke, forever, the previous, public mould of relegating anyone *not* socially acceptable (not to overstate the obvious observation) as sub-human — or, *if* a compensatory *savant,* treated like a circus freak. Our science-fiction writers have long realised it is the compensatory latent savant powers which are markers towards what nature has in store for mankind, but...

12. *Handbook for Psychiatric Nurses*. Ed. Dr. Brian Ackner. Published by Balliere, Tindall & Cox. Ninth Edition.1964.
13. *Textbook of Medical Treatment*. By Dunlop. 11th Edition. 1968.
14. Emil Kraepelin (1856-1926.)
15. Eugene Bleuler (1857-1939.)
16. Ackner. Ibid. 1964. See Chapter 16.
17. Ibid.
18. Ibid.
19. *Pragmatics of Human Communication* by Paul Watzlawick, Janet Helmick Beavin, and Don D. Jackson.
20. Kraepelin. Ibid.
21. Acker, Ibid. 1964. p.138.
22. Jonathan Swift (1667-1745)... satirised in his 1743 edition *Tale of A Tub* : ... *A Digression*, &c. p121-122.
23. Ackner. Ibid. 1964 pp 320-335.
24. Charles Dickens (1812-1870). *Oliver Twist* By Charles Dickens 1838. The book was published shortly after the passing of 1834 *Poor Law Amendment Act*. The Victorian parish officers *Relieving Officer* and *Beadle* were men with much power — as Dickens acknowledged in his first work, Boz.
25. *Sketches of Boz,* By Charles Dickens. Published 1836. See Chapter One the first page.
26. *Put Away. A Sociological Study of Institutions for the Mentally Retarded*. By Pauline Morris. Foreward by Peter Townsend. Published . London. Routledge & Kegan Paul.1969.
27. *Mental Health Act* 1959, Form 2.
28. Lord Chief Justice Widgery. Mr Basil Boxall (aka Admin Baz) remembered his participation in this event with Dr. Brian Joyce (not his real name). I have been unable (to date) to trace this case in writing. Likely, it was to be a 1973 MH Act.

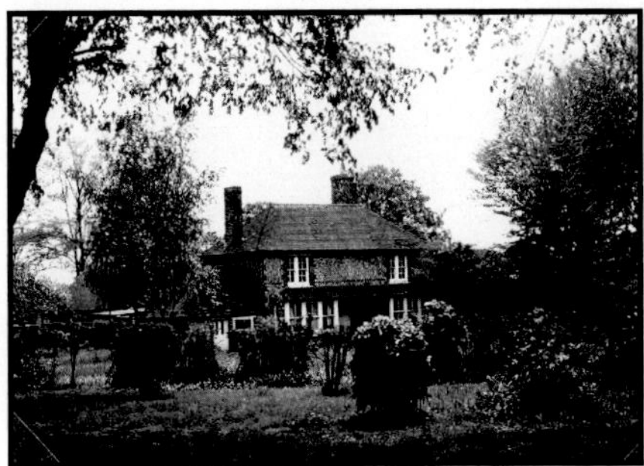

1980. St Martins Farm

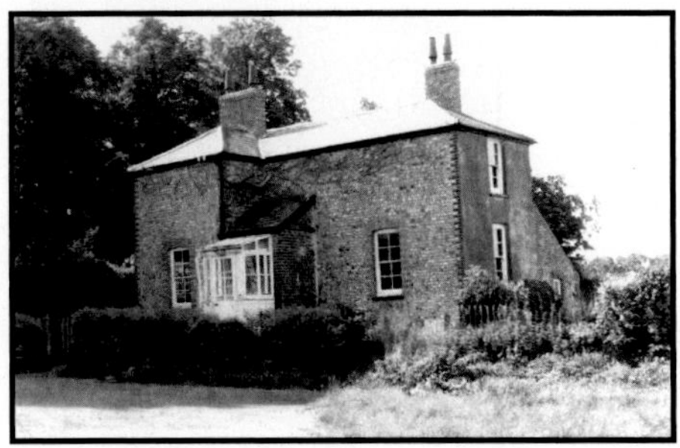

1980. Stockman's Cottage

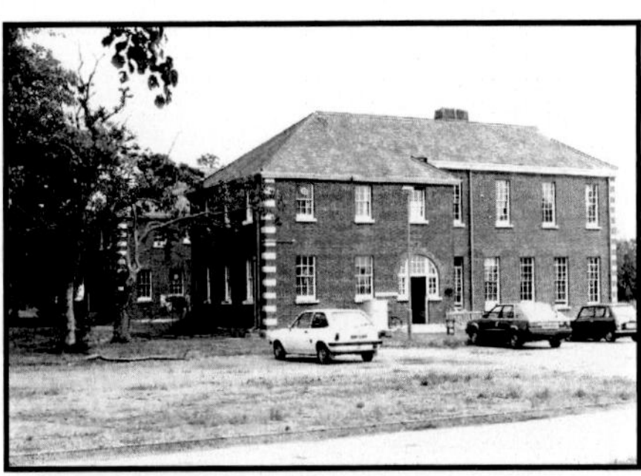

1990. Kingsmead Villa (built 1933)

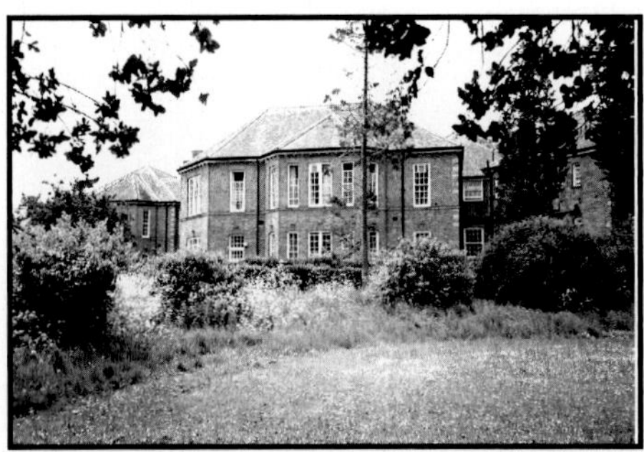

1990. Richmond Villa (Gordon House) built 1933.

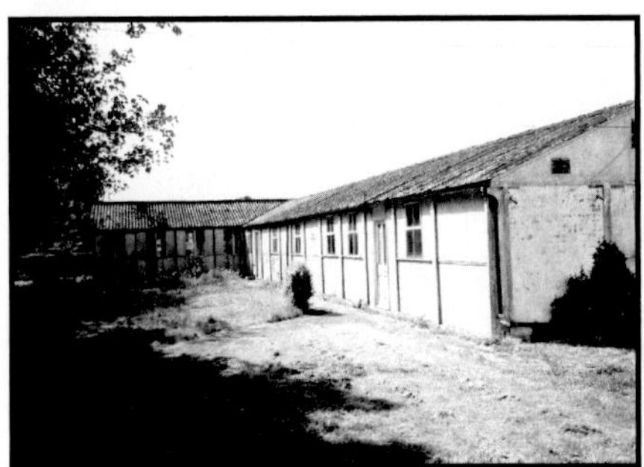

1980. Nurse Training prefabs, built early 1950s

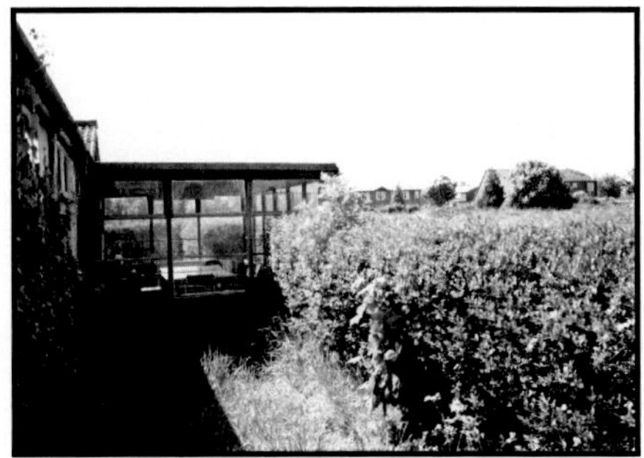

1980. Nurse Training prefab annexe.

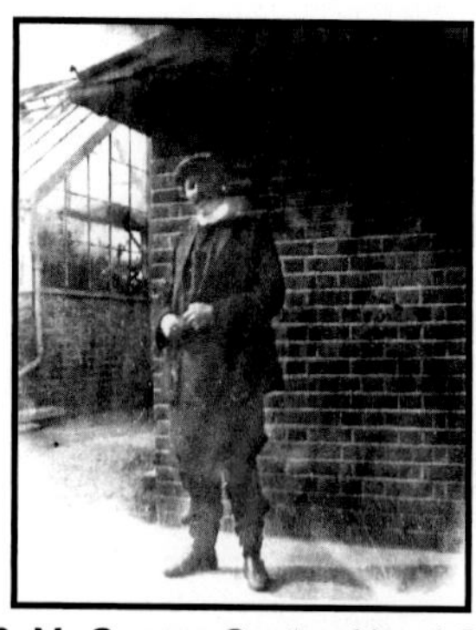

1909. Mr George Souter, Head Gardener and propagator at Graylingwell.

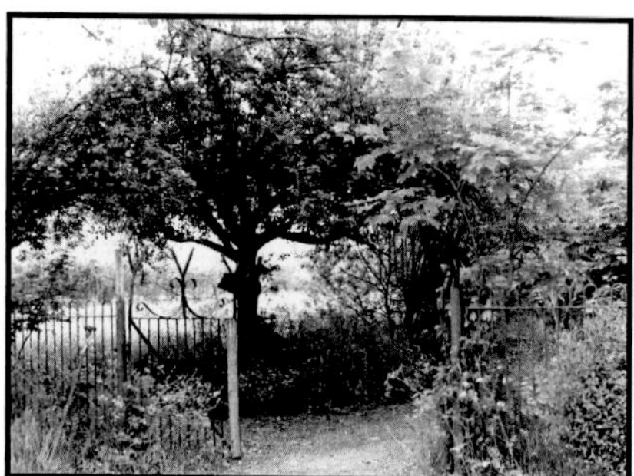

1990. Entrance to Graylingwell Orchard and kitchen garden, no longer in use for hospital.

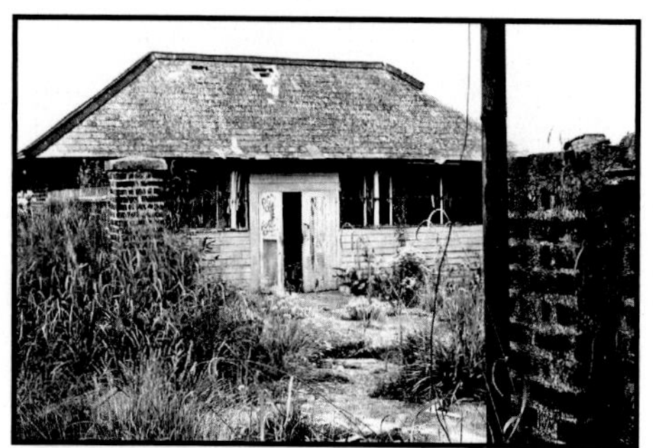

1980. Remains of Gardening Unit.

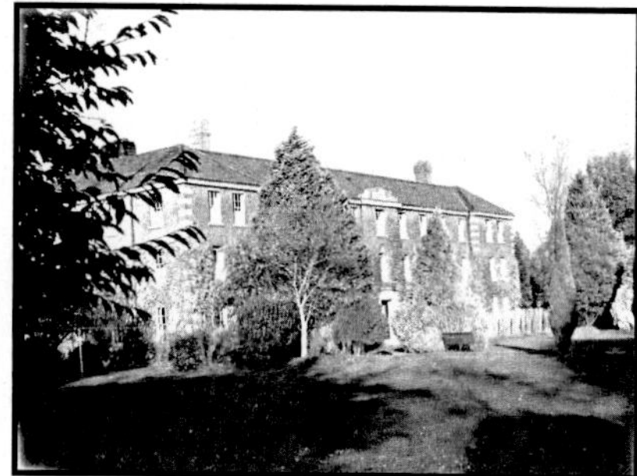

1980. Pinewood Nurses Home, built 1933.

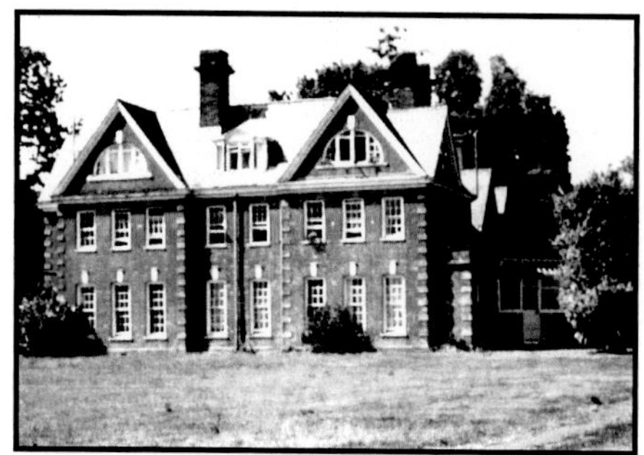

1980. Graylingwell House. Residence of the Superintendents, until 1959.

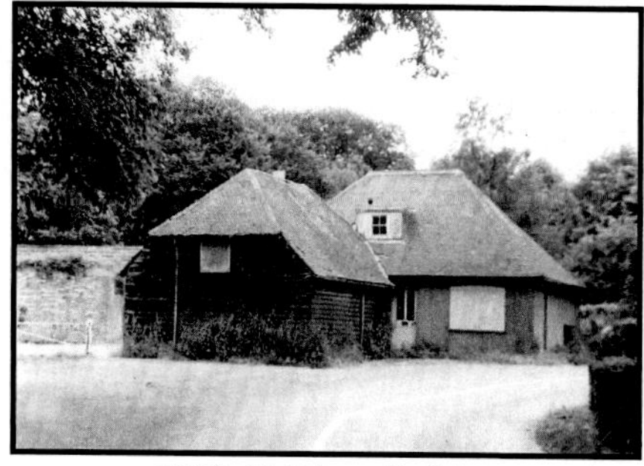

1980. Old Farm Buildings.

(Photos by author.)

Notes, References and Sources. Chapter Six.

1. Jean Cocteau. (1889-1963). *Paris Album. 1900 - 1914.* Translated by M.Crosland. Published. W.H.Allen 1956. See *Introduction.*
2. Jean-Paul Sartre (1905-1980). *La Nausee.* (Nausea) French 1938. *The Diary of Antoine Roquentin. A novel.* Published (English) London. John Lehmann. 1949. *Nausea* by Jean-Paul Sartre. Penguin pb. 1965. It was the Penguin pb that I was to read many times, over the coming years. My first reading was, in retro, far too negative. All refs come from the Penguin edition:

   > 'My Thought is *me* ... but I hate existing' (p145).

   Most profound, I read that he is only *pure,* and himself, when he rejects any contact with his flesh...

   > '... this cold is pure, this darkness is so pure; am I myself not a wave of icy air? To have neither blood, nor lymph, nor flesh. To flow along this canal towards that pallor over there. To be nothing but coldness.' (pp43-44.)

   He (reads) is with in the wind, but exists (it seems), imagines, or feels, paradoxically, *only* when he really has no body... and is disengaged. Hardly a nihilistic statement. Unless an oxymoron.... Yet, surely, source of Sartre's tangible nausea.
3. Bertrand Russell (1872-1970). *A History of Western Philosophy.* By Bertrand Russell. Published by George Allen & Unwin Ltd. Simon & Schuster, Inc. 1945.
4. Enid Blyton (1897-1968). Enid Blyton's *Sunny Stories* was the title of a series of small, thin, red-covered booklets (mags), published in the 1940s. As an infant, I recall being read to from these short stories, whilst taking refuge in various air-raid shelters, Anderson and Morrison, and down our Orphanage cellars — hiding, during the loud noisy cacophony and lightning flames of numerous air raids about us.
5. Colin Wilson (b.1931). *The Outsider.* By Colin Wilson. Published. London. Gollancz. 1956.
6. Carl Jung (1875-1961). *Psychology of The Unconscious.* 1912.

7. Franz Kafka (1883-1924). *Metamorphosis* (1915). Penguin Modern Classics.
8. Jean-Paul Sartre. *Playboy*. May 1965. Interview. pp.69-76.
9. Sartre. *Nausea*. Penguin. pb. ed. (!978 reprint.)
10. Ibid. p.22.
11. Ibid. p.27.
12. Ibid. p.52.
13. Ibid. p.82.
14. G.K. Chesterton (1874-1936). Books of Essays. *Heretics* (1905). *Orthodoxy* (1908).
15. Ibid. *Orthodoxy.*
16. Len Deighton (b.1929) *Billion Dollar Brain.*1966. Penguin pb. (*The Ipcress File*. 1962 and, *Funeral in Berlin*. 1964.)

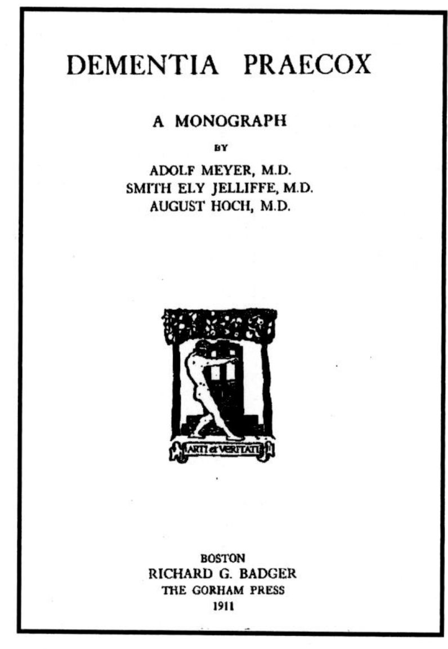

DEMENTIA PRAECOX

A MONOGRAPH

BY

ADOLF MEYER, M.D.
SMITH ELY JELLIFFE, M.D.
AUGUST HOCH, M.D.

BOSTON
RICHARD G. BADGER
THE GORHAM PRESS
1911

1911. Described by Kraepelin, 'Dementia Praecox' was an earlier attempt to describe symptoms of intellectual impairment observed in young patients; in fact, it wasn't dementia (as such), but a loss of integration of the various mental functions, especially of affect and thinking, descriptive of Schizophrenias (Acker, 1964. p138) — whatever its source.

Mental Health Act. Compulsory 72hrs Admission Paper.

Form 2

MENTAL HEALTH ACT, 1959

Emergency Application for Admission for Observation
(Section 29)

(1) Name and address of hospital or mental nursing home

TO THE MANAGERS OF (1)..

....

(2) Name and address of applicant

1. I (2).. of ....

....hereby apply for the admission of

(3) Name and address of patient

(3).. of ....

....to the above-named hospital for observation in accordance with Part IV of the Mental Health Act, 1959.

(4) State relationship (see section 49 overleaf)

2. (a) I am a relative of the patient within the meaning of the Act, being the patient's (4)..........................

Delete (a) or (b)

OR

(5) Name of local social services authority

(b) I am an officer of (5).. appointed to act as a mental welfare officer for the purposes of the Act.

3. I last saw the patient on ....19........

4. In my opinion it is of urgent necessity for the patient to be admitted and detained under Section 25 of the Act, and compliance with the requirements of the Act relating to applications for admission other than emergency applications would involve undesirable delay.

5. This application is founded on the medical recommendation forwarded herewith.

(6) If the medical practitioner who has made the recommendation had no previous acquaintance with the patient, the applicant should state here why it is not practicable to obtain a recommendation from a practitioner having such acquaintance

6. (6)..

....

....

....

Signed..

Date ....

RECORD OF ADMISSION *(This is not part of the application, but is to be completed later at the hospital or mental nursing home.)*

(7) Name of patient

(a) (7)..was admitted to

(8)..in pursuance of

this application at (9)..........................on..........................19..........

Delete (a) or (b)

OR

(b) (7)..was already an in-patient

(8) Name of hospital or mental nursing home

in (8) ....

on the date of this application and the application was received by me on behalf of the managers

(9) Time and date

at (9)..........................on..........................19..........

Signed.. on behalf of the managers

Date ....

The 1959 Mental Health Act (7 and 8 Eliz. Lic. 72) included a Section 29 for Emergency Observation (for 72 hours), and a Section 26 for up to one year care and treatment. All compulsory sections could be reversed — and often were.

The word 'lunacy' inferring not-normal in (then) mind and body was on statute in the 16th century and, since that date, legislation to attend persons putting themselves, or others, At Risk (life threatening) because of their disorder, has been available in one form or another (as it still is today....)

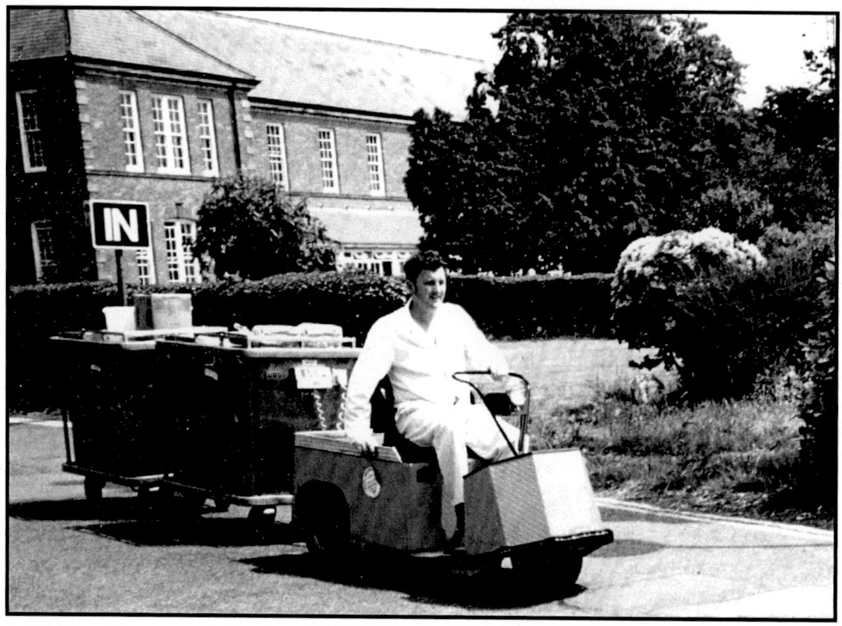

1980. Electric motorised trolley with hot food containers en-route for Graylingwell wards.

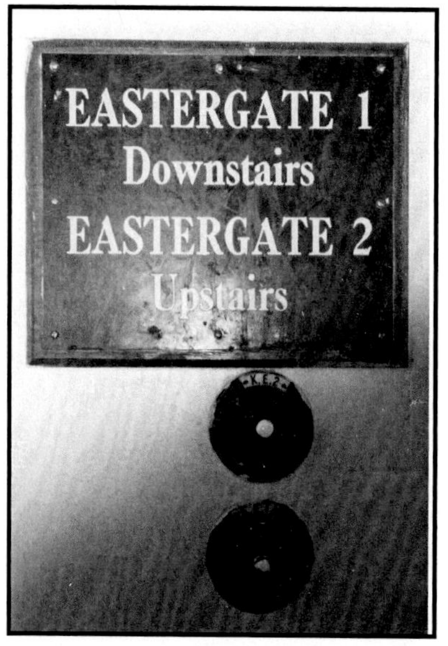

Old Eastergate Block. Note round nipple bells for KE1 & KE2 from 1914-18 war. K for King's side vis the Male side wards of the hospital (Q was for Queen's Female wards).

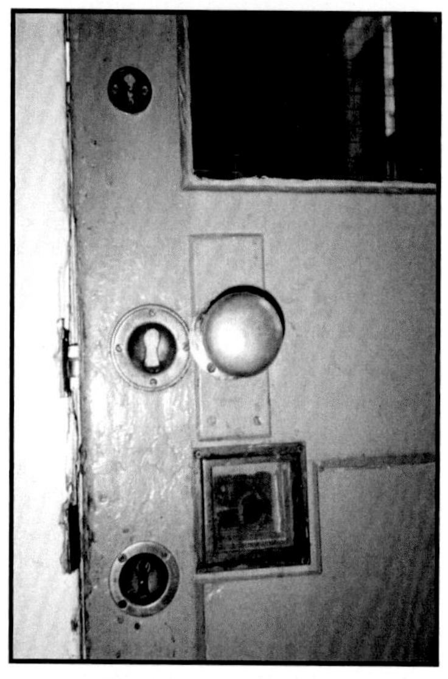

Old entrance to Eastergate block, evidence at least of four-5 previous safety lock fittings from earlier years.

(Photos by author.)

Notes, References and Sources. Chapter Seven.

1. Sholem Asch (1880-1957). *The Nazarene*, By Sholem Asch. Translated from the Yiddish, by Maurice Samuel. Published. London. Routledge.1939. See. Chapter One. The opening line....
2. Jean Cocteau (1889-1963). *Round The World Again In Eighty Days*, By Jean Cocteau. Translated by Stuart Gilbert. Published. London. Routledge.1937. See. p.148.
3. Charles Chaplin (1889-1977). *My Autobiography,* By Charles Chaplin. Published. London. Bodley Head 1964. See. p.418
4. Language of ... In the 1960s and Seventies, I read a modest amount of Charles Darwin, Ivan Petrovich Pavlov, H.J.Eysenck, Nikolaas Tinbergan, Konrad Lorenz, B.F Skinner and others, on latent imprinted biology, cellular memory, instinct and, the breadth and *limitation* of known, robot human senses — so far.

   Vitus B. Drosher (*The Magic Of The Senses. New Discoveries In Animal Perception*. Published. W.H.Allen. London. Transl.1969 p.3.), said:

   > 'the human eye, optically speaking, is a piece of bad workmanship. If the image projected onto the retina by the 'camera', our eye, were examined by an optician, used to high standards, he would be disgusted.There is more blurring, at the edges, than with a cheap pair of child's binoculars; straight lines look curved, and the outlines fade away under iridescent haloes. The *nervous system corrects* these faults so perfectly, that we perceive a technically flawless image of our surroundings.'

   One can speculate on becoming blind through trauma, or being born blind, and how ambiguous *insight* and dream images are to then be explained. And, inevitably, how man may manipulate one's own, and all, or any others' senses, consciously, or by using the unconscious brain and cellular records — latent within.

   Lucian Freud (b.1922), painter and grandson, of Sigmund Freud, said, in *Some Thoughts On Painting*. (Published. *Encounter.* Periodical. July 1954. pp.23-24):

   > 'My object in painting pictures is to try and *move the senses* by giving an *intensification of reality.*'

Another artist, Pablo Picasso (1881-1973), quizzed in an interview about the meanings or intensions motivating his different periods of art works - about the famous *Guernica* painting, and its particular image of a bull, 'was it symbolic', based on his thoughts upon the Spanish Civil war and Franco's collusion with Nazi Germany and Fascist Italy....

> "No ," said Picasso, "the bull is not fascism, but it is brutality and darkness."... "My work is not symbolic, " he answered. "Only the *Guernica* mural is symbolic. But in the case of the mural, that is allegoric. ... I *paint this way*," he replied, "because it's a *result of my thought. ...* I express myself through painting and I *can't explain through words*, I can't explain why I did it that way ... I see every detail. I see the size, the thickness, and I *translate it in my own way.* " (Source, *The Penguin Book Of Interviews*. Edited by Christopher Silvester. Published. Viking.1993 pp.369-375: Pablo Picasso. Interviewed by Jerome Seckler. *New Masses*, 13 March 1945.). ... My use of italics.

In film, the use is made of multi-linked pictures and mobile projected film images, as made by Eisenstein (1898-1948), through his *creative editing*. I read this in a revelation of his Koestler-like *matrix*. Of Sergei's use and appreciation, of the *Synchronisation of Senses* and the reality, that *what* we *initially* see and interpret in rank experience is *often* completely false. For *Things are not necessarily what they seem.* One may manufacture mould and shape selected film images, using a *matrix* of all the senses — including the emotions — and, like Ivan Pavlov, predict an outcome. Source, See *The Film Sense*, By Sergei Eisenstein. Translated, edited by Jay Leyda. Published. Faber & Faber. London. 1943. Chapter II pp.60-91. And also refer to *Film Technique* By Pudovkin. Newnes. London.1935 edition p.45:

> 'There is a law in psychology that lays it down that if an emotion give birth to a certain movement, by imitation of this movement the corresponding emotion can be called forth.'

The English Poet Ted Hughes interviewed in 1970 about the origins of his metaphorical poetry, after a detailed answer to the popular misconception that his subject matter was all about violence, said,

> 'it was *not* about being a fascist or a symbol of some horrible totalitarian genocidal dictator – what I had in mind was that this hawk *Nature* is thinking. Simply Nature.'

Hughes said, *Crow* reflected the non-romantic facts of life, and death, not just the ideal, cosy rosy, pretty pretty images as the norm ideal. Hughes chose the claws of The Crow (an ideal of style) rather than The *Eagle,* in his work. And, as to his inner and supposed metaphorical historic models for the shape and content of his verse, Donne, Shakespeare et cetera:

> 'this business of influences is mysterious. Sometimes it's just a few words that open up a whole prospect. They may occur anywhere. Then again the influences that really count are most likely not literary at all.' And finally pertinent. He says, on his *wordcraft*. "I think it's true that formal patterning of the actual *movement of verse* somehow includes a mathematical and a musically deeper world than free verse can easily hope to enter. It's a mystery why it should do so." (*London Magazine*. January.1970. See.Interview. Egbert Faas. *Ted Hughes and Crow*. pp.5-20.) ... Again, my use of italics.

5. *The Paris Review*. Writers at Work. 3rd Series. Penguin.1977 ed. See. 3. *Jean Cocteau*. pp.57-81. Quote. p.73.)
6. Jean-Paul Sartre. *Existentialism. By Jean-Paul Sartre. Translated by Bernard Frechtman*. Published. Philosophical library. New York. 1947. See for e.g.; p.18:

> 'Atheistic existentialism, which I represent, is more coherent. It states that if God does not exist, there is at least one being in whom existence precedes essence, a being who exists before he can be defined by any concept, and that this being is man or, as Heidegger says human reality.'

7. Colin Wilson (b.1925). *Introduction To the New Existentialism.* Hutchinson.1966 His definition of Existentialism.
8. William James (1842-1910).
9. Darold A.Treffert (b.1932) *Extraordinary People. Understanding Savant Syndrome*. By Darold A.Treffert M.D. Published (as) An Authors Guild Backprint com Edition. iUniverse, Inc. Printed in USA. *Extraordinary People. An Update*. 2006.

10. William James. *Brief Course of Psychology*. Published. Holt.1892.
11. Rider Haggard (1856-1925). *The People Of The Mist*. 1894.
12. G.K.Chesterton (1874-1936). *Heretics*.1905. *Orthodoxy*. 1908.
13. Ouspenky's *New Model of The Universe* was published, in English, in 1931. O was a contemporary of Chesterton, Shaw and Wells.
14. P.D.Ouspensky's Russian *Tertium Organum* was first printed, in English, in 1922. I was well acquainted with the Second Edition of this book. (*Tertium Organum*. By P.D.Ouspensky. Translated from the Russian by Nicholas Bessarabov and Claude Bragdon. Published. Second Edition. London. Kegan Paul, Trench Trubner.1924.) Ouspensky's work detailed human existence being located during *a moment of consciousness*, to quote William James, its mathematics and deduced geometry unseen but realised in time & space. The title followed Aristotle and Roger Bacon. ... Roger Bacon (1214-1294). Author of *Novum Organum* (which I was *not* familiar with. Nor was I acquainted with Aristole's (384-322 B.C.) earlier Greek *Organum*). Bacon, the medieval philosopher & scientist (in my gross ignorance), from the outset presented THE conundrum. In a science of and value of rank Experience (vis-a-vis application and observation of any experiment ...). Since it is the *retrospect* of said experiment, and whoever (by whatever limited tangible means) gathers memories, as traces of that event. As experience infers the precise and passed *moment*. The very word EXPERIENCE infers a contradiction in abstract and physical terms ...Erm! Peter Ouspensky had provided an excellent lucid introduction on this subject.
15. Ouspensky. *A New Model of The Universe,* Ibid 1931. p19.
16. Arthur Koestler.*The Spanish Testament*. Gollancz. pb. 1937.
17. Andre Gide (1869-1951).
18. Jean-Paul Sartre. *Playboy* magazine. May 1965. Interview.
19. G.K.Chesterton. *Orthodoxy*. 1908. See. Chapter. *The Eternal Revolution*.
20. *Nausea*. Sartre. Ibid.
21. F.Molina. *Existentialism as Philosophy*. Published. Spectrum pb. 1962.
22. H.J.Blackham. *Six Existentialist Thinkers*. Published. Routledge pb. 1961.

23. Sartre. *Being and Nothingness* by Jean-Paul Sartre. Translated by Hazel Barnes. Published by Philosophical Library New York.1956.
24. Heideggar. (1889-1976). *Being and Time* by Martin Heideggar. Translated by John Macquarrie & Edward Robinson. Published. Oxford. Basil Blackwell.1967.
25. Peter Hays. *New Horizons in Psychiatry.* By Peter Hays. Published. Pelican (Original) pb. 1964.
26. Dr. Russell Barton. *Institutional Neurosis* By Russell Barton M.B., B.S., FRCP (London) ... Fwd by Noel Gordon Harris, M.D., ...Published. John Wright & Sons. Bristol. (First Edition.1959.) Third Ed. pb. 1976.
27. Dr. Joshua Carse.(d.1971) *Graylingwell Hospital* Medical Superintendent from 1938-1963.. Well known for his backing for the *Worthing Acre Experiment* 1956-7.
28. Dr. James Boswell's *Life of Johnson.*(1791). See. (Johnson) Age 54...
29. On *Parallel Worlds.* ... But *not* in our possible mortal perspective.
30. P.D Ouspensky. ... with disapproval
31. *Nausea* ... Sartre's seminal book enlarged upon this spatial aspect of special interest to me — moments of *self-observation* — and so in observing Others.
32. J.P.Sartre. *The Diary of Antoine Roquentin.* London. Lehmann.1949 ed.
33. Arthur Koestler. *The Ghost In The Machine.* London. Hutchinson.1967. See. Picador pb. (Pan Books). 1975. Chapter. XIV. *The Ghost In The Machine.* pp.197-221.
34. Word-play Sole and Soul. Piscean theology. Or Lewis Carroll' philosophy...
35. Judith Groch. *You and Your Brain.* Published. Harper & Row. New York. 1963. See... Pan-piper Science series pb.... On words — see p147.
36. *Nausea...* Ibid. pb. See. p182.
37. H.G. Wells (1866-1946). *The Man Who Could Work Miracles.* Published.1900. Short story, made into a G.B. b&w film, title of that name, directed by Alexander Korda, and released in 1936. Beware of what you wish for....
38. J.P. Sartre. ... Ibid. pb. p.189.

39. A. Koestler. ...Ibid, *The Spanish Testament*. 1937 pb..
40. P.D. Ouspensky.... *A New Model Of The Universe*. 1931. Chapter III *Superman* pp. 113-148. ... *Superman as a Higher Being*. Not - the exact opposite and abased brutish Nazi genetic images - *deliberately* taking out of context Nietzschean Superman - and Western beloved graphic schoolchild comic-book heroes, depicted as Superman, Captain Marvel (SHAZAM) and the Marvel Family. (All other cultures too have similar moral heroes.)
41. Friedrich William Nietzsche (1844-1900). *Thus Spake Zarathusa*.1883. ... See. *Thus Spake Zarathusa. A Book For All And None*. First Translation 1899. Second Impression Translated by Alexander Tille. Published by T.Fisher Unwin. London. 1908.
42. Max Muller (1823-1900). *Zend Avesta*: aka Avesta (text — Vid or Veda abasta Law) Zend (commentary)... based on the ancient sacred writings of (Parsees), the good historical Persian, (Zarathusa) Zoroaster & his disciples. *Collected Works of F.Max Muller. iv. Theosophy or Psychological Religion.1893*. Published by Longmans, Green and co. London.1917 ed. ... See. *Zend Avesta* pp.35-43.
43. Albert Camus (1913-1960). *The Outsider.* 1942. ...
44. English *Punch* magazine. Date 2.9.67
45. Carl Jung. Ibid. *Psychology of the Unconscious*. Heideggar on individual utility...
46. P.D. Ouspensky. ... *A New Model Of The Universe*. !931. See Chapter VII, p271.
47. L.P.Davies. (1914-1988) ... *Twilight Journey.* 1967.
48. Chuang Tsu (aka *Zhuagzi,* 369-286 BCE), a Chinese Taoist Philosopher also a known Meng official given the name Zhou.
49. Ray Bradbury (b.1920). *A Sound of Thunde*r, first appeared in Collier's magazine in 1952, and re-printed among a collection of short stories in *The Golden Apples Of The Sun*. By Ray Bradbury. Published. Rupert Hart-Davis. London. 1953.
50. Robert Heinlein (1907-1988). *By His Bootstraps,* first published in 1941....
51. Stephen Baxter (b.1957). A teacher in Mathematics & Physics. Baxter's *The Time Ships* (1995) was an authorised sequel to H.G. Wells *The Time Machine* (1895). Wells died in 1946. Stephen Baxter

has also co-written several books with Arthur C. Clarke, doyen writer of Science Fact and Science Fiction exploratory works.

52. Henry James (1843-1916). Brother of psychologist William James. Henry James novel, *Sense Of The Past* (1917), was incomplete at the time of his death in 1916 though, I understood, he had made further notes on this subject matter. I notice that literary commentators refer to the novel as Romantic Fiction, (not psychological science-fiction); though there does seem to be coincident (to me), a correlation with Matheson's fantasy *Bid Time Return* (1975) where its hero, a playwright, is able to return, from the 1970s, to 1912, falls in love and motivates his mortal death, returning back into the past, to complete a *hidden* life, re-uniting with his loved one, using his unconscious life span... such a power, perhaps, of true romantic love... And surrender to divine love.
53. Richard Matheson. (b.1926). His novel, *Bid Time Return,* was published by Viking Press in 1975. The novel was also called *Somewhere in Time* (Tor Books, New York.1980), after the title of a feature film of that name. A subsequent novel, *What Dreams May Come* (Putnam. New York.1978), was also made into a feature film. The theme and *substance* of these inner works reminded me of certain New Psychology, Clinical Abreaction, Occult and Jungian psychoanalysis explorations. But, most, like the under-estimated good humane wartime work of Lord and Lady Dowding, for the wartime bereaved, reflected in the brief writings in five or so books and pamphlets by the Air Chief Marshal Lord Hugh Dowding (of Battle of Britain fame). The delightful Powell & Pressburger 1946 GB film, *A Matter Of Life And Death,* its US title *A Stairway To Heaven,* appeared (to me) to be a gentle reflection on this spiritual side, and allusion to the Dowding's little appreciated therapeutic family-work.
54. P.D. Ouspensky. *A New Model Of The Universe*.1931. See previous note 46.
55. Koestler's *The Spanish Testament* 1937. And *Act of Creation.* Hutchinson 1964.
56. Ibid.1937.
57. Sir A.J.Ayer (1910-1989). *Philosophical Essays*. by A.J.Ayer. Published. London. Macmillan. 1954.

58. P.D.Ouspensky. *A New Model Of The Universe*. 1931. See p.308....
59. Peter Hays. *New Horizons In Psychiatry*. 1964. Pelican pb The Causation of Schizophrenia p56.
60. David Cooper (1931-1986). *Psychiatry and Anti-Psychiatry*. By (Dr.) David Cooper. Published. Tavistock. London. 1967. See also. *The Dialectics Of Liberation*. Edited by David Cooper. Pelican Original pb 1968. And, *The Grammar Of Living*. Pelican pb 1974.
61. Ronald Laing (1927-1989). Dr. Ronald Laing. A colleague of Dr. David Cooper. Dr. Laing was an enormous influence on changing psychiatry, in the 1960s and Seventies.
62. William Shakespeare (1564-1616). Play the *Tempest*. iv.i.48.
63. P.D. Ouspensky. *A New Model Of The Universe*.1931. See. Chapter VII.
64. Other. E.g.; defs of Shaman — *A priest or priest doctor* .... & Shamanism. See, The OED ...Onions 1933. Vol 2. p.1864 (1952 ed).
65. P.D. Ouspensky. *A New Model Of The Universe*. 1931.
66. Robert Sheckley (1928-2005). *Untouched By Human Hands*.1945. See. London Four-Square pb.ed.1967.
67. Shakespeare. *King Lear*. 1.1... *Nothing will come of Nothing*. An easy example of philosophers and scientists who insist no human emotion is real, it never scientifically exists, if *it* cannot be *observed* by (their) five senses: only *afterward,* behaviour *(a word, not a solid) can* be confirmed...
68. Sartre. ... *Nausea* pb. See. p189.
69. Ibid. See. p190.
70. Ibid. See. p192.
71. Ibid. See. p
72. Professor C.S.Lewis See the introduction to his 1942 essay, on *Miracles*.
73. Jean-Paul Sartre.
74. *Every thing must be right*. Like a key for a singular lock fitting. A jigsaw.
75. The 1935, infamous, German Nazi mandatory Race Laws.
76. (See cross-ref previous, *Chapter Two*. Notes and Ref. No.57.) Watershed. Bedlam USA 1946. Years off, into retirement, collating these memoirs, related to *Better Court Than Coroners,* I discovered

the new electronic web, and its temporary computer global research resources. I learnt of Albert Deutsch, and the (later submerged) USA 1940s journalist explorations into existant, yet *hidden,* most dire conditions of neglected (then) State *Veteran* (owed duty of care ex-servicemen) Hospitals, and of many civilian *State Psychiatric Institutions,* found throughout the United States Of America. I was horrified by what I learned. Much of the book's documentary evidence, on the gross neglect of the country's own armed service veterans and mental patients in state hospitals during the war years *and* early postwar years made grim reading. Within his book *The Shame Of The States* By Albert Deutsch. (Published. New York. Harcourt, Brace And Company 1948) .

On page 49 of Deutsch was a selection of captioned photographs; one photograph titled BYBERRY (taken in the *Philadelphia State Hospital for Mental Diseases, Byberry);* this showed a number of naked men in one "Incontinent Ward", *among three hundred others*, all naked, with no clothes supplied *because* financial resources were so sparse, and the number of patients in the hospital so huge — more than 6,100 Byberry patients in situ. Such pithy, actual resources, were denied their charges by the state, as there was insufficient qualified staff to properly attend patients' basic needs, eating, medicines, and clothing. Deutsch, and his colleagues, witnessed all very basic material needs of hundreds of innocent disabled mental patients proven to be neglected. Fortunately, America duly responded to Deutsch, and conditions began to improve.... Progress.

In the grounds of one *massive* American mental hospital, *The Pilgrim State at Brentwood*, New York, with a capacity for 10,000 patients in 1943, several hospital buildings (closed down 1947), built in its grounds, were provided for the US Army for up to 1,500 wounded (including shell shock) psychiatric patients, known as *The Mason General.* Deutsch (Ibid.1948) reported that:

> "Upward of 33,000 mentally ill soldiers were treated from its opening in June, 1943, the event (was) kept secret from the public — during the war years."

77. *Sans Everything. A Case to Answer*. By Barbara Robb, on behalf of AEGIS. Published. London. Nelson.1967. N.b. Contributors included Brian Abel-Smith, Russell Barton and C.H.Rolph.
78. *Report of the Committee of Inquiry into Whittingham Hospital.* (Payne Report). Published. 1972. Chairman, Sir Robert Payne. Terms of Reference (1971) : *To inquire into the administration of and conditions at Whittingham Hospital and to make recomendations.* The Payne Report published in *Documents on Health and Social Services. 1834 to the present day.* By Brian Watkin. Published, Methuen. pb.1975. *See*. pp.402-409.
79. Kathleen Jones. *Asylums and After. A Revised History of the Mental Health Services: From the Early 18th Century to the 1990s*. By Professor Kathleen Jones. Published. The Athlone Press. 1993. (And see *Documents on Health and Social Services 1834 to the present day.* By Brian Watkin. Published Methuen & Co Ltd. 1975.)
80. Dr. Maurice Nicholl. *Psychological Commentaries. On the Teaching of GI.Gurdjieff. and P.D.Ouspensky.* Published. London.Vincent Stuart. 1952. See.Vol.1. The opening Letter (17th March, 1941):

> 'All the articles that were written in the last war are just the same as the articles written in this war, and will be for ever and ever. ...'

About man's progress (problems), as a *self-developing organism.*

81. P.D.Ouspensky. *Tertium Organum* appeared, in English, in 1922. And *A New Model of The Universe,* in English, in 1931.
82. George Gurdjieff (1878-1949) *All and Everything or Beelzebub's Tales to his Grandson. 'An Objectively Impartial Criticism of the Life of Man.'* was not published till 1950 — one year after Gurdieff's death. J.G.Bennett, with Gurdjieff's approval, had much to do with this publication, as I understood its history.
83. Abraham Maslow (1908-1970). The Pyramid of Needs demonstrated five ascending human needs; at base (i) The Physiological (metabolic) body needs. (ii) Safety needs (stasis) — to feel and be secure. (iii) The need to Belong, as HG Wells amplified, homo-sapiens is a gregarious creature, a need to love and be loved, by mortal and divine. (iv) Self-esteem. And respect of others. To possess a sense of worth, a meaningful life. Of purpose. (v) Self-actualisation. As much as possible, to achieve a maximum of one's human potential.

To engage the capacity of which is, in proper context, the good Superman mortal within us (innate savant). Of course, this is my adaption of Maslow's model.

Reading about the history of medicine, nursing and psychology, back as it was in the early 1900s, I learnt of the growth in a *New Psychology* (viz Psychotherapy), and the clinical use of Mesmerising (aka hypnosis), hypnotic-suggestion; and of auto-suggestion in early treatment of shell-shock (ether) abreaction. And a growing acceptence of *some* Nervous Disorders as *not* Malingering. But there was a tumour — *too much* was only about the study of the *angst,* abnormal human phenomena — as litmus of the accepted normal. But, at last, some physicians and psychologists were responding to the study of The Normal — *what is* naturally, actually, Good (aka *New Existentialism)*, and how to achieve betterment, in the 1960s and Seventies; Abraham Maslow (and Carl Rogers) was one of them. See, for e.g.; *Toward a Psychology of Being* (1968) and *Further Reaches of Human Nature* (1971).

84. Barbara Robb. *Sans everything, A Case To Answer*. Presented by Barbara Robb. Published. Nelson. London.1967.
85. Sartre. ... *Nausea* pb. See. p.220.
86. J.C.Powys (1872-1963). *Autobiography.* (First published in 1934.) Refer. A New Edition, with an Introduction by J.B.Priestley. Published, Macdonald: London.1967. See Chapter Eight. *Burpham.* p.381.
87. P.D.Ouspensky. *A New Model Of The Universe*. 1931. See Chapters X and XI.
88. Hunter. ... *Memory. Facts and Fallacies*. By Dr. Ian M.L. Hunter. Pelican pb.
89. P.D.Ouspensky. *A New Model Of The Universe*. 1931. See p.480.
90. Ibid. 1931. See. Chapter III *Superman*. pp.113-148.
91. Ibid. 1931. See. Chapter XII *Sex And Evolution*. pp.513-541.
92. 1960s and Seventies, the *International Times* (aka IT) was an English newspaper, mostly for late teens and twenties, '*with it'* youth, of both sexes. *Playboy,* an imported American monthly periodical for all ages, but predominantly male. I extracted some interviews (e.g.; Sartre and Graves) from these *Playboy* magazines.
93. Graylingwell *Annual Report*.

94. George Crabbe (1774-1843). *Poems*. By The Rev.George Crabbe, LL.B. In Two Volumes. Published. London. Hatchard.1809. Fourth Edition. See.Vol.1. *The Village*. pp.16-17:

> 'Their's is yon House that holds the Parish Poor, Whose walls of mud scarce bear the broken door ; ... The Lame, the Blind, and far the happiest they! The moping idiot and the Madman gay.'

95. *Holloway Sanatorium*. Virginia Water. Egham. Surrey. A private resource, built for persons of the middle class, afflicted with mental disease, after 1879, at the instigation of the Victorian philanthropist Mr Thomas Holloway. The Gothic style palace provided for 100 male and 100 female patients. (See *Illustrated London News*. August 16, 1879. pp.161-162.) The Entrance Hall, alone, was high ceilinged, magnificent, with its ornate shaped arches and wide carpeted staircase — as can be seen in 20c. picture postcards of the building.
96. *Craiglockhart Hospital*. Little known, in the 1960s, *Craiglockhart,* in Edinburgh, was used, during 1916-1919, for Officers suffering shell shock (aka war neuroses) — as a rehabilitation convalescent unit. It had previously been an Hydropathic (medical treatment by external & internal application of water) health facility. The large palatial building's early history had been in private estate ownership; owned by the Munro family, since the Eighteenth century, until sold off in 1877 to the *Craiglockhart* Hydropathic Company. After the Great War, it would later survive as part of Edinburgh's Napier University. *Craiglockhart War Hospital* is presently known for its brief, but prominent, association with the well known war poets, Siegfried Sassoon and Wilfred Owen, and their psycho-therapeutic treatment by Dr. W.H.Rivers and colleagues. And, more recently, by the excellent fictional novel *Regeneration,* by Pat Barker (Published Viking. London.1991) and subsequent feature film, in 1997, of the same name.
97. Thomas Carlyle (1795-1881). The quote, I believe, came from Carlyle's *On Heroes And Hero Worship* (1841).
98. Barbara Robb... *Sans everything*. 1967.
99. Robert Burton (1577-1640). *Anatomy of Melancholy.* Published 1621.
100. Gustav Fechner (1801-1887). Founder of Psychophysics.

'The theory that to every psychic occurrence there corresponds a physical occurance in the material world, that "self-perceptibility" is the spiritual aspect of matter, matter being the element through which alone, inward spiritual occurances can be observed by other spiritual beings.' (*Religion of a Scientist. Selections from Gustav.Th.Fechner.* Edited and translated by Walter Lowrie. Published. Pantheon Books. USA. London. Kegan Paul, Trench, Trubner. 1946. See p.78). *On Life After Death.*(1836) *From the German of Gustav Theodor Fechner.* By Dr. Hugo Wernekke. Third Edition. Published. Chicago & London.1914.

A problem for any modern reader, in debate, I reckon, for any closed-mind or flat-earther, that revolts against *any* mention, in *any* context, of just the generic word psychic — spiritual — or with human being.

101.F.Molina. *Existentialism as Philosophy.* 1962 pb.

102.Colin Wilson. *The Outsider Cycle* (1955-1965), a series of six non-fiction books, with their central theme of then topical Existentialism. Wilson would later explore a New Existentialism and non-angst practioners, like Abraham Maslow, Rollo May, and Carl Rogers.

103.Martin Heideggar, *Being and Time.*

104.Man and His Being. *Being and Time.* (Heidegger, 1967). *Being and Nothingness.* (Sartre 1956). *The Mystery of Being.* (Marcel 1951). *Being and Having* (Marcel 1957). *The Difficulty Of Being.* (Cocteau.1966). ... The dates refer, mostly, to English Translations, and NOT the dates the books were written, or first published. I do not pretend to have read aforesaid in their entirety, or fully comprehend the texts and contexts but, where as in the 1960s I was convinced such titles and substance were nihilistic, I later realised how *very* wrong I was, in my initial dipping and obsession, wanting to explore my human self and others (its) mortal existence — how, why, what, when and where. I found, albeit in retrospect, such philosophical utterings were actually profoundly religious; whatever synopsis the authors and commentators declared to the contrary. All good stuff.

105.Heideggar's classic was not translated into French till 1978 — I read *Being And Time* by Martin Heidegger (1962 ed). See. pp.13-35. Esp intro footnote:

'.. horizon is used with a connotation ... something which we can neither widen nor go beyond, but which provides *limits* for certain intellectual activities performed 'within it'....'

106. Existential Dave told me he'd read Kafka, *many* times.
107. Louis Pauwels (1920-1997), a French journalist. Pauwels was a member of a Gurdjiff's Work Group for 15 months, from 1948. He wrote a book on *Gurdjieff,* published in 1954. A glossy English translation (Times Press) appeared in 1964, with a number of Surrealist illustrations. It was a second-hand edition, copy of the 1964 ed., that attracted my eye. It was purchased in Meynells, of East Street Chichester (the contents, surrealist illustrations, I discussed with the proprietor). A little later another more general, and more occult, popular book was published, called *The Dawn Of Magic,* in 1960, co-written with Jacques Bergier — published in English, in 1963, of which I purchased an English pb. in a later edition. But, it was the former *Gurdjieff* work, with credit and debit contributors reflections on Gurdjieff and Ouspensky et al, which I found more helpful.
108. Jean Cocteau. See *The Difficulty Of Being*. (Owen. London.1966). And see, especially, *Diary Of An Unknown* (these memoirs started in 1951) published in 1953. *See*. (Paragon. USA.1988 ed. *On Distances*. pp.163-187.) Fascinating interviews, with artists, doctors, philosophers, mathematicians, and leading scientists, in his lifetime, including Picasso, Einstein and Poincare. My humble opinion; Cocteau's honest Essays and Journals appear, in the media, as grossly under-rated.
109. Colin Wilson. *Necessary Doubt*. Fiction.1964.
110. Colin Wilson. *Mind Parasites*. Fiction.1967.
111. Colin Wilson. Note added to... Wilson was prolific, a good communicator. He published over one hundred lucid non-fiction, and fiction books, from 1956: translated into many languages.
112. William James. The abridged edition. *Briefer Course. Psychology.* London Macmillan. Holt.1892. (pp.468) ... 'Things have been doubted, but thoughts and feelings have never been doubted. The outer world but never the inner world..... of who the knower really is ...' (p467).

113. William McDougall (1871-1938). I read *An Outline of Psychology* (1923). And *Abnormal Psychology* (1926). But only dipped into his earlier *An Introduction To Social Psychology* (1908). Very much reflecting the temper of the early Twentieth Century, its merits and retrospective demerits. As Nietzsche's Superman (and Darwinism) and other evolutionists too — all were utterly abused by Hitler's (and Stalin), misuse of all studies, in human ethology. Genocide. One *major abuse,* was the deliberate adoption of Galton's Victorian (Charles Darwin and Herbert Spencer; 'survival of the fittest') Eugenics. The summary breeding out of all, deemed (political *and* handicapped disabled) weaker of our homo-sapien species, under the man-made dictator's race laws. The focus, survival of the strongest, being found among many Psychologists and Psychiatrists (even as Emil Kraepalin. See. For e.g.. *Forgotten Lunatics of the Great War*. Peter Barham. 2004. Chapter 7. How the weak progress. pp139-149) and, especially in Politics (dissenters) on designating who, or what, is *Abnormal* too, I reflected, was a weeding, often amoral, elitist trend set, experienced well into the early post-war watershed years of 1946.

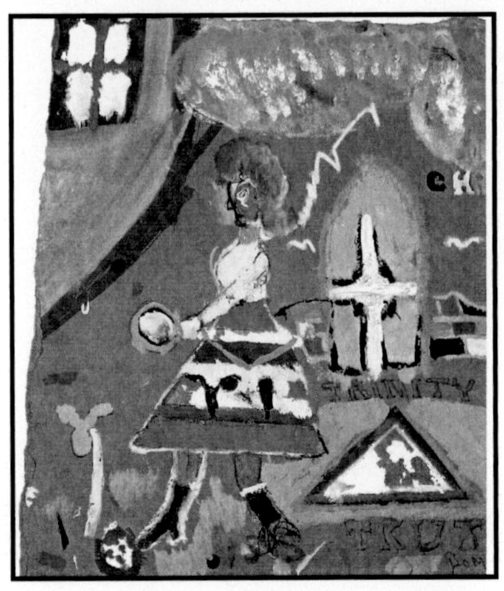

Picture of Isis on oil painting executed by temporary resident on Bramber Two ward by Will P. (aka signed Dominus). Given to author by Will on May 15th,1968.

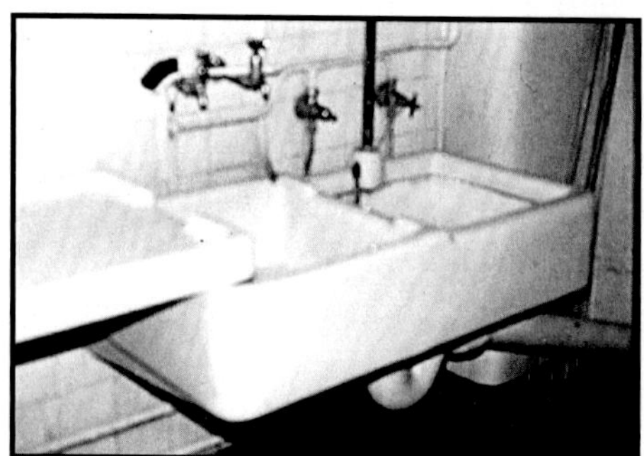

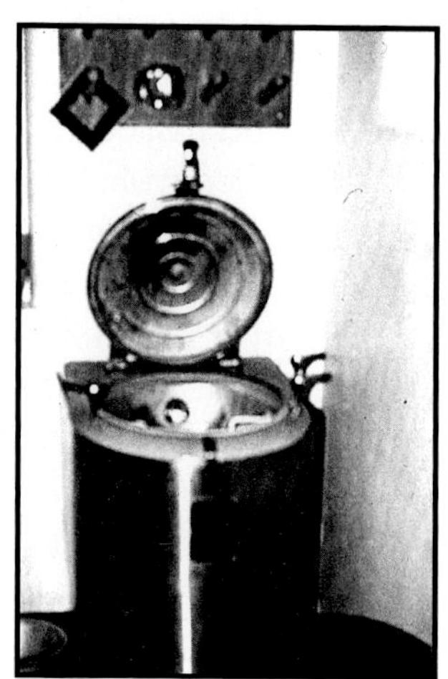

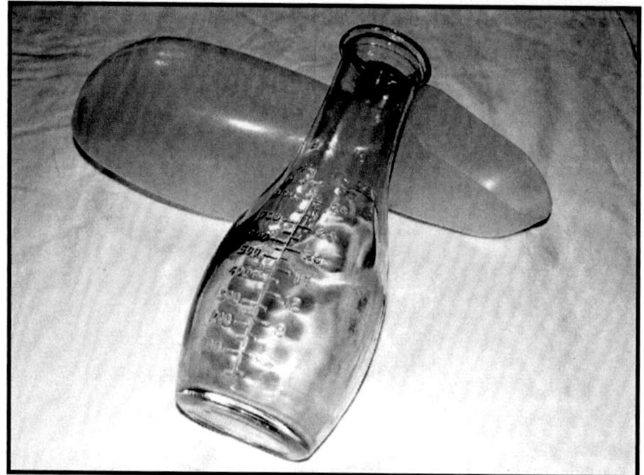

1969. Sluice Room of Chilgrove Ward and England (Sick) Ward. Thick glass urine bottles, soon replaced by plastic ones, for both males and females; boiling instruments for sterilisation replaced by CSSD supplies. Photos by author.

Notes, References and Sources. Chapter Eight.

1. T.S.Eliot (1888-1965). *The Complete Poems and Plays of T.S.Eliot.* Faber & Faber.1969. See. Play. *The Cocktail Party.* p.410. Act Two. Reilly to Edward.
2. *Outline and Recommendations of the Committee on Senior Nursing Staff Structure.* London, HMSO. 1966. (Reprinted 1969.) Aka *The Salmon Report.*
3. Anna Sewell (1820-1878). Author of *Black Beauty*, Published in 1877.
4. This new Poor Law amendment introduced, as such, *The Mental Treatment Act* of 1930, a supplement to the still valid *1890 Lunacy Acts.*
5. Mary Jane Ward (1905-1981). Mary Ward, novelist and journalist, in a USA 1946 austere book, *The Snake Pit*, based its content on her admission, whilst suffering from a schizophrenic breakdown (this seems unclear), into *Rockland State Hospital,* New York, in 1941. (This would have been well within the wartime lack of resources, and abuse in lack of essential facilities — found by fellow journalist, Albert Deutsch (1948). See Notes and refs, in Chapters Two and Seven). This was one of four believed admissions. I couldn't find any mention of Mary Jane Ward's early years, from 1905 to 1941. She was re-admitted in a further breakdown in 1957, and another in 1969, dying in 1981. The substantial gaps, between given acute episodes, are probably a good indication of support, her active lifestyle and talent. She had eight published novels, three of which were on mental illness. *The Snake Pit* was made into an Oscar winning film in 1948. (See also Ch.2, Note 57)
6. T.S.Eliot... *The Complete Poems and Plays of T.S.Eliot.* 1969. *See.* p.172. Poem *The Four Quartets.* Burnt Norden. 1.
7. William Seabrook (1886-1945). Travel writer and alcoholic, Seabrook wrote a non-fiction book called *Asylum* (1935), based on his voluntary admission into a hospital in USA, during the 1930s. The book an auto-biographical account of his treatment.
8. Magic Roundabout (English TV 1965-1977). Originaly created for French Children's television, in 1963, by Serge Danot. In Britain, it appeared to evolve, and be more for an avant garde adult audience with somewhat underground, satirical undertones of Zen and

P.J.Travers' Mary Poppins — about The Swinging Sixties. Beatles and colour of Psycheldelia:

> 'Remember the swinging Sixties, 'said Zebedee. 'A time when anything was possible; you could do your own thing, or even somebody else's thing if you wanted to.' ... 'The funny thing was, the wilder things got the more popular we became. The BBC were furious!' said Mr Rusty.' (*Zen and the Magic Roundabout Maintenance. A Brief History of Time (for Bed).* Published. Penguin. Fantail Books.1992. See. Chapter. *Peace, Love And Merchandising*.)

9. In the 1960s and Seventies, *Bob Dylan* (b.1941), *Joan Baez* (b.1941), and *Donovan Leitch* (aka *Donovan*. b.1946), were all young postwar songwriters, folk-singers, rank political activist supporters of the Civil Rights movement, anti-war, anti-Vietnam and, anti-nuclear disarmament campaigners and, supporters of exiled Russian dissenters: all sympathies reflected in their own created tuneful lyrics. And whose music was replete on Amberley and Summersdale Wards, where young patients were being admitted. Good stuff.
10. Arthur Murray's Dance Inc (See Note & Reference...)
11. *Cheque Book of Bank of Faith.* By C.H.Spurgeon. Published in 1893. Charles Haddon Spurgeon was the Baptist 1865 founder of one of the Orphan Homes Institutions in which I spent six years of my childhood, between 1944 and 1951.
12. Frank Leonard. *City Psychiatric* by Frank Leonard. Published. Ballantine Books USA 1965. And, by New English Library as pb.1966. See *Preface* of pb..
13. Ken Kesey (1935-2001). The 1975 USA film '*One Flew Over The Cuckoos Nest*' was based on a Beat novel by Ken Kesey, first published back in 1962. He'd worked awhile as an orderly, at a mental hospital in California. The male only Mental Hospital in the film was based on then Pendle Oregon Asylum (presently called East Oregon Correctional Institution). Kesey appears to have been a firm advocate in recreational drugs, including liberal use of (then fashionable) LSD. But he was, it seemed, against psychiatric patients taking *prescribed* medication. Anti-authority was the focus of the film's content; as seen in defiant main anti-hero, petty-criminal Randle McMurphy (well played by Jack Nicholson).

"Before I took drugs." said Kesey, "I didn't know why the guys in the psycho ward at the VA Hospital were there. I didn't understand them. After I took LSD, suddenly I saw it. I saw it all. I listened to them and watched them, and I saw what they were saying and doing was not so crazy after all." Slowly his first novel, *One Flew Over The Cuckoo's Nest*, came to him. (At one Trips Festival, staged by Kesey and his Merry Pranksters Jan 1966 - late 1966, the free use of the drug LSD was made illegal.) So.... at one point Kesey flashed, from a projector, "Anyone who knows he is God, please go up on stage." (*Acid Dreams. The CIA, LSD, And The Sixties Rebellion.* By Martin A. Lee and Bruce Shlain. Published. Grove Press, New York. pb. 1985. See. Chapter 5. *The All-American Trip*, pp.119-138.)

In Kesey's book, it's Columbian Indian patient Chief Broom who is the main focus. I found the Oscar winning film most entertaining. But it, in retrospect, appeared, to me, to have added to the cherry-picking (viz better patients) of political motivated anti-psychiatry, as well as advocating the closure of mental hospitals — discharging many unhappy acute disturbed pauperised patients back onto the streets, or into already filled prison wards. Only where sufficient state funds and qualified caring nursing-staff, et cetera, was in evidence — could better duty-of-care prevail. In the USA, albeit in principle, anywhere, according to its own writers and graphic documentaries, evidence of attendents, aides, wholly untrained, and even reported armed guards, stationed in some American State Hospitals.

Not many years later, in the early 1980s, as a professional, visiting one very good Mental Health Hostel in the community, I learnt that a recently taken on temporary member of staff, a University Psychology Student, had been freely giving hallucinogenic Magic Mushrooms to one of the vulnerable residents — whilst enthusiastically, privately, encouraging all the patients *not* to take their prescribed medication. The absolute incongruity of this staff member's actions appeared to be beyond him. He was dismissed, as soon as his dangerous irresponsibilties were discovered.

14. Tony Hancock (1924-1968). I was first endeared to the dour comic genius, when listening to Hancock in a BBC Radio show called

Educating Archie, in 1951. And was well hooked after 1954 when, along with loveable irascible South African Sid James (1913-1975), he appeared on the BBC in *Hancock's Half Hour.* This was heard first on radio, but then appeared, as a comedy sit-com, on BBC black and white television. *The Blood Donor* was one hilarious sketch seen during this period.

15. Tarot Cards.... Playing cards and Tarot origins have been dated back to the days of the ancient Egyptian Priests, when a Pack of Three Card sets *might* have been derived from written sets — hieroglyphic symbols, giving mystical, hidden (to the unread) information, on the three seasons (Spring, Summer, Winter) on the rize and fall flooding of the life-giving River Nile. Later history amplified the fortune and gambling playing cards of the ancient Priests (also known esoteric systems to the ancient Chinese, Indians, Jewish Cabbala, and wandering Gypsies) into European four card sets; four seasons (Spring Summer Autumn and Winter) mystical and known tangible natural (now known as scientific) predictions: if you play your cards right — and have direct computer-like brain access, to latent knowledge of the universe. (See. *A New Model of the Universe* by P.D.Ouspensky, 1931. Chapter V. *The Symbolism of the Tarot.* pp.207-241. Written. 1911-1929.)
16. Maurice Nicoll, Dr. (1884-1953). Son of Sir William Nicoll. Dr. Maurice Nicoll was friend, and close colleague, of Dr. Carl Jung and Dr. Ernest Jones. A First World War Captain in the RAMC, serving in Mesopotamia, and, back home, an associate of Dr. W.H.Rivers. Dr. Nicoll worked with injured servicemen suffering from shell-shock (aka war-neuroses). He met Ouspensky and Gurdjieff in 1921, attending their school at Fontainbleu, in France. After 1931, Dr. Nicoll adopted the ideas behind O and G's work and, till his death in 1953, taught *The Work,* based mostly in Southern England. I was acquainted with the East Sussex school, at Upper Dicker.

    (See. *Psychological Commentaries on the Teaching of Gurdjieff and Ouspensky.* By Maurice Nicoll. Published. in Six Volumes. Five on the Commentaries. (1766.pp.) by Vincent Stuart. London. (From 1952). ... and a Sixth volume, an *Index,* in 1996 by Samuel Weiser, Inc. (USA).

17. Dr. Carl Jung (1875-1961). Psychiatrist. See *Synchonicity, An Acausal Connecting Principle.* By Dr. C.G.Jung. (First published in an essay, in 1951.) Published. Routledge. London. pb.1999 ed. See. *Resume.* p.144-145. In the divine (aka Nature) sense, Jung said:

> 'By synchronicity I mean the occurrence of a *meaningful coincidence in time. ...'*

An event which I might deem an accident or fate, which cause is unknown to me, maybe influenced by a sequence or specific singular other, events and natural circumstances: but this, I appreciate, is to greatly *understate* Jung's explanation. That there is no such thing, *in reality,* as an absolute accident — in life.

18. Colin Wilson. *Mysteries. An Investigation into the occult, the paranormal and the supernatural.* By Colin Wilson. Published by Hodder and Stoughton. London.1978 *see* Appendix pp.631-633.
19. Ibid...
20. B.F. Skinner (1904-1990). Behavioural Psychologist. Following J.B.Watson and Ivan Pavlov's works on conditioning animal reflex experiments (including rats and human beings), Skinner developed *Operant Conditioning*. See, for e.g., '*Beyond Freedom And Dignity.*' Published. Jonathan Cape. London.1972 (pp.214-215).

> 'What is Man? ... An experimental analysis shifts the determination of behaviour from autonomous man to the environment ... It is autonomous inner man who is abolished ...'

21. *The Times* 6th May 1966.
22. *England and Wales. Sexual Offences No2. Bill.1967.*
23. *Journal.of Abnormal and Social Psychology*, (1963) 67, 371-378. ... See '*Progress in Behaviour Therapy. Proceedings of a Symposium.*' Edited by Hugh Freeman. Published. Bristol. John Wright & Sons. 1968. This book contained *considerable* material on (then) *Aversion Therapy* — which I had personally seen being accepted voluntarily by patients (there was *no* malpractice in Graylingwell) in practice. See, especially, *The Treatment of Homosexuality by Aversion Therapy.* M.P.Feldman (pp.59-71). This was the mid-sixties. See,

also, 'Milgram, Stanley. 1974. *Obedience to Authority: An experimental view.* Published. New York: Harper & Row.

24. The Hill, 1965. *The Hill* was the title of a 1965 GB film, the whole plot located in an army prison (glasshouse) located in the Libyan Desert of North Africa, in WW 11. Sean Connery plays the role of Roberts, an ex-Squadron Sergeant Major leader (with a duty of care for his men) of an Armoured Division, who strikes a superior officer who was ordering him, and all his men, into an obviously tactical, totally fruitless, suicide battle. And, removed from the field on his arrest, as predicted, the entire squadron are decimated. Lone survivor Roberts is branded a coward, which clearly, on the evidence supplied, he was not.
25. *The Daily Sketch,* of March 16th 1967, had reported a '*Shock Cure for a shoplifting wife.*' I expect wags had a field-day, commentating on that tit-bit of information.
26. Altshul. ... *Neurology for Nurses* by A.Altschul. Published 1965.
27. Bickerstaff. ... *Psychology for Nurses* by Bickerstaff. Published.1965.
28. John Buchan (1875-1940). ... *The Thirty Nine Steps,* by John Buchan. Published. Blackwood. Edinburgh and London. 1915. Scudder, an American journalist, after being assaulted by foreign spies and dying, gives Hannay a laconic message: *Thirty-nine steps. I counted them. High tide.10.17pm.* (Hannay is accused of the murder, and flees to search out the true killers.) The message referred to the amount of seaside steps leading up to the level of a hideaway house, from where the spies were, and would be, waiting to be picked up by enemy submarine.
29. William Sargant (1907-1988). On the Treatment of War Neuroses, also known as Battle Fatigue. See, for example, Sargant.W. and Slater. E. (1940) Acute War Neuroses. *Lancet,* 2 1.-181. And see *An Introduction To Physical Methods of Treatment in Psychiatry,* by William Sargant and Eliot Slater (1944). Published. Edinburgh: E & S Livingstone. And. Sargant.W. and Shorvon, H.J. (1945) Acute War Neuroses. *Arch, neurol, psychiat.(Chic.),* 54, 231- 181.. Most relevant. See (An illustrated American report, in an un-named USA hospital), *Battle Exhaustion. A Technique of War-time Healing that will be Useful in The Peace.* Picture Post. July 28th 1945. pp.15-18 .... See Sargant's book. *Battle For The Mind. A Physiology Of*

Conversion And Brain-Washing. By William Sargant. Published. Heinmann. London. 1957. ... And. ...*The Unquiet Mind. The autobiographiy of a Physician in Psychological Medicine*. By William Sargant. Published. Heinmann. London.1967. (My own signed, *not* to me, copy, says Will Sargant.) ... I was unclear in social history exactly what dates Dr. Sargant worked, over in the former EMS Summersdale military quarter of Graylingwell Hospital, in the 1940s. The hospital also, apart from sharing its limited accommodation with evacuated homeless civilians, maintained therapeutic and custodial care work with its full psychiatric population. I noted Dr. Ernest Jones, Freud's friend and biographer, in the 1940s, also worked with the Hospital Medical Superintendent, Dr. Joshua Carse, and his excellent staff — as *Annual Records* affirm.

30. Len Deighton (b.1929). Novelist. *The IPCRESS file*. By Len Deighton. Published. Hodder & Stoughton. London.1962. As a National Serviceman in the RAF, he'd worked as a photographer for the Special Investigation Branch, which one may infer, inevitably, made him privy to considerable, albeit classified, secret information. Deighton's detailed background research for his writings reflected real life, in wartime and postwar years into the 1960s.
31. Martin Thomas (Thomas Martin). ... A fiction writer, contributing to an historic popular genre, of hundreds of past and present detective Sexton Blake novels, written by numerous authors which date back to 1893 and *The Missing Millionaire* by Harry Blyth (Hal Merith): Sexton Blake (with his assistant Tinker), often refered to as the working-man's Sherlock Holmes. See *Sexton Blake Brainwashed. (An ex-vietnam prisoner, threatens the entire defence structure of the West.)* By Martin Thomas. The Sexton Blake Library. 5th Series. Novel 42, May 1968. Published. London. Fleetway Publications. Mayflower Paperbacks. (Mayflower 0763-8.)
32. Len Deighton. The IPCRESS file was also the title of a GB film in 1965, unbeknown to myself, and our general populace, minutiae within the fictional book and film was actually based on then still classified American CIA facts. Also, the book and film are quite different!

33. Richard Condon (1915-1996). See. *The Manchurian Candidate* by Richard Condon. Published. McGraw-Hill Book Co. USA. 1959. ... Filmed with the same title *The Manchurian Candidate* in 1962 in the USA starring Frank Sinatra. ... The novel and film drew heavily (like Len Deighton), on first-hand knowlege of wartime North Korean (imported Manchurian-Chinese psychologists) enemy, brainwashing and planting of false memories — *and* implanting sublimated new data in captured prisoners. The American CIA, in response to this fact, commenced their own experiments in brainwashing, practising on its own native people, and involuntary selected citizens using, or rather abusing, with excess LSD and other hallucinogenic drugs and wilful abuse of physiological treatments, by illegal Operant Conditioning methods (The Black Arts, sometimes called Black or Bad Science).
34. Carl Jung. ... *Synchronicity. An Acausal Connecting Principle.* 1951.
35. Tweedledee and Tweedledum. ... Tradition has it that the origin of the old nursery rhyme on the odd robust twins dates back to an earlier epigram by John Byrom (1692-1763), which included ... 'Twixt Tweedle-dum and Tweedle-dee.' In Lewis Carroll's (Charles Dodgson) book *Through The Looking Glass And What Alice Found There* (1872), the two rotund characters T and T squabble and sing the old nursery rhyme, then agree to have a battle, but never do — and go off into the wood. Updating. Perhaps like the stalemate of Nuclear opponents West versus East (Russia) and the squabble is the babble of the sterile Cold War (Jaw Not War). Tweedledee and Tweedledum prefering, rightly, the rattling of the sabres, to the prattle of a battle.
36. Australia and White only policy; now defunct since 1973 and ratified by the *Racial Discrimination Act* of 1975 (which said racially-based selection criteria was illegal). In a *pre-war* Travel Book on Australia (my father, though I have no memories of him, was of Australian birth), I read of the White policy which was *not* itself apparently based on one of superiority, but echoed a longstanding fear of an *invasion* by masses of Asians — particularly Japanese. (Refer to *The Menace of Colour*, by W.Gregory. Seeley Service & Co., London.1925. ... And. *Australia's Empty Spaces* by Sydney Upton. London. Allen & Unwin.1938. p.26.) Before the second world war,

Upton estimated that only 60,000 full-blooded aborigines, 20,000 half-castes, and 27,000 coloureds existed, in the whole of Australia. Yet, as an indiginous people, they had suffered abominably through the formal Government legislation, as exampled by the 'Stolen Generations' eugenics generation — which had, for decades, forcibly removed innocent aboriginal children from their parents, to *improve* their prospects; that policy existed from late 19th century into the 1960s — now properly defunct.

37. Bohumil. Bilek.... *Fifth Column at Work.* By B.Bilek. Published.Trinity Press. London.1945. A book replete with hundreds of items of documented forensic evidence, on the effect of wilful Fifth Column Heinleinist Storm Troopers within Czechoslovakia.
38. John Marks. See *The Search For The 'Manchurian Candidate. The Story of the CIA's Secret Efforts To Control Human Behaviour.'* By John Marks. Published. Allen Lane. Penguin Books. London.1979. Most Scientific Research (stating the obvious) is about Trial & Error and Correction. Research (e.g. MRC) involving experiments on human beings was, *ideally,* morally controlled according to the Geneva Convention, Nuremberg Code, Statutory Laws and, of course, Mother Nature's Laws. But, sadly, Social History is replete with examples of treatments given in rank *abuse* of this guiding ethic to people (with or without advocates for the vulnerable), who have not willingly submitted to such maltreatment. Marks' book had, at its core, examination of an American CIA 'Ultra Secret" ongoing project designated MKULTRA, the content of which was exposed by him after the project became declassified, revealing apparent, seen in retrospect, wanton abuse of otherwise well-intended, good standard psychiatric and psychological methods of clinical (aka medical) forms of treatment.
39. Len Deighton. (See above notes 32 & 38) *IPCRESS FILE.* First Edition.1962.
40. Martin Thomas. (See above note 31.) *Brainwashed Sexton Blake.*1968.
41. Bertrand Russell (1872-1970). *Bertrand Russell's Dictionary of Mind, Matter and Morals.* Edited, with an Introduction by Lester E. Denonn. Published. Philosophical Library. New York. 1952. See p.194..

42. Len Deighton. *The IPCRESS File* the 1965 GB film starring Michael Caine.
43. Ted Hughes (1930-1998). See *In a Piece for Radio*, printed in the monthly Journal *Encounter* of July 1965, extracted from his work, *Eat Crow*.
44. William James. *Brief Course of Psychology*. Published. Holt. 1892.

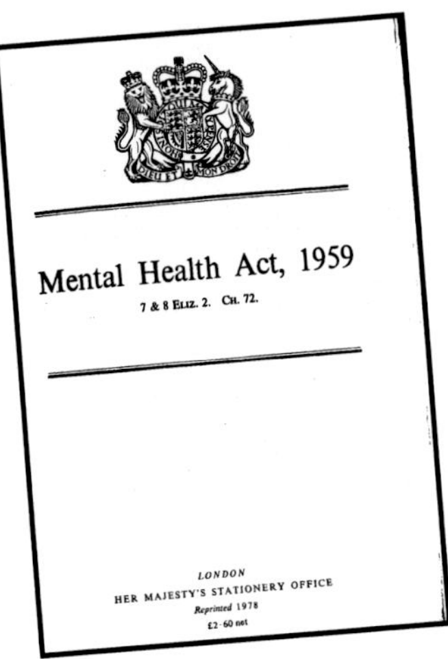

Mental Health Act, 1959

7 & 8 Eliz. 2. Ch. 72.

LONDON
HER MAJESTY'S STATIONERY OFFICE
Reprinted 1978
£2·60 net

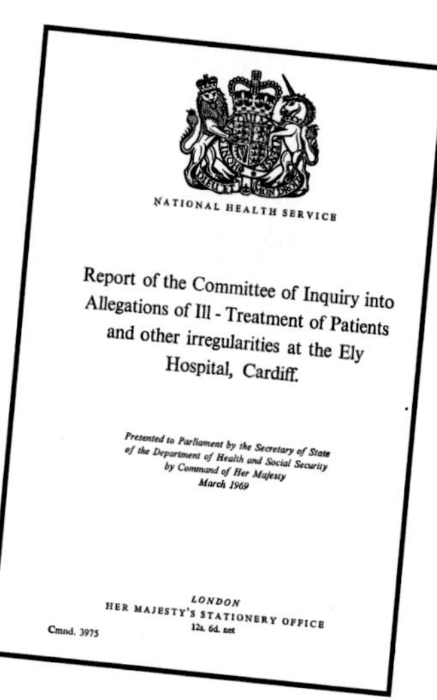

NATIONAL HEALTH SERVICE

Report of the Committee of Inquiry into Allegations of Ill - Treatment of Patients and other irregularities at the Ely Hospital, Cardiff.

Presented to Parliament by the Secretary of State of the Department of Health and Social Security by Command of Her Majesty March 1969

LONDON
HER MAJESTY'S STATIONERY OFFICE
12s. 6d. net

Cmnd. 3975

HMSO Reports. For centuries, government reports, and urgent public enquiries, pre-dated new laws and facilities, for disabled, mentally ill, and feeble minded.

Art. VII. *Observations on Madness and Melancholy, including practical Remarks on those Diseases, together with Cases; and an Account of the morbid Appearances on Dissection.* By John Haslam, late of Pembroke Hall, Cambridge; Member of the Royal College of Surgeons, and Apothecary to Bethlem Hospital. The Second Edition. 8vo. pp. 352. London: Callow. 1809.

Pinel's Treatise on Insanity. By Dr. Davis. 8vo. Sheffield. 1806.

Cox's Practical Observations on Insanity. Second Edition. 8vo. Lond. 1806.

Arnold on the Management of the Insane. 8vo. Lond. 1809.

1809. Reports, detail published, in *The Quarterly Review*; their remarks pre-dated a number of the new Acts/Laws of the 19th Century — and the coming of the mandatory County Asylums throughout Great Britain.

A COMPARATIVE VIEW OF THE CURES OF CASES OF INSANITY IN DIFFERENT INSTITUTIONS FOR LUNATICS.

No.	PUBLIC ASYLUMS.	Period	Aggregate of Cases.	Centesimal Proportions. Recent Cases.	Old Cases.	Recent and Old Cases.	Complicated Cases.
	BRITISH.						
1	*Aberdeen*	1814-15	21	—	—	—	33
2	*Bedford*	1812 to 1819	176	—	—	—	37
3	*a* Bethlem, (London) *Cured and discharged*	1684 to 1703	1,294	—	—	69	—
	b Ditto *Ditto*	1748 to 1784	8,874	—	—	29	—
	c Ditto *Ditto*	1784 to 1794	1,664	—	—	34	—
	d Ditto *Ditto*	1799 to 1814	4,830	—	—	39	—
	e Ditto *(Treatment completed)*	1817 to 1820	364	—	—	54	—
4	*Cork*	1798 to 1817	1,431	—	—	—	40
5	Exeter	1801 to 1819	615	—	—	57	—
6	*Glasgow*	1814 to 1819	457	50	13	—	41
7	Hereford	1817 to 1819	47	—	—	49	—
8	*Lancaster*	1816 to 1819	2.1	—	—	—	25
9	Leicester	1794 to 1819	483	—	—	66	—
10	*Liverpool*	1816 to 1819	135	—	—	—	30
11	Manchester	1766 to 1819	2,415	—	—	39	—
12	*Montrose*	1805 to 1818	154	—	—	—	22
13	*Newcastle* and *Durham*	1806 to 1817	402	—	—	—	40
14	*Norfolk (cured and discharged)*	1814 to 1819	243	—	—	—	48
15	Norwich . . Bethel	1813 to 1819	260	—	—	52	—
16	*Nottingham*	1812 to 1819	336	—	—	—	33
17	*Retreat* . . . (York)	1796 to 1819	253	83	35	—	44
18	St. Luke's, (London) *(Treatment completed)*	1751 to 1819	10,641	—	—	48	—
—	Ditto *(Ditto)*	1751 to 1800	5,735	—	—	49	—
—	Ditto *(Ditto)*	1800 to 1819	4,906	—	—	46	—
19	*Stafford*	1819	116	—	—	—	26
28	*Wakefield*	1819	138	—	—	—	19
21	York	25 years	2,445	—	—	45	—
—	Ditto	1815 to 1819	134	45	12	33	—

No.	PUBLIC ASYLUMS.	Period	Aggregate of Cases.	Centesimal Proportions. Recent Cases.	Old Cases.	Recent and Old Cases.	Complicated Cases.
	FRENCH.						
22	*a La Salpetriere*	1804 to 1813	2,749	—	—	62	43
—	*b* Ditto	1806 to 1807	——	86	—	—	55
23	*Bicetre*	1807 to 1813	1,196	—	—	—	45
24	*a Charenton*	1803	499	—	—	—	36
—	*b* Ditto	1806	363	—	—	—	42
25	*Armentieres* . . *(Maison de Detention)*	1811	94	—	—	—	3
26	*Lille* . . *(Ditto)*	1811	88	—	—	—	1
	ITALIAN.						
27	*Genoa*	1816	138	—	—	—	2
	GERMAN.						
28	*Vienna* . . *(Joseph's II.)*	1803 & 1804	1,116	—	—	—	36
29	*Berlin* . . *(La Charite)*	1806 to 1818	2,190	—	—	—	43
30	*Sonnenstein* . (Saxony)	1814 to 1816	189	24	—	—	12
31	*Celle* . . (Hanover)	1816 to 1818	204	—	—	—	32
	PRIVATE ASYLUMS.						
	BRITISH.						
32	*Laverstock*	1817 to 1819	150	71	—	—	51
33	*Droitwich*	to 1816	619	76	17	—	45
34	*Spring Vale*	to 1816	144	84	35	—	60
	FRENCH.						
35	*a Dr. Esquirol's* . . (Paris)	1801 to 1813	335	—	—	—	52
—	*b* Ditto		66	—	—	—	62
36	*Dr. Dubisson's* . . (Ditto)	to 1816	300	—	—	—	59

(1) Parl. Rep. 1816. App. p. 41. (3) *a* Stow's Survey of London, chap. 26. *b* Haslam's Observ. &c. p. 245. *c* Ibid. p. 249. *d* Parl. Rep. 1815, p. 131. *e* Ann. Rep. (4) Hallaran on Insanity, edit. 2. p. 34. (5) Ann. Rep. (6) Ibid. (12) Parl. Rep. 1816, App. p. 21. (16) Ann. Rep. (18) Ann. Rep. (21) *a* Hist. York Asylum, App. p. 6. (22) *a* Rap. sur l'etat des Hopitaux, &c. a Paris. *b* Carter's Acc. of Foreign Hosp. 1819. (23) Rapport, &c. (24) *a* Dict. Scien. Medic. tom. xvi. p. 204. *b* Compte rendu de l'Admin. centr. en 1807. (25) Annuaire statistique du Depart. du Nord, annee 1813, p. 184 et suiv. (26) Ibid. (27) Fodere, Traite du Delire, tom. i. p. 588. (28) Ibid. p. 587. (29) Report of La Charite, 1818. (30) Dr. Pienetz's Rep. (Nasse's Journ.) Nov. 1818. (31) Dr. Bergmann's Rep. April, 1819. (32) Dr. Finch's Private Commun. and Parl. Rep. 1815, p. 50. (33) Parl. 1816, p. 45, 51. (34) Ibid. 1815, p. 128. (35) *a* Dict. des Scien. Medic. tom. xvi. p. 201. *b* Esquirol sur les Passions, &c. p. 22. (36) Du Buisson, Traite des Vesanies, p. 38.

*** The Return for Liverpool (No. 10) is very variable: when a sufficient number of pauper lunatics is received into this Asylum from the neighbouring parishes to fill a public conveyance, they are transmitted to Lancaster County Asylum. This practice equally affects the results of both Institutions.

ART.

1821. Quarterly Review, Statistics. Bethlem and St. Lukes served a number of Sussex patients — but, no deemed incurable (after 2 years) who were returned to their parish workhouse, or alternative facility. Under the old Poor Law their care paid for by their local parish poor law, contributed by relatives where possible.

Statistics — In Great Britain only Bethlem and St. Lukes were known in art and literature: in France — Charenton.

LECTURES ON CONDITIONED REFLEXES

Brainwashing. A few works read, or consulted specifically, on brainwashing in BCTC - mostly negative accounts - **mostly about gross and wanton abuse of otherwise valid psych treatments used for betterment of ill patients.** .....

1. *Ward 6.* Dr Anton Chekov. 1892.
2. *Lectures on Conditioned Reflexes.* Prof. Ivan Pavlov. 1928.
3. *World Film News.* August 1937.
4. *Fifth Column At Work.* B.Bilek. 1945.
5. *Night and Fog.* Resnais. Film.1955.
6. *Mental Seduction and Menticide. The Psychology of Thought Control & Brainwashing.* Joost A.M. Meerloo. 1957.
7. *Battle For The Mind.* Dr. William Sargant. 1957.
8. *The Manchurian Candidate.* Richard Condon. 1959.
9 *IPCRESS File.* Len Deighton. 1962.
10. *Ward 7.* Valery Tarsis. 1965.
11 *The Unquiet Mind,* Dr. Williiam Sargant, 1967.
12. *Sexton Blake.Brainwashed.* Martin Thomas. 1968.
13. *Beyond Freedom and Dignity.* Prof. B.F.Skinner. 1972.
14. *Obedience To Authority.* Prof. Stanley Milgram. 1974.
15. *Russia's Political Hospitals.* Vladimir Bukovsky. 1977.
16. *Operation Mind Control.* Walter Bowart. 1978.
17. *The Search For The Manchurian Candidate.* John Marks, 1979.
18. *Acid Dreams, The C.I.A., L.S.D., and the Sixties' Rebellion.* Martin Lee and Bruce Shlain. 1985.
19. *A Russian Madness.* John Collee. Article, *Observer Magazine.* 28 June 1992
20. *Eye Of Vichy.* Film. Chabrol. 1993.
21. *Brainwash. The Secret History Of Mind Control.* Dominic Streatfield. 2006.

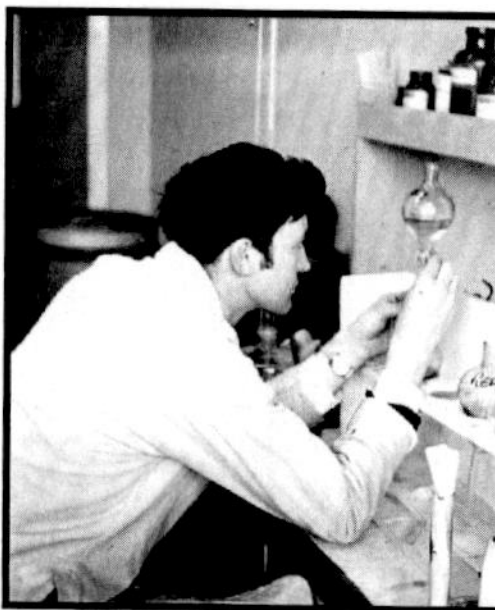

Notes, References and Sources. Chapter Nine.

1. Dr. Maurice Nicoll. *'Psychological Commentaries.'* 5 Vols. Published. London. Vincent Stuart.1952. See. Vol.Three. Quaremead, Ugley. June 1, 1946. See. *Commentary On Memory*. p902.
2. See *Volume II*. Paperwork. Lists & Forms.
3. Ibid.
4. Ibid.
5. *The Mysteries Of Purity*. Al-Ghazzali. Translated by N.A.Faris. Published. Lahore. 1966. ... A Holy book on Good Hygiene. As a centuries earlier historic Persian *Zend Avesta*.
6. Houghton. ... *Practical Nursing*. By M.Houghton & M.Whittow. Published. London. Balliere, Tindall and Cox. pb. 1965.
7. Karl Jaspers (1883-1969). Philosopher and Psychiatrist. (See notes 8 &10 below.)
8. Jaspers. ... *The Future of Mankind*. By Karl Jaspers. (1958.) Translated by E.B.Ashton. Published. Phoenix books. The University of Chicago Press. pb. 3rd impr 1963:

   > 'World peace rests on two premises: First, on *free* will — right and justice are to rule instead of force. Second, on *reality* — the human world is not and will never be one of right and perfect justice, but man can strive to make progress on the road to justice.' (p.17.)

9. H.G. Wells (1866-1946). *Mind At The End Of Its Tether.* Published 1945. Wells' last published book during his lifetime.
10. Karl Jaspers. ... *General Psychopathology.* A seminal psychiatric textbook, on the aetiology of human emotions. Published in German in 1923 and 1946. And published in English (my second-hand copy) in 1963 by the Manchester University Press. Translated by J. Hoenig, M.D., D.P.M.. and Marian W, Hamilton, B.A. Oxon. (See note 7 & 8 above.)
11. Rumi (1207-1273). ... known also as Jalal ad-Din Muhammad Balkhi-Rumi. Persian poet.
12. Acronym PTSD ... post traumatic stress disorder. See. *Shell Shock to PTSD. Military Psychiatry from 1900 to the Gulf War.* By Edgar Jones And Simon Wessely. Published. The Maudsley Monagraphs. Psychology Press. Hove. 2005. PTSD, originally termed Post-Vietnam Syndrome, was formally defined in 1980. See *Glossary of*

Diagnostic and Other Terms, (under) *post traumatic stress disorder (PTSD)* on p.234.

13. Colin Wilson... *Introduction Of The New Existentialism* (1966). London. Hutchinson. ... See also *New Pathways Of Psychology* (1972).
14. *The Great Escape*. By Paul Brickhill. Published. Faber And Faber.1951. The true life wartime episode took place on September 23, 1944. Seventy-six allied airmen prisoners escaped from a 120 foot tunnel from Stalag Luft III, located in Eastern Germany at Sagan in Silesia; only three escaped, the rest were recaptured. Although known *not* to be spies, fifty of the caught escapees were murdered by the Gestapo, on direct instruction from Hitler. Of the ill-fated fifty, 28 were non-British, including several Poles, Australians, New Zealanders (one - a Maori), Canadians, Czechs, Norwegians, South Africans, A Frenchman, A Greek, and a Lithuanian. Of the 76 but three escaped recapture - two Norwegians and a Dutchman. Four Brits escaped again later on. An epic tale. (See update. Letter. *The Guardian*. April19th 2008 p.29.) I had no idea what connection our exhausted dying man, k/a Colonel (not a RAF rank) to us, had with the *aftermath* of the 1944 incident. Subsequently, I never made any enquiries. It was unlikely that our bedded patient the ex-Major, located only yards away from him, had any inkling of this sad silent terminal 1968 drama of a fellow wartime survivor.
15. Dr. A.J.Cronin (1896-1981). Book, *The Citadel*. Published. Gollancz.1937. Film *Citadel,* starring Robert Donat in 1938. And, later, author of books on Dr. Finlay's Casebook.
16. The following list of bibliography suggests past reccommended introductory textbooks for all RMPA student nurses existent in the 1940s and early postwar years; the works indicate a wartime emphasis on Physical Treatments for Mental Illness. ... *Modern Mental Treatment. A Handbook for Nurses*. By E.Cunningham Dax M.B., B,S., B.Sc. Lond., D.P.M. Medical Superintendent Netherne Hospital, Coulsdon (Surrey). Published. Faber & Faber, London.1947. ... See also, *Physical Methods of Treatment in Psychiatry*. By (Drs) Sargant and Slater, Published. E & S Livingstone, Edinburgh.1944 (For senior nurses). ... *Shock Treatment in Psychiatry,* By Jessner

& Ryan. Heinmann. London.1942 (Advanced details on convulsion therapy and insulin coma treatment). ... *A Study Of Hypoglycemic Shock Treatment In Schizophrenia,* by Isobel G.Wilson. H.M.Stationary Office. London.1937. ... *Psychosurgery.* By Freeman & Watts. Chas.H.Thomas. Baltimore. (On prefrontal leucotomy). ... *Psychiatric Nursing.* By K,N. Steele. Publ. F.A.Davis Co. Philadelphia. 1944. (American textbook on hydrotherapy and other treatments.) ... *Psychiatry. Theory and Practice for Students and Nurses.* By (Dr.) H.C.Beccle. London. Faber & Faber.1947. (For English students of psychiatry.)

17. See *Appendix. Appendix One*. Annual Reports.
18. Therapeutic. ... E.g.., *Family Psychiatry* By John G, Howells. M.D.. D.P.M. Published. Oliver & Boyd. London. 1963.
19. West Sussex County Asylum (Graylingwell) Hospital *Regulations* 1897.
20. *Modern Mental Treatment. A Handbook for Nurses*. By E.Cunningham Dax. Faber & Faber. 1947. (And enclosed hand-written notes on CO2 Therapy, for patients in early neuroses)...
21. *Picture Post*. 4th June 1949. See article on p.29. *I worked in a Snake Pit* by Joan Skipsey, a journalist for the *Topeka State Journal.*
22. Carl Soloman (b.1928). ... His father was the successful publisher of USA *Ace Books*. ... See *The Beat Generation & The Angry Young Men*. Edited by Gene Feldman and Max Gartenburg. Published by the Citadel Press. New York. 1958. The Beat Generation were a group of young American postwar writers and Angry Young men (Part Two) included a number of English postwar writers. Part Three included literary *critics* from both sides of the water. ... See. Part One pp.153-163. *Carl Solomon. Report From The Asylum.*
23. *Neurotica* magazine, published by Jay Landesman 1948-1951. See Spring ed 1950. Allen Ginsberg (1926-1997) at one time spent eight months in *Rockland* Mental Hospital, where he met Carl Soloman (where he, too, was then a temporary patient). Ginsberg's long poems *Howl* (1956) and *Kaddish* (1961) reflected considerable compassion for his sick mother suffering from mental illness, and recorded in his writings. Subsequently, Ginsberg's long-poem *Howl* was dedicated to his new friend, Carl Soloman.

    The first line of *Howl*, often quoted, said:

> I saw the best minds of my generation destroyed by madness, starving, hysterical, naked, dragging themselves through the negro streets at dawn looking for an angry fix, angelheaded hipsters burning for the ancient heavenly connection to the starry dynamo in the machinery of night...'

Ginsberg's well chosen metaphor of *madness* and *heavenly connection (*initially through dangerous, and destructive, drugs and false prophets of *angry fix* but, later, more mature, by Yogic Meditation and Zen Buddhism) was concrete *and* multi-layered. His mother, and some of his Beat writer friends (or close relatives) suffered from bouts of diagnosed mental illness, and admission into Psychiatric Hospitals, sometimes, a result of illicit drug-taking. At the end of 1954, Ginsberg met Peter Orlovsky, a high school drop-out who was in the Korean conflict as an Army medic, and became his lifelong friend. Peter's brother, Lacifado was, like Ginsberg's mother, suffering from a mental illness. (Sources. *City Light Books*. *Howl* and *Kaddish*. The Pocket Poets Series. San Francisco. 1956-1968. And.... update. *Google & Safari* Search Engine. Biographies of Allen Ginsberg and Carl Soloman. 19.04.2008.)

But, in the 1960s and Seventies, few of my known contemporaries had experienced, read or ever heard of the middle-class Beat, University graduate (or drop outs) writers — until Ken Kesey's *One Flew Over The Cuckoo's Nest* (Beat book 1960, but as happy Hippy film 1975). The USA recorded *Woodstock,* a three day Music Festival August 1969 (film 1970), of Peace *Man*, Music and Love, with lots of cannabis and LSD tabs and free love (if you could afford it), this introduced the new Hippy Movement, of the Sixties and early Seventies — which appeared to have replaced the angst Beatniks with the happy Hippies. But, again, at first, the Jazz Beat and happy Hippy movement firmly identified with Bob Dylan, Donovan and Joan Baez and this more monied, optimistic, postwar generation of university students as well as easier accessible illicit hallucinogenic drugs, related psychedelic rock music and protest folk songs against Vietnam and, worse, potential nuclear war. Exit World War Two.

24. Kalinowski ... *Shock Treatment,* initially called Electo Shock Therapy (EST) had an element of risk — not just a temporary loss of memory — but back or other muscular injuries could be side-effects, in the

simulated convulsion. This was later solved when Scoline (curare), a muscle clinical control drug, was introduced to the treatment, which itself was renamed Electro Convulsive Therapy (ECT). It would remain a controversial treatment — though, as I witnessed, ECT, in moderation, was quite successful in reducing rank idiopathic (clinical) depression. Reactive depression, by definition, needed time, possible psychotherapy. Talking out, how to what when and where so, conceptually working on its probable aetiology.

I soon realised that to a *well* member of our community, any and *all* forms of physical attempts at treating sympathetically *any* form of diagnosed mental illness is suspect. Unlike any physical affliction (fracture, etc.) or clinical disease (measles, etc.), when a remedy is accepted. There can *never* be a *total* quick fix for *all* Mental Illness, no more than one specific *elixir* will cure every sickness.

25. *Illustrated* magazine. 1947.
26. *Illustrated* magazine, February 8th, 1947.
27. Limbo 90. ... *Limbo 90*. By Bernard Wolfe. Published. Penguin pb.1952. A graphic novel depicting a future imagined pessimistic science-fiction world, forty-years on, made *possible* by its robot electronic, cybernetic operators in 1990.
28. Norman Weiner (1894-1964). After the war, Weiner refused to do any further research work for government (with its ongoing destructive interference), especially on Military Projects — on ethical grounds. See. Cybernetics: *Or the Control and Communication in the Animal and the Machine*. Published. Cambridge, MA: MIT Press.1948. ' The first (known) *digital* computer was built in 1944, and started working at Harvard University.' See the futurist non-fiction. *The World In 1984. Volume 1 (of two). The Complete New Scientist Series*. Edited by Nigel Calder. A Pelican Original pb. Published (1964). Penguin pb 1965... *A World Dominated By Computers?* by Dr. M.V.Wilkes, FRS. University Mathematical Laboratory, Cambridge. pp.147-150. ... Weiner's 1948 book was much used by Wolfe, in Limbo 90. Progress.

'A man-made *man* was unveiled at a research laboratory in Azusa, California, today. It can breathe, blink, open its jaws (revealing a fine set of teeth), react to drugs, and move its tongue. "Sim I." first of a series of "human simulators"...' (*Daily Express*. Saturday March 18 1967. p2.)

A mechanical robot - a zombie of the future to be, I thought, when I read this report. In the 1960s I recall computers were also known as *electronic morons,* whatever prospect of motorised AI — artificial intelligence envisioned: a new abacus in the making. Machines being built to run a lazy world. Wells and Asimov had it well sussed.

29. *Limbo 90*. ... See p.6 and back page of the 1952 Penguin pb edition.
30. *Picture Post*. Letters ...
31. *Picture Post*. December 1946. ... *Grateful Reader*. Name and address supplied.
32. *Picture Post, John Bull* and *Illustrated*. 1930s-1950s weekly magazines.
33. Herbert Spencer (1820-1903). English Philosopher and contemporary of Charles Darwin's (1809-1882) *Origin Of Species* (1859). Herbert Spencer's *First Principles* (1863). I recall little of Spencer and his, what seemed obvious, survival of the fittest species, through *force*, whether it be divine (aka nature biology and botany) or human influence; it seemed more *political* than Darwin — the latter absorbed me for sometime in the early 1960s..
34. Dr. A.J.Cronin (1896-1981). (Refer above note 15). Dr. Cronin served as a Royal Navy surgeon, during World War One. And spent sometime working as a young physician, in a Glasgow Private Lunatic Asylum, which greatly and sypathetically served him well, in the years ahead. See. *Adventure In Two Worlds*. Autobiography. Published.1952. ... Dr. Finlay was originally written as a rural Scotland family doctor, in the 1920s village of Tannochbrae. Remodelled for BBC television (1962-1971) as Dr. John Finlay (known as an ex-Major RAMC of 1946) and viewed, I believed, as warm but vulnerable, sometimes volatile and quixotic, but always sincere. This became a very popular soap series, *Dr. Finlay's Casebook,* eagerly watched on the hospital wards of Graylingwell Hospital, in the 1960s and early Seventies. See, *On Call with Doctor Finlay*. By Peter Haining. Published. Boxtree.pb.1994.
35. *Adventure in Two Worlds*. (Autobiography). Published. 1952. See above note.
36. *Strand* magazine collection, 1895.

GRAYLINGWELL HOSPITAL - CHICHESTER
(NB: ALL FIGURES FROM OFFICIAL ANNUAL REPORTS AND RECORDS)

YEAR	BEDS		YEAR	BEDS		YEAR	BEDS
1898	452		1936	1055		1974	641
1899	478		1937	1064		1975	654
1900	505		1938	1065		1976	602
1901	544		1939	1063		1977	572
1902	699		1040	1051		1978	587
1903	695		1941	1042		1979	583
1904	727		1942	1074		1980	591
1905	751		1943	1053		1981	562
1906	767		1944	1056		1982	519
1907	770		1945	1056		1983	504
1908	766		1946	1080		1984	486
1909	796		1947	1062		1985	461
1910	763		1948	1101		1986	436
1911	676		1949	1105		1987	431
1912	777		1950	1117		1988	367
1913	816		1951	1124		1989	309
1914	795		1952	1123		1990	299
1915	WHP		1953	1129		1991	264
1916	WHP		1954	1149		1992	247
1917	WHP		1955	1167		1993	???
1918	WHP		1956	1140		1994	273
1919	WHP		1957	1092		1995	258
1920	538		1958	1061		1996	266
1921	602		1959	1022			
1922	665		1960	1016			
1923	740		1961	1055			
1924	738		1962	1061			
1925	746		1963	1039			
1926	750		1964	1022			
1927	787		1965	1030			
1928	843		1966	1038			
1929	877		1967	1020			
1930	882		1968	964			
1931	913		1969	892			
1932	941		1970	827			
1933	962		1971	768			
1934	997		1972	732			
1935	1023		1973	643			

STATISTICS: NOTE: **WHP** = WAR HOSPITAL PERIOD

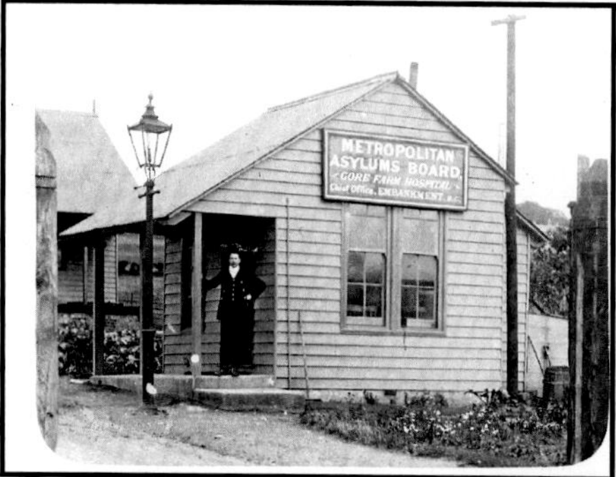

M.A.B. (Metropolitan Asylums Board (London)), Gore Farm, Established 1878. Training colony for young feeble minded — Pre WWI. Photo PC nd.

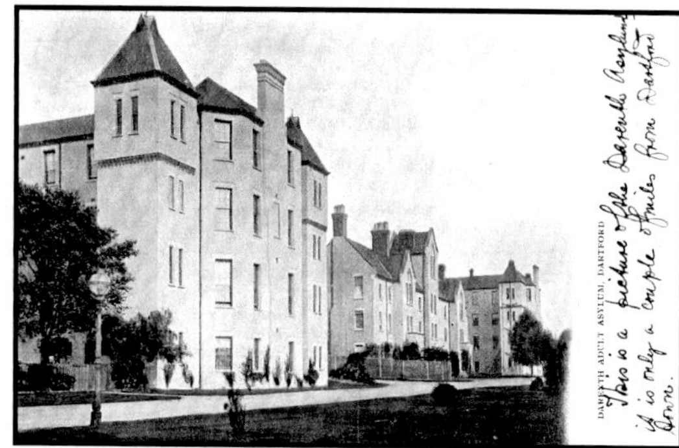

Darenth Adult Asylum, Dartford. Established in 1878, in 1967 Darenth Park recorded 1,868 MS beds. It was closed and demolished in 1988. Photo PC 1904.

On a routine home visit to Worthing, in the 1980s, to a Mrs T. (who was then in her late seventies) she told me, that: 'Sixty years or so ago, when 18 years old, I worked at Darenth Asylum. Most of the Mentally Handicapped were so bad that they were incurable. And we fed them in cells, with a slot at the bottom, where we put the food in — and pushed it in.' 'Surely', I asked, 'they must have been only for the very bad — dangerous?' 'No', she replied. 'Most of them (severely mentally handicapped adults in asylums) were like that — then.' On further enquiry, she did not recall any deliberate cruelty in the 1920s and thirties — but conditions and facilities were quite austere. I compared the memories of Mrs T. with my 1970s visit to Coldeast — and Highdown, Worthing (for example): and excellent published, compassionate, pictures by Lord Snowdon: Conditions of the mentally subnormal, persons with learning difficulties, in the 1980s; much improved. (In the UK, we knew very little of treatment for the Mentally Handicapped, in the 1920s.)

Notes, References and Sources. Chapter Ten.

1. Dr. Harold Kidd. Medical Superintendent. *West Sussex County Asylum* (Graylingwell Hospital). See. *Annual Report.*1905.
2. Reverend George Crabbe (1754-1832). Cleric-poet *and* pre-Dickens. Crabbe exposed the horrific living conditions for far too many of the nation's post-Napoleonic sick, lunatic, poor and unemployed — during an inevitable economic crisis, cost of the long wars, during his lifetime. (See also Chapter Seven, Note 94.)
3. Ibid. Crabbe k/a *Letter 18.*
4. Ibid.
5. *Sussex Daily News,* 29.11.1893. One notable 'of Selhurst' published, in a letter, an oblique objection to the Chichester Architect's proposed sum of £7,000, estimated for the new *West Sussex County Asylum*'s staff and patients detached stone church. It would eventually be opened, led by The Bishop of Chichester himself, in full pomp and ceremony.
6. Bob Dylan ... *The Times They Are A'Changin'* (1964). Title of one of his topical songs, in the Hip 1960s.
7. *Sunday Times. Supplement.* 29.09.1968. The excellent article was entitled *Mental Hospitals. A Suitable Cause For Conscience. Report D.A.N. Jones. Photographs; Snowdon.*
8. Dr. Samuel Johnson (1709-1784). *A Dictionary Of The English Language* (1755). See, The Twelfth Edition. London.1807.
9. RMPA. *Handbook for Psychiatric Nurses* (Red Handbook). Ninth Edition. Edited by (Dr.) Brian Ackner. Published. Bailliere, Tindall & Cox. 1964. ...
10. Nigel Walker. ... *Crime and Insanity In England.* Vol.1. The Historical Perspective. by Nigel Walker. Published. Edinburgh Paperbacks. Edinburgh University Press.1968. p.25.
11. *Cases Of The House Of Lords.* Published in a large Folio dated 1769.
12. Ibid. The case was about innocence and *idiocy* and of the *Royal Prerogative* Statute, which protected the inheritance of an idiot to be managed by whoever was properly *entitled* and protected by law, and owed a supposed duty of care to the so named.
13. In a *Google* Search, 28.8.2006. for a *Sutherland Clan* family tree.

14. The Law then stated that No woman could legaly inherit a title, only the eldest son, but Elizabeth was an only *surviving* child. Hence the legal conundrum.
15. Ibid.
16. Latin text. See. *Appendix* of *Breave,* (1769) No iv.
17. *Mental Deficiency Acts,* Implemented 1914, and its *Amendments*, 1925, 1927 and 1930 Acts. Considerable delay in improvement of real resources was unhelped by the events of the *First World War,* and many wrongful diagnosed *moral idiots,* uncounted shell-shock NYD casualties, placed in local parish workhouses; in epileptic and lunatic *(Insane)* wards. There was also a mis-directed classification in a jaundiced, so-called scientific Darwinian eugenics policy, still practised during the 1920s. In between the two world wars, poor social conditons existed for the deemed mentally subnormal, with a termed learning disability. Yet; *The Royal Prerogative* duty of care statute, prevailed. Presumably *only* for those who *owned* property — not humane reasons; ergo, there were insufficient funds under the existing Poor Laws.

    See. *Royal Commision On The Law Relating To Mental Illness And Mental Deficiency.* 1954-1957. HMSO. Report, and *Report of the Committee of Inquiry into Allegations of ill - treatment of Patients and other irregularities at the Ely Hospital, Cardiff.* (Wales). March. 1969. HMSO. And. *Put Away. A Sociological Study of Institutions for the Mentally Retarded.* By Pauline Morris. Foreward by Peter Townsend. Published. London. Routledge & Kegan Paul. 1969. Of special interest see. *Forgotten Lunatics of the Great War.* By Peter Barham. Published. by Yale University Press. 2004.
18. See. Graylingwell Hospital *Annual Reports* of the 1960s.
19. *The Hollies.* American music pop group of the Sixties and Seventies. *He Ain't Heavy, He's My Brother,* was a Single Ballad, record released in the UK, September 1969.
20. Ibid.
21. William James (1842-1910). ... (See also Chapter Seven. Note 10):

> 'Our non-sensational, or conceptual, states of mind, on the other hand, seem to obey a different law. They present themselves immediately as referring beyond themselves. Although they also possess an immediately

given 'content' they have a 'fringe' beyond it, and claim to 'represent' something else beyond it....' See *Psychology*.1892. p.465.

22. Robert Graves (1895-1985). One of several letters I received from him, and his wife Beryl Graves in 1971.
23. Henry Gray (1827-1861). British anatomist cartographer. *Gray's Anatomy* 1858.
24. William Harvey. (1578 -1657). *On the Motion Of The Heart And The Blood In Animals*. Published.1628.
25. Maurice Merleau-Ponty (1908-1961). French existential philosopher, who wrote against behaviourism in psychology. See.*The Structure of Behaviour* (1942).
26. Maurice Merleau-Ponty. *The Visible And The Invisible*. 1968. (See. *Working Notes*. December 1960.)
27. Jean Cocteau (1889-1963). Cocteau's classic French film *Orphee* (1950) was a modern adaption of the Greek myth of *Orpheus and Eurydice*. A second film, *Testament d'Orphee* (1959), was also made on this theme. In death does dream become the reality or reality is it but a brain in a dream — a polemic on after-death, and possible rebirth. 'Alice' and Cocteau as shadows 'through the looking glass', et cetera.
28. Dr. Samuel Johnson (1709-1784). One oft quoted origin of the metaphor Black Dog, certainly known by poet William Cowper and Dr. Johnson, was from a classic Latin myth, quoted by Roman poet Horace Flaccus (65-8 BC), in which a sighting of a *black dog* with pups was an unlucky omen. An image much used in future horror books (the devil in the shape of a black dog in Goethe's *Faust*) and film scenarios. Johnson described his melancholia (depression as), 'The Black Dog I hope always to resist ...'
29. Winston Churchill (1874-1965). Churchill referred to the Black Dog, as metaphor for his bouts of depression.
30. William Cowper (1731-1800). ... Probably much closer to biological truism (to the black dog), are references to the presence of *black bile* issued by the spleen, To Robert Lloyd. 1754. ... 'Are gloomy thoughts led on by Spleen,' during bouts of suicidal melancholia, as described in autobiographical poems of William Cowper. ... He'd private means to fund his occasional acute admissions into the St. Alban's Private Madhouse owned by Dr. Nathaniel Cotton. (1705-

1788.) (See. *The Correspondence of William Cowper*. By Thomas Wright. In Four Volumes. Published. London. Hodder and Stoughton. MCMIV. See esp Vol.One. 1763, p.11 & p.22 - incl footnote)

31. Ibid.
32. *Life And Letters*. September 1930. Vol V. No 28.
33. Antonia White (1899-1980). ... A pseudonym for Eirene Adeline Botting.
34. Antonia White. *Beyond The Glass,* by Antonia White. Eyre & Spottisworde.1954.
35. Ibid.
36. Ibid.
37. *Life And Letters*. Sept..1930.
38. Dr. Oliver Sacks (b1933). English neurologist. (A Brothers Grimm fairy tale (1812-1815) called *Sleeping Beauty,* a long sleeping Princess is awakened suddenly, by a handsome Prince's loving kiss. Another fictional variant was Washington Irving's (1783-1859) comatosed time traveller, Rip Van Winkle (1820). There are many other such stories.) See non-fiction *Awakenings* by Oliver *Sacks.* Published. London. Gerald Duckworth.1973 ... Film starring Rober De Niro and Robin Williams *Awakenings* USA 1980.
39. Antonia White. ... *Beyond The Glass*. 1954.
40. Watkins of 19 & 21 Cecil Court, off Charing Cross Rd. London.
41. Upper Dicker studies. For serious students interested in *The Fourth Way.*
42. Horatio Bottomley (1860-1933). Politician, businessman, orator, petty criminal and imprisoned swindler. But he was also the founder, in 1888, of the *Financial Times* and one time owner, from 1914, of the English patriotic weekly magazine *John Bull*, of which as child and young adult, I was a much later, avid reader. (See *The Rise and Fall of Horatio Bottomley.* By Alan Hyman. Published. London. Cassell.1972.) The popular magazine, *John Bull,* was added to my early reading, the *Illustrated* and *Picture Post* — as well as my wartime and postwar children's comic heroes, in the *Champion, Hotspur, and Wizard* and, *Captain Marvel (Marvel Family)*, and The Hulton Press early 1950s comic, the *Eagle*. By the time of the late 1960s most, if not all, of the previous listed 40s and 50s comics and weeklies had folded, and departed, like the *Boy's Own Paper*.

And, of course, deceased, like versatile rogue MP Horatio Bottomley. *His* ashes were scattered nearby Alfriston, on gallops of the Sussex Downs. He'd kept race horses in stables in the grounds of his estate at *The Dicker* (Upper or Lower Dicker) in East Sussex.

43. P.D. Ouspensky (1878-1947). See *The Fourth Way A Record of Talks and Answers to Questions based on the Teaching of G.I.Gurdjieff.* Published. Routledge & Kegan Paul. London.1957.
44. Miss Marjorie Incledon (1899-1973). .... ' *A Pupil's Postscript. Beryl Pogson teaching the Fourth Way.*' By Bob Hunter. Published. Eureka Editions pb.1998. See p.441, about Prof Tolkien's *Lord of The Rings:*

> 'A cousin of the author, Marjorie Incledon, was in The Dicker group, and she seemed to me to have an affinity with Tolkien's turn of mind and humour.' (I agree.)

See also. *Work Talks at The Dicker* 1966. By Beryl Pogson. Booklet. Quack Books. York. pb. (Re-published 1994.)

45. John Locke (1632-1704). ... Philosopher. (See note 46 below.)
46. John Locke. ... *An Essay concerning Human Understanding.* Published in Four Books. Written by John Locke, Gent. The Fifteenth Edition. 1760. (Two Vols). See. Vol. One - Book.2. p.121 on *Discerning.*
47. Plamil. Mechanical Cow. ...*Typescript* of B.B.C. T.V.1. Broadcast on April 3rd 1968, in TOMORROW'S WORLD. Speaker: Raymond Baxter.
48. Lord Sir Hugh Dowding (1882-1970). ... Known as Hugh Caswall Tremenheere, later, 1st Baron Dowding of Bentley Priory (1943), from where near Stanmore in Middlesex he'd directed RAF fighter command in the Battle of Britain, from 10th July to 12th Oct 1940, as the British Air Chief Marshal of the Royal Air Force. *The Battle Of Britain* and Lord Dowding's *world of experience* greatly affected my grandparents, parents, and my own recent wartime generation, to a very high degree.... From all that I read and heard about him, from those that knew him (and his good lady), this so-called 'stuffy' man, all was good and kindness, and of humility and greatness in substance. But I had some difficulty in comprehending his 'Spiritual' side, its love rays (so Christian it appeared) and description of giving that love to many war victims, civilians and servicemen, and of

true mediumship (many survivors suffering *mental illness* as a result of the war) in application. It became self-evident that this faith was not only part of the man - it was *the man* with absolute integrity.

See. *Leader Of The Few.* (Preface By Lord Dowding.) By Basil Collier. Published. Jarrolds. London.1957. And also. *Dowding And The Battle Of Britain.* (Foreward by Lord Dowding). By Robert Wright. Published. Macdonald. London. 1969. Of special interest. Dowding's own writings. *Twelve Legions Of Angels* by H.C.T.Dowding. Published. Eyre and Spottiswoode. London.1941. (Ref. The *Star* newspaper. 28.10.1941). *Many Mansions.* By Air Chief Marshal. Lord Dowding. Published. Psychic Book Club. Rider & Co. London (nd).... *Lynchgate.The Entrance To The Path.* By Air Chief Marshal. Lord Dowding. Published. Rider & Co.1945. ... *The Dark Star.* By Lord Dowding. Published. Museum Press. London.1951 .... *God's Magic. An aspect Of Spiritualism.* By Air Chief Marshal. Lord Dowding. Published. The Spiritualist Association Of Great Britain. London. (nd). ... And see his wife's. ... *The Psychic Life of Muriel, The Lady Dowding. An Autobiography.* (Formerly published under the title *Beauty Without Cruelty.*) A Quest Book USA.1982 pb. Originally published as *Beauty - not the beast.* Spearman 1980. Lord Dowding (she wrote, see pp.92-93) was instumental in repealing through the House of Lords, a defunct Witchcraft Act of 1735, and introducing a *Fraudulent Mediums Act* in 1951, which meant proving wilful fraud (this motion would have pleased Conan Doyle and Harry Houdini). A film called *The Battle of Britain* was released in 1969 starring Sir Lawrence Olivier as Lord Dowding, for which Olivier met the ex-RAF Air Chief Marshal, then aged 87 years.

49. John Cowper Powys (1872-1963). ... *Autobiography* 1934. By John Cowper Powys. ... See 1967 reprint. Published. Macdonald: London. (intro by J.B.Priestley.) See Chapter Eight. *Burpham.*
50. Bertrand Russell (1872-1970). ... *The History of Western Philosophy* (1946).
51. P.D.Ouspensky. ... *In Search of the Miraculous* by P.D.Ouspensky. Published. Routledge & Kegan Paul.1950. I wonder if Dave ever found and read a copy of this work.

52. George Gurdjieff ... Mancurian Dave was referring to the body of The Work.
53. Arthur Koestler (1905-1983). ... *The Ghost in the Machine* 1967.
54. *The Champion*, a children's wartime comic, with its hero, an RAF *Spitfire* boxer and pilot called Rockfist Rogan (like Biggles), who fought in the Battle of Britain.
55. Dr. Ernest Jones Psychoanalyst. See Graylingwell's *Annual Report.*1943.
56. Brenda Wild, a Graylingwell Staff Nurse RMN colleague, recalled the incident.
    (Years later, in 2010, Dr Joyce's (Dr Vawdrey's) son, David Vawdrey, would tell me details of this on the ward incident, and how dramatic it really was.)
57. Mary Jane Ward's 1947 USA book & 1948 fictional film of *The Snake Pit.*
58. *The Picture Post*, May 21, 1949. See page 23.
59. Boys Own Paper (aka BOP)...
60. *Practical Mechanics* magazine.. Published. Newnes. January 1937 edition. A then very popular English schoolboy's monthly magazine.
61. Science Fiction pulp magazines. *Astounding Science. Weird Tales. Galaxy.* See. *Astounding Days: A Science Fictional Autobiography.* By Arthur C. Clarke. Published Gollancz,1989.
62. Robert Heinlein (1907-1988). The script of the 1950 film *Destination Moon* was written by Robert Heinlein; its semi-documentary style was intended to be as realistic as was possible, without the visual benefits of advanced technology, available in future film-making; as in A.C. Clarke and Stanley Kulbrick's GB 1968 film scenario of *2001: A Space Odyssey.*
63. Arthur C.*Clarke* (1917-2008). See non-fiction *The Explorations of Space.* By Arthur C.Clarke. Published. Temple Press Ltd. London. 1951.
64. Ibid. ...*The Explorations of Space.* See pic. facing p.87. (Lord The Air Chief Marshal Sir Hugh Dowding and Flight Lt. (Sir) Arthur C. Clarke served in the RAF and contributed much towards the factual and futuristic science-fiction, of radar; about ideas on terrestrial and outer-space tele-communications potential, based on existent *rays* of radar. ... See. Short story, *Sentinel of Eternity,* by

Arthur C. Clarke (this submitted to The BBC in 1948, and rejected). First published in a science-fiction pb. magazine, in *10 Story Fantasy.* Spring 1951.Vol.1. (as) *Sentinel of Eternity.*

65. *Another World or The Fourth Dimension* by A.T.Schofield, M.D. Sonnschein. 1890. *Four-Dimensional Vistas* by Claude Bragdon. Routledge 1916. Einstein's *Theories of Relativity* 1905 & 1915. Ouspensky's *Tertium Organum.* 1922. Hinton - & others. There were (are) many writings, indeed experiments, realised in order to find and define existent territory, anticipated as 'beyond' the known present chemical elemental table. Elements we humans have realised, in biology, alchemy chemistry and Kabbalah form; from the nanotechnology lightest atom in gas and heavenward *en soph,* down to the most heavy, seen (there's an oxymoron) and detected. All elements are designated in a space lexicon as separate, singular *and* generic classification in geometry and physics. *The Fourth dimension*, as fact and metaphor, therefore includes, in past time; aether, ectoplasm, rays, traces, threads, strings; whatever metaphors in a lexicon, which in truth recognises abstract and elemental constructs — as yet exact *beyond* human knowledge.
66. Bertolt Brecht (1898-1956), and Frank Wedekind (1864-1918). Two German dramatists who defined, in their writings, an honest vision of social reality in their country.
67. Lulu ... The principal tragic heroine in Wedekind' s play *Pandora's Box* (1903), later made into a graphic silent film released in 1929. ... See. *Lulu in Hollywood.* By Louise Brooks. Published. London. Hamish Hamilton.1982. ... And. *The Threepenny Opera* 1931 film, by the German director G.B.Pabst (who also directed Pandora's Box) from a stage play by Bertolt Brecht (1928), a grim social satire, updating John Gay's 1728 *The Beggar's Opera* into an ugly European post-war economic poverty, depravity and madness, caused by the late unfinished Great War and immediately prior to the worse horrors to come with the rise of Adolph Hitler, in the early 1930s. (As an anti-nazi, Brecht fled Germany for Scandinavia and the USA in 1933). See *Three-Penny Novel.* By Bertrolt Brecht, Translated from German by Desmod I. Vesey. Verses translated by Christopher Isherwood, Published by Bernard Hanison Limited. London I958.

In Brecht's opening Chapter, *Survivor, he* aptly sets the tone in this graphic work:

> 'A soldier, by the name of George Fewkoombey, was shot in the leg in the Boer War, so that the lower half of his leg had to be amputated in a hospital in Cape Town. When he came back to London he received £75, in return for which he signed a paper stating that he had no more claims on the State. ...'

The British Pension system, for war veterans, had little changed in the aftermath of *The Great War* (only 100 years before had been the Napoleonic Wars) and the abject poverty for war-wounded and their families under the Parish Poor Law is well documented. (See above, in an already classic study e.g.., Peter Barham's, *Forgotten Lunatics of the Great War.')*

68. Film ... *See. Singin' in The Rain USA* 1952, starring Gene Kelly, Donald O'Connor and Debbie Reynolds. ... There was a title song, with the same name, in a *Hollywood Revue Of 1929* - released in 1929.
69. Antonin Dvorak (1841-1904). Whilst for years I recognised the music of *The New World Symphony,* I certainly had no idea what it was called. ... And as for *Goin Home ...*

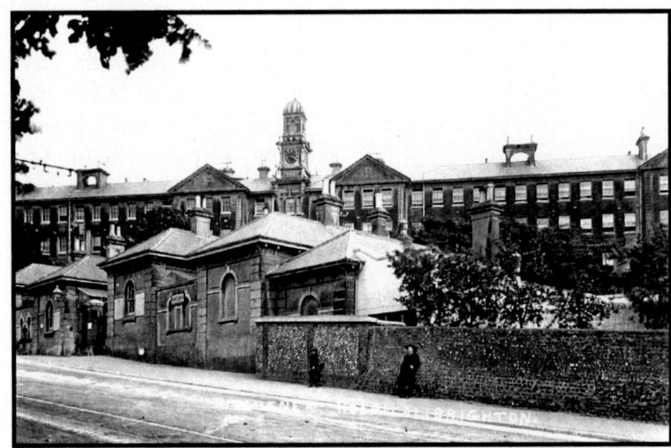

Brighton Workhouse at the top of Elm Grove, a workhouse, from 1865; later, Brighton General Hospital. In the 1960s (and afterwards) I introduced ex-patients, and helped them to 'move on' to this casual ward (such as Vagrant Joe, see C.4); here you can see it adjacent to the road. I visited, and found the unit excellent in every way — still, an old workhouse ward.

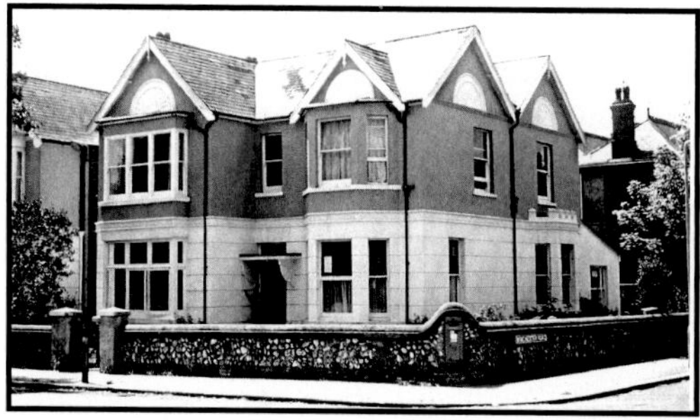

Left: 1980s. The Shakespeare Road Mental Health Hostel, Worthing. Overseered by Stonham and a local Management Committee (professional and voluntary agencies). I was a Chairman of this facility for several years, in the early 1980s.

Right: Hostel stall at Charity Fete, in Courtlands grounds, Worthing. Local MIND and Stonham Staff, and hostel residents around the food stall, during Summer 1985. Centre right is a picture of Joy King, then manager of Shakespeare Road Hostel; left, centre is Mr. Cyril Grant, who supported the charity of Stonham by helping to fund the Hostel.

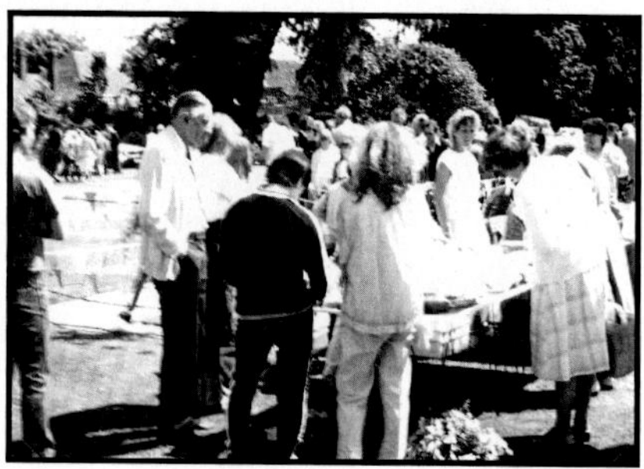

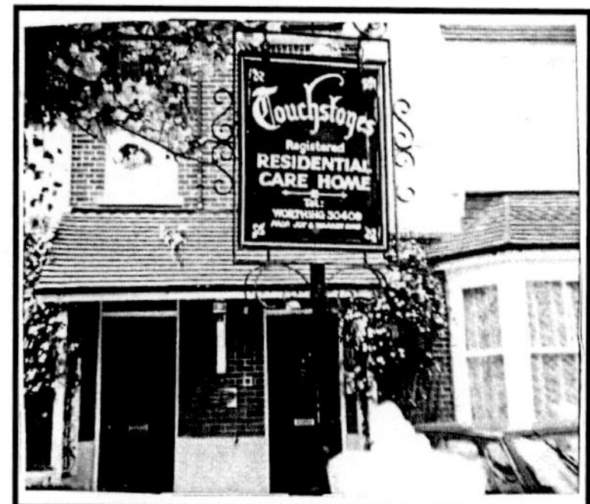

Left: Touchstones Rest Home, situated in Worthing; one of a number of registered rest homes that took discharged patients from Graylingwell. Joy later left the Stonham Charity facility, and founded her own down the road, an excellent private facility; very successful. I placed a number out of Graylingwell — my patients still there, more than 10 years later.

Above, are examples of Community Care facilities, in the early 1980s, for ex-Graylingwell patients, who were in need of continuing care (but free to come and go, at will); they were funded (at least in part) by the local authorities, and DHSS benefit agencies — including pocket money. I regularly visited both Shakespeare Road , and Touchstones (as well as many others) until my retirement in 2000. Photos by author.

Notes, References and Sources. Chapter Eleven.

1. Charlotte Bronte (1816-1855). Aka Currer Bell. See. Mrs. Gaskell.1810-1865. See. *The Life of Charlotte Bronte* by Mrs. Elizabeth C. Gaskell. 1857... Published by Smith & Elder.1900 edition. p595.) From a letter by Charlotte Bronte dated February 15, 1853, to Martha Brown.)
2. *Mikado 1885* ... lyrics by Sir W.S.Gilbert (1836-1911) :

   ' As some day it may happen that a victim must be found. I've got a little list — I've got a little list.'

3. The DRO ...The Disablement Rehabilitation Officer established a formal link, working with the DHSS unemployment bureau. *Egham* was one of the rehab re-training centres which ran set training courses, with a view to preparing attenders with newly acquired industrial skills in order to gain full or part-time paid employment. One DRO worked regularly with Graylingwell Hospital IT unit. I knew him quite well, as a liaison with *Hago Products* of Bognor Regis — an excellent local employer.
4. Probation Officers ... The government Probation Service (pre-war and wartime, sometimes known as *Police Court Missionaries*) would experience many radical changes, in the years ahead. At this time in the 1960s and early Seventies, their officers, in addition to following up discharged prisoners welfare, also did considerable *preventative* work in the NHS and in the Community Social Services, with recovering Mentally ill and, Handicapped children, adults and families. I became a great admirer in the high quality of their often *Sisyphus* Welfare Work, and would befriend one dedicated Senior Probation Officer and his family, during the 1970s.
5. MS (*not* psychiatric) was the acronym for Mentally Subnormal. See *The Hospitals Year Book* 1967 (published annually for the NHS and other caring profession administrators). This reflected firm divisions in the various *diagnosed* patient categories of that time; thus *Graylingwell* listed as 1,200 beds for *Mental Illness; Roffey Park* Rehabilitation Centre, a small unit, in Horsham, West Sussex, with 117 beds for *Neurosis* patients; *Worthing* (*General*) *Hospital,* designated for 197 *acute* beds; *Royal Earlswood Hospital,* Surrey, for 675 beds *MS* (Mentally Subnormal). The foregoing, but

a small sample of the many which were divided. There were collective thousands of filled beds in Mental Illness (long-stay Psychiatric) and, collective thousands in separate large Mental Subnormal Hospitals and ESN (Educational Sub-Normal) institutions, and local Day Centres.

6. *St.Lawrence ... St Lawrence's Hospital*, Caterham, in Surrey, had austere provision for 2,218 MS beds. *Coldeast Hospita*l, Nr Southampton, had provision for 622 MS beds.
7. Lord Snowdon (b.1930). During the early 1960s he became a picture Editor for the *Sunday Times,* and rightly established as a renowned documentary film photographer. (Photographer. Anthony Armstrong Jones e.g.; *London*. Published by Weidenfeld & Nicolson. London.1958.) See the compassionate report published in the *Sunday Times Supplement* of Sept. 29th 1968.
8. I gained an academic post-registation *'Diploma in Psychiatric Care of Children*' from this unique unit - Dr. Chris Haffner its Head of Department. I attended *Portsmouth Polytechnic* during 1971-1973 whilst working at St James' Hospital Children & Parents Unit. Subsequently, I gained promotion to Charge Nurse, working for a period as a Night Superintendent at *The Wessex Unit*. Then, moving on to the Worthing Social Services Department, in Crescent Road, for the West Sussex County Council; first qualifying as a generic social worker, later as a specialist Social Worker in Mental Health.
9. Group Captain Leonard Cheshire, VC. OM. (1917-1992). ... In 1948, he founded the charity *Cheshire Foundation Homes For The Sick.* An early Home was *Le Court,* at Liss in Hampshire. My Graylingwell colleague, Admin Baz, recalled the hospital giving a large donation, including surplus beds stored after the closure of the wartime EMS Summersdale Hospital military unit, to help establish Gp Captain Cheshire's first Home.
10. Dr. Maurice Nicholl (1884-1953). ... *Dream Psychology.* By Maurice Nicoll. Published. Hodder & Stoughton. 1917. (See Second Edition.1920 p.ix. Footnote. (See. Symposium in *Journal of British Psychology,* 'Why is the "Unconscious" Unconscious?' by Maurice Nicoll, W.H.R.Rivers, and Ernest Jones, vol.ix, part 2, October 1918.) Dr. Nicholl had said, 'I believe that dream symbolism is a *primary* form of expression, ...' (1920 ed. p.ix) To date (early 2008,

finishing this manuscript), I'd been unable to track down a copy of this incredible (to me) worded Symposium.

But. A postscript. At long last, after years of wanton search for a copy of the 1918 Nicoll, Rivers & Jones, 'symposium' transcript, and Dr. Nicholls written reply to the 1918 Question as to " Why is the 'Unconscious' Unconscious? " After one of my routine visits to *Watkins* in Cecil Court during the early 2000s, I obtained a pb copy of Beryl Pogson's (she'd been his secretary for fourteen years) *Maurice Nicoll. A Portrait* - first printed in 1961. In this biography (p.57) she recorded:

> 'On 16th July 1918 Dr. Nicoll contributed to a symposium held at a Joint Session of the British Psychological Society, the Aristotelian Society and the Mind Association. To the question — 'Why is the "Unconscious" Unconscious?' Dr. Nicoll's reply was summarised thus: 'Because life is a process of progressive evolutions, and the context of the healthy conscious mind requires to be closely adapted to reality if the individual is to be successful. Therefore, the progressive transmutations of psychic energy are carried out at levels beneath consciousness, just as the progressive transmutations of the embryo are carried out in the womb of the mother, and it is only the comparitively adapted form that is born into waking life. Thus from this point of view we must regard the unconscious as the inexhaustible source of our psychic life, and not only as a cage containing strange and odious beasts.'

In May of this year (1918), Dr. Nicoll gave a course of lectures at the University of Birmingham, on Psychotherapy, at a post graduate course in Crime and Punishment. In the autumn, Dr. Nicoll was appointed to the staff of the Empire Hospital for Officers in Vincent Square, where he had begun his work on shell shock. (See also. *Better Court Than Coroners*. Chapter One. Notes & References. No.7.)

11. Mr and Mrs. Maclintock's surname is a *pseudonym;* like his popular wife (our Aggie aka Mrs. Mac), her husband was an RMN, formerly employed at this hospital.
12. Dr. A.J.Cronin (1896-1981). See *On Call With Doctor Finlay*. By Peter Haining. Published. Boxtree. London. pb. 1994.
13. The Brown Family. Brown, an obvious pseudonym of the *Green* family; Uncle Cecil Green (Farm foreman), Father (Shepherd and dairyman) Ronald Green; Mother Nellie Green. And their two daughters - *Shirley Wingham* nee Green and a Graylingwell long-serving Staff Nurse RMN

and here, as yet, un-named. The dialogue in this book is extracted from a lengthy Chichester video film transcript, (dated 1st February 1995) taken for me by a colleague, CPN John Donnabie; with myself interviewing Mr & Mrs. Green and their married daughter Shirley. It was also the occasion of Mr & Mrs. Green's Golden Wedding anniversary. The family were all well aware I was collecting first-hand information from staff and ex-staff employed at Graylingwell Hospital for a history, yet to be written at sometime or other. It was a delightful, informal, event, in which I gathered some wonderful warm-hearted Graylingwell memories, photos and ephemera, of the family, their hospital patients and other staff, dating back through and before the war, and (via Uncle Cecil) back into the late 1920s.

14. Shirley Wingham, nee Green. Daughter of shepherd Ronald & Nellie Green.
15. National competitive Prize winning dairy and other Graylingwell farm stock.
16. From tape recording of the Green Family, dated 1st February 1995.
17. See *The Woman who wrote Black Beauty,* by Susan Chitty. Published by Hodder and Stoughton, London.1971. pp123-124.
18. See. *The Life and Letters of Mrs. Sewell* by Mrs. Bayly. Published. James Nisbet. London.1889. Third Edition, pp 127-129. Anna's Mother, Mrs. Sewell, was a published writer and a charitable *District Visitor* (Church social-worker). Daughter, Anna, then aged 37 years, in 1857. Her leg injury was sustained when 14 years old, this physical disability worsening (later to contract tuberculosis, phthsis) was away in a sanatorium, and due to return home to Grayling Wells after treatment for her condition:

> 'Anna's back and chest are better, feet quite lame, and her head not much better. I expect she will return in May (1857).'

On one of my frequent visits to second-hand bookshops I purchased a gem of a find. It was a small green paperback of poetry by Mrs. Sewell called *Children of Summerbrook.* Five Scenes of Village Life. Described in Simple Verse. Published. London. Jarrold And Sons. (nd.) Tenth Edition. Sixty-Fourth thousand. The copy has an inscription to: 'Ada Ford, from Miss Bryant. Dec. 21st 1869.' At the rear of the book is printed a full page of seven previous literary works of Mrs. Sewell as read to Ragged Child Schools. First verse of *Summerbrook.* (Read):

> *'Away from all the noise and air Of cities and of towns, A little village lay concealed Amongst the Sussex Downs....'*

On examination of the little green book's content, there was little doubt that the verses described Chichester's *Summersdale,* and the vicinity of *Grayling Wells* in the mid-1850s or so. Certainly her mother's good books were well read by Anna Sewell, as she grew up.

19. Anna Sewell (1820-78). With her Quaker parents resident in *Grayling Wells,* north of Chichester (there were *at least* two nearby farm wells in use). After living in Sussex, and latterly in Chichester awhile in the mid-1850s (and, a year abroad for treatment), Anna moved to *Blue Lodge* Wick In Gloucestershire for six years (1858-64). Her home dwelling ... 'stood within a drive of Bath and Bristol between the mining villages of Liston and Wick ... on a high hill .' (*Chitty.* Ibid p129.) Anna, now quite infirm, finally settled up north in Norwich from 1867-77 where, mostly house-bound, she composed her only but profound (in its care and charity towards the duty of care towards animals — horses in particular) novel. The work was written whilst resident in *The White House,* at Old Catton in Norwich. The full title of the published First Edition of her book was, '*Black Beauty : his grooms and companions. The autobiography of a horse....*' Published by Jarrold & Sons in 1877; twenty years after she'd left Graylingwell. Anna died shortly after its publication, in 1878.
20. See. *Better Court Than Coroners. Volume II.* Forms & Lists.
21. Ibid.
22. *See.* A GB monthly magazine. *World Film News.* August 1937 p.9 and p.23.
23. Frank Capra (1897-1991). The pre-war adventure film, *Lost Horizon,* USA 1937, was directed by Frank Capra, but much ' re-cut' (to Capra's chagrin) before distribution. I wonder what substance was removed by the censors, rather than copy editors, in social comment that *might* have reflected that awesome pre-war time.
24. John M. Huston (1906-1987), son of actor and producer Walter Huston. Two gritty wartime made documentary films directed by John Huston,

The Battle of San Pietro (1944) and *Let There Be Light* (1946), were banned during the war from the general public, and the latter classified by the USA, for thirty-five years. The film, San Pietro, is a record of the USA 143rd of the 36th Infantry Division. It's a bloody 30 minute record of battle for the control of the Liri Valley in Italy, in late 1943. On completion, in 1944, the film was first banned, even to the military, but in 1945 General George C. Marshal reversed the ban for viewing by the US military in training. The second film, completed in 1946 as *Let there be Light,* was ordered by the Government (Top Secret) and directed by John Huston. A select team of cameramen, of the US Signal Corps, were drafted in to a Rehabilitation Unit in the *Mason General Hospital,* on Long Island in New York. Mason's patients, war wounded survivors, were initially diagnosed with psychological, psychosomatic symptoms but, as the cameras recorded, these were not symptoms of abnormalities, but the result of attrition. What in the Great War had been experienced as war neuroses, shell shock; the *unendurable* horrors of war. *Let there Be Light* was eventually de-classified in 1980.

25. See. *Volume II*. Graylingwell Hospital. *Social History*. 1897-2008.
26. My Mikado forensic List, of *anti-war* documentary films, included the following printed films — but I was aware that, in censorship, the cuttings floor was replete with deemed *not pretty* footage. And sanitised versions were often the norm, for destined public viewings:

1945. April. *A Painful Reminder,* a British Army Documentary, filmed in the German *Belsen* Concentration Camp (Film advised by Alfred Hitchcock) after its capture. The film was banned from the public for forty years, as being too factual and too horrendous for public consumption. (Shown as sequel to English ITV3 television showing of the mammoth 1973 World At War series, in 1985.)

1955. *Night and Fog*, An half hour authentic documentary on The Camps by the French Director Alan Resnais and collated for the French Archives.

1964. *The Great War. 1914-1918.* A series of global stitched documentaries, produced and collated by the British Broadcasting Corporation television network.

1969. *The Sorrow And The Pity.* A Documentary by French director Marcel Ophuls which was banned from French television for many years, though available elsewhere.

1973. *The World At War. 1939-1945.* Another global stitched series of documentaries for British television, this great work narrated by Sir Laurence Kerr Olivier.
1985. *Shoah* . A documentary by Claude Lanzmann on the Nazi extermination of the European Jews in Poland.
1993. *Eye Of Vichy.* A Documentary by French director Claude Chabrol, composed solely of original propaganda films made during the war; and released in Vichy occupied France for public consumption at the total and ultimate direction of Nazi Dr. Paul Joseph Goebbels, Propaganda Minister of The Reich government of Vichy occupied France.

27. One Nation decrying another for its racial policies of genocide, whilst practising its own duplicity, deceitful brand of being an *Exclusive Club.* In truth, with all outside others being deemed second-class citizens or, worse, unwanted foreigners as aliens. And combined within all of this material, I found considerable commercial media presented buckets of crocodile copy, in a lucrative World Of Entertainment scenario. The handicapped, physical and social, disabled on display. Racial. *Miscegenation Laws,* against mixed marriage, long abounded throughout the world and, *sans* charity, restricted many health and social services to but a few. Not preach but matter of fact to live and deal with.
28. *Introduction to the New Existentialism.* By Colin Wilson. Published by Hutchinson. 1966. see p27.
29. For one long, but brief moment, I had, *had,* an inner vision of a medieval Boar's head with an apple in its mouth being served at a frolicsome banquet; and envisioned a Biblical *Salome* looking up at the severed head of *John the Baptist*; even a rich cooked Christmas turkey. Worse, momentary... I thought of Pierre Boulle's *Planet Of The Apes* debating, perhaps, the animal parts of the less-than-apes humans; and, converting humans from slaves into food or soap, perfume, shoes... or other gross products. But, I couldn't hack this range of insights for too long, and slipped back into my trace normalities. Though, as this anecdote describes, I, too, store and submerge such images; rather than erase, and drop them down-and-out, on to my inner cuttings floor. And my sympathy to John, Jean Paul Sartre *and* for too many other war-time captives, found in where-ever occupied countries; it was, is, *their* living *ironic* reality.... as concentration camp survivors, like Primo Levi....

30. Max Muller (1823-1900). ... See. *Theosophy or Psychological Religion. (Collected Works of Max Muller.* Vol 4 *The Gifford Lectures 1892.)* Published. Longmans, Green and Co. London. 1917. .. .See. *Lecture VI.* on *The Problem of the Origin of Evil. (The eschatology of the Avesta.) See* pp.177-205.
31. Max Muller. Ibid. See p.184.
32. Advocates of anti-psychiatry, like writings of Foucault. Goffman and Szsaz.
33. Colin Wilson. *Introduction To The New Existentialism.* By Colin Wilson. Published. Hutchinson. London. 1966.
34. Jack Kerouac (1922-1969). On the Beat. (See. Chapter Eight. Notes & Refs. No.13. and. Chapter Nine. Notes & Refs. No.22)
35. Colin Wilson. *Introduction To The New Existentialism.* 1966.
36. Abraham Maslow (1908-1970). Pyramid of Needs. (See. Chapter Seven. Notes & Refs. No.83.)
37. John G. Howells (b.1918). ... See *Family Psychiatry.* By John G. Howells M.D., D.P.M Published. Oliver & Boyd, Edinburgh and London.1963. (A copy of which was presented to me as a prize by Graylingwell Hospital Chichester Management Committee for. Progress 2nd Year 1968 / 1969.)
38. *Playboy* magazine. *Interview* with Jean-Paul Sartre. May 1965.
39. *Playboy* magazine. *Interview* with Jean-Paul Sartre. January 1966.
40. Jean-Paul Sartre. Essay 1944. *La Republique du silence.*
41. Arthur Koestler (1905-1983). *Spanish Testament* by Arthur Koestler Published Gollancz. 1937.
42. Norberto Bobbio (1909 - 2004) . *The Philosophy Of Decadentism. A Study In Existentialism.* By Norberto Bobbio. Translated by David Moore. Published. Oxford. Basil Blackwell 1948. See. Bobbio's book's *Appendix. The Decadentism Of Sartre.* pp 53-60.
43. Bobbio. Ibid. p56. ... See also. *The Feast of Unreason.* By Hector Hawton. Published. Watts & C0. London.1952 p 7, & p151:

> ' Professor Noberto Bobbio was too harsh when he described Sartre as "the perfect incarnation of the decadent intellectual," but I can sympathize with such an outburst.'

44. Jean-Paul Sartre (1905-1980). See *Being And Nothingness* (1956 ed):

> 'Nothingness does not itself have Being, yet it is supported by Being. It comes into the world by the For-itself and is the recoil from fulness of self-contained Being which allows consciousness to exist as such.' (p.632).

Erm! A vacuum doesn't have Dr. Brian Joyce consciousness, or does it? I only *know* of my Human awareness — I *know* nothing, of no-one or anything else, Being but a metaphor.

45. Norberto Bobbio. Ibid. (See. Note & Refs 42 and 43)
46. Dictionary dated 1684. *An English Expositour Or Compleat Dictionary Teaching. The Interpretation of the hardest words, and most usefull terms of Art, used in our Language. First set forth by J.B. Dr. of Physick* ... Seventh time revised. ... By a Lover of the Arts. Cambridge. Printed by John Hayes, Printer to the University, and are to be sold by H. *Sawbridge* at the Bible on *Ludgate*-hill, *London.* 1684. In the *Preface to the Reader,* it states the earlier and first edition (no date given) was 'begun by Dr. John Bullocker', a practising physician, presumably, during the mid and early Seventeenth century. I often dipped into this gem, which I found in a secondhand Chichester bookshop in the 1960s. And, yes, it existed during my London ancestor Dr. Thomas Manton DD's family's lifetime. I was aware that the First Edition, its author Dr. J.B., had lived before the Plague and Great Fire of London. The 1684 English Dictionary and an authentic lexicon, a worthy original trace.
47. Oliver Cromwell (1599-1658). ... (See. *Oliver Cromwells Letters & Speeches with Elucidations*. By Thomas Carlyle (1846). Three Volumes Complete In One. Published. Ward Lock & Co. London. (n.d.) pp.727-729.) At *the* formal declaration of the new Protectorate, Dr. Thomas Manton, in 1653 was reluctantly 'persuaded' – *or else* – by militant Oliver Cromwell himself, to clarify the new Protectorate's (1653-1658) parliament by formal prayers. Subsequently, Mr Manton was elected as one of Cromwell's (the King's) chaplains. Despite being a non-conformist, Manton was not only *against* the recent Regicide, but supported bringing back from France of King Charles (King Charles the Second) – having demonstrated this loyalty in attending the earlier 1651 execution scaffold of his Puritan friend Christopher Love, and his funeral, despite open hostile threats of Cromwell's troops. Dr. Manton was (again, or else) to attend all future parliamentary sessions.

> " And Mr Manton by prayer, recommended his Highness, the Parliament, the council, the Forces by land and sea, and the whole Government and people of the The Nations, to the blessing and protection of God." (See. *Cromwell's Letter* CCIII. Friday, 26th June. 1657.)

48. Dr. Thomas Manton DD. (1620-1677), also known as Mr Thomas Manton. Puritan Divine, Cromwellian dissenter and later in service to Charles the Second. (See Note & Reference No. 47 above.) What is a Puritan. What is it to be pure and untarnished? Just what is Purity — its implications as a concept, and impossibilities.
49. The absolute. Purity and its designated names. See Frederick Nietzsche's ass, in 1899 *Thus Spake Zarathustra.* And his *A Book For All And None.* And, also, Arthur.C.Clarke's 1953 *The Nine Million Names of God.* Invented words, ciphers literary symbols, icons in recognition of existential unknown, and its hidden elements.
50. Emil Kraepalin (1856-1926). Affective (emotional - nervous) disorder by definition, *swings of mood,* as a sympton of being unstable; going-up in elation, or of going-down in depression. In psychiatry known as mania when on a high, or diagnosed as depressive (melancholic) when *abnormally* low. Kraepelin in 1896 grouped this tendecy to experience *excess* in - both margins, labelled it as Manic-depressive Disorder - aka Manic-depressive Psychosis. The word psychosis a pseudonym for madness - ergo *out-of-control.* Kraepelin believed they (the symptoms) were caused by a singular *disease* process. (See. *Handbook for Psychiatric Nurses.* Brian Ackner. 1964. pp. 118-119). During the Great War (later parlance - Bipolar disorder):

> 'Kraepelin detected a grim justice in the mortality statistics, believing that the " iron fist of war" had managed to stem the degenerate tide and, for the time being, ease the economic burden posed by incurable patients.'

It appears that German military Dr. Kraepelin believed that shell-shocked survivors, and many of the dead and dying, were from a naturally *degenerate* stock. (*Forgotten Lunatics of the Great War.* By Peter Barham. Published. Yale. 2004. See. Part iii Revolting Psychology. Chapter 7. *How the Weak Progress.* p.45.)

51. Dr. R D Laing. (1927-1989). *R.D.Laing. A biography*. By Adrian Charles Laing. Published. Peter Owen.1994. See, Chapter Eleven. *Early Days of Kingsley Hall,* pp.101-117.
52. Dr. R.D. Laing. *R.D.Laing. A Divided Self.* By John Clay. Published. Hodder & Stoughton.1996. ... See.p.42. Karl Jaspers, who shared Laing's view that schizophrenics had exceptional insights which they could not express intelligibly. *Book Reviews* by Dr. R.D. Laing. Review of *General psychopathology* by Karl Jaspers, International Journal of Psychoanalysis, vol.45, no.4, 1964. See Clay pp.298-299.
53. See. *Forgotten Lunatics of the Great War,* by Peter Barham. 2004.
54. William James (1842-1910). See. *The New Psychology:*

    > ' People talk triumphantly of " the New Psychology, " and write " Histories of Psychology," when into the real elements and forces which the word covers not the first glimpse of clear insight exists.' *Psychology*. By William James. London. Macmillan. 1892. See p.468.

    And, for e.g., *Miracles and The New Psychology. A Study in the Healing Miracles of the New Testament*. By E.R.Micklem. Published. Oxford University Press. London. 1922. ... In years ahead I became puzzled as I met new psychology students (in the Seventies and Eighties), who dismissed any and *all* of William James, and anything on Psychotherapy writings as too metaphysical; and out-of-hand, being unfashionable; and *only* giving favours to current *clinical* behavioural operant psychology. Why must it be Either Or?
55. Colin Wilson's St Neot's Margin (a place in Cambridgeshire). A metaphor Wilson called 'the indifference threshold,' he said:

    > 'In psychology, a threshold, means a level at which some stimulus becomes noticeable.' (See. *Dreaming To Some Purpose. An autobiography*. By Colin Wilson. Published. Century. London. 2004. p102.)

56. Karl Jaspers ... *General Psychopathology* (1923). By Karl Jaspers. Translated by J.Hoenig and M.W.Hamilton. Published by Manchester University Press. 1963. See p368.
57. Ibid Jaspers 1963 ed. p.368. ... See Jaspers own ref., 'of a South American *earthquake'* given as (Kehrer, Bunke's Handbach, vol.1, p337)'.

58. See. *Better Court than Coroners'*, Volume II.
59. Aleister Crowley (1875-1947). ... See, for e.g., *Magick in Theory and Practice,* by Aleister Crowley, 1929. Crowley became dependent overdosing on illegal drugs; see *Diary of a Drug Fiend* (1923). He'd been an onetime member of an Occult and Theosophy study group in the early 1900s, called the *Golden Dawn.* 'Do what thou wilt shall be the whole of the law' taken from his *Book of the Law.* Published in 1909, which lead to many mishaps.
60. Aldous Huxley (1894-1963). See *The Doors of Perception.* Published 1954. Huxley took part in a tightly controlled experiment with the hallucinogenic drug Mescalin.
61. IT and OZ, two 1960s and Seventies popular psychedelic, designated (but not banned) underground alternative magazines; for the younger generation of its time.
62. Aldous Huxley *Doors of Perception* 1954. See p10
63. H.G. Wells (1866-1946). *The Man Who Could Work Miracles.*1936.
64. Sorcerer's art. ... (See above note, No. 46) The 1684 *English Dictionary* defined *Sorcery,* as:

> ' Sorcery or Sorcellery, (contracted from sorsilegium). Divination by lots; all vulgarly taken for inchantment or Witchcraft.'

I noted that the same dictionary had no separate entries for Inchantment or Witchcraft; but there was, 'Wizard... A Wise man, a witch, a cunning man.' Which suggests that even then, different definitions of imitation (fraud) and, possible (real) Man or Woman could aso possess *true* wisdom. But Statutes remained in force on prosecuting Witches, as fraudulent mediums, (science-fiction, indeed science-fact, was *then* unknown... erm!) up until the mid-twentieth century, when the *Witchcraft Act of 1735* was finally repealed, and replaced by the *Fraudulent Mediums Act,* in 1951.

65. Mary Anne Attwood (b.1817); nee Mary Anne South, daughter of Thomas South, of Bury House, Gosport, Hampshire. ... See, ' *Suggestive Inquiry into the Hermetic Mystery. With a dissertation on the more celebrated alchemical philosophers being an attempt towards the recovery of the ancient experiment of nature.* ' (Published William Tait, Belfast. (And.) London. J.M.Watkins, at 21 Cecil Court. 1918

ed.) This loaded Magnum Opus was first published anonymously, in 1850, by publishers Trelawney Saunders, its author a young Mary Anne South. She married the Reverend Alban Thomas Atwood, Vicar of Leake, near Thirsk, Yorkshire. The alchemic cum philosophical work, was subseqently published under her married name.

I found, in reading (dipping into) the *Inquiry,* practically all modern commentators address Alchemy as either philosophical nonsense, or alchemy as being of 'vulgar metal into transmuted gold' (chemistry). Or metaphysical, embracing all life and whatever by the use of symbol, algebra, mathematics and theology (psychology and theosophy in its day), as Dr. Carl Jung. As the 1850 work quotes:

> '*Every one must seek it for himself*; it behoves us not to break the seal of God, for a fiery mountain lieth before it at which I myself am amazed and must wait whether it be God's will.' (23rd Epistle.1649 edition.) See. p.49.

The foregoing quote reminded me of writings of Jacob Boehme (1575-1624). But, far more pertinent, of JRRT Tolkien's (1892-1973) learned, talented cousin Marjorie Incledon's (1891-1973), *same quote,* to me, in that 1970 postcard from The Dicker. (See also, Chaper Ten. Note & ref.44.) And, of course, to young aspirants Marc and Jean, attending OT and IT in the old Farm Yard at Graylingwell Hospital in 1970. They, too, had to seek out the mysteries of life for themselves as pure of heart and bereft of toxin as possible.

66. Lady Dowding. See, *The Psychic Life of Muriel, The Lady Dowding. An Autobiography* 1980. (See, *Better Court Than Coroners.* Chapter Ten. Note & ref. No.48.)
67. Lord Dowding. (See, *Better Court Than Coroners.* Chapter Ten. Note & ref. No. 48.)
68. Basil Collier (See, *Better Court Than Coroners.* Chapter Ten. Note & ref. No 48.)
69. A.E.Waite (1857-1942). *The Turba Philosophorum or Assembly of the Sages.* (aka The Epistle of Arisleus). Translated, by A.E.Waite, from the Latin (Editor 1896). Published. London Rider.1914 edition. I found a second-hand copy, purchased in a bookshop off the Charing Cross Road, was much *scored* and clearly much studied, its advocate owner well versed in chemistry and astronomy.

70. Jean Cocteau's seminal *Orphee* (1950). .... All psychotherapy, post-shell shock, and PTSD abreactive treatment, life-saving nostalgic explorations - are aspects of *retrieval* (back to a conscious life), - in this context.
71. Bob Dylan ... *Gotta Serve Somebody,* from Dylan's album *Slow Train Coming* 1979.
72. See, *Better Court Than Coroners. Volume II.* Forms & Lists. Psychological Tests used in the 1960s and Seventies.

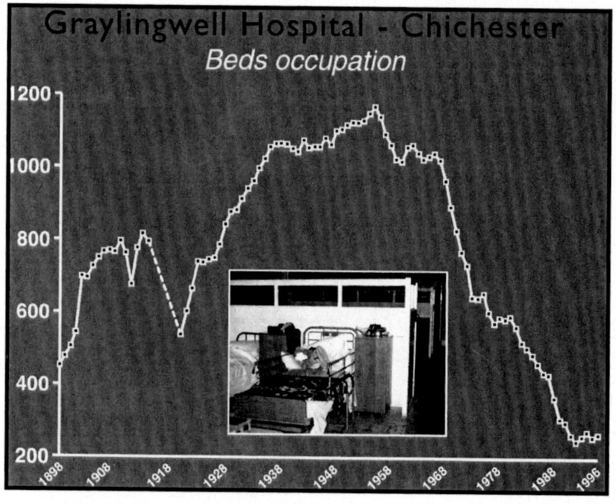

Graylingwell Hospital Bed Statistics Chart, 1898-1996. Graph contributed by social worker Mrs Cath Vandercamman (insert pic by author). Sad, the bed picture is that of my 1968 patient, and colleague, of years before; Epileptic John, of Chilgrove Ward. He died not long afterwards — full of dignity.

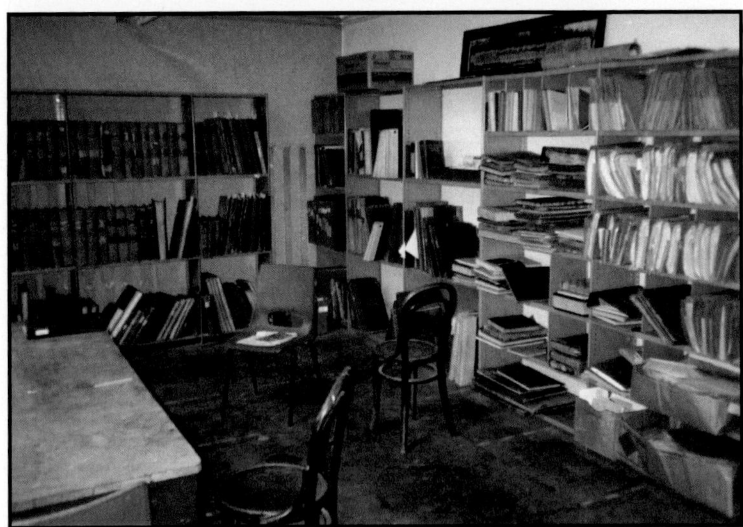

1980. Archives in the loft of *Patients' Affairs Dep't* housed thousands of Case Files and ephemera. Some archives were already stored at Chichester County Hall. Much of my own material came from purchases at local bookshops, contributions from past serving staff, and a considerable amount rescued from discarded rubbish. But most data in the narrative came from my own personal memories and recordings.

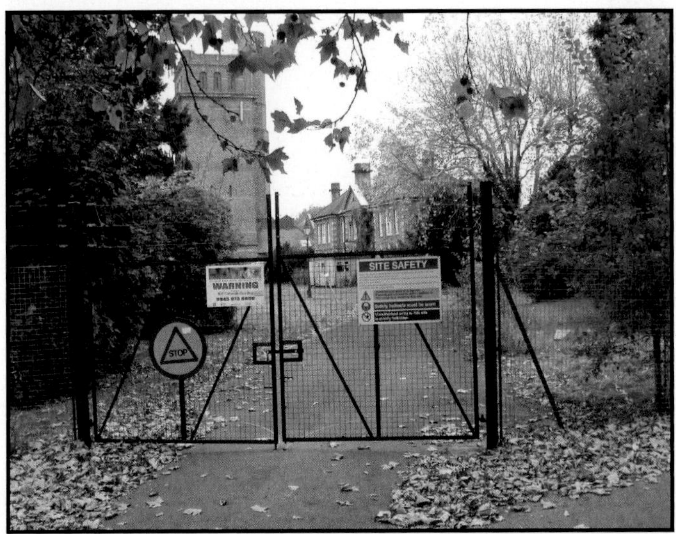

2007. *The Front Entrance* of the Main Building. Graylingwell *Hospital Closed.*

Photos by Author

General Subject Index.
And Bibliography book titles (in Italics).

A

B

C

D

E

F

G

H

I

J

K

L

N

O

P

T

U

General Index. Proper Names.

N

O

P

R

S

T

V

W

Z

Glossary of Abbreviations

AKA	Also Known As
AM	ante meridiem (morning, before noon)
ASW	Approved Social Worker
AWRE	Atomic Weapons Research Establishment
B1	Bramber One
B2	Bramber Two
BBC	British Broadcasting Corporation
BD	bis in die (twice daily)
Bro	Brother
C patrol	Chilgrove (block)
Chi	Chichester
CIA	Central Intelligence Agency
COHSE	Confederate of Health Service Employees (union)
COS	Charity Organisation Society
CPN	Community Psychiatric Nurse
CQSW	Certificate of Qualification in Social Work
CSSD	Central Sterilised Supplies Department
DA / da	Drug Addict
DD	Doctor of Divinity
DDA	Dangerous Drugs Act
DGO	Dressing Gown Order
DHSS	Department of Health and Social Security
Dip. PsyCC	Diploma in Psychiatric Care of Children
Dip. SW	Diploma in Social Work
DOC	Duty of Care
Dom	Dominus (master)
DPM	Diploma in Psychological Medicine
Dr	Doctor
DRO	Disablement Rehabilitation Officer
E2	Eastergate Two
ECT	Electro Convulsive Therapy
ECY	Electroplexy
EEG	Electroencephalogram
EMI	Elderly Mentally Ill
EMS	Emergency Medical Services
EN	Enrolled Nurse
ep	Epileptic
ESN	Educated Sub-normal
ESP	Extra Sensory Perception
EST	Electro Shock Therapy
GITM	Ghost In The Machine
GNC	General Nursing Council
GPI	General Paralysis of Insane
H bomb	Hydrogen Bomb
HM Forces	His/Her Majesty's Forces
HMC	Hospital Management Committee
HMSO	His/Her Majesty's Stationery Office

IM	Intramuscular
IPCRESS	Induction of Psychoneuroses by Conditioned Reflex with Stress
IQ	Intelligence Quotient
IRA	Irish Republican Army
IT	Industrial Therapy
IT	Information Technology
IT	Intermediate Treatment
IT	International Times
KE1/2	Kings E (Eastergate) Wards 1 and 2
KGB	Komitet gosudarstvennoy bezopasnosti or Committee for State Security
LSD	Lysergic Acid Diethylamide
Lt	Lieutenant
MA1	Male Admission 1
MA2	Male Admission 2
MAB	Metropolitan (London) Asylums Board
MAO	Mono Amine Oxydase - Inhibitor
MASH	Mobile Army Surgical Hospital
MC2	Male Chilgrove 2
MD	Doctor of Medicine
MHA	Mental Health Act
MKULTRA	M-K-ULTRA: An American Secret Service experimental brainwashing project
MO	Medical Officer
MRC	Medical Research Council
MS	Mentally Subnormal
MWO	Mental Welfare Officer
NASA	National Aeronautics and Space Administration
NCO	Non Commissioned Officer
NHS	National Health Service
NUPE	National Union of Public Employees
NVC	Non Verbal Communication
NYA	Not Yet Admitted
NYD	Not Yet Diagnosed
NZ	New Zealand
OGPU	State Political Department, a forerunner of the KGB
OT	Occupational Therapy
P & I	Press and Information
PAI	Public Assistance Institution
PIO	Principal Information Officer
PN	Pupil Nurse
PNO	Principal Nursing Officer
POS	Place of Safety
POW	Prisoner of War
PRN	pro re nata (as occasion requires)
PSW	Psychiatric Social Worker
PTSD	Post Traumatic Stress Disorder
QDS	quater die sumendus (four times a day)
QE1/2	Queens E (Edgeworth) Wards 1 and 2
RAF	Royal Air Force
RAFVR	Royal Air Force Voluntary Reserve
RAMC	Royal Army Medical Corps

Rev.	Reverend
RMN	Registered Mental Nurse
RMPA	Royal Medico-Psychological Association
RNMH	Registered Nurse Mentally Handicapped
RSM	Regimental Sergeant Major
RSPCA	Royal Society for the Prevention of Cruelty to Animals
SEN	State Enrolled Nurse
SEO	Senior Executive Officer
SNO	Senior Nursing Officer
SRN	State Registered Nurse
SS	Schutzstaffel (German Secret Service)
TAVR	Territorial Army Volunteer Reserves
TB	Tuberculosis
TLC	Tender Loving Care
TPR	Temperature, Pulse and Respiration
TTOs	To Take Out (wards)
TV	Television
UK	United Kingdom
USA	United States of America
USSR	Union of Soviet Socialist Republics
VA	Veterans Affairs
VAD	Voluntary Aid Detachment
VD	Veneral Disease
VIP	Very Important Person
WD	War Department
WSCC	West Sussex County Council
WSG	West Sussex Gazette
WW1	World War One
WW2	World War Two

West Sussex Asylum.—Appointment of MEDICAL SUPERINTENDENT.—The Visiting Committee appointed by the West Sussex County Council for providing an Asylum are desirous of receiving applications from duly registered and qualified Medical Practitioners for the office of Medical Superintendent. The Asylum, which is in course of erection, is within a mile of Chichester and will, in the first instance, accommodate 450 patients. The salary will be £450 a year, with unfurnished house (the Committee paying rates and taxes), light, washing, coals, and vegetables. The gentleman appointed will be required to enter upon his duties on or about the 1st July, 1896, and to give up the whole of his time to the duties of his office, and not to attend to or engage in any professional or other business or employment except that of the Asylum, and not to have any interest, direct or indirect, in any establishment or house for the reception of any lunatic or other patient.

Applications, stating age, qualifications, and experience, accompanied with copies of testimonials (not exceeding five, and which will not be returned), to be sent to me endorsed "Medical Superintendentship," on or before the 25th March, 1896. Personal canvassing is strictly prohibited.

ERNEST H. BLAKER, Clerk to the Committee.
West Pallant, Chichester, Sussex, 25th February, 1896.

Advert for 1st Medical Superintent 1896. (to be Dr. H.A. Kidd)

West Sussex County Asylum.—Appointment of ASSISTANT MEDICAL OFFICER. The Visiting Committee are desirous of receiving applications from duly registered and qualified medical practitioners for the office of Assistant Medical Officer.

The salary will be £150 a year, with board, lodging, washing, and attendance.

Candidates must be under thirty years of age and unmarried.

Applications, stating age, qualifications, and experience, accompanied with copies of not more than three testimonials, to be sent to me, endorsed "Assistant Medical Officer," on or before the 5th April, 1897.

Personal canvassing is strictly prohibited, but candidates may send copies of their testimonials to the Committee, whose names and addresses may be obtained from me.

ERNEST H. BLAKER, Clerk to the Committee.
West Pallant, Chichester, March 15th, 1897.

Advert for 'Assistant Medical Officer' 1897 (to be Dr.Steen)

DOMESTIC.

WEST SUSSEX COUNTY ASYLUM, CHICHESTER.

WANTED, at once, a FEMALE COOK. Must have had previous institution experience. Salary to commence £[illegible] per annum.

Also KITCHENMAID, commencing £18; SCULLERY-MAID, commencing £16; LAUNDRESS, commencing £30; and LAUNDRYMAID, commencing £16: all with board, lodging, washing and uniform.

Applications, stating age and full particulars, to be sent to THE MEDICAL SUPERINTENDENT.

Advert for Domestic Staff c. 1898

DOMESTIC.

WEST SUSSEX COUNTY ASYLUM, CHICHESTER.

WANTED, a FEMALE COOK. Must have had previous Institution experience. Salary £35 per annum, with board, lodging, washing, and uniform.

Form of application can be obtained from THE MEDICAL SUPERINTENDENT.

Advert for Domestic Staff c. 1898

Early Job Adverts for Graylingwell Staff.